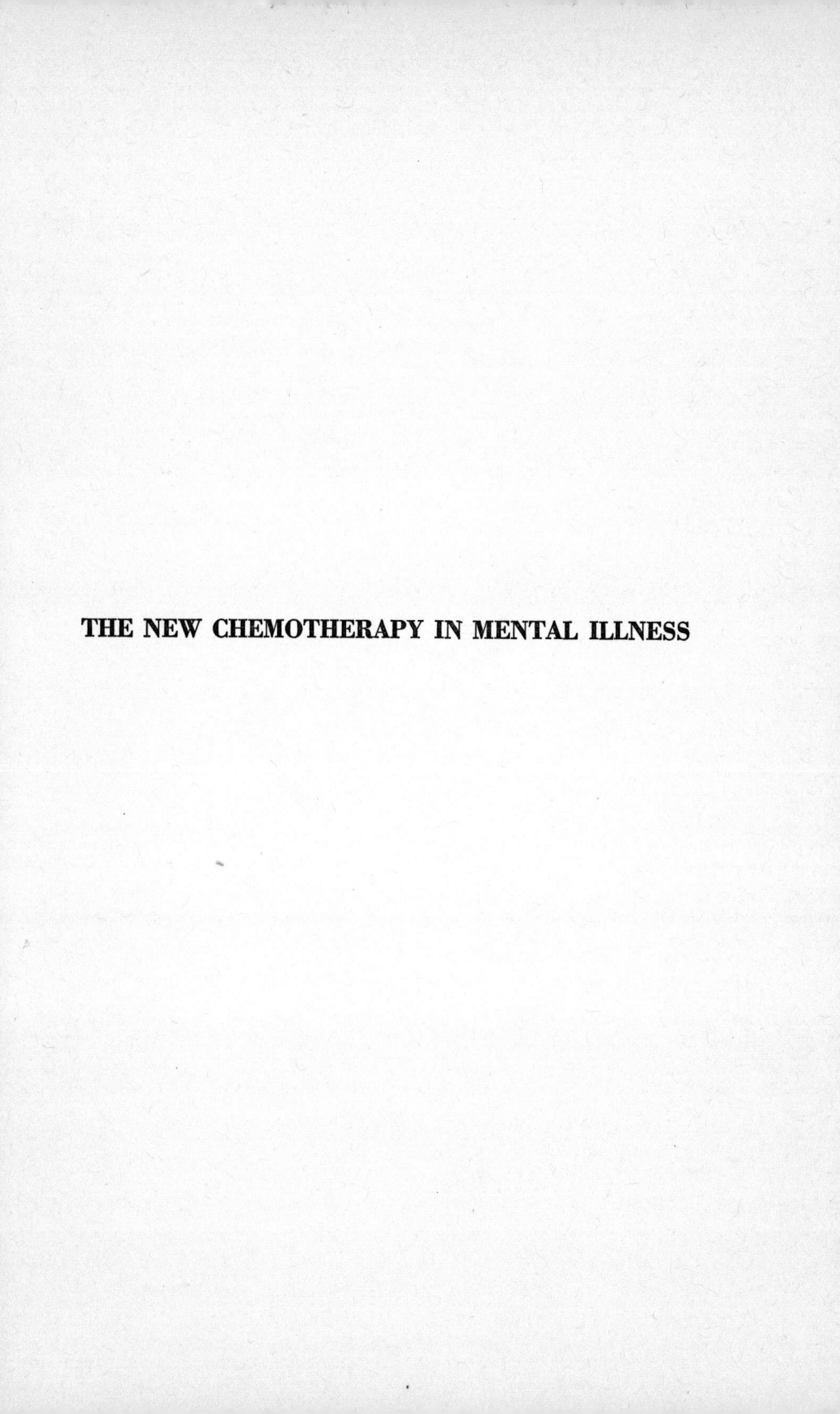

THE NEW CHEMOTHERAPY IN MENTAL ILLNESS

THE NEW CHEMOTHERAPY IN MENTAL ILLNESS

THE HISTORY, PHARMACOLOGY AND CLINICAL
EXPERIENCES WITH RAUWOLFIA, PHENOTHIAZINE,
AZACYCLONOL, MEPHENESIN, HYDROXYZINE AND
BENACTYZINE PREPARATIONS

EDITED BY

Hirsch L. Gordon, M.D., Ph.D., F.A.P.A.

Department of Psychiatry, New York Medical College
Metropolitan Medical Center
Associate Psychiatrist, Metropolitan Hospital, N. Y. C.

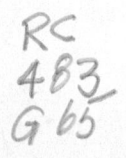

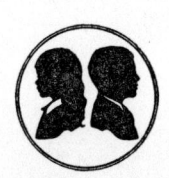

PHILOSOPHICAL LIBRARY
NEW YORK

Copyright, 1958, by Philosophical Library, Inc.
15 East 40 Street, New York 16, N. Y.
All rights reserved

Printed in the United States of America

CONTENTS

Introduction *by* Hirsch L. Gordon, M.D. — xi
Ataractic Drugs — xix

Part One: GENERAL SURVEYS

"The Tranquilizing Drugs" *by* Morris Fishbein, M.D. — 3
"Pharmacology of the Ataractic Drugs" *by* Edward B. Truitt, Jr. Ph.D. — 6
"The Ataractic Drugs: The Present Position of Chlorpromazine, Frenquel, Pacatal, and Reserpine in the Psychiatric Hospital" *by* H. Angus Bowes, M.D. — 10
"Prospects in Psychopharmacology" *by* Harold E. Himwich, M.D. — 23
"The Ataractic Drugs: Their Uses and Limitations in Psychiatry" *by* Howard D. Fabing, M.D. — 36
"Ataractics in Medical Practice" *by* Joseph F. Fazekas, M.D., James G. Shea, M.D., and Paul D. Sullivan, Jr., M.D. — 42
"What's New and Usable in the Chemical Treatment of Abnormal Behavior" *by* John T. Ferguson, M.D. — 50
"Drugs Recently Introduced in the Treatment of Psychiatric Disorders" *by* Irvin M. Cohen, M.D. — 60
"Evaluation of the Therapeutic Effects of Drugs in Psychiatric Patients" *by* Lincoln D. Clark, M.D. — 67
"New Drug Therapies in Psychiatry" *by* F. A. Freyhan, M.D., Patricia Turner, M.D., and Rita Stenzler, M.D. — 74
"Progress in Psychiatric Therapies" *by* Paul H. Hoch, M.D. — 82
"A Comparative Study of Various Ataractic Drugs" *by* Paul E. Feldman, M.D. — 91
"Some Observations on the Use of Tranquilizing Drugs" *by* Thomas S. Szasz, M.D. — 100
"A Review of the Newer Drug Therapies in Psychiatry" *by* Vernon Kinross-Wright, M.D. — 107

Part Two: CLINICAL EXPERIENCE: (A) IN PSYCHIATRY DISEASE

"Use of the Tranquilizing Properties of Reserpine" *by* J. Campbell Howard, Jr., M.D., and Frank J. Vinci, M.D. — 114
"The Use of Reserpine in an Acute Psychiatric Treatment Setting" *by* Garfield Tourney, M.D., Emil M. Isberg, M.D., and Jacques S. Gottlieb, M.D. — 122
"Use of Reserpine in Chronic Non-Disturbed Psychotics" *by* James Boudwin, M.D., and Nathan S. Kline, M.D. — 127
"Observations During the Treatment of 175 Psychotic Patients with Reserpine *by* Rudolf B. Freund, M.D. — 135
"Reserpine in the Treatment of Patients with Chronic Mental Disease: A Controlled Study" *by* Lawrence Koltonow, M.D. — 142

"Reserpine in Hospitalized Psychotics: A Controlled Study on Chronically Disturbed Women" *by* Arthur Lemon Arnold, M.D., and Harry Freeman, M.D. — 146

"Behavioral Changes of Chronic Schizophrenics in Response to Reserpine" *by* Roy E. McDonald, M.D., Robert B. Ellsworth, Ph.D. and Jane Eniss, R.N. — 151

"Reserpine (Serpasil) in the Management of the Mentally Ill" *by* Robert H. Noce, M.D., David B. Williams, M.D., and Walter Rapaport, M.D. — 156

"Effect of Reserpine and Open-Ward Privileges on Chronic Schizophrenics" *by* Allen S. Penman, Ph.D. and Thomas E. Dredge, M.D. — 164

"Short-Term Treatment of Psychiatric Patients with Reserpine" *by* Stephen B. Payn, M.D., and Fred V. Rockwell, M.D. — 174

"Use of Reserpine on an Admission Service" *by* Ernest Gosline, M.D., and Nathan S. Kline, M.D. — 181

"A Controlled Study of Reserpine on Chronically Disturbed Patients" *by* M. Duane Sommerness, M.D., Rubel J. Lucero, M.A., John S. Hamlon, M.D., J. L. Erickson, M.D., and R. Matthews, R.Ph. — 191

"Improved Behavior Patterns in the Hospitalized Mentally Ill with Reserpine and Methyl-Phenidylacetate" *by* John T. Ferguson, M.D. — 196

"Treatment of Two Hundred Disturbed Psychotics with Reserpine" *by* Joseph A. Barsa, M.D., and Nathan S. Kline, M.D. — 204

"Has Chlorpromazine Inaugurated a New Era in Mental Hospitals?" *by* Winfred Overholser, M.D. — 212

"An Evaluation of Promazine Hydrochloride in Psychiatric Practice" *by* Stanley Lesse, M.D. — 218

"A Clinical Study of Mechanisms of Action of Chlorpromazine" *by* Erwin Lear, M.D., Albert E. Chiron, M.D., and Irving M. Pallin, M.D. — 224

"A Case of Corticotropic Hormone-Induced Psychosis Treated with Promazine Hydrochloride" *by* Dean J. Plazak, M.D. — 236

"Chlorpromazine, New Inhibiting Agent for Psychomotor Excitement and Manic States" *by* H. E. Lehmann, M.D., and G. E. Hanrahan, M.D. — 240

"Large Doses of Chlorpromazine in the Treatment of Psychiatric Patients" *by* Frank J. Ayd, Jr. M.D. — 251

"Psychiatric Experience with Chlorpromazine" *by* Willis H. Bower, M.D. Mark D. Altschule, M.D., and Leonard Cook, Ph.D. — 255

"Effects of Chlorpromazine in Psychiatric Disorders" *by* Irvin M. Cohen, M.D. — 261

"Thorazine in the Treatment of Acutely Disturbed Psychotic Patients" *by* Gordon R. Forrer, M.D. — 269

"Effects of Chlorpromazine on Chronic Lobotomized Schizophrenic Patients" *by* Harry Freeman, M.D., and Herbert S. Cline, M.D. — 273

"The Influence of Chlorpromazine on Psychotic Thought Content and Mechanism" *by* Douglas Goldman, M.D. — 282

"Clinical Trial of a New Phenothiazine Compound: NP-207" by Vernon Kinross-Wright, M.D. — 286

"Chlorpromazine Treatment of Mental Disorders" by Vernon Kinross-Wright, M.D. — 292

"Office Treatment of Pain and Psychic Stress: The Use of a New Tranquilizing Agent" by Jack R. Wennersten, M.D. — 300

"Promazine Hydrochloride in the Treatment of Chronic Catatonic Schizophrenics" by Clarke W. Mangun, M.D., and Warren W. Webb, Ph.D. — 305

"The Use of Chlorpromazine in Psychotherapy" by H. L. Newbold, M.D., and W. David Steed, M.D. — 310

"Preliminary Report on Five Hundred Patients Treated with Thorazine at Rochester State Hospital" by Benjamin Pollack, M.D. — 317

"Chlorpromazine in the Treatment of Neuropsychiatric Disorders" by N. William Winkelman, Jr., M.D. — 332

"Chlorpromazine and Reserpine, and Their Relation to Other Treatments in Psychiatry" by Lothar B. Kalinowsky, M.D. — 343

"A Critique of the Tranquilizing Drugs, Chlorpromazine and Reserpine, in Neuropsychiatry" by Harry Freeman, M.D. — 351

"The Use of Chlorpromazine and Reserpine in Psychological Disorders in General Practice" by H. Azima, M.D. — 361

"Use of Chlorpromazine and Reserpine in Mental Disorders" by Mark D. Altschule, M.D. — 366

"Experience with the Use of Chlorpromazine and Reserpine in Psychiatry" by George W. Brooks, M.D. — 375

"Ambulatory and Comparative Treatment of the Anxiety Neurosis Syndrome with Chlorpromazine, Phenobarbital and Dimethylane" by Wallace Marshall, M.D. — 382

"Thorazine and Serpasil Treatment of Private Neuropsychiatric Patients" by Frank J. Ayd, Jr., M.D. — 388

"Chlorpromazine (Thorazine)—Rauwolfia Combination in Neuropsychiatry" by Harold B. Eiber, M.D. — 397

"Use of Chlorpromazine and Reserpine in the Treatment of Emotional Disorders" by William W. Zeller, M.D., Paul N. Graffagnino, M.D., Chester F. Cullen, M.D., and H. Jerome Rietman, M.D. — 401

"Chlorpromazine and Reserpine" by Francis N. Waldrop, M.D., and F. Regis Riesenman, M.D. — 410

"Effect of Chlorpromazine and Reserpine on Budgets of Mental Hospitals" by Werner Tuteur, M.D. — 416

"Chlorpromazine Alone and with Reserpine" by Leo E. Hollister, M.D. Kenneth P. Jones, M.D., Bernard Brownfield, M.D., and Franklin Johnson, M.D. — 419

"Reserpine in the Treatment of Disturbed Adolescents" by George T. Nicolaou, M.D., and Nathan S. Kline, M.D. — 425

"The Use of Reserpine (Serpasil) in Three Hundred and Fifty Neuropsychiatric Cases" by Veronica M. Pennington, M.D. — 435

"Drug Therapy—Clinical and Operational Effects: Changes in the Mental Hospital Resulting from the Addition of Chlorpromazine to the Total Therapeutic Program" by Benjamin Pollack, M.D.   442
"Use of a Chlorpromazine-Dextro-Amphetamine Combination in Anxiety Neuroses" by Thomas M. Hart, M.D.   448
"Clinical Study of Proclorperazine, a New Tranquilizer for the Treatment of Nonhospitalized Psychoneurotic Patients" by Thomas J. Vischer, M.D.   452
"The Use of Azacyclonol and Pipradol in General Practice" by Thomas G. Allin, Jr., M.D., and Raymond C. Pogge, M.D.   457
"Frenquel" by Richard C. Proctor, M.D., and Theodore Odland, M.D.   464
"Azacyclonol (Frenquel) in the Treatment of Chronic Schizophrenics" by Joseph A. Barsa, M.D., and Nathan S. Kline, M.D.   469
"The Effect of Meratran on Twenty-Five Institutionalized Mental Patients" by J. W. Schut, M.D., and H. E. Himwich, M.D.   470
"Clinical Studies on a-(2-Piperidyl) Benzhydrol Hydrochloride, a New Antidepressant Drug" by Howard D. Fabing, M.D., J. Robert Hawkins, M.D., and James A. L. Moulton, M.D.   475
"Meprobamate, Its Pharmacologic Properties and Clinical Uses" by F. M. Berger, M.D.   483
"Treatment of Anxiety States with Meprobamate (Miltown) by Walter A. Osinki, M.D.   495
"Meprobamate in Anxiety Reactions Involving Depression" by Abraham Ruchwarger, M.D.   502
"Clinical Study of a New Tranquilizing Drug: Use of Miltown" by Lowell S. Selling, M.D.   506
"Preliminary Study on the Use of Hydroxyzine in Psychosomatic Affections" by Luis Farah, M.D.   511
"A Clinical Trial of Benactyzine Hydrochloride ('Suavitil') as a Physical Relaxant" by Anthony Coady, M.B., and Eric C. O. Jewesbury, D.M.   522
"Suavitil in the Treatment of Psychoneuroses" by Olaf Ostergaard Jensen   529
"A New Drug Effective in the Central Nervous System" by E. Jacobcen   535
"Modern Drug Treatment and Psychotherapy" by Alexandra Adler, M.D.   537
"Psychotherapy and Ataraxics: Some Observations on Combined Psychotherapy and Chlorpromazine Therapy" by Stanley Lesse, M.D.   541

Part Three: CLINICAL EXPERIENCE: (B) IN RELATED CONDITIONS

"Miltown as a Tranquilizer in the Treatment of Alcohol Addicts" by Joseph Thimann, M.D., and Joseph W. Gauthier, M.D.   550
"The Use of Chlorpromazine Hydrochloride in the Treatment of Barbiturate Addiction with Acute Withdrawal Syndrome" by William Brooks, M.D., Lawrence Deutsch, M.D., and Robert Dickes, M.D.   553
"Use of Chlorpromazine in the Withdrawal of Addicting Drugs" by Charles E. Friedgood, M.D., and Charles B. Ripstein, M.D.   556

"The Use of Chlorpromazine in the Treatment of Acute Alcoholism" by Salomon N. Albert, M.D., Edward L. Rea, M.D., Cecil A. Duverney, M.D., James Shea, M.D., and Joseph F. Fazekas, M.D. ... 560

"Use of Chlorpromazine in Chronic Alcoholics" by James F. Cummins, M.D., and Dale G. Friend, M.D. ... 563

"Meprobamate (Miltown) as Adjunct in Treatment of Anogenital Pruritus" by Oscar J. Sokoloff, M.D. ... 567

"Use of Tranquilizers in Diseases of the Skin" by Paul LeVan, M.D., and Edwin T. Wright, M.D. ... 571

"Therapeutic Process in Electroshock and the Newer Drug Therapies" by Leo Alexander, M.D. ... 574

"Treatment of Depression with Meratran and Electroshock" by Henry E. Andren, M.D. ... 581

"Chlorpromazine and Reserpine as Adjuncts in Electroshock Treatment" by Merritt W. Foster, Jr., M.D., and R. Finley Gayle III, M.D. ... 584

"Drug Therapy in the Emotionally Disturbed Aged" by Sol Levy, M.D. ... 592

"The Treatment of Anxiety, Agitation and Excitement in the Aged: A Preliminary Report on Trilafon" by Frank J. Ayd, Jr., M.D. ... 596

"Improving Senile Behavior with Reserpine and Ritalin" by John T. Ferguson, M.D., and William H. Funderburk, Ph.D. ... 601

"Hydroxyzine: A New Therapeutic Agent for Senile Anxiety States" by Mervin Shalowitz, M.D. ... 611

"Chlorpromazine (Thorazine) Treatment of Disturbed Epileptic Patients" by Vincent I. Bonafede, M.D. ... 616

"Meratran with Reserpine: Adjunctive Use in the Treatment of Parkinson's Disease" by John C. Button, B.Sc. ... 623

"Combination Reserpine-Methylphenilacetate in Epileptics with Psychosis" by G. Donald Niswander, M.D., and Earl K. Holt, M.D. ... 627

"Use of Meprobamate (Miltown) in Convulsive and Related Disorders" by Meyer A. Perlstein, M.D. ... 633

"Reserpine (Serpasil) in the Management of the Mentally Ill and Mentally Retarded" by Robert H. Noce, M.D., David B. Williams, M.D., and Walter Rapaport, M.D. ... 640

"Some Considerations on the Use of Chlorpromazine in a Child Psychiatry Clinic" by Herbert Freed, M.D., and Charles A. Peifer, Jr. ... 646

"Chlorpromazine for the Control of Psychomotor Excitement in the Mentally Deficient" by Judith H. Rettig, M.D. ... 651

"Potentiation of Hypnotics and Analgesics: Clinical Experience with Chlorpromazine" by Robert Wallis, M.D. ... 657

Part Four: SIDE EFFECTS

"Complications and Concomitants" by Otis R. Farley, M.D. ... 662

"Ineffectiveness of Chlorpromazine and Rauwolfia Serpentina Preparations in the Treatment of Depression" by Lawrence H. Gahagan, M.D. ... 667

"Discussion of Dr. Gahagan's Paper" by Edwin J. de Beer, Ph.D. ... 672

"Complications of Chlorpromazine Therapy" *by* Irvin M. Cohen, M.D.   673
"Complications During Reserpine Therapy" *by* C. H. Cahn, M.D.   682
"Adverse Reactions to Meprobamate" by Henry T. Friedman, M.D., and Willard L. Marmelzat, M.D.   684
"Inherent Dangers in Use of Tranquilizing Drugs in Anxiety States" *by* Herman A. Dickel, M.D., and Henry H. Dixon, M.D.   668
"Edema and Congestive Failure Related to Administration of Rauwolfia Serpentina" *by* George A. Perera, M.D.   696
"Recurrent Thorazine Induced Agranulocytosis" *by* Benjamin Pollack, M.D.   698
"Drug-Induced Blood Dyscrasias" *by* Stuart L. Vaughan, M.D.   701
"Hematemesis and Melena Complicating Treatment with Rauwolfia Alkaloids" *by* Leo E. Hollister, M.D.   709
"Agranulocytosis While Receiving Combined Reserpine-Chlorpromazine Therapy" *by* Joseph A. Barsa, M.D., and Nathan S. Kline, M.D.   714
"Jaundice Caused by Chlorpromazine (Thorazine)" *by* Lawrence R. Loftus, M.D., Kenneth A. Huizenga, M.D., Maurice H. Stauffer, M.D., Howard P. Rome, M.D., and James C. Cain, M.D.   718
"Liver Function and Hepatic Complications in Patients Receiving Chlorpromazine" *by* Irvin M. Cohen, M.D., and John D. Archer, M.D.   725
"Fatal Acute Aseptic Necrosis of the Liver Associated with Chlorpromazine" *by* R. N. Elliott, M.D., A. H. Schrut, M.D., and J. J. Marra, M.D.   730
"Psychosis and Enhanced Anxiety Produced by Reserpine and Chlorpromazine" *by* G. J. Sarwer-Foner, M.D., and W. Ogle, M.D.   732
"Undesirable Effects and Clinical Toxicity of Chlorpromazine" *by* Irvin M. Cohen, M.D.   744
"Fatal Hyperpyrexia During Chlorpromazine Therapy' '*by* Frank J. Ayd, Jr. M.D.   754
Bibliography   757

INTRODUCTION

By Hirsch L. Gordon, M. D.

The use of drugs to allay emotional upheavals is as old as medicine itself. Anything that reduced pain from the somatic sphere was also employed to allay anxiety in psychogenic disturbances. We therefore utilized the pharmacopoeia related to central nervous system depressants and stimulants. The autonomic drugs: sympathomimetic (adrenergic), sympatholytic (adrenergic blocking), parasympathomimetic (chlinergic) and parasympatholytic (cholinergic blocking), proved in many instances efficacious.

However, sedation brought somnolence, dulling of the psyche and arresting of the thought processes. This was undesirable. One can therefore appreciate the favorable reception given to a new type of pharmaceutical preparation which apparently has as its site of action the hypothalamus, where the two divisions of the autonomic nervous system integrate. In this respect it manifests a significant difference from sedatives such as phenobarbital, sodium bromide, myanesine and others. It does not act on the cortex as do the barbiturates but affects deepseated brain centers.

The first of many so-called "tranquilizing" drugs of recent years possesses a romantic, almost legendary history. While known for centuries in India for a variety of healing powers for the body and the mind, this plant was first described by a botanist, Dr. Leonard Rauwolf of Augsburg, Germany (1582) and named after him Rauwolfia Serpentina by Plumber (1703).

After two and a quarter centuries we hear of it again when Drs. Salimuzzaman Siddiqui and Rafat Hussain Siddiqui isolated from its roots five alkaloids used with disappointing results (1931). At the same time two other Hindu physicians, Drs. Gananath Sen and Kartick Chanra Bose, claimed that it reduced high blood pressure and controlled "insane mania." In 1941 Sir Ram Nath Chopra and associates suggested "unknown factors" responsible for the activities of Rauwolfia. In 1944 the Gupta group traced the major activity to a resin fraction of the root. Ciba started its Rauwolfia research in 1947 and a year later it sent one hundred grams of Ajmaline (prepared by the Siddiquis) to Sir Robert Robinson in Oxford for further study. In 1949 Rauwolfia first appeared in a publication outside of India when Dr. Rustom Jal Vakil published a report of its clinical trial in the British Heart Journal. In 1950 Drs. Emil Schlitter and Hans Schwartz isolated Serpentine. In 1952 Robert W. Wilkins of Boston University reported on Rauwolfia in hypertension and in September of the same year Emil Schlitter (Basle) and Johannes Miller of the Ciba Laboratories announced their identification of reserpine. H. J. Bein of Ciba experimenting on rabbits found that reserpine has an anti-hypertensive and sedative action, but the animals could easily be aroused. A year later (1953) Robert W. Wilkins reported on reserpine in hypertension and in 1954 at a symposium held in the New York Academy of Medicine he reported that it relieves psychoneurotic symptoms. Since then the derivatives of the ancient Hindu drug Rauwolfia Serpentina Benth, known in medical practice by such trade names as Serpasil (Ciba), Serfin (Parke-Davis), Reserpoid (Upjohn), Rau-Sed (Squibb), Rauwiloid (Riker), Moderil (Pfizer), and Raudixin (Squibb), occupy their well-deserved place in psychopharmacology. The other similar drug groups known as tranquilizers followed.

Professor Alister Cameron suggested for these drugs the word "atarax." When we consult Greek lexicons we find that it was used by the classical writers Epicurus, Hipparchus, Xenophon and Plato in the sense of "peace of mind," "perfect composure" and "without confusion." In similar sense it is found in the Septuagint version of the Book of Esther 3:13; 8:13.

The Rauwolfia Serpentina blockades the sympathetic and causes the parasympathetic predominance. Its curative effects are divided into three phases: (1) Sedation. It sets in immediately or after several days, decreasing agitation and turbulence. It is particularly effective in hospitalized, restive, overactive and incoherent patients, many of whom become pleasant and co-operative. (2) The turbulent period. It lasts from several hours to several weeks. Patients' behavior appears to have worsened. They complain of dizziness, their impulsiveness is sometimes beyond control and there is an increase in delusions and hallucinations. Latent psychotic manifestations "break wide open"; however the drug is not reduced. (3) Integration finally takes place and turbulence subsides. The Rauwolfia derivatives lack anticonvulsive properties but antagonize audiogenic seizures. The effects of reserpine become manifest after a period of latency which varies with the route of administration and dose. Parenteral administration reaches the maximal effect in three hours, apparently because reserpine had first to be converted into another compound.

It has been reported that it will reduce anxiety and obsessive-compulsive drives and will overcome excessive inhibition and reticence. It eliminates the hyperirritability and insomnia of hyperthyroidism. The reduction of hypertension may be due to decreased responsiveness to emotional environmental stress. There is a marked improvement in patients who manifest excited, combative, frankly manic states. In catatonic excitement it improves communicability, lessens impulsive behavior. Assaultive episodes become reduced and restraints are not needed as before. Many patients become co-operative, sociable, friendly and amenable to psychotherapy. In addition, craving ceases without withdrawal symptoms. The delirium of alcoholics is of short duration. In sexual pathology it reduces craving and frigidity. It diminishes the hyperkinesia of Huntington's Chorea. It quiets overactivity, reduces epileptic seizures (?) in children and allays tension headaches. In dermatology it affects severe chronic pruritis and in allergy it potentiates the effects of other antihistaminic agents. Those suffering from cerebral palsy and other brain injuries who show psychomotor overactivity can also be helped in part. Children who are disturbed and are behavior problems and the agitated and confused seniles are improved.

We must not overlook the side effects such as nasal stuffiness, tremulousness, mild gastrointestinal disturbances, edema of face and feet and somnolence. Parkinsonian-like syndrome and convulsion also occur, but are more rare. The drug is considered to be contraindicated in states of depression, which may increase and even result in suicide.

The claims for the therapeutic effect of the Rauwolfia Serpentina derivatives are numerous and occasionally exaggerated not only in the literature of the pharmaceutical houses (Ciba, Parke-Davis, Riker, Squibb, Upjohn and others), but also in the reports of more optimistic authors. Yet we do not discard any claim as it may become confirmed by future clinical experience.

The phenothiazine compounds were discovered in France and as 4560 R. P. (Largactil) it was developed in the Rhone-Poulenc Special Research Laboratories. It was described in a monograph prepared for the Archives Internationales de Pharmacodynamie in 1952 and published in 1953 by five French physicians: S. Courvoisier, J. Fournel, R. Ducrot, M. Kolsky and P. Koestchet. Phenothiazine compounds are assumed to exercise a depressant action at the myoneural junction and directly on the muscle, an inhibiting action on the diencephalic centers and a dampening effect on the arousal mechanism in the reticular substance. In the experimental stage it has already been noted that they exert a curare-like action on the neck muscles, retard motor activity and reduce aggressiveness. They have a selective depressant action on the central nervous system, acting primarily at the subcortical level in cerebrum, diencephalon, medula and, to a lesser extent, on the peripheral autonomic system. Peripherally they have minor antispasmodic, anticholinergic, antihistaminic and adrenolytic action. Their antiemetic effect is believed to result from blocking emetic impulses at the chemoreceptor trigger zones and vomiting center in the medulla.

Here are a number of phenothiazine compounds used as psychopharmacological agents: Amazine (USSR), Avomine (Phenergan, Lysivane), Deparcol, Megaphen (Germany) Largactil (Chlorpromazine—Canada, France, England and Italy), Pacatal (Warner-Chilcott), Proclorperazine (Compazine, SKF), Promazine (Sparine, Wyeth), Thorazine and Trilafon (Schering). It is interesting that chlorpromazine was first developed by French physicians in 1950 in their search for a better antihistaminic, in which they failed.

But it proved later to be of tremendous benefit in major psychotic disorders among hospitalized patients. The phenothiazine preparations have shown themselves to be of great value in a number of nervous conditions. They achieved a calming-down effect in the acute stage of schizophrenia and a diminution of psychomotor activity without abolishing contact. There is also a disappearance of hallucinations and delusions. It produces a tranquilizing non-hypnotic sedation, in chronic schizophrenia, in which remissions were until now a rarity. Improvement is now common. In the acute manic phase of manic depressive states the change is particularly dramatic. The hyperactivity subsides completely in most patients. As to depressive states, opinions vary. In fact, many failures resulting in suicides have been reported. This development reminds us of diabetes, for which insulin is a Godsend in hyperglycemia, but in hypoglycemia it is a menace to life. Phenothiazine reduces hyperactivity, but where it is already reduced, it may cause depression and lead to suicide. In the senile, psychotic agitation and belligerence are calmed down, as is the psychomotor agitation and delirium tremens of the acute alcoholic. In chronic alcoholics it reduces the tension that finds release in inebriety. Withdrawal symptoms in drug addiction, such as nausea, diarrhea, insomnia and restlessness are abolished. Even the step-children of mental illness, as are those suffering from general paresis, mental retardation and mental defects have obtained through the phenothiazine preparations substantial relief. Neurological disorders like epilepsy, chorea and spastic states have been greatly benefited, though some doubt its effects on convulsive disorders.

We must not overlook the possibility of unpleasant side effects: local irritation (vomiting, burning in the mouth) autonomic disturbances (nasal congestion, pallor, hypotension, tachycardia, constipation), interference with central regulatory mechanism (hypothermia, fever, increase in appetite, somnolence, inhibition of drives), sensitivity reactions (jaundice, dermatitis, photosensitivity), reactions of unexplained origin (vivid dreams, tremor, parkinsonanism, confusion and engorgement of the breast), agranulocytosis and hypoplastic anemia.

In the mentioned complications, antihistamine is indicated for allergic skin reactions and Parkinsonianism is diminished if dosage is decreased. If the latter persists, one mg. of cogentin 2 or 3 times daily should be administered. Jaundice is more dramatic and quite alarming to the uninitiated. It is often signaled by fever and pruritis and progresses to yellowing of the skin and sclera attributed to obstruction in the smaller biliary radicles. Some withdraw the drug and put the patient to bed. Lately, since the true nature of the jaundice and its reversibility have become known, the drug is continued and a high protein and high carbohydrate diet given. ACTH or cortisone may shorten its duration. While no permanent liver damage is discovered, jaundice, nevertheless, lasts from 2 days to 3 months in 14 out of one thousand patients. Undernourished patients or those suffering from a wasting disease or with a history of biliary involvement are subject to this non-serious but unpleasant complication. Agranulocytosis that is ushered in with a sore throat and stomatitis occurs between 20 to 60 days after beginning of therapy. It is detected by white blood counts. It is claimed by some that phenothiazine is also helpful in neuroses of various etiologies, as it is in free floating anxiety or aggression, in which psychotic excitement or agitation are prominent.

Both the phenothiazine and the Rauwolfia preparations are supposed to give a sense of well-being, emotional equilibrium and a more resilient response to stress. It affords a detached serenity without clouding of consciousness or impairment of mental faculties. However, many private practitioners have had limited or no success with these drugs in their private practice and they assume that the phenomenal results obtained in the treatment of mental cases as reported in the psychiatric press refer mostly to psychotic patients on the hospital wards. But even if this be the case, its benign effects in numerous authenticated cases merit the close attention of the medical profession.

Azacyclonol hydrochloride is known also by the names of its preparations: Frenquel in the gamma isomer of Meratran (Merrell). While Meratran increases activity in laboratory animals, Frenquel diminishes it. In 1954 it was demonstrated that pipradrol (Frenquel) blocked the LSD-255 psychosis and helped in schizophrenic dissociation syndromes. It has no effect on normal people and is not indicated in minor neurotic disturbances. It is confined to schizophrenic disorders and confusional states. Some cases of acute schizophrenia, alcoholic hallucinosis, senile and arteriosclerotic hallucinosis respond to oral administration of the drug, according to some observers. It promotes cooperation and facilitates psychotherapy and ward adjustment. When used with electroconvulsive therapy it reduces the required number of treatments. This is a new type of antihallucinatory and anticonfusion drug; it neither sedates nor stimulates and has no adverse effect on the pulse rate, blood pressure and respiration. Frenquel may have a synergistic action with chlorpromazine, and when each one of them used separately shows no results, they may be effective in combination. However, its chemical action in blocking hallucinations has not been studied sufficiently.

In 1946 F. M. Berger and W. Bradley described the pharmaceutical properties of mephenesin which has been widely used in conditions of muscle spasm. However, its action was of short duration, caused by the rapid oxidation of its hydroxyl groups. A related compound, propanediol dicarbamate (meprobamate), proved to be a muscle relaxant, an anticonvulsant and tranquilizer. Known under the trade names, Miltown (Wallace) and Equanil (Wyeth), and first synthesized by B. J. Ludwig and E. C. Piech in 1950, it is distinguished by its effects on voluntary muscle only. This drug, however, has no influence on the diaphragm and does not impair respiration. It has a marked blocking action on interneurons. The knee jerk (which has a reflex arc with no interneurons) is not affected by the drug. The drug does not affect the peripheral nerve, but its effect on the myoneural junction is debatable. The drug has a selective action on the thalamus which is its unique property. It does not seem to affect the autonomic nervous system and thus differs from other ataraxics which have potent adrenalytic, atropine-like and antihistaminic action. It relaxes muscular tension associated with anxiety and hyperemotionalism and returns the patient to social productivity. It induces sleep by removing physical and emotional tension. Unconsciousness does not set in suddenly and one can be awakened easily. The drug is therefore indicated in insomnia. Its emotional and muscular relaxing qualities are useful in headaches due to severe nervous tension and resulting in sustained contraction of posterior muscles of head, neck and shoulders. It is claimed the drug facilitates alcoholic withdrawal, menstrual stress, neurodermatitis and the reaction to pain. It diminishes the pre-electroshock anxiety and is efficacious in petit mal epilepsy. It is not certain whether it controls the spasticity in cerebral palsy but is apparently ineffective in Parkinsonianism and in grand mal. Some have reported relief in the glosus feeling in the throat, palpitation, heavy feeling in the chest, air hunger, anorexia, digestive disturbances, urinary frequency and turbulence of thought and mood.

Drowsiness is controlled by amphetamine. Allergic reactions: Erythematous rash, fever, fainting spells and the angioneurotic edema of bronchial spasm are easily relieved by epinephrine and antihistaminics. It may be said that the drug has no contraindications, but all of these drugs must be used with caution in schizophrenics who require alertness to maintain reality contact.

Recently a new drug has been added to the family of the ataraxics which J. B. Roerig & Company has named Atarax. It is a hydroxyzine hydrochloride. Its sedative properties are greater in intensity than the common side effect of antihistaminic drugs. It modifies psychosomatic manifestations when they were caused by an increase in emotional tension. In states of excitation, anxiety neurosis and arteriovisceral conditions the therapeutic results are particularly effective. Neuroleptic treatment can be safely carried on for several months with hydroxyzine since it is low in toxicity. If treatment is interrupted after a period of one or two months, manifestations of the disease reappear with less intensity. It has proven to be helpful in patients with various dermatoses in which emotional stress was thought to be a factor. The drug was found to potentiate Rauwolfia Serpentina.

According to some workers, Benactyzine Hydrochloride ("Suavitil"), by blocking certain nerve pathways in the hypothalamus, aims to protect the higher cerebral centers from environment disturbing stimuli. In human subjects Suavitil reduces autonomic reaction to undue emotion.

It is a cholinergic substance. Therapeutic doses are eliminated from the body within a few hours. There are no euphoria or withdrawal symptoms. It raises the threshold for external stimuli and acts like a pharmaceutical "curtain" between the subject and his annoying problems. In certain doses it blocks thoughts, conscious and subconscious. Muscular relaxation follows. There are no hallucinations. It is helpful in cases of psychoneurosis with anxiety repression and obsessive compulsive anxiety, also in compulsive reactions including compulsive alcoholism. It does not replace psychotherapy. The drug may also be used in conjunction with barbiturates, reserpine and chlorpromazine.

In the short period of three years since the ataraxics have appeared on the therapeutic horizon, they have created a prolific literature. These drugs became very popular and the warnings sounded against their indiscriminate use were of little avail. It has been estimated that 30 million prescriptions for them were filled in 1956 at a cost of one hundred million dollars. They are manufactured under 42 trade names by 36 pharmaceutical companies.

It is almost impossible to convince the public and even the general practitioner that in many cases psychotherapy, shock therapy and hospitalization cannot be replaced by pills. When such replacements are attempted they fail to reach their target because the dynamics and motivation of our behavior are ignored. Under some circumstances results may be tragic and General Maxwell D. Taylor, Army Chief of Staff, was justified in decreeing (April 21, 1957) that any pilot using the tranquilizing drugs is barred from flying until four weeks after he has stopped using them.

Many of the general practitioners who could no longer deny the existence of emotional disturbances among their patients, found in the tranquilizers a pharmacotherapy that is a panacea for all mental illnesses.

However, the mood-changing drugs have outgrown their period of sensation and fad. It may be admitted that many hasty workers have been overenthusiastic in their evaluation of the results obtained where evidence was not conclusive. But many other reliable practitioners have offered undeniable proof of the efficacy of these new drugs. We shall let the clinicians have their say as to the therapeutic actions and their undesirable side effects.

ATARACTIC DRUGS

Rauwolfia Serpentina Benth

Deserpidine	
Raudixin	(Squibb)
Rau-Sed	(Squibb)
Rauwiloid	(Riker)
Reserpine	
Reserpoid	(Upjohn)
Serfin	(Parke-Davis)
Serpasil	(Ciba)
Moderil	(Pfizer)
Sandril	(Lilly)

Phenothiazine

Avomine	(Phenergan, Lysivane, RP. 4560)
Dartal	(Searle)
Deparcol	
Largactil	(Chlorpromazine—Canada, England, France and Italy)
Megaphen	(Germany)
NP-207	(Sandoz)
Pacatal	(Warner-Chilcott)
Proclorperazine	(Compazine, SKF)
Promazine	(Sparine, Wyeth)
Thorazine	(SKF)
Trilafon	(Schering)
Vesprin	(Squibb)

Azacyclonol Hydrochloride

Frenquel	(Merrell)
Mer-17	
Meratran	(Pipradrol)

Mephenesin

Equanil	(Wyeth)
Miltown	(Wallace)
Propanediol Dicarbamate	(Meprobamate)
Phenaglycodol	(Ultran, Lilly)

Hydroxyzine Hydrochloride

Atarax	(Roerig)

Benactyzine Hydrochloride

Suavitil	(Medicinalco)

THE NEW CHEMOTHERAPY IN MENTAL ILLNESS

Part One

GENERAL SURVEYS

THE TRANQUILIZING DRUGS

Morris Fishbein, M.D.

When William Osler made his valedictory address to the University of Pennsylvania in 1889, he chose the subject "Aequanimitas." He said, "In the physician or surgeon no quality takes rank with imperturbability." Then he defined the word: "Imperturbability means coolness and presence of mind under all circumstances, calmness amid storm, clearness of judgment in moments of grave peril, immobility, impassiveness, or, to use an old and expressive word, *phlegm.*" He was doubtful that it could be acquired except by inheritance and he thought that some of his students, "owning to congenital defects," might never be able to acquire it. He counseled, nevertheless, that education with practice and experience might help to attain imperturbability in fair measure.

The doctor, Osler felt, should develop an "inscrutable face by education of his nerve centers." In concluding this discussion of imperturbability he said: "Cultivate then, gentlemen, such a judicious measure of obtuseness as will enable you to meet the exigencies of practice with firmness and courage without, at the same time, hardening the human heart by which we live."

The mental equivalent to imperturbability which Osler called "a bodily endowment," is a calm equanimity. He considered one of the first essentials in securing it is "not to expect too much of the people amongst whom you dwell." Osler recognized that prosperity is an aid to equanimity and enables us to bear with composure the misfortunes of our neighbors.

At the most recent meeting of the Society of Biologic Psychiatry, the president, Dr. Harold E. Himwich, said "A few short years ago it would have been impossible to read a paper on the new tranquilizing drugs, but now we know that chlopromazine and reserpine are valuable in the treatment of disturbed psychotic patients." Since that paper was read, other drugs have been added to the list, notably Frenquel, Miltown and Equanil. These are the drugs which affect the brain. Both reserpine and chlorpromazine depress the hypothalamic mechanisms, particularly that part concerned with the patterns for emergency, for fight and flight. Chlorpromazine depresses not only these mechanisms but also the sympathetic and parasympathetic nervous systems. Other research has indicated that chlorpromazine prevents the awakening, alerting or arousal reaction, producing what is in effect a pharmacologic lobotomy. Frenquel, according to Himwich, depresses neither the hypothalamus nor the activating system and is still a tranquilizing drug.

The mechanism by which these drugs have their effect is not clearly established. However, some evidence indicates that a neurohormone called serotonin is involved. When it is insufficient in amount to produce its normal effects, abnormal behavior may be observed. In concluding his address Himwich wrote, "These new drugs are not a flash in the pan, but their therapeutic values have been widely corroborated. However, they are not a complete answer to our therapeutic problem, because no one drug is able to ameliorate the condition of all of the patients and none of them is as efficacious for melancholia as is electric shock."

The discovery of new drugs of this type invariably sets off a chain reaction in which new fields are investigated and various combinations of new and old drugs are tested for specific effects. Already there are combinations of reserpine with various sedative drugs of the barbiturate series and with other active ingredients. In one study reserpine and chlorpromazine were given in combination and the combination was said to have certain advantages over therapy with reserpine alone. Indeed, the authors say that chlorpromazine seemed to potentiate the clinical effects of reserpine. "The course of combined therapy," say Drs. J. A. Barsa and N. S. Kline, "was less stormy and less distressing to the patient because of the milder and shorter turbulent period." Already these drugs are said to have worked miracles in state institutions for the mentally disturbed, permitting great numbers of patients to be discharged to their homes beyond what might have been possible in previous years. Dr. A. E. Bennett says that "both drugs have facilitated psychotherapy through physiologic relief of anxiety, tension, insomnia or somatic symptoms in some cases."

In addition to the drugs already mentioned, consideration must be given to the pharmacologic properties of Miltown which is a meprobamate, a drug which is related to mephenesin and which was found in a study of such preparations to be the most potent anticonvulsant in the series and also to possess a muscle-relaxant action of considerable intensity and long duration. Dr. J. C. Borrus found that it was most effective in anxiety and tension states through a lessening of tension, reduced irritability and restlessness, more restful sleep, and generalized muscle relaxation. Chiefly in its favor is an absence of toxicity both subjectively and objectively as compared with other drugs, and "there were no withdrawal phenomena noted on cessation of therapy." Dr. Lowell S. Selling confirmed its non-habit-forming character and found it of must value in the so-called anxiety neurosis syndrome, especially when the primary symptom is tension. His studies and other studies made since his first publication indicated a special value to Miltown in accomplishing withdrawal from alcohol with a minimum of discomfort. Among the special qualities listed for this drug, based on clinical studies, are as an agent in anxiety and tension states; as a muscle relaxant, particularly in fibrositic rheumatic disorders; an agent in such conditions as torticollis and back pain; for control of spasticity in such conditions as cerebral palsy, and as a somnifacient of a different order than the hypnotics or sedatives. Few allergic reactions have been reported and all of them responded to therapy with antihistamines. In a new series of studies by Dr. F. Lemere this drug proved effective in 70 per cent of a group of 250 non-hospitalized patients and he considers it "the drug of choice for the relief of tension, anxiety and insomnia."

Another discovery has reported this drug selectively effective in a high percentage of cases of petit mal. Further, several reports by general practitioners have indicated its desirability in what are commonly called tension states but which might include psychoses, psychoneuroses and personality disorders, as well as a wide variety of conditions classified en masse as psychosomatic, including headaches, dysmenorrhea, hypertension, motion sickness, peptic ulcers and a variety of dermatologic disorders.

One wonders what Sir William Osler might have said had he had available in 1889 such aids to imperturbability and equanimity as have come with the new tranquilizing drugs. This is in the nature of a medical revolution. Ten years hence statistics of institutions for the mentally disturbed and for the alcoholic may indicate the results of administration of these and other new remedies which are bound to come. Already the great progress that has been made is an indication of the future.

PHARMACOLOGY OF THE ATARACTIC DRUGS

Edward B. Truitt, Jr., Ph.D.

Associate Professor of Pharmacology, School of Medicine,
University of Maryland, Baltimore

ATARAXIA, or peace of mind, has been claimed for a growing list of compounds labeled the tranquilizing drugs. These agents belong to 4 groups with divergent chemical and pharmacologic properties. An arbitrary classification is as follows:

1] *Rauwolfia alkaloids*: reserpine (Serpasil), rescinnamine, recanescine
2] *Phenothiazines*: chlorpromazine (Thorazine), promazine (Sparine) mepazine (Pacatal) proclorperazine (Compazine), perphenazine (Trilafon)
3] *Propanediol dicarbamate*: meprobamate (Miltown, Equanil)
4] *Diphenyl methanes*: azacyclonol (Frenquel), benactyzine (Suavitil), hydroxyzine (Atarax).

These drugs resolve into similar groupings based upon the type of action on the Siamese fighting fish *(Betta splendens)*.

How these diverse agents calm maniacal states, reduce anxiety, and produce sedation without cortical depression is only partly known. Their modes of action are being explored by many avenues, including neurophysiologic, biochemical, and psychiatric as well as pharmacologic methods. Unfortunately, with some of these drugs the evidence for their tranquilizing action rests mainly on clinical observations, with very little experimental data.

ACTION OF SERPASIL

The unusual depressant action of the Rauwolfia root and its alkaloids has long been known in India, but it was in this country that wide-spread use in neuropsychiatric conditions evolved from observations of patients taking the drug for hypertension. This sedation can be seen in animals, especially wild, jungle-bred monkeys. When Serpasil is administered, the biting, tooth-baring reaction to the approaching human being is replaced by a calm, unafraid, curious attitude. The monkey will accept food from the hand and may even be led around the cage by the hand. With large doses, the animal may appear to be asleep but is easily aroused and is responsive to the environment. Accompanying this mental change are other signs: miosis, bradycardia, hypotension, hypothermia, hyperperistalsis, ptosis of the eyelids, and relaxation of the nictitating membrane. All of these latter effects are attributable to depression of the sympathetic autonomic nerve supply to the respective organs. An autonomic imbalance exists in which the unopposed parasympathetic innervation becomes dominant. This depression of the sympathetic system occurs centrally, since the end organs still respond to epinephrine.

Attention was directed to the hypothalamus as the central site of Serpasil action by the similarity of the effects in animals to those of lesions in the posterior hypothalamic sympathetic center. Evidence that Serpasil interferes with the metabolism of 5-hydroxytryptamine or serotonin in brain cells has suggested that its action may be connected with the function of this substance as a neurohormone in the hypothalamus. It is interesting that only three of the many alkaloids from Rauwolfia—reserpine, rescinnamine, and recanescine—have an action on serotonin and are the only ones with tranquilizing effect.

The electroencephalogram shows a distinct difference in the action of Serpasil compared to that of barbiturates and bromides. In contrast to the sleep pattern produced by the latter, Serpasil evokes an alertness pattern in the record. This is reflected in some of the pharmacologic actions of the agent: it facilitates the convulsant action of cortically acting stimulants such as caffeine and Metrazol and antagonizes the effectiveness of antiepileptic drugs such as Dilantin. These effects are probably related to the stimulant action of Serpasil on the reticular activating system of the mesodiencephalon, but the correlation between this and its action in the hypothalamus is still unclear.

Many side effects preclude the acceptance of Serpasil as an ideal agent. Nasal stuffiness is distressing to many patients. Drowsiness, hypotension, parkinsonian tremor, miosis, and facial edema offset the benefits.

Action of the Phenothiazines

Thorazine can be considered as the prototype of the phenothiazine tranquilizers. It is an outcome of investigations into a number of phenothiazine derivatives with antihistaminic action. With Thorazine, this effect is weak and far overshadowed by strong central sedation. In addition, other minor actions make it a polypharmacologic drug. It possesses, in some degree, adrenergic and cholinergic blocking actions, antiemetic effects, and hypothermic action.

Contrasted to Serpasil, the central sedation produced by Thorazine is almost immediate in onset, an advantage in combating anxiety, tension, and extreme agitation initially. Also, with Thorazine, the nature of the central depression is characterized more by drowsiness; the drug may produce alarmingly extended periods of coma when given to patients receiving ordinary therapeutic doses of barbiturates and opiate analgesics. The drug can depress the reticular activating system and may so insulate an animal from external—and perhaps internal—stimuli that conditioned reflexes are lost.

Less is known of the fundamental neurochemical effects of Thorazine. It has a sparing action on adenosine triphosphate breakdown, especially in subcortical areas such as the thalamus and hypothalamus. Its neural action has also been explained as a cerebral manifestation of its adrenolytic action.

Even more than Serpasil, Thorazine must be used with caution and discretion because the manifold actions give rise to a variety of sometimes dangerous side effects. Severe blood dyscrasias may occasionally result from strenuous therapy. Jaundice of the retention type may be caused by a depression of the motility of smooth muscle in the biliary system. Parenteral administration is often accompanied by distressing orthostatic hypotension by reason of the drug's action on the sympathetic control of vasomotor tone. Like Serpasil, a parkinsonian tremor may arise after prolonged therapy. Other side effects include dry mouth, photosensitivity, tachycardia, dermatitis, and occasional neurologic manifestations.

SPARINE is claimed to produce less hypotension and allergic skin reactions. Jaundice and parkinsonism are so far unreported in limited trials with this drug. One instance of agranulocytosis occurred with overdosage. Although therapeutic potency is difficult to assess from clinical reports, apparently the lack of the chlorine atom on the phenothiazine ring in Sparine slightly diminishes potency as well as toxicity.

PACATAL does not differ strikingly from either Thorazine or Sparine.

ACTION OF MEPROBAMATE

Meprobamate is the dicarbamic ester of a propanediol compound related to mephenesin (Tolserol, Myanesin). Esterification with carbamic acid blocks the rapid metabolism of these compounds by the body, which is responsible for the transient action of mephenesin. Like mephenesin, meprobamate depresses multineuronal reflexes in the spinal cord and lower brain centers. Complex reflexes with a large number of interneurons are sensitive to depression by the drug, while simpler two-neuronal reflexes such as the knee jerk are unimpaired.

The depression of interneurons blocks the development of excessive skeletal muscle tone, commonly called tension, either from reflex origin locally caused by irritation or from higher centers of psychic origin. With large doses, a taming effect can be produced in wild monkeys, similar to that described for Serpasil. An electroencephalogram made with subcortical electrodes demonstrates sensitivity of thalamic centers to the drug.

Though it is lacking in potency compared to Rauwolfia alkaloids and phenothiazines, meprobamate is almost devoid of side effects. Drowsiness and muscle weakness have been reported, but the former can be offset by stimulants and the latter may be avoided by reduction of dosage. Recently, several reports of allergic skin reactions have appeared, but the number is small, considering the widespread use of the drug.

ACTION OF THE DIPHENYL METHANES

The drug FRENQUEL has an unusual origin. It is a position isomer of a closely similar compound, Meratran, a potent central nervous system stimulant. However, like Thorazine and other ataractics, Frenquel lengthens the sleeping time of barbiturate-treated animals. The agent combats effectively the drug psychoses produced by lysergic acid diethylamide (LSD) and mescaline. This appears to correlate well with its sole clinical action as an antihallucinogen, mostly in schizophrenia. The side effects and toxic effects are few in doses up to 400 mg. orally and parenterally. In animals, very large doses induce toxic effects similar to Meratran overstimulation.

SUAVITIL was made in Europe in 1936 and was first recognized as an atropine-like and local anesthetic drug useful for parkinsonian tremor. It bears close structural relationship to Artane and Trasentine. Of late, it has been recognized to have unusual central actions on associative processes and time awareness in human beings. In large doses of 4 to 10 mg., Suavitil may produce a state of absent-mindedness and confusion. It has been demonstrated to repair the tension and anxiety reactions produced in rats and cats by frustration and conflict-producing situations. At present, the drug is devoid of the more serious toxic effects of the phenothiazine group. It has some atropine-like side effects and may produce drowsiness, since, like all ataractics, it synergizes barbiturates and opiates.

ATARAX is another mild tranquilizing drug lacking the serious toxic hazards of the phenothiazine group and has been more widely explored in Europe than in this country. Chemically, the structure is closely similar to chlorcyclizine (Di-paralene). Drowsiness is the only side effect.

SUMMARY

It seems likely that the chemical interrelationships of the many antiparkinsonian and the antihistaminic agents possessing drowsiness as a side effect with the milder peace-of-mind drugs will prompt a reevaluation of many drugs formerly overlooked for ataraxia.

Although the peripheral effects of the ataractic drugs are well understood as to site and mechanism of action, the effects in the brain on emotions, memory, motivations, ego, conditioned responses, and other higher functions are yet to be unravelled. For this reason, one must urge great caution in the use of drugs that so significantly affect these functions while we still lack a rational basis for their actions. Certainly, the greatest admonition for the proper use of tranquilizing drugs is the suicidal tendency that may be activated in depression states.

THE ATARACTIC DRUGS: THE PRESENT POSITION OF CHLORPROMAZINE, FRENQUEL, PACATAL, AND RESERPINE IN THE PSYCHIATRIC HOSPITAL

H. Angus Bowes, M.D.
Clinical Director in Psychiatry, Ste. Anne de Bellevue Veterans Hospital, Ste. Anne de Bellevue, Quebec, Canada

The desire to take medicine is perhaps the greatest feature which distinguishes man from animals.

—Sir William Osler

Perhaps never before in the field of emotional conflict have so many medicines been consumed by so many patients with so many diverse results as in the psychiatric hospitals of North America during the past 2 years that have seen the birth of the ataractic era. It has been a painful period of parturition for those of us who are reluctant to reformulate our psychiatric concepts at the sensationalistic behest of ill-advised and overoptimistic publications. Some enthusiastic members of our own fraternity have not been completely free from criticism in this respect. I have attended conferences on these drugs where the atmosphere approached that of a revivalist meeting.

Chlorpromazine and reserpine have been advocated for the treatment of every condition from anxiety to zoophobia. No wonder that there is chaos in this field, with many psychiatrists doubting what are the real indications for these drugs and, perhaps, pondering their own inability to confirm the optimistic claims advanced by research workers whom they trust, admire, and respect.

We have all heard so many panegyrics on these drugs individually that an attempt at their collective appraisal might help to clarify the present position. In giving you an account of our own experiences with these ataraxics, I hope to act as a purveyor of ataraxy itself and that, in medical terminology, means "freedom from confusion and anxiety." In my Oxford dictionary it is defined as "stoic indifference"—you may need that as well!

We have a small modern veterans psychiatric unit of 550 beds; 200 for senile and failing psychotics and 350 for the admission and active treatment cases. During the past 5 years we have had just over 1,100 admissions (31% return cases) and over 1,000 discharges. We have only a small staff of 8 psychiatrists, half of whom are still in training. However, we receive many of our admissions directly from the armed services shortly after their symptoms develop and, in addition, we offer rehabilitation services, including job-replacement, outpatient support, and financial aid to many of our discharged patients, for, with commendable foresight, our Canadian cousins have given pensions only to psychotics, whom they help, and not to neurotics, whom they hinder. I think that this eulogy of our psychiatric facilities is important in the objective assessment of what these new drugs will do and will not do. Here is no static, custodial backwater in which the administration of new drugs to a mass of patients might draw attention to the overlooked fact that many of them had spontaneously improved during the years.

In this optimistic and busy setting we started using chlorpromazine over 2 years ago. We were early in this field as we were fortunate in having Dr. Hanrahan, who with Dr. Lehmann, did the original North American research on chlorpromazine, as a frequent visitor to our staff conferences and his experience and advice were of considerable help in starting our work with this new drug. Our results were so encouraging that we started to use reserpine as soon as it became available.

Now, what did we learn from these 2 drugs? First, that in chlorpromazine we had, for the first time, a drug that would tranquilize without stupefying. It was more effective than electrotherapy in aborting manic attacks and could replace much of the maintenance electroconvulsive therapy which we had been using extensively to prevent the regression of chronic schizophrenics. It was also much more effective than any sedatives we had in the symptomatic control of excitement, aggression, destructiveness, and restlessness. Given in conjunction with ECT it shortened the course of treatment and either prevented the postconvulsive confusion frequently encountered after long courses of treatment, or, if it did develop, helped its resolution.

This reduction in the number of electric treatments and the confusions usually accompanying them enabled us to shorten the patient's hospitalization by applying supportive psychotherapy, with emphasis on complete honesty and the reality situation, at a date earlier in the acute psychoses than would formerly have been possible. We did not find chlorpromazine to be as good a tranquilizing agent as reserpine in the elderly patients because of the development of orthostatic hypotension, confusion, and mild pyrexia.

In treating schizophrenics we were able to confirm Kline's findings of a period of sedation followed by turbulence and reintegration with large doses of reserpine, and we used this method of treatment in acute psychoses showing withdrawal and apathy. We reserved chlorpromazine for the agitated schizophrenic but found that often ECT had to be used as well before the patient became amenable to psychotherapy.

Emboldened by these findings we discontinued insulin coma therapy on July 1, 1955, and substituted intensive group therapy using chlorpromazine and reserpine as adjuvants. This new project rejoiced in the singularly cacophonous designation of "The Ataraxic Push Group"—but it worked.

Personally, I have long regarded insulin merely as an adjuvant to group psychotherapy, but it is a messy form of treatment, expensive, time-consuming, and, with a 0.6% mortality rate and prolonged comas, it is frequently shock therapy not only for the patients but for the staff as well. So I was strongly motivated for the change.

At the beginning of the "Ataraxic Push Group" the nurses were quite re sentful of their altered role and, at first, the patients were also. Many patients sat around with the wooden expression of the early stages of Parkinsonism, with pieces of tissue stuffed into their mouths to absorb the saliva—reserpine has such aesthetically unpleasant side-effects—or restlessly tottered around the room in a state of emotional turbulence. However, they did become amenable to psychotherapy and the physician in charge of the group, who has had considerable experience with insulin, is firmly convinced that this is a better form of treatment. His very enthusiasm must have made a significant contribution to the success of the project.

Let me give you some figures. In 1954, 26 patients received insulin coma therapy with a 90% remission rate; in the last 6 months of 1955, 30 patients were treated in the ataraxic group—all have been discharged from hospital and are fully employed and adjusting satisfactorily.

The modifications we have learned from experience are that there is no need to have the unpleasant side-effects mentioned earlier. We have gradually used reserpine less and less and replaced it with chlorpromazine. The Parkinsonian symptoms that still occur are controlled by Cogentin. The indication for inclusion in this group has also changed. At first it was merely a continuation of insulin coma group. Now we can include patients whose physical condition would have contraindicated that form of treatment and those schizophrenics who fail to respond to supportive psychotherapy given in conjunction with ECT or ataraxics or both.

There are 3 small, closed, side-room sections that used to be filled to overflowing with disturbed patients requiring isolation. Five years ago, with the aid of ECT, I was able to empty one of these sections and use it as a probation ward. Last July, we decided to do something about the hard core of disturbed and aggressive patients who still haunted the remaining 2 sections and to attempt to reintegrate these 15 rugged individualists into the large wards.

With the help of large doses of chlorpromazine and reserpine we were soon able to reduce them to a state of benevolent stupor. The nursing orderlies became less afraid of them and more accepting. They were then transferred with their orderlies to a room on the admission ward. A period of laissez-faire then followed in which the whims and caprices of these tranquillized patients were indulged as far as possible and they were quite literally fussed over and petted. They were taken for walks, encouraged to play cards and games and to participate in occupational therapy. Within 2 months they were all transferred to other wards where they remained docile and pleasant.

The nursing staff, as in most periods of laissez-faire in psychiatric therapy, were much more disturbed than the patients and were fearful of their reverting to their former behavior. However, when they remained quiet and pleasant in their new surroundings, the tension of the nursing staff gradually relaxed and they learned to accept the change. One of the sections thus liberated has become an honor ward for a modified therapeutic community who receive just sufficient chlorpromazine to take the edge off their psychotic drives. Seclusion has thus been reduced to less than one-tenth and for days on end the remaining side-room section remains empty.

So much for chlorpromazine and reserpine. The promise of these 2 drugs had gradually converted me from a dubious dilettante to an avid enthusiast in the ataraxic field. It was with real enthusiasm that I commenced research on 2 new ataraxics: Frenquel and Pacatal.

Frenquel, which was given to 50 acute and 80 chronic psychotics, is the gamma isomer of Meratran, a central nervous stimulant without autonomic side-effects. In the course of toxicity studies it was discovered that this new compound made laboratory animals quiet and tractable. In 1954, Fabing noted that it would prevent the development of experimental psychoses if given before LSD-25 or mescaline and would relieve the subjective symptoms of psychosis produced by these phantasmagorics. These dramatic results stimulated interest in the application of this new drug to the treatment of schizophrenia and in May 1955 Rinaldi *et al.* presented a most encouraging report of the efficacy of Frenquel in the treatment of 39 disturbed patients with psychoses of long duration.

The following month I was able to obtain supplies of the new drug and proceeded to investigate its potentialities. At first we gave half our acute admissions, irrespective of diagnosis, Frenquel tablets alone with supportive psychotherapy. When injectionable material became available this was used at hourly intervals in quite high dosages.

In addition, 30 patients on a 59-bed ward of chronic disturbed patients, mostly severe schizophrenics who had failed to respond to any physical methods of treatment, were given 40 mg. t.i.d. To secure their cooperation in taking the tablets, I told the entire ward that we had a new drug that might help them to get out of hospital and that we were going to give it to the patients whose names began with the letters A to K and asked the L's to Z's to watch for the difference. This directive group therapeutic session was quite an experience.

Within 2 weeks of commencing treatment a striking change had taken place. The patients on Frenquel had become more sociable, they were neater, cleaner, and tidier. They looked better. Some chronic eczematous rashes cleared up. All their skins looked healthier and their eyes clearer. They gained weight. They stopped responding to their hallucinations. This was so encouraging that all the patients on the ward were given 40 mg. t.i.d. and within one week the ward became quiet and orderly. For the first time the patients would read books and magazines instead of tearing them apart. Curtains could be left up instead of being pulled down. Pictures were no longer destroyed and flowers could be left untouched in their vases. Yet there was no oversedation seen in the patients. They played cards together and appeared much more sociable and interested in their environment. Some who had previously banged their heads against the walls and covered their heads with their coats stopped responding to their hallucinations. It was most impressive.

It had been my plan to put half of these patients on placebos, but, as the delivery of these was delayed and we were running short of tablets, all the medication had to be stopped. Within 4 weeks the ward gradually regressed to its former state. Fights again became frequent, complexions muddy and eyes lack-lustre. Hallucinations returned; no improvements were maintained. When the placebos, identically flavored and disguised arrived, they were given to the first 30 patients by the nursing staff who did not know of the substitution.

The patients responded almost exactly as in their previous reaction to the genuine tablets. Had they been conditioned? Was this merely suggestion? It was all quite intriguing.

Meanwhile, the other patients, forlorn and dejected, rather pathetically held out their hands for the tablets and crept away dejected when refused them. So, we gave them the genuine tablets and they improved even more dramatically than the other 30 on placebos, some of whom had retained their hallucinations.

At present we are running a "double blind" study on 10 patients who appeared to benefit from Frenquel but who failed to maintain their improvement on placebos. Apparently 4 patients benefited.

To return to the admission cases. At first we appeared to be obtaining some very significant results but they were transient. Apparently the tablets, even in large dosages, were not effective. The intravenous injection of 20 mg. repeated half-hourly, produced a few slight improvements but they were not maintained. The 100 mg. injection, repeated hourly, helped a few patients to reorientate. One elderly schizophrenic complained bitterly that following the injection he felt lonely as his voices stopped talking to him; however, his loneliness lasted only half an hour. A few patients with senile confusional states became lucid for a few minutes after the injection. It was also possible to discuss delusional material fairly objectively with a few patients after injecting 100 mg. without their becoming as disturbed as they would have done previously. These positive results were obtained only by those physicians who still retained some enthusiasm over the new drug. Some skeptical colleagues obtained no results at all. What positive results we obtained could be duplicated by sodium amytal, chlorpromazine, or reserpine and we were having such encouraging results with Pacatal that our investigation was discontinued. However, we shall always be grateful to Frenquel for its complete lack of toxicity and the very forceful demonstration it gave us that we can never discount interpersonal relationships, emotions, and enthusiasms in psychiatric treatment.

The success of Phenergan, Diparcol, and chlorpromazine in pharmacology has focussed much attention on the phenothiazines and in 1954, a synthetic derivitive, N-methylpiperidyl-(3)-methylphenothiazine, was first tested and discovered to resemble closely chlorpromazine in its pharmaceutical action but to be much less toxic. Horatz has reported on over 5,000 cases of the use of Pacatal, as the drug is now called, as a premedication in surgery. Kleinsorge has used it with barbiturates in "therapeutic sleep," a modification of continual narcosis being extensively developed in Europe. We were fortunate in being the first hospital in Canada to be given supplies of Pacatal for clinical assessment of its place in psychiatry, and our studies started in June 1955.

After an initial personal test to make sure that the new drug could safely be administered, half the patients on chlorpromazine had Pacatal substituted in the same dosage and it was also given to one-third of the new admissions. Toxicity studies had shown a wide margin of safety, but for the first 3 months all the patients on the new drug had a weekly battery of liver, urinary, and blood tests and their temperatures, pulse and respiratory rates, and blood pressures were recorded thrice daily and they were weighed weekly.

In our experience with 250 cases to date we have found no evidence of liver or kidney damage; the pulse rate, blood pressure and temperature remain constant on normal dosage and though the white cell count fluctuates we have had no cases of agranulocytosis. Two patients have developed leukopenia; in one we discontinued the drug as at the time we had little experience of it; in the other we persisted with Patcatal as it was helping the patient and the white cell count gradually returned to normal. We now restrict our laboratory studies to a weekly white cell count and differential for the first month and monthly thereafter unless the white cell count is abnormal. A careful physical check is kept on the patients and this is much more valuable than any laboratory studies.

There is always the danger that a noisy and aggressive patient who has forcibly been drawing attention to himself may become quiet and uncomplaining when put on the drug and so may be overlooked and may develop serious complications. This happened to 2 of our patients. The first, a veteran of 83, made a remarkable recovery from a recurrent manic episode in 5 days when we discovered that he had an atonic bladder and he required an in-dwelling catheter for one week. The second was a deteriorated young schizophrenic who developed severe constipation and a paralytic ileus that lasted 4 days.

The complications that occur with Pacatal are associated with the drug's parasympatholytic effects. Nearly all the patients developed dry mouths and half of them had difficulty in accommodation. Their pupils became dilated and they had trouble in reading small print. This was generally associated with high dosages but did occur in a few patients on only 150 mg. daily. It affected younger patients more than the elder. We subsequently learned that if chlorpromazine were substituted for half the dosage of Pacatal, the symptom frequently cleared up. Constipation occurred in 10% and if this was overlooked the patients became quite toxic and starting vomiting. We now prevent the development of eliminatory complications by the routine use of laxatives and have prostigmine available for obstinate constipation and oliguria.

There were no cases of jaundice or extra-pyramidal syndrome. In fact we found that Pacatal, substituted for half the dosage of chlorpromazine, cleared up the symptoms of Parkinsonism which frequently occur with chlorpromazine. This was presumably attributable to the atropine-like effect of Pacatal. No allergic reactions such as edema or rashes occurred though several patients had previously experienced such reactions on chlorpromazine. We found that the large dosages we used at first produced tremors, orthostatic hypotension, and mild pyrexia in elderly patients, who became quite confused and toxic. We now find that between 75 and 150 mg. daily will make these disgruntled and irascible old hypertensives much more pleasant and cooperative. One paranoid, resentful veteran of the Boer War, who had long been an administrative thorn in the flesh of our hospital, became pleasant and friendly within one week of treatment and has been maintained in a reasonable frame of mind on 100 mg. Pacatal daily for the past 9 months, despite an alcoholic cirrhosis.

We were unable to confirm Kline's unfavorable report on the toxicity of Pacatal and we can only presume that he was investigating impure material[1].

---

[1] This has since been confirmed in a personal communication.

The method of administration was to give those patients who would cooperate 100 mg. tablets thrice daily. The dosage was then adjusted up or down till the desired degree of tranquillization was obtained. We found this varied between 75 and 900 mg. daily at first, when we were using rather high dosages. We now find that 600 mg. daily is sufficient to render the most excited patients quiet in 2 or 3 days. Intramuscular injections of the acetate are supplied in 2 cc. ampules containing 50 mg. This is diluted to 5 cc. with sterile water as saline precipitates it and is much less painful than an injection of chlorpromazine. I have given it intravenously in the pure form with no adverse results. We have given between 50 and 200 mg. daily by injection. It does not flatten the patient the way chlorpromazine does and he remains ambulatory but tranquil. We found Pacatal the treatment of choice in manic excitement and schizo-affective psychoses. Like all the other ataraxics, it is not indicated in depressions of the intensity encountered in psychiatric hospitals though it will help to calm the agitation of the involutional depressive and is an excellent adjuvant to ECT, shortening its course and preventing the development of postconvulsive confusion or aiding its resolution if it does arise. In the more chronic patients Pacatal was most effective in the symptomatic treatment of aggression, destructiveness, restlessness and insomnia.

In comparison with chlorpromazine it was found by both patients and volunteers alike to be almost twice as strong a tranquillizer and to have a slightly euphoriant effect. One patient said it was "like champagne after beer." The volunteers stated that it did not make them feel as heavy and drowsy as chlorpromazine but that it cut down their drive more and reduced their tension and hostility to the point that they were unable to enter into arguments. It was found to produce a vague feeling of restlessness and uneasiness when given to chronic severe anxiety neurotics whose reactions were characterized by palpitations and tremors, in other words, sympathetic overactivity. Apparently the parasympatholytic effect of Pacatal had still further increased their autonomic imbalance. We subsequently learned through experience that patients of pyknic build, who generally tend to show a para-sympathetic responses to anxiety by sweating and gastro-intestinal upset, benefited more from Pacatal than the asthenics, who respond better to chlorpromazine.

This was well demonstrated by 6 recurrent manics, all of whom had previously been treated in our hospital for manic episodes with chlorpromazine. They were all of pyknic build and responded more rapidly to treatment with Pacatal. Two recurrent manics of asthenic build were given Pacatal during the manic phase and though they improved gradually, their remission was much more rapid on changing to chlorpromazine. These results were confirmed by our experiences with acute schizophrenic psychoses, which characteristically occur in asthenics; these responded more rapidly to chlorpromazine than to Pacatal.

We are now obtaining excellent results in the treatment of severely disturbed psychotics by using Pacatal and chlorpromazine in equal dosage. Not only do the 2 drugs appear to act synergistically to each other's complications. Perhaps the Funkenstein test might be a further help in deciding which drug to use or in what proportions. Certainly the alliterative aid "Pyknic-Pacatal," "Asthenic-Thorazine" (or "Lean-Largactil") has become a helpful guide in our application of this most promising new ataraxic.

It is my impression that the ataractic drugs work centrally by depressing the autonomic outflow and thus reducing the physical concomitants of anxiety. The patient, now freed from his sweating tremors, palpitation, and gastrointestinal upset, is able to take a more objective view of his emotional problems with which he may now cope with the aid of psychotherapy. In addition his drive is so much reduced that the fear of losing self-control is markedly diminished. Chlorpromazine, as a predominantly sympatholytic drug, is indicated in the asthenic who is prone to feel anxiety at an adrenergic level. Pacatal, a more vagolytic drug, is helpful to the pyknic, whose anxiety is frequently cholinergic in character. A combination of both drugs would seem to be indicated in those patients who lie somewhere in between these extremes.

After this review of the accomplishments of the ataraxics, it is time to take an objective view of their place in the psychiatric hospital. In their favor, let us say that for the first time our discharges outweigh our admissions, that the hospital atmosphere is calmer and more optimistic, seclusion is down to below one-tenth of its previous rate and ECT to one-third.

However, not one single deteriorated schizophrenic has been discharged as a result of these drugs. They just will not touch the hard bedrock case. This near-miracle, in our experience, can be accomplished only by lobotomy when the indications for this last-resort treatment are overwhelming. Now, before we submit any of our patients to lobotomy, we first try them on intensive courses of these drugs and a few patients show just sufficient temporary improvement to make us hold up their operations for a further period of reassessment and observation. This has significantly reduced the number of lobotomy operations in the last 2 years.

The general acceptance of these "wonder drugs" by the lay press and our own specialists has considerably stimulated the enthusiasm of our medical and nursing staff. In the course of research work on the back wards, we have come to take an unusual interest in the legacy of chronic schizophrenics bequeathed us by former therapists. An infectious air of optimism has been created in the increased interest that research causes the staff to show in them. Even such mundane procedures as the estimation of blood pressures, pulse and temperature rates achieve an added significance when they are taken by an enthusiastic nursing sister, who, unconsciously, is anxious to give the research physician just what she thinks he ought to want and is equally as eager to obtain it from the patient by cajolery or flattery. It makes their work more interesting and adds a sense of achievement to what has often become a dull and monotonous task.

We, ourselves, objective though we think we are, by our very interest bring a feeling of sympathy and understanding to those chronic patients who have been doubly condemned for their failures firstly, to adjust to society and secondly, and much more heinous still, to respond to the treatment we had to offer.

These factors of interest, expectancy, optimism and enthusiasm must not be underrated in our appraisal of these new drugs. If they have done nothing else, the ataraxics have spurred us on to new efforts. In this age of anxiety, when the social acceptance of the material accomplishments of the individual far outweighs his psychic needs, we are likely to become dependent upon ataraxics more and more. The "emotional aspirin" is likely to become just as much a part of our way of life as the epileptic's anticonvulsant, the alcoholic's amphetamine, the executive's anatacid, the salesman's hip-flask, and the socialite's sedative.

Summary

The ataractic drugs are so called from their ability to produce ataraxy: freedom from confusion and anxiety. In a veterans' psychiatric unit of 550 beds with a high rate of admissions and discharges, chlorpromazine and reserpine have been intensively studied during the past 2 years and since June 1955, Frenquel has been given to 130 patients, and Pacatal to over 250, in an effort to clarify the indications for these ataraxics in the treatment of acute and chronic psychoses.

Our experiences with Frenquel are described in some detail as the originally hopeful and eventually disillusionary results obtained may explain many ambiguous findings in this complex field of research. Frenquel appears to have antihallucinatory and physically tonic effects in a small minority of regressed schizophrenics but to be of no value in the treatment of acute psychoses. Reserpine has also failed to fulfill earlier expectations. It is now reserved for the tranquillization of arteriosclerotics and as an adjuvant in the psychotherapy of some withdrawn schizophrenics.

Pacatal, a phenothiazine derivative recently developed in Europe, and chlorpromazine are virtually interchangeable and synergistic. Pacatal is almost twice as strong a tranquillizer but a weaker hypnotic. It is mildly euphoriant and strongly parasympatholyitc unlike chlorpromazine, a sympatholytic and depressant. Both are indicated in the symptomatic relief of psychomotor excitation, aggression, destructiveness, restlessness, and tension in acute and chronic psychoses. A combination of both, in which their mutually antagonistic autonomic effects reduce the incidence of complications and abolish the Parkinsonian syndrome, is yielding promising results.

In this study these drugs have significantly reduced the need for ECT and lobotomy without replacing these valuable methods of treatment. The seclusion of disturbed patients has been reduced to one-tenth. Since July 1955, insulin coma therapy has been replaced by group psychotherapy using ataraxics as adjuvants. Over twice the number of patients can be treated, so far with better results. Our discharges during 1955 outnumbered our admissions; the hospital atmosphere is calmer, and there is increased confidence and optimism. These latter factors cannot be ignored.

Alone, ataraxics merely modify symptoms but in conjunction with psychotherapy they open up wide vistas of therapeutic promise.

Discussion

Gordon O. Patton, M. D. (Ste. Anne de Bellevue, Quebec).—In discussing the position of ataraxic drugs in the psychiatric hospital, Dr. Bowes has already stressed the importance of interpersonal relationships, emotions, and enthusiasms. I would like to suggest a slightly different emphasis on these factors by reference to the "hard core of disturbed and aggressive patients" and "the substitution of the ataraxics for insulin coma therapy."

Last summer 10 cases were selected solely on the criterion that they had the longest continuous terms in our side-room section, varying from 2½-77 months. Ataraxics were administered for 4 days. The patients were then moved to a large dormitory on our admission ward. Two nursing orderlies were with them. When the move was completed, a nurse aptly described the situation in these words: "It is peculiar to see all the patients so relaxed, while the orderlies look as if they are sitting on the edge of a volcano waiting for it to erupt." Fortunately no major eruption occurred and the tension subsided. The nurses responded to the challenge and rendered invaluable aid in assisting the orderlies to develop a variety of methods to control aberrant behavior. On a few occasions orderlies were transferred off the project in order to avoid the use of locked doors or any kind of physical force.

Six weeks later these 10 patients were distributed to various wards throughout the hospital. Subsequent reassessment of each patient's behavior indicated definite improvement in 5, slight or no improvement in the other 5. It seems that these last 5 were maintained out of seclusion more as a result of change in staff attitude than because of a change in the patients. Change in staff attitude had been made possible by feeding ataraxics to the patients.

Support for this view is the fact that two weeks later, the 5 remaining secluded patients were transferred out of the side-room section with no special program or preliminary medication. Tolerance for aberrant behavior had increased as the staff had learned new methods of control. They had witnessed the demonstration that such things could be done. They now had the responsibility of maintaining their own prestige and self-esteem. The ataraxic drugs still play an important part, but this change in staff attitude seems equally important in keeping our side-rooms almost empty.

Last summer I was quite enthusiastic about the change from insulin coma therapy to the ataraxic push group. It certainly made work more pleasant and less rigorous in many ways. Great feelings of security are afforded both patient and staff when the most disturbed admission cases can be controlled on chlorpromazine within a few hours. At an early stage the patient can be given to understand that the controls will be returned to him as soon as he has the ability to use them. This is an excellent start in personal relationship therapy. But at present I find a definite lack of evidence that the duration of treatment or quality of recovery has been essentially different for our patients in these 2 groups.

I have the impression that during treatment the following differences have existed:

1. Some patients seem to reach a degree of improvement short of readiness for discharge, but then stagnate for weeks in a quiet, contented, seclusive state. In the ataraxic-push group I have yet to find a method to break up this stagnation. With insulin coma therapy the patient could usually be stimulated to further improvement by discussion or interpretation of his actions or his semistuporous remarks, at the time of awakening from comas. Analytically orientated interpretations flowed freely on such occasions.

It may be that insulin coma therapy is the treatment of choice for the quiet withdrawn patient, lacking gross physical evidence of tension.

2. There has been a change in themes of conversation during group therapy. In the insulin group the patients frequently ventilated their feelings of loss of self-confidence, inadequacies, past history, and various personal conflicts, with frequent reference to their experiences associated with the comas. In the ataraxic group a patient may use one session for such ventilation, but in general there is more emphasis on the theme that he was sick, is now better, almost ready to leave hospital and go to work.

This change of emphasis seems to suggest a somewhat different process of recovery, namely: (1) On insulin coma therapy, conflict material brought vividly into consciousness each morning may result in desensitization, so there is less need for psychotic defenses, and recovery ensues. (2) In the ataraxic group the emphasis may be on repression and reintegration. This very process of recovery may explain my difficulty in disturbing a plateau during therapy. The situation is very different when the patient's defenses are weakened each morning by comas.

In summary, I see some of the important functions of these drugs as: (1) An improved method of control of disturbed patients. This may create new feelings of security for both patient and staff, thereby making possible or even initiating a different type of therapeutic community. (2) They make the patient more accessible to a therapeutic milieu.

BENJAMIN POLLACK, M. D. (Rochester, N. Y.).—The concentration on steroid chemistry, the investigation of the pituitary-adrenal axis, the indole and trytophane derivatives, and the investigation of the metabolism of phosphorus show both consistent and varying results. The relationship of these substances to mescaline, lysergic acid, and other substances indicates that many of these products can produce grossly similar biochemical changes in the body and, according to their concentration, varying reactions in the human organism. This has opened wide speculation and hope that through biochemical and physiological means, the key to the mystery of the causation of mental illness may be solved. It must, however, be emphasized that mental illnesses, particularly schizophrenia, seem to be due to many causes and they show varying changes in the body, particularly in the responses of the adrenals, hypothalamus, and metabolites, not only among different schizophrenics but also in the same schizophrenic from day to day. Although many of the hallucinogens and psychomimetic drugs can produce some of the symptoms of schizophrenia, namely, hallucinations and depersonalization, it must be emphasized that these are only a small picture of the altered behavior and do not necessarily have the same fundamental implication of similar etiology. The studies of the effect of such drugs on serotonin have indicated some exciting possibilities, but its specificity and possible relationship to mental phenomena remain to be further investigated. Biochemical interaction and changes are findings in various forms of mental illness, but unfortunately are not consistent even in the same illness or in the same individual.

It is quite obvious that mental illness is the product of multifactorial changes which seem to be related to an interference with the major enzyme systems.

It is quite evident that concentration on a unitarian approach will end in failure. It has been readily demonstrated that reversal of the chronic schizophrenic psychosis cannot be produced by the substitution or, indeed, the inhibition of a single factor found in research. The attempt to restore such autonomic control of the body by the use of parasympathomimetic or sympathomimetic drugs has ended consistently in failure.

Our experience at the Rochester State Hospital comprises 2 years' observation with over 1,500 patients given chlorpromazine, several hundred with reserpine, and smaller numbers given other drugs such as Meratran, Frenquel and promazine. It is interesting to note that the 2 original drugs, chlorpromazine and reserpine, still seem to have the greatest appeal and acceptance. The great variety of other drugs which have been produced in an attempt to mimic the action of these drugs have failed to produce higher therapeutic benefits. It is still our finding that chlorpromazine appears to produce the greatest benefits followed closely by reserpine. Frenquel (400 mgm.), Meratran, and similar drugs seem to be without value in the treatment of psychotics and we have abandoned their use entirely.

The foregoing papers report a wide variety of results from the use of other drugs such as Pacatal and promazine. It is important to remember that patients improved before electroshock and drug therapy were available. In estimating the results of treatment one must be aware of the statistical expectancy of spontaneous improvements without the use of such treatments. Thus the results here reported seem to indicate extreme therapeutic variations from the use of these products, from almost universal success to that of minimal or no results. It must be pointed out that the use of such drugs has been associated with an increased use of other factors which may play a fundamental role in the enhancement of the effects of such products. We have been impressed with the increase of good results when drug therapy has been considered as only one of a multitude of treatments in which psychotherapy and a total push program play a major role.

The use of terms such as antihallucinatory is to be deplored. It would, indeed, be naive to think of treating a single symptom of mental illness as if this were a unitary and unrelated finding. The exploitation of drugs based upon such expectancy has led to failures which should have been obvious.

One is impressed with the great variation in the therapeutic evaluation of these drugs. Since this field seems to hold hope, it would appear appropriate for this organization to appoint a committee to delineate certain clinical symptoms and changes in the body which can be evaluated and compared by various investigators. The need for the inclusion of similar factors appears obvious and would increase the comparative validity of reported results. The papers here presented indicate a feeling of encouragement and hope that perhaps organic and clinical research may hold the key to the future control of mental illness. It must always be remembered, however, that many of the reported findings are not the cause but the result of mental illness and that a single biological or chemical change is not primary but secondary. The resurgence of such investigation and the great emphasis upon the medical treatment of the psychotics is, indeed, an encouraging hope for the future.

Reply to Foregoing Discussions

H. Angus Bowes, M. D. (Ste. Anne de Bellevue, Quebec).—In answer to the many remarks that have been made concerning the toxic effects of Pacatal I am deeply sympathetic with the discussants. I went through the same phase last summer and at one time became so discouraged as nearly to give up my research with this powerful new drug, but we weren't killing anybody and we were doing some patients a lot of good, so I decided to deal with complications as they arose and was fairly successful in that we had only two major complications which never recurred.

They say that beauty is in the eye of the beholder; perhaps the observation of symptoms carries with it this projective implication. In the investigation of new drugs one goes through phases of enthusiasm and frustration. We are looking for the universal panacea—the magic bullet. Here we have a new drug —it may be the answer to our problems—our enthusiasm mounts despite our superficial attempts at objectivity. Our results are proportionately better and then along comes a damning pronouncement by an authority as eminent in the ataractic field as Dr. Kline. It deals a severe blow to our confidence. We start looking for trouble and we find it. Mentally sick people are very much like children in their ability to sense indecision, fear and anxiety in their parent surrogates, which is the role that therapists and nurses play.

Of course, there are some unpleasant side-effects such as dryness of the mouth and failure of accommodation. However, the patients themselves, in my experience, regard this as a trivial price to pay for the ataraxy they are experiencing. This symptom can be ameliorated by an old-fashioned combination of glycerine and lemon juice. At least it means that most of them will take in adequate fluids because of their intense thirst.

With regard to the eliminatory complications, some of our patients are so regressed that they are unable to give any account of their excretory processes. It is an unjustifiable intrusion to have our nurses and orderlies checking on their toilet activities all the time. However, we did give them laxatives as a routine and in cases of suspected severe constipation, however dynamically oriented you are, do not hesitate to slip on a rubber glove, insert a digit and see if there is any obstipation there. It is better to risk the exacerbation of a psychosis than to invite a paralytic ileus.

With regard to atonic bladder—these patients are thirsty, give them lots of fluids and if anything goes wrong don't hesitate to discontinue or reduce the medication and try prostigmine; you will get some results with that. Above all, realize that laboratory reports are inadequate and tardy substitutes for clinical observation, though it is much easier to read a green slip from the laboratory than to go up and look at a patient. I think we must have confidence in our clinical judgment to cope with emergencies as they arise and to prevent their recurring. Lack of clinical acumen will only lead to the misuse of what appears to be a most promising ataraxic.

PROSPECTS IN PSYCHOPHARMACOLOGY

Harold E. Himwich, M.D.

It is true that medications have been used for a long time for brain diseases, but now we are developing pharmacological agents that influence the mind as well. Against such a dichotomy between brain and mind we have the idea that any sharp delimitation between these two aspects of behavior is not possible; on the contrary, we have a continuous spectrum. For example, though we prescribe atropine and atropine-like drugs against Parkinsonian and the new tranquilizing drugs to mitigate hallucinations and delusions, atropine does affect the mind and can even bring on an organic confusion while Parkinsonism is one of the side reactions of the new drugs. Therefore, one term to include the entire gamut of such drugs would be preferable. The descriptive designation of neuropharmacology is acceptable. Yet on an operational basis, because some are more interested in the practice of neurology and others in psychiatry, it seemed advisable to use the name *psychopharmacology* to emphasize the new direction taken by pharmacology.

Pharmacological treatments for the mind are not new. They have been employed for a long time. In the past we have gradually developed methods to deal with disturbed, hallucinating and delusional patients. Barbiturates bring surcease to the patient and to the physician who attends him, but the results are relatively ephemeral. Electroshock is also widely used to maintain feasible interpersonal relationships in an otherwise disturbed ward. Now, however, violent patients can be managed in an open ward by methods which are less drastic than electroshock and with more enduring results than those of the barbiturates. The new pharmacological agents appear to be of a different order so that a term is now applied to drug action with new meaning, that is, *tranquilization* to connote sedation without hypnosis. Fabing has suggested the term *ataraxia*, denoting peace of mind, to describe the action of the new psychopharmacological agents.

What are these drugs? What have they accomplished? What are their mechanisms of action? What is in store for the future?

CLINICAL EVALUATION

The two new drugs have had many names attached to them, but the accepted generic nomenclature refers to them as chlorpromazine and reserpine. Though the effects of these drugs are still under active investigation, we already have a considerable body of knowledge on the clinical actions of these drugs, and they will be referred to briefly.

Reports reveal that patients with schizophrenic reactions in catatonic or paranoid excitement, manic depressives in the hypomanic or manic stage, patients with agitated senile reactions, acute obsessive states, tension states and acute anxiety are helped by chlorpromazine. In fact, a component of overactivity in the patient suggests a favorable usage of these drugs, and for that reason, the more disturbed the patient, the more dramatic are the results obtained with this tranquilizing drug. In contrast, patients with burnt out schizophrenic processes who are regressed and without active hallucinations and delusions are not as favorable subjects for this form of therapy. Patients with depressive reactions without anxiety and tension, patients who suffer from chronic anxiety neurosis with extensive somatization are not likely to be helped.

In general, the same therapeutic delimitation has been reported for reserpine. Patients who had been assaultive, resistive, raving and denudative were so improved that they were able to return home. Disturbed, psychotic patients could be removed from maintenance electroshock treatment. Even some of those who had responded poorly to electroshock could be sent home after receiving reserpine.

The distinction between the results obtained on excited patients and those with apathy is again seen in the effects of reserpine on geriatric disorders. The proportion of elderly psychotic patients who were irritable, quarrelsome and apprehensive, revealing improvement on reserpine, was greater than that of the patients who showed chiefly depression, negativism, apathy and withdrawal. In fact, the chronic administration of reserpine may produce such untoward response as withdrawal, lethargy and unhappiness but not anxiety. Chlorpromazine, too, may evoke depression with obsessive features.

The advantages of these two drugs are not limited to the hospital and a greater number of discharged patients, but are also extended to the physician's office because more psychotics can now be treated on an ambulatory basis. Neuroses have also been satisfactorily managed. Patients with stubborn anxiety and signs of tension are rendered relaxed and comfortable and are able to go about their daily duties with less effort. There are other than therapeutic advantages involved. Whether in private practice or in the hospital these treatments are less expensive than the standard ones, and the factor of economy is a large one. The highly trained personnel required by the standard treatments will form a smaller factor for consideration in the future. Among the benefits afforded by these drugs must be included a better atmosphere on the ward, affecting both patients and personnel.

My experience, gained in association with Doctors L. H. Rudy and F. Rinaldi, is concerned with approximately 40 patients on whom the effects of Frenquel, a more recent advance, as well as of reserpine and chlorpromazine have been evaluated in turn on the same group of patients. At this time I would simply like to point out briefly some clinical differences among these three drugs, keeping in mind the fact that our conclusions apply to the small number of patients we have studied. Both reserpine and chlorpromazine were effective in the treatment of patients with paranoid reactions. We, however, regarded chlorpromazine as better for this clinical category and especially so because reserpine activated the symptomatology of two of our patients. In the tranquilization of patients with schizoaffective reactions chlorpromazine also appeared to be the drug of choice. On the other hand, the patients with hebephrenic reactions, as well as those with mixed hebephreno-catatonic reactions, benefited more from reserpine. Though the members of the last two groups exhibited better ward adjustment and management with chlorpromazine, they did so at the price of aggravation of the symptoms of withdrawal, apathy, passivity and seclusiveness. Similarly, reserpine produced an improvement in one patient with involutional depression, yet on chlorpromazine his condition became worse. Taking into consideration all the clinical categories we found that reserpine produced a greater number of improvements in our moderately disturbed and chronically ill patients.

Frenquel, too, was of value and induced beneficial effects on our patients with schizophrenia. Some of these belonging to the paranoid group revealed a moderation in the intensity of their hallucinatory and delusional experiences with resulting improvements of behavior. Ward adjustment became better as hostility and overactivity diminished.

More appropriate behavior was also observed in the hebephrenic and hebephrenocatatonic patients as their thought processes and speech became more comprehensible and logical while catatonic features were rendered less prominent in intensity and duration.

In a comparison of the effects of Frenquel with those of reserpine and chlorpromazine, a difference was noted in so far that one or the other of the latter two induced in some patients of each clinical category a degree of improvement greater than that attained by any patient under Frenquel. Thus the modifications of behavior induced by Frenquel were neither so extensive nor so marked as were those observed following the use of reserpine and chlorpromazine. Yet when weighing Frenquel on the balance, its greater safety and freedom from side effects are arguments in its favor. Certainly this tranquilizing drug was valuable in the treatment of our moderately disturbed and chronically ill patients.

Physiological Analysis

Experience has taught us that drugs have multiple sites of action, each with different thresholds of susceptibility. This aphorism applies not only to the various organs of the body but also to the component parts of the brain. Though the final effect of a drug must be defined in terms of its integrated action on the entire body, yet for the sake of convenience the influence of chlorpromazine and reserpine on different brain structures will be considered separately.

The consensus in regard to both drugs is that they depress the hypothalamus, the portion of the brain which as demonstrated by Cannon and his students, notably Bard, contains the patterns for mobilizing the organism for the fight and flight reactions. In this area are found centers for the control of basal metabolism and temperature, the sleep-wakefulness cycle and blood pressure. In addition the hormonal balance is changed as the support afforded to the anterior pituitary gland is reduced by hypothalamic depression. The amount of gonadotrophic hormones released by the anterior pituitary is decreased, and for that reason menstrual disturbances are observed. The anterior pituitary is rendered less susceptible to stimulation, and that has an effect similar to that evoked by a lowered production of ovarian hormones, a phenomenon which brings on lactation. Chlorpromazine influences hypothalamic functions in such a manner that basal metabolism is decreased and body temperature lowered. Blood pressure falls, and sleep is facilitated as barbiturates and other hypnotic and narcotic drugs are potentiated. Most important for the treatment of disturbed patients is the fact that the posterior hypothalamus, containing sympathetic centers, is so affected by chlorpromazine that patterns for emotional expression tend to be inhibited. The central action which serves to diminish blood pressure is greatly enhanced by the chlorpromazine blockade of the sympathetic ganglia. Heart rate is increased, in part due to an atropine-like action but also in response to a fall of blood pressure. This drug-induced fall of blood pressure, in addition to the depression of metabolism and of temperature, explains why chlorpromazine is an essential part of the hibernation cocktail. With a fall in basal metabolism temperature and blood pressure, the blood supply dwindles and operations are rendered relatively bloodless. Such a change, favorable for surgical procedures, should, however, be carefully controlled so that systolic pressure does not fall below 55 to 65 mm. Hg. For brain operations the patient should be kept in the Trendelenberg position as elevation of theh head to reduce bleeding further can produce permanent cerebral damage.

Reserpine, like chlorpromazine, depresses hypothalamic mechanism and

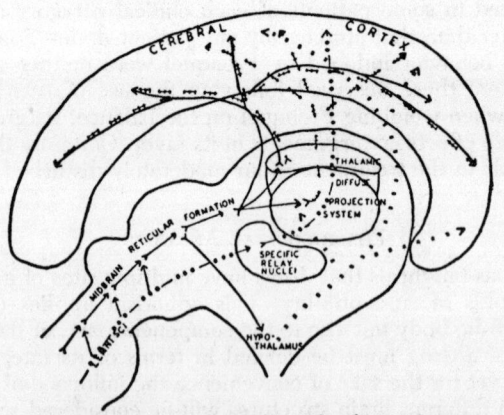

FIG. 1. Mesodiencephalic activating system

Stimuli from the periphery of the body evoke impulses which travel via the lemnisci through the specific relay nuclei of the thalamus and thence to specific sensory areas of the cerebral cortex. The lemnisci send collaterals to the mid-brain reticular formation, and by these paths impulses advance through that formation to the thalamic diffuse projection system, which in turn arouses the cerebral cortex in a diffuse manner. Collaterals from the mid-brain reticular formation also pass to the hypothalamus and carry impulses from that area by way of the diffuse system to the cerebral cortex.

like chlorpromazine does exert direct effects on peripheral nerve structures. The inhibition of the sympathetic representation in the hypothalamus explains the fall in heart rate, the drop in blood pressure, the constriction of the pupils, and the increased intestinal activity. These parasympathomimetic effects, however, are not caused by peripheral stimulation of parasympathetic nerves but by peripheral inhibition of sympathetic nerves.

NEUROELECTRICAL ANALYSIS

Dr. Franco Rinaldi and I, working on rabbits, reported another central site for the action of these drugs, namely the mesodiencephalic alerting system. Historically this system is built up of two portions, the reticular formation of Moruzzi and Magoun and the thalamic diffuse cortical projections of Jasper (fig. 1). The two parts may, however, be regarded as acting together, and for brevity they will be termed simply the activating system. Probably collaterals

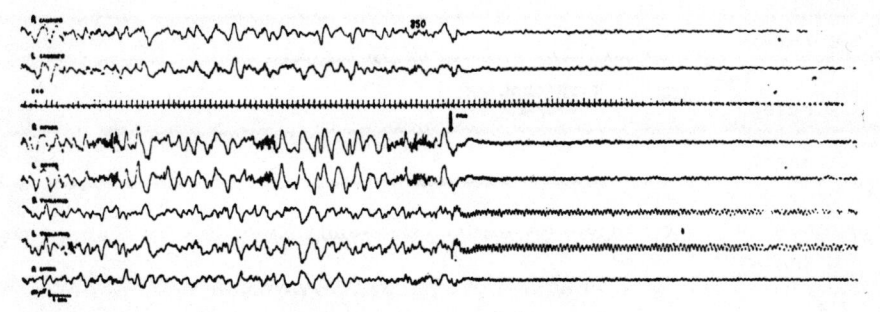

FIG. 2. Peripheral stimulation arouses activating system

An impulse from the periphery evoked by pain activates the alerting mechanism and changes the drowsy pattern to one of alertness. The left part of the figure reveals the resting pattern of high voltage slow waves and 14 per second spindles. The right part of the record shows cortical fast low voltage activity and 4 to 7 cycles per second rhythm of thalamic origin.

Records are derived bilaterally from the limbic cortex, the motor cortex, the caudate nucleus and the thalamus. In addition an ECG record is presented.

from the lemnisci carry afferent impulses to the reticular formation. The hypothalamus is involved in the function of the activating system as the excitatory process is conducted from the reticular formation to the subthalamus and hypothalamus in turn and thence back to the cortex either directly or via the thalamus. When this system undergoes stimulation, the altering, arousal or awakening EEG pattern is produced. As, however, excitation diminishes or ceases, the sleep or drowsy pattern is observed. The drowsy pattern is characterized by slow waves of high amplitude interrupted by 14 per second spindles, and the alert pattern, by low amplitude rapid waves in the cortex between 20 and 30 per second as well as a continuous repetition of 4 to 7 per second waves in the thalamus (fig. 2). Not only is the arousal reaction evoked by nervous stimuli, but it is facilitated by central nervous system stimulants, for example, amphetamine or Meratran (fig. 3). In contrast, drugs inducing sleep like the barbiturates are associated with the drowsy pattern. An early effect of barbiturate depression is the development of high voltage fast frequencies, but the latter give way to slow delta waves as presented in figure 4. Though there are exceptions to the rule, in general it may be said that behavioral arousal is associated with stimulation of this activating system and behavioral sleep with its depression. The effect of a pain stimulus to evoke the arousal reaction is seen (fig. 2), but chlorpromazine in small doses blocks such a response. For example, the pain stimulus no longer is capable of producing the alert state. This drug therefore diminishes the inflow of stimuli to the cortex, and we observe an inhibitory action (fig. 5). Thus in addition to the depressant effect of chlorpromazine on the hypothalamus we find a second site for depression in the activating system.

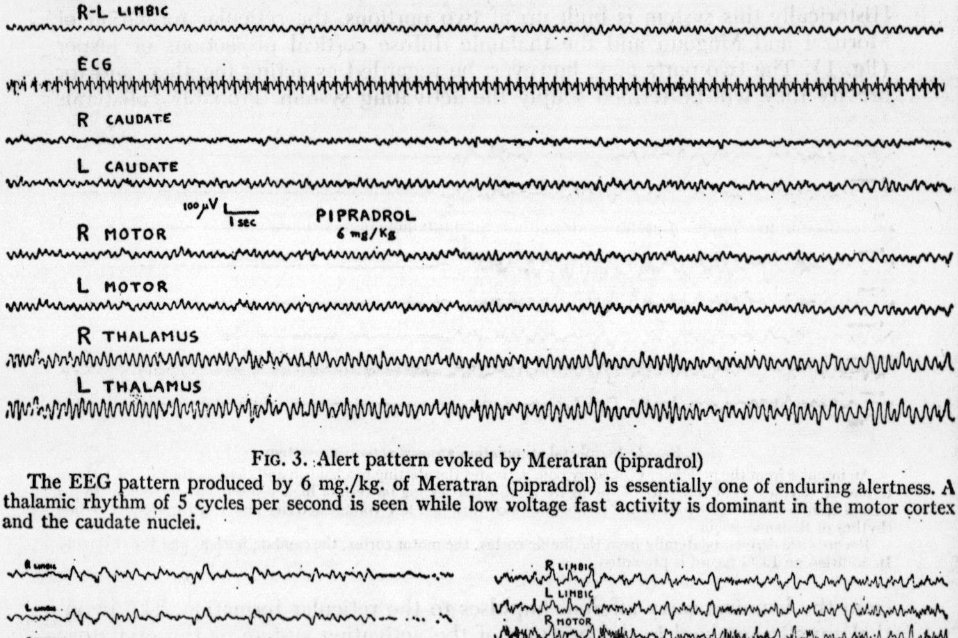

FIG. 3. Alert pattern evoked by Meratran (pipradrol)

The EEG pattern produced by 6 mg./kg. of Meratran (pipradrol) is essentially one of enduring alertness. A thalamic rhythm of 5 cycles per second is seen while low voltage fast activity is dominant in the motor cortex and the caudate nuclei.

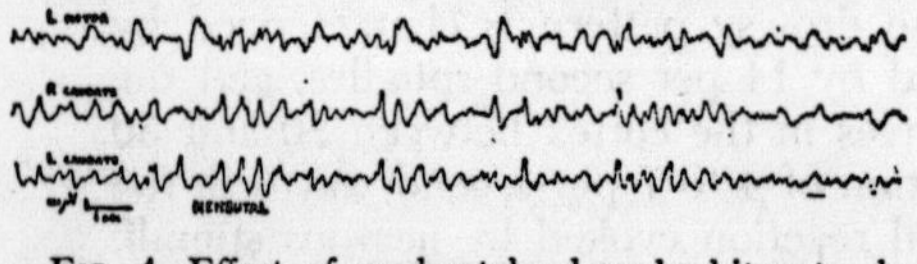

FIG. 4. Effect of moderately deep barbiturate depression on brain waves.

Slow, 1 to 3 cycles per second, waves become diffusely dominant over the entire record as the activating system is depressed by pentobarbital (Nembutal).

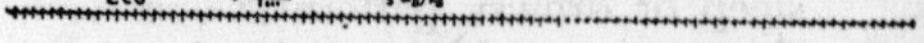

FIG. 5. Alerting effect of stimulus prevented by 5 mg./kg. of chlorpromazine.

Note the absence of the alerting reaction to pain due to comparatively low doses of chlorpromazine. Comparison with the control record (fig. 2) reveals the similarity of the chlorpromazine-produced pattern to the normal sleeping picture.

According to Gellhorn the latter is involved in a diminution of the affect.

Reserpine, in comparatively small amounts, stimulates this activating system (fig. 6). With doses of 0.5 mg./kg. or less little change is seen, from 0.5 to 1.0 mg./kg. alerting is facilitated, while from 1.5 m./kg. upward a persistent alerting response is elicited. Even though the injection of reserpine was made into the carotid artery, arousal followed only after a latent period of from 20 to 30 minutes. This alerting response may be involved in the tranquilizing effect of reserpine. The same dose which depresses the hypothalamus may also stimu-

FIG. 6. Enduring alert pattern induced by reserpine

The resemblance of this picture to the normal alert pattern is due to the absence of high voltage slow activity and sleep spindles. Instead we observe low voltage fast waves in the cortex and a regular 4 cycles per second thalamic rhythm. Note bradycardia induced by reserpine.

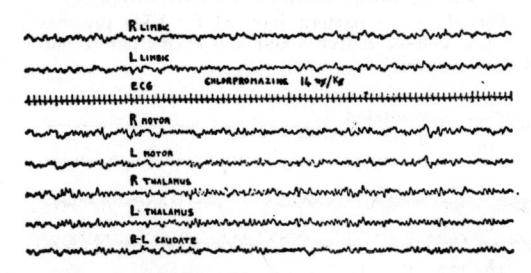

FIG. 7. Enduring alert pattern induced by large doses of chlorpromazine.

A continuous arousal pattern with low voltage rapid waves in the cortex and 5 cycles per second in the thalamus is observed.

late the activating system, and thus the sleep which would be facilitated by hypothalamic depression is counteracted by the arousal reaction. Chlorpromazine, when given in large doses, also evokes the alerting response (fig. 7). Thus in quantities greater than those required to depress the activating system chlorpromazine exhibits a reversal, and the activating system is stimulated. Large doses of chlorpromazine act like reserpine to evoke arousal.

A side reaction of the arousal state is the production of Parkinsonism. As discussed by Magoun the activating system possesses centrifugal effects as well as centripetal ones. The reticular formation and the reticulo-spinal tracts carry the main motor outflow of the extrapyramidal system. Experiments of Ward, McCulloch and Magoun and of Folkerts and Spiegel show that the overactivity of this system is responsible for the characteristic tremor of Parkinsonism. Stimulation of the activating system by these drugs may therefore produce a Parkinsonian picture just as well as by the liberation of this system from cephalad control due to lesions in the basal ganglia or the substantia nigra.

Are the two central sites of action on the hypothalamus and the activating system the only cerebral areas influenced by reserpine and chlorpromazine? Such a statement would be rash in the present state of the rapid development of this subject. For reserpine, Schneider *et al.* find a facilitation of synaptic transmis-

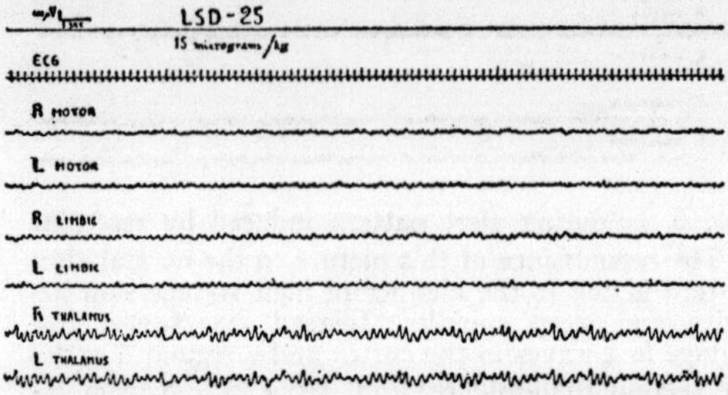

FIG. 8. LSD evokes alert EEG pattern

The abnormal pattern induced by LSD presents fast low voltage activity and 4–6 cycles per second thalamic waves.

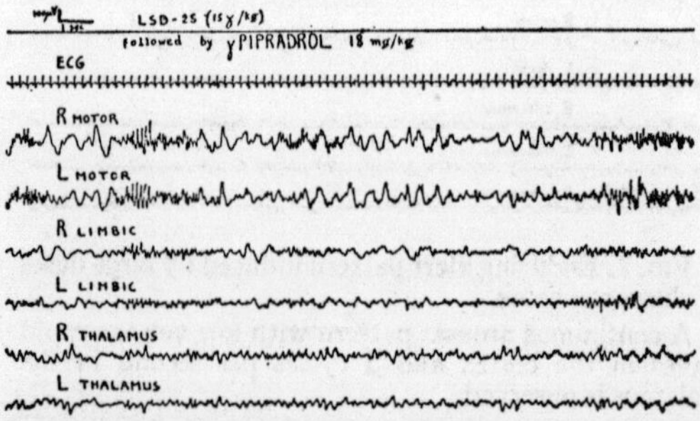

FIG. 9. Frenquel (gamma-pipradrol) eliminates abnormal EEG pattern induced by LSD.

The slow waves and 14 cycles per second spindles, abolished by LSD (see fig. 8), reappear on the normal drowsy electrical pattern restored by Frenquel (gamma-pipradrol).

sion in the cord. They suggest that if a similar facilitation occurs in the cortex, we may have an additional explanation for the hypothalamic depression induced by reserpine as the cortical inhibition of the hypothalamus is strengthened. For chlorpromazine, too, may augment the cortical inhibition exerted upon the hypothalamus.

I feel sure that we have not completely elucidated actions of these drugs on the brain. The importance of the activating system may not be limited only to the prevention of such hypnotic effects as can be evoked by the barbiturates or by the production of the side reactions of Parkinsonism. It is probable that depression of the hypothalamic sympathetic mechanisms mitigates the severity of the psychotic symptomatology. The present observations, however, do not extend the action of these drugs to the cortex which presumably is involved in hallucinatory and delusional experiences. Still another site is suggested by Frenquel which does not depress the hypothalamus and yet appears to be effective therapeutically. In a group of patients with acute psychotic episodes, Fabing has obtained striking results. In our series of moderately disturbed delusional and hallucinatory patients we have also seen some improvements.

How then are we to explain the salutary action of Frenquel on the psychotic patient? The only hints that we have are suggested by the observations of Fabing that Frenquel benefits model psychosis induced either by LSD (d-lysergic diethylamide) or mescaline. In animal experiments we observed that LSD or mescaline induced the arousal reaction. This is not characteristic of hallucinogenic drugs only because many central nervous system stimulants like amphetamine and Meratran (fig. 3) can also evoke the arousal responses. When Frenquel is injected subsequent to either amphetamine or Meratran, it does not reverse the arousal response, but when Frenquel is administered after LSD or mescaline, the alerting reaction is eliminated from the EEG and the resting pattern is restored (figs. 8 and 9).

The lead afforded by Frenquel is suggestive because the low amplitude rapid frequency waves produced by LSD and mescaline are also found in untreated human subjects. Though such waves have been reported in but few so-called normal individuals, they occur in about one-third of the patients with schizophrenia, manic-depressive reactions, psychoneurosis, and more than half of the patients with involutional psychosis exhibit such waves. The mechanism for bringing about this low amplitude fast activity is unknown. It may be due in the first place to a disorder of the cerebral cortex. Another suggestion is that it represents the effects of an overactive alerting system upon the cortex. It is hardly likely that a peripheral stimulus is the cause of such overactivity. We must therefore seek for a central site in some structure of the brain, perhaps in the cerebral cortex. Under such conditions we might have a positive feedback. Not only does the cortex stimulate the activating system, but the activating system in turn stimulates the cortex, and so we have a vicious cycle. One way to test such susceptibility is to administer Frenquel to patients with low amplitude fast activity and see whether or not it can be eliminated. If Frenquel is successful in reducing fast activity, it may not be impossible that there is an association between the electrical hyperactivity of the brain and the psychotic process and that both are inhibited by the action of Frenquel.

NEUROCHEMICAL ANALYSIS

I have briefly reviewed some of the behavioral results obtained by the use of Frenquel, reserpine and chlorpromazine. The alterations produced by these drugs, the clinical improvements, are explained in part by the observations made on animals as well as human subjects, including such pharmacological effects as depression of hypothalamic mechanisms. The observations made with the aid of the EEG were also helpful, for they disclose additional aspects of drug action on the activating system. But what are the biochemical changes which are the source of the pharmacological actions inducing alterations in behavior? Experiments of Grenell and associates revealed that when chlorpromazine was injected into rats and brain tissue was analyzed, changes in oxidation of the excised cerebral tissues were not observed. These results are in agreement with others on cerebral metabolic rate obtained in the human subjects who had received reserpine or chlorpromazine. However, a significant alteration was observed in excised cerebral tissues, an accumulation of energy rich phosphates

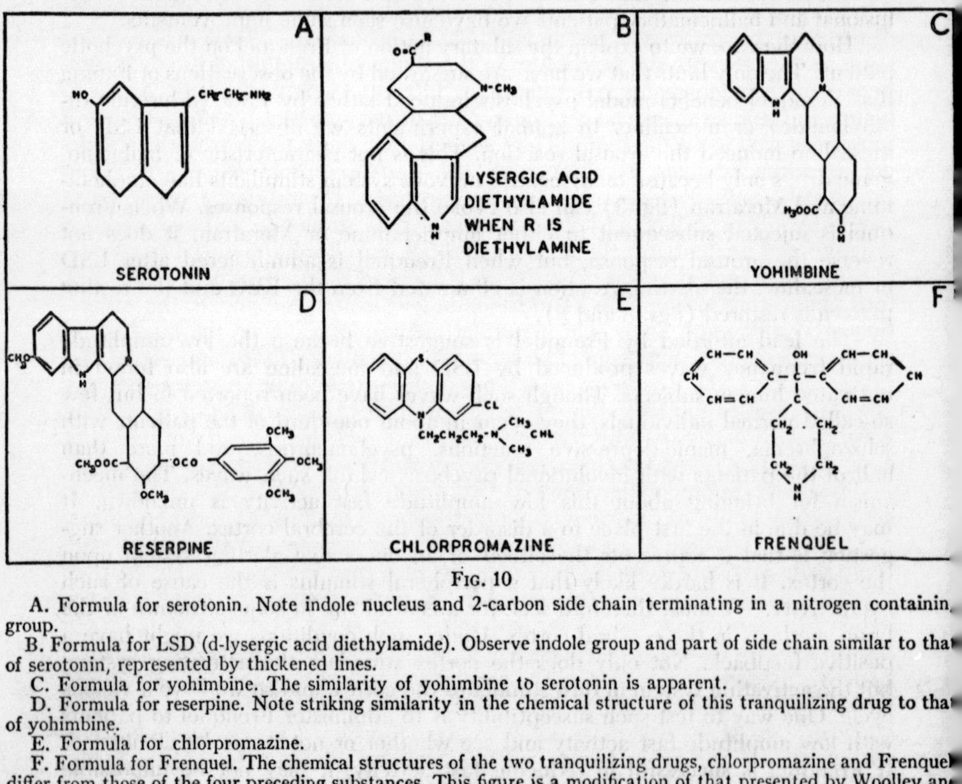

FIG. 10

A. Formula for serotonin. Note indole nucleus and 2-carbon side chain terminating in a nitrogen containing group.
B. Formula for LSD (d-lysergic acid diethylamide). Observe indole group and part of side chain similar to that of serotonin, represented by thickened lines.
C. Formula for yohimbine. The similarity of yohimbine to serotonin is apparent.
D. Formula for reserpine. Note striking similarity in the chemical structure of this tranquilizing drug to that of yohimbine.
E. Formula for chlorpromazine.
F. Formula for Frenquel. The chemical structures of the two tranquilizing drugs, chlorpromazine and Frenquel, differ from those of the four preceding substances. This figure is a modification of that presented by Woolley and Shaw.

in the form of adenosinetriphosphate (ATP). This accumulation could be due either to the accelerated production of ATP or its slower utilization. According to the authors the latter is the correct interpretation. It may be of some importance that the midbrain region of the rat containing the thalamus and hypothalamus showed a greater increase of ATP than any other cerebral part as a result of chlorpromazine.

The next step in our inquiry is to determine the cause of these changes in brain metabolism, and the answer to this question may involve the neurohormones of the brain. In that regard the experiments of Hoffer, Osmond and Symthies on a breakdown product of adrenaline should be considered. These workers observed that a substance contained in a pink or deteriorated adrenaline solution evoked hallucinations. They believe that the hallucinogenic substance includes the indole nucleus as part of its chemical structure, and also pointed out that some hallucinogens like LSD, harmine, medmain, yohimbine contain this indole nucleus (fig 10). In fact Rinkel *et al.* have suggested that LSD may influence the enzyme system concerned with the metabolism of adrenaline. Marrazzi and Hart as well as Liddell and Weil-Malherbe emphasize disturbance of an adrenergic neurohumoral mechanism. Woolley and Shaw were also struck with the similarities in the chemical structure of the hallucinogens, but their viewpoint was somewhat different as they stressed the resemblance to the neurohormone serotonin (5-hydoxytryptamine) found in smooth muscle as well as in the brain. They suggest that these pathogenic substances act as antimetabolites, combine with the same receptors as serotonin, but prevent the normal response elicited by serotonin. In addition, evidence in a paper by Shore, Silver and Brodie reveals that serotonin in large doses is sedative and pontentiates the action of Evipal, an ultrashortacting barbiturate, in mice. This central action of serotonin is blocked by pretreatment with LSD, thus implicating serotonin in brain function and lending support to the suggestion of Woolley and Shaw that abnormal mentation is due to the blocking of serotonin receptors. Reserpine, like serotonin, potentiates Evipal, an action also prevented by LSD. Reserpine, which resembles serotonin in chemical structure (fig. 10), causes the liberation of serotonin. The evidence for this conclusion was obtained partly on dogs, for reserpine increased their urinary excretion of a metabolic product of serotonin, namely 5-hydroxyindoleacetic acid (5 HIAA).

Further experimentation showed that reserpine has a bi-phasic action on serotonin, not only an early and temporary increase but also a late and enduring diminution. Perhaps the continued injections of reserpine would prevent serotonin from attaining normal values, and in that case the benefit derived from reserpine lies in a decrease of serotonin. If these results yield a clue to the action of reserpine on the brain, and this is yet to be proved, then I would like to offer a tentative explanation for the therapeutic effects of reserpine, namely, that the abnormal activity of disturbed psychotic patients is associated with an excess of serotonin and that under continued dosage of reserpine the concentration of serotonin in the brain is reduced. In accordance with this speculation the lag in the clinical effects produced by reserpine represents the time necessary for the elimination of serotonin from the body and perhaps lowering its concentration in the brain. Furthermore, the continued pharmacological action of reserpine after that drug is withdrawn may indicate the period necessary for the restoration of the serotonin depots.

It is of interest that both chlorpromazine and Frenquel potentiate Evipal though Frenquel is weaker than chlorpromazine in this regard. The administration of chlorpromazine does not, however, increase the excretion of 5 HIAA. It would appear that these drugs act like serotonin. They are serotoninmimetic and go to the same receptors as serotonin, thereby reducing the effectiveness of that neurohormone. This viewpoint is the opposite of Woolley and Shaw and suggests that abnormal mentation is associated with an excess of serotonin while a reduction in the concentration of serotonin is therapeutically beneficial.

Recent experiments, performed in our laboratory by Dr. E. Costa, have yielded additional evidence for such a conception. Using the rat uterus as a test object he observed that the uterine contraction produced by serotonin is blocked by each of the three tranquilizing drugs. The block evoked by Frenquel is of shortest duration, that induced by chlorpromazine lasts for a longer time, while the effect of reserpine is the most enduring of the three. Perhaps that is the reason why reserpine is the most effective of the three agents in causing the release of serotonin and the excretion of 5 HIAA. Furthermore, Dr. Costa has found that LSD and mescaline potentiate the uterine contraction caused by *minimal* doses of serotonin. This observation does not contradict that of Gaddum and Hameed who found that LSD inhibits the *maximal* contraction induced by serotonin. Thus, at least for the rat uterus, the three tranquilizing drugs reduce the effect of serotonin, while in contrast LSD and mescaline augment its action. Though these experiments are suggestive, their significance in regard to the function of the brain will require further work.

The Future

What has the future in store? Before making an attempt to define the paths of further progress, it is well to examine our present position. Most physicians who have tested these drugs are convinced that they are a great step forward. The beneficial effects are not a "flash in the pan" but have been widely corroborated. We can therefore look with satisfaction at the progress we have made. Do we cure our patients? Until we have unearthed the roots of schizophrenia, the answer to this question remains a semantic one. But now the psychiatrist has at his command drugs which are of aid in wiping out the symptoms of psychotic patients just as the internists can use insulin for the elimination of the symptoms of diabetes.

Added to our armamentarium are drugs which aid in the control of disturbed psychotic patients. These drugs are effective not only for disturbed patients with psychomotor overactivity but also for emotionally tense ones with acute anxiety. The value of these drugs is being tested for various clinical categories, and in general one might predict that in many conditions for which bromides were formerly used and now barbiturates are prescribed, the new drugs will receive preference.

Therapeutic evaluations reveal that they are not the complete answer for our problem. All these drugs are tranquilizers. Though they are used successfully against depression associated with anxiety and tension, we still await the pharmacological agent that is as effective as electroshock for melancholia. The plans for the immediate future also involve a consideration of some of the inadequacies of these drugs. Both chlorpromazine and reserpine exhibit undesirable side reactions, and efforts are now being bent toward their alleviation.

More important is the observation that not all patients were helped equally by any one of these three drugs and those of some clinical categories are benefited more than others by each of them. The discovery of additional pharmacological agents therefore becomes imperative. The suggestion from reserpine and chlorpromazine that drugs must depress the hypothalamus to be effective should be considered as it is apparent that such a depression will mitigate the severity of emotional expression both in somatic and mental terms. A second site of action is found in the activating system. Frenquel suggests the possibility of still other loci. One way to attain this goal of discovery of new therapeutic agents is indicated by past experience. Variation in chemical structures of the drugs now used may induce new and unexpected actions, and such variants should and will be evaluated clinically. But drugs of entirely different chemical constitution must be produced, perhaps with specific affinities for the receptors of neurohormones in the brain. Recent evidence from Brodie's laboratory, as well as our own, indicates that the tranquilizing drugs alter behavior by their influence on serotonin.

We are living in a moment of excitement, rich in potentialities that can be realized by increased interaction between psychiatrists and pharmacologists. We cannot help but feel that the advances made by chlorpromazine and reserpine, important as they are, represent only the initiation of a new era in psychiatry. The advent of Frenquel may be regarded as another harbinger of such an era. The science of psychopharmacology has come to stay!

THE ATARACTIC DRUGS:
THEIR USES AND LIMITATIONS IN PSYCHIATRY

Howard D. Fabing, M.D.

A group of drugs which sedate in a selective kind of way, which quiet certain overactive patients, and which tranquilize some of the disturbed, have appeared over the medical horizon in recent years. Intensive activity in pharmaceutical research circles here and abroad gives every indication that this list will become longer rapidly.

A year ago, when there were fewer of these drugs, I suggested that a new word be devised to classify them pharmacologically. Leaning on the erudition of my friend, Alister Cameron, Professor of Classics in the College of Liberal Arts of the University of Cincinnati, I proposed that they be labelled *ataraxics*, or that these compounds be called *ataractic drugs*, if an adjective were made out of the new word. It comes from the Greek noun *ataraxia*, which means "freedom from disturbance of mind or passion." Epicurus, the famous Greek philosopher, was especially fond of this word, and *ataraxia*, the state of being *a tarache*, or without confusion and mental turmoil, and therefore calm, was one of the prime goals of Epicurean philosophy. I remember my first discussion with Cameron about this word. He was amazed that the medical profession, which steals words right and left from Greek and Latin, had not scooped this one up in its basket before.

As the inventor, or part-inventor, of a word, I feel a sense of responsibility. The term was proposed in order to clarify our thinking about a new group of drugs, but I am beginning to wonder whether it has done so. As the list of these compounds grows, and as more people use the word for more things, it becomes less clear in definition and in outline. Perhaps this is a reflection of the general vagueness of our present state of knowledge about these new compounds. Whom are we trying to tranquilize, and with what drug? What do we mean by *tranquilize*? Are these "don't-give-a-damn" pills as some headline writer has called them? Will an enemy drop a ton of them in the water supply of our major cities and then march triumphantly through our streets and conquer us while we sit in a rocking chair at the window, not lifting a finger in our own defense because we are too listless and inwardly peaceful to get up on our feet and fight for our freedom? I heard an imaginative disc jockey talking like this on my automobile radio one morning a few weeks ago. I disagree, emphatically. These drugs have limited uses and different indications. They are not immediate in action, and as a group some have small effect while others have no effect on the so-called "normal" segments of the population.

It would probably be helpful to divide these drugs into two groups in discussing their uses. The first are those which have been used primarily in major psychiatric disorders, or the psychoses, and the second are those which are suggested for trial only in the minor psychiatric disorders, or the neuroses. This is an oversimplification of the matter, but it may help to bring us closer to the general area of usefulness of the drugs. Thus far there are three compounds which fall generally into the first class—those used in the major psychoses. They are reserpine, chlorpromazine and azacyclonol.

RESERPINE

Reserpine has a long and romantic history in the herbal medicine of India. The snakeroot plant from which it is derived was named after Leonhart Rauwolf, a 16th century botanist, and is called *Rauwolfia serpentina.* Reserpine is its most active fraction. Small doses were noted to have a beneficial effect in lowering the blood pressures of hypertensive patients. The extensive work of Dr. Nathan Kline and his associates at the Rockland State Hospital, N. Y. plus that of other investigators, has yielded the clinical knowledge that reserpine is of value in improving the symptoms of a majority, but certainly not all of the overactive, destructive, noisy disturbed psychotic patients one encounters on the back wards of a large hospital for the mentally ill.

For the most part these patients have schizophrenia, perhaps the most sinister of all sicknesses of the mind. These patients live within a shell of their own detached daydreamy thoughts. They do not think and talk and behave logically and consecutively. There is a constant intrusion of clashing ideas which block the normal flow and progression of speech and thought which we expect in one another. They may hear imaginary sounds and voices and they may see imaginary things which to them have a reality more real than the real things about them, and they may respond to the bidding of these hallucinations, even if the hallucinations urge them into acts of violence. They often develop delusions that they are being persecuted, or that they are persons other than their normal selves, and they may come to look on the people around them with suspiciousness and fear. Sometimes the detached inner world of their thoughts and visionary experience may appear ludicrous and funny to them, and they giggle and shout and sing inappropriately as they respond to this jumbled mixup in their minds. Sometimes they become wrapped up in study and contemplation, it seems, and sit expressionless and mute for hours and days in their catatonic stupor.

Schizophrenia is anything but peace of mind. To me it seems to be its very opposite—mental turmoil compounded. Reserpine is capable of reducing the explosive outbursts of antisocial behavior in these patients, of bringing more order into their thinking, of reducing the compelling drive of hallucinations and delusions, and of bringing them closer to contact with your world and mine—the world they knew before they got sick. On occasion reserpine appears to be capable of bringing the whole schizophrenic process, with its rich and variable cluster of symptoms, to an end, and may permit the patient to resume a life in the world of his fellows. This is more likely to occur if the patient is overactive and restless than if he is retarded and mute, and is much more likely to occur if he has been ill for a year or less. The road back to mental health is difficult for those who have travelled far along it in the other direction.

It appears that reserpine can bring some measure of relief to about 60 percent of these patients. Life in mental hospitals is much less hectic when it is used, and the need to give this group of violent patients repeated electroconvulsive treatments to control outbursts of aggressive behavior has diminished greatly. The number of patients capable of discharge from mental hospitals has been relatively small thus far. Other overactive psychotic patients, especially those with senile and arteriosclerotic dementia, and those with paresis, or syphilitic infection of the brain, can also be made less disturbed by the drug on occasion. Some serious epileptics, mental defectives, cerebral palsied and other brain-injured patients who exhibit this same type of psychomotor overactivity can also be helped by this drug, at least in part. It is also of value in delirium.

Recently it has become apparent that reserpine can cause mental difficulty as well as alleviate it. A growing number of observations reveal that patients on this drug may get morbidly depressed, and may even attempt suicide. This kind of drug-induced melancholia calls for immediate withdrawal of the medication, the use of mood-elevating drugs, and, if necessary, electroconvulsive treatment to cope with these serious depressive reactions. This teaches, too, that reserpine is contraindicated in that other large group of mentally ill patients, the depressed. Here, rather than produce peace of mind, or tranquility, it may have the opposite effect. Other side-reactions of the drug are nasal stuffiness, dizziness, somnolence and Parkinsonism. These can be quite troublesome in office practice despite measures to get around them. Although reserpine has been advocated for certain symptoms of the minor psychiatric disorders of neurotic type, it is not easy to use over a long period, and many of my colleagues find that either they or their office patients give up the drug in an appreciable number of cases.

Chlorpromazine

Chlorpromazine[1], the next drug on the list of those ataraxics which may be of value in the major psychoses, was developed for study as an antihistaminic. The French physicians who investigated it some six years ago did not find it a very effective antihistaminic agent, but soon learned that it was of value in the vomiting of pregnancy, in psychogenic digestive disturbances, in various pain syndromes, and in major psychiatric disorders. A great deal of study of this compound has been undertaken in the countries of Western Europe, Canada and the United States in recent years. As with reserpine, the largest investigations have been made in hospitals for the mentally ill and have involved thousands of patients. Again, the schizophrenic group has been studied most widely, and they receive the same order of benefit as do those under reserpine therapy. The overactive schizophrenic gets the most benefit, and his chances for alleviation of his symptoms to the degree that he may be discharged from the hospital are much better if he has been sick less than one year.

Chlorpromazine dosage has gone to great heights in the hands of some

---

[1] Chlorpromazine is 10-(3-dimethylaminopropyl)-2-chlorphenothiazine.

investigators. Patients have received more than 4000 mg. daily in the study of this drug's effectiveness on occasion. One of the most earnest students of chlorpromazine is a colleague of mine in Cincinnati, Dr. Douglas Goldman. He is the medical director of a very large, overcrowded, understaffed state institution, Longview Hospital. He has taken a new lease on life lately. The reduction in assaults, the lessened use of restraint, the increased granting of privileges to locked-ward patients, the lessened need for repeated electroshock treatment to control explosive behavior, and the beginnings of an improved discharge rate of patients from the hospital all stem from the use of this drug in his hands and parallel the kind of improved state of affairs which Kline reports with reserpine at Rockland.

Goldman likes to tell the story about Willie. Willie was a dishevelled, mute, untidy schizophrenic who had to be spoon-fed and who managed to tear off just about all the clothes anyone tried to put on him. Willie received an eight-weeks' trial with chlorpromazine, but at the end of that time Goldman was not greatly impressed with his improvement. He announced that he was going to withdraw Willie's drug, whereupon an orderly raised a clamor, pleading for its continuance, insisting that Willie was much better. He said, "Wait a minute. I'll prove it to you. I'll get Johnny." In a moment he returned with Willie's identical twin. "See, they were both alike two months ago," he said. They stood side by side. Johnny's hair fell in his face, he was soiled, his pants were torn, and he was barefoot. Willie was fully clothed, barbered, shaved, clean, and wore shoes. The difference was obvious. Instead of taking a patient off chlorpromazine, he put another on.

AZACYCLONOL

The third drug which belongs in the list of the ataraxics which may be tried in the major psychiatric disorders is azacyclonol[2]. This drug has no effect whatever in the "normal" population, and is not indicated in the minor neurotic disturbances. Its action is confined to the schizophrenic disorders and to acute confusional states. It may be used intravenously as well as orally. In a small number of acute schizophrenic syndromes it has been dramatic in its efficacy. It has been less valuable in the chronic cases. We have found that it will block the development of an LSD or a mescaline psychosis when given as a premedication in a small number of experiments, and will abort these reactions when given intravenously. Some investigators have confirmed this, whereas others do not agree. A larger number of experiments will probably prove that Frenquel has this blocking effect in some cases but not in all of them.

Azacyclonol has been almost uniformly good in relieving approximately 100 cases of post-operative confusion. Other confusional states respond nicely, too. We have had dramatic success with a small group of cases of delirium tremens. Proctor at the Bowman-Gray School of Medicine in Winston-Salem has relieved 16 of 19 cases of delirium tremens quickly with Frenquel. Senile patients often go through troublesome confusional periods. Frenquel has helped us with these on many occasions, too. Our best friends in this have been the nurses. They

---

[2] Azacyclonol is alpha-(4-piperidyl) benzhydrol hydrochloride.

run a quieter hospital and require less restraint for disturbed patients. One nice advantage of this drug is that it produces no side-reactions.

We now come to a consideration of the ataractic drugs which appear to have no value in the psychotic patient, but which are suggested in the treatment of the psychoneuroses. Ever since their introduction about forty years ago, physicians have used small doses of phenobarbital and other barbiturates in caring for these cases, and these drugs continue to be used profitably and widely, alone and with psycho-therapeutic measures. More recently a new group of drugs for the management of these symptoms have been developed in Europe, and one in this country.

MEPROBAMATE

Meprobamate[3], a derivative of mephenesin, has been used widely in the United States during the past year for the control of nervous tension, or "jitteriness," along with its accompanying bodily reactions of tension headache, globus sensation in the throat, palpitation, heavy feeling in the chest, air hunger, anorexia, digestive disturbances, "butterflies" in the abdomen, urinary frequency, muscle tension and tremor, and the other disturbing subjective accompaniments of anxiety which all of us have experienced at one time or another. With most of us these reactions come and go, and we shrug our shoulders and say that we "sweated out" a stressful situation. When these symptoms persist, along with the turbulence of thought and mood which accompanies them, an anxiety neurosis is present.

Meprobamate is no cure-all for these symptoms, but is worthy of trial for the relief that it may bring. The only side-reaction I have observed is a kind of excessive relaxation of the musculature which the apprehensive patient may consider to be an alarming weakness, and occasionally a complaint of dizziness. It is too early to assess the value of this drug critically. It seems to be of most value in cases where the patient has good insight into his condition, i.e., when he knows that his disorder is of nervous origin, and when he is aware of the situation which produced the stress which led to his symptoms. The relief of the somatic components of his anxiety state by meprobamate will bring a dramatic end to his troubles on occasion in cases of this type.

Other compounds have been made available in Europe in this therapeutic area, and will probably be proposed for distribution here later. Jacobsen, who developed Antabuse in Denmark, has introduced *Suavitil*[4] in the treatment of these cases. A Danish medical friend writes me that he has used it on himself when he is under stress. "Perhaps you will understand something of its action if I tell you that when I am all tensed up, it seems to permit me to do what I want to do," he reports. This is subtle pharmacological action, indeed. The Belgians have been studying another compound of this type which they call *Atarax*[5], and the Italians are working with a procaine antagonist, *diethylammonium para-aminobenzoate*, for which similar action is claimed.

You will note in the foregoing discussion that none of these compounds

---

[3] Meprobamate is 2-methyl-2-n-propyl-1, 3 propanediol dicarbamate.
[4] Suavitil is benactyzine HC1.
[5] Atarax is 1-p-chlorobenzhydryl-4, 2-(hydroxethyoxy) ethyldiethydiamine HC1.

seem to be of benefit in the depressed, melancholy, slowed up states of partial mental clouding and disordered mood which are so common in the clinical practice of psychiatry. Another group of drugs, which are cerebral stimulants or mood-elevators (euphoriants or analeptics) have been used rather than the ataraxics in these depressive disorders. Drugs of the amphetamine series have been used to elevate mood for many years. Recently pipradol HL1[6] and methyl-phenidylacetate HC1[7] have been added to the list. These drugs are of value in mild depressive reactions, but electroconvulsive therapy becomes necessary if this complaint is at all serious. Further research in this area, leading to knowledge of the disturbance of body chemistry which undoubtedly occurs in melancholia, and to an improved pharmacologic attack upon it, is needed urgently.

STATUS

Where, then, do we stand today in the field of the so-called tranquilizing or ataractic drugs? First of all, a group of them are pointing their guns at major psychiatric illnesses, the schizophrenic and confusional psychoses. None as yet seem to be able to claim sure victory in this field, but clinicians are excited at two thoughts: (1) that a breach has been made in the wall, and (2) that the biochemists and the pharmacologists are finally turning their attentions to this vast field of medicine. The second group of drugs, just beginning to be tested, report therapeutic effectiveness in some of the neuroses. We call these the minor psychiatric disorders, but this is an euphemism. They are minor because they are not such severe illnesses. They are certainly major when we consider the distress, the anguish and the economic toll they cause.

If the people in the scientific laboratories keep working and producing as they have been doing lately, is the millennium just around the corner? Are the mental hospitals to be emptied out soon, and will the new drugs produce in us the serene peace of mind and tranquility that the followers of Epicurus searched for in their philosophy? Let's not kid ourselves about these things. There are many chronic neurological and psychiatric diseases, and although we talk a great deal about their etiology, we know practically nothing about the cause of many of these conditions which fill half our hospital beds. Rational therapy will come after we gain this knowledge. Furthermore, as we empty a few beds occupied by the psychotics who are young, we fill them up immediately with the aged. The geriatric problem is a monstrous one. As for the tranquillity business, let me remind you that about 2200 years ago Aristotle said, *"anthropos politikon zoon,"* which means that man is a political animal, which is another way of saying that we struggle constantly to maintain ourselves as individuals in a group. This will always produce stress as long as human beings rub elbows together.

We have almost exhausted ourselves striving for a vague thing we call "security" during the last quarter-century, and we seem no closer to it than when we started. Let us not add another unattainable goal of dubious value, i.e., "serenity," pills or no pills.

---

[6] Pipradol HL1 is alpha-(2-piperidyl) benzhydrol HC1.
[7] Methyl-phenidylacetate HC1 is methyl a-phenyl-2-piperidineaceate HC1.

ATARACTICS IN MEDICAL PRACTICE

Joseph F. Fazekas, M.D., James G. Shea, M.D., and Paul D. Sullivan, Jr., M.D.

THE MANAGEMENT of functional disturbances of the central nervous system, as manifested by increased psychomotor activity, constitutes a difficult problem in medical practice. The more common of these disturbances include the acute anxiety states, the several syndromes resulting from the ingestion of alcohol, and the agitation associated with the various psychoses.

Heretofore, the only agents readily available for the management of these hyperexcitable states were the aliphatic depressants, such as barbiturates, chloral hydrate, and paraldehyde, and the bromides. The chief disadvantage of these preparations was that in effective doses they commonly produced such a deep state of sedation that the patient was rendered useless and helpless in his environment. Furthermore, because of their primary cortical site of action, they may well have perpetuated the underlying psychoneurologic disturbance, even though temporarily masking its overt manifestations (*Figure* 1).

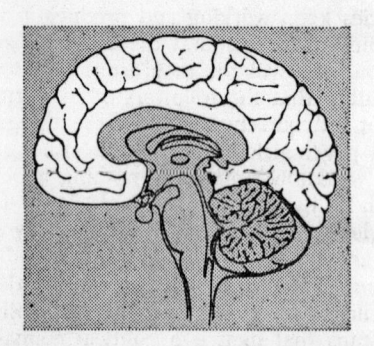

Figure 1. *Cerebral cortex. The primary locus of action of aliphatic depressants.*

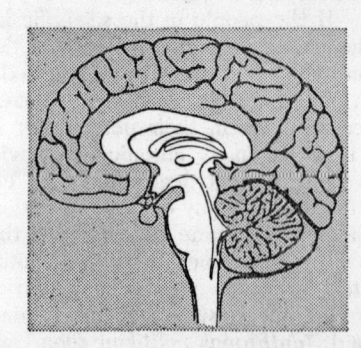

Figure 2. *Subcortex. The primary locus of action of ataractics.*

The failure of hypnotic doses of the above drugs to control the overly excited patient suggests that brain structures other than the cerebral cortex may well be important in the etiology of the disturbed state. In other words, lack of synchronization, or impaired transmission of centripetal impulses from subcortical areas may make impossible their proper integration at cortical levels. Treatment of the latter areas alone could hardly be expected to control the disturbed patient.

It is well known that the aliphatic depressants, in larger doses, cause a descending depression of the neuroaxis beginning with the phylogenetically higher centers. With high doses of these drugs, subcortical areas are undoubtedly also depressed. In certain clinical states such as delirium tremens, a regenerative cycle may be operating in which centripetal and centrifugal impulses constantly activate both cortical and subcortical areas. There is diffuse excitation of the central nervous system.

Recently, chlorpromazine, promazine, reserpine and meprobamate, which selectively influence various subcortical areas, have been used for the management of patients with anxiety reactions and increased psychomotor activity (*Figure 2*). The present discussion is concerned with an evaluation of the comparative effectiveness of these drugs. It may be worthwhile to begin this discussion by reviewing briefly some of the known physiologic and pharmacologic effects of the subcortical tranquilizing agents.

PHARMACOLOGY OF ATARACTICS

In contrast to the barbiturates, the subcortical depressants, even in large therapeutic doses, do not reduce the total cerebral oxygen consumption (*Figure 3*). This is an important consideration, particularly in the management of those states in which there may be a depression of oxidative metabolism.

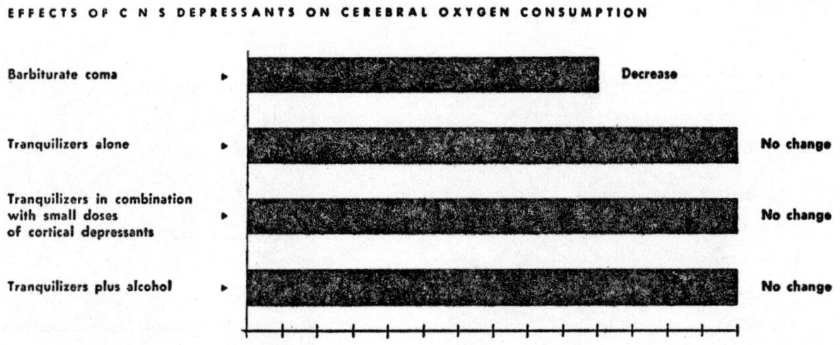

EFFECTS OF C N S DEPRESSANTS ON CEREBRAL OXYGEN CONSUMPTION

Barbiturate coma	Decrease
Tranquilizers alone	No change
Tranquilizers in combination with small doses of cortical depressants	No change
Tranquilizers plus alcohol	No change

Figure 3. *Chart showing the effects of central nervous system depressants on cerebral oxygen consumption.*

Clinically, a dramatic potentiation of the action of relatively small doses of barbiturates or analgesics occurs when they are administered simultaneously with most of the tranquilizing agents. Even such combinations do not cause an appreciable reduction of cerebral oxygen consumption. This lack of additive depression may be ascribed to the different loci of action of the two groups of drugs.

Since cerebral oxygen consumption appears to be uninfluenced by subcortical depressants in therapeutic doses, an explanation of their action must be sought in disturbances of either the utilization or transmission of the energy derived from oxidative reactions. The work of Grenell indicates that chlorpromazine in some manner interferes with the utilization of adenosinetriphosphate (a high energy phosphate compound). It is interesting that he observed this inhibition to be greatest in the reticular formation, the area in which the phenothiazine derivatives presumably exert their maximum effect.

Marazzi and Hart have noted that drugs such as epinephrine, mescaline and lysergic acid diethylamide, which cause anxiety or hallucinations, produce an increase of synaptic resistance (as evidenced by a diminution of trans-synaptic electrical potential). This change was reversed by the administration of chlorpromazine. It was also suggested by these authors that serotonin, which causes the most pronounced increase in synaptic resistance, may act as a humoral inhibitor in the natural function of the central nervous system.

Pletscher, Shore and Brodie have shown that reserpine lowers the concentration of serotonin in the brain and intestine, and that following its administration, there is a marked increase of the breakdown product of serotonin, 5-hydroxyindole acetate, in the urine. The implication is that reserpine competes with serotonin for cerebral end-organs, and that serotonin may play a role in the development and perpetuation of abnormal mental states.

Rinaldi and Himwich have demonstrated electroencephalographically that chlorpromazine depresses the alerting pattern in the reticular formation; whereas reserpine, although stimulating the reticular formation, apparently inhibits the activity of the hypothalamus (*Figure* 4).

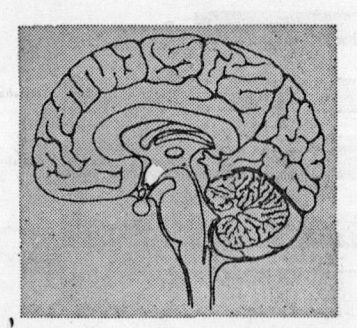

Figure 4. *Hypothalamus. Probably the primary site of action of reserpine.*

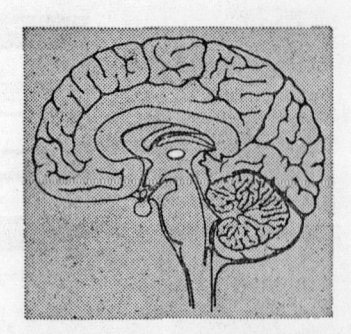

Figure 5. *Thalamus. Probably the primary site of action of meprobamate.*

Studies by Berger demonstrate that meprobamate (Equanil, Miltown) appears to have a central depressant action upon the thalamus and peripherally causes muscle relaxation (*Figure* 5).

Clinically the pharmacologic effects of these drugs also indicate their varied subcortical sites of action. *Table* 1 illustrates some of their major pharmacologic effects. It is evident that these drugs must exert their primary actions on dif-

Effects of Various Tranquilizing Agents

	Reserpine	*Chlorpromazine*	*Promazine*	*Meprobamate*
Body temperature	Fall	Fall	Unknown*	No change
Metabolic rate	Fall	Fall	Unknown*	No change
Barbiturate potentiation	Yes	Yes	Yes	None
Antiemetic action	None	Yes	Yes	None
Blood pressure	Fall	Occasional vascular collapse	No significant change	No change
Pulse rate	Bradycardia	Tachycardia	No change	No change
Intestinal motility	Increase	No change	No change	No change
Induction of sleep	Yes	Yes	Yes	Moderate
Muscle relaxation	None	None	None	Yes

Probably the same as chlorpromazine because of structural similarity.

Table 1.

ferent subcortical areas. The effects of reserpine on blood pressure, pulse rate, intestinal motility and pupillary size suggest the posterior hypothalamus as its primary site of action since it does not antagonize the effects of sympathomimetic substances such as epinephrine or norepinephrine, nor does it potentiate the effects of acetylcholine. Chlorpromazine must also exert an inhibitory effect upon the hypothalamus, as well as the reticular formation, since it produces a fall in body temperature and a decrease in metabolic rate.

Chlorpromazine differs from reserpine in that the autonomic changes following its administration may be ascribed to its adrenolytic effects, a possible ganglionic-blocking action and to its atropine-like properties. The locus of action of promazine has as yet not been determined, but it is probably the same as that of chlorpromazine.

It is possible that the loss of the chloride radical may be responsible for the relative absence of peripheral autonomic effects.

Meprobamate apparently blocks long internuncial neuronal circuits between the cortex and thalamus. It apparently does not influence autonomic activity. However, in large doses, it abolishes certain reflexes, and in therapeutic doses produces relaxation of skeletal muscles.

The following discussion will consider the indications for and contraindications to the use of the tranquilizing agents for the management of various clinical conditions encountered in medical practice.

Anxiety States

Perhaps the largest group of patients to whom the practitioner would have occasion to administer the tranquilizing agents are those suffering from acute and chronic anxiety states. (The patient who is subject to acute anxiety attacks usually suffers from an underlying chronic anxiety state.) In acute attacks, there is evidence of overstimulation of the autonomic nervous system, and the patient may complain of palpitation, nausea, frequency of urination, paresthesias and feelings of choking or suffocation and of impending death. In such situations, the administration of 50 to 100 mg. orally or intramuscularly of promazine or chlorpromazine will usually be effective in inducing a state of sleep from which the patient may awake free of the acute anxiety reaction.

Many of the patients, even without acute reactions, frequently complain of nervous tension, as well as subjective somatization of their chronic anxiety state. In such conditions it has been shown that the phenothiazine derivatives (promazine and chlorpromazine), reserpine and meprobamate may be useful in reducing the severity of the disorder (the last-named drug presumably being more specific in its effect). The dosage of meprobamate, usually 400 mg. three times daily, must be individualized and subsequently adjusted to obtain the desired clinical response. Complications associated with long-term therapy are probably seen in lowest incidence with meprobamate.

Somatic Disturbances

The emotional detachment and relaxation induced by the ataractic drugs makes them extremely useful in the management of anxiety states associated with somatic diseases. The psychologic stress frequently accompanying various disease states in many instances retards recovery, and may create difficulty in the hospital management of such patients. There is hardly an organic disturbance in which the administration of a tranquilizing agent would not be beneficial. We have found promazine to be particularly useful in the management of patients with terminal disease states due to malignant neoplasms and renal failure. In addition to inducing a relaxed state and an attitude of detachment from their environment, the antiemetic properties of the drug have proven extremely valuable. Promazine has also been useful in the management of asthmatic patients; the tremendous psychic component accompanying this disease is generally recognized.

The effective dose in organic illness should be determined by beginning with 25 to 50 mg., administered every four to six hours, and increasing the dose gradually until the desired response is achieved. We have used doses of promazine as high as 800 mg. a day to manage patients with intractable pain due to cancer. The route of administration will obviously depend on the condition of the patient.

In those diseases associated with pain, it is important to remember to reduce the dose of analgesic to approximately one-half to two-thirds because of the potentiating effect of the ataractics.

Because of its predisposition to cause vascular collapse, chlorpromazine should not be used in conditions such as acute myocardial infarction, or cerebral thrombosis, where even temporary acute reduction of pressure may be harmful. Furthermore, in clinical disorders in which vascular collapse may be a complication, it is inadvisable to administer reserpine since we have observed that this drug tends to block corrective hemostatic circulatory mechanisms, e.g., compensatory tachycardia. However, it has been observed that anginal symptoms may be alleviated by the administration of reserpine. It is difficult to state whether this effect is due to improved coronary circulation secondary to bradycardia, or to reduction of chronic anxiety with consequent indifference to minimal symptoms.

Alcoholic Syndromes

The practitioner is not infrequently called upon to assist in the control of the combative and assaultive acutely inebriated individual. The phenothiazine derivatives (promazine and chlorpromazine), because of their immediate onset of action, are most suitable for the management of such patients. They may be administered orally, intramuscularly or intravenously, depending on the cooperation of the subject. These drugs are effective within approximately 45 minutes after oral therapy, 30 minutes after intramuscular injection, and 5 minutes following intravenous administration. Dosage should be relatively small (25 to 50 mg.) because of the potentiating effects of these drugs on the depressant action of alcohol. The duration of sleep may be six to ten hours, probably depending greatly upon the alcohol concentration in the blood.

The majority of patients suffering from the after-effects of continued overindulgence in alcohol require treatment for insomnia, anxiety and tremors. Here again the immediate control of the disorder is best accomplished by one of the phenothiazine derivatives. Sleep will be induced within 30 to 45 minutes by 100 mg. given orally (or intramuscularly if necessary), thereby relieving the overt manifestations of this condition. Following the initial doses, smaller doses, may be given repeatedly, usually every four to six hours, as long as signs and symptoms persist. Because of the unpredictable duration of the syndrome (one to seven days), we do not advocate the use of reserpine, which has a delayed onset of action even when administered intravenously, and whose action may persist for some time after spontaneous recovery from the alcoholic syndrome. Many alcoholic patients, because of acute gastritis, are unable to retain either food or fluids. The blocking effect of the phenothiazines on emetic centers is extremely helpful in such cases.

Because of difficulty in management and precariousness of the condition, patients with hallucinatory post-alcoholic syndromes (acute hallucinosis and delirium tremens) should be hospitalized. Intravenous medication is required because of the urgency of the situation. Promazine is probably the drug of choice because of its rapid action and apparent relative freedom from liability to induce vascular collapse. An initial dose of 200 mg. is usually effective in inducing sleep. However, in severe cases, larger doses may be required (300 to 400 mg.), or the initial dose of 200 mg. may have to be supplemented with 100 to 200 mg. of pentobarbital (Nembutal). Doses of promazine (200 mg.) are repeated when necessary, usually at four to six-hour intervals. Supplementary use of the barbiturate is discontinued as soon as promazine alone is found to be effective.

The effects of intramuscular administration of 2.5 to 5 mg. of reserpine in such patients are manifested after eight to 24 hours. Sleep induced by this amount appears to be more profound and longer lasting than with the phenothiazines. Reserpine may be continued in these doses every 12 hours. Here again because of the unpredictable duration (one to seven days) of this syndrome, we prefer to use the phenothiazines rather than reserpine. An unfavorable deterrent to the use of reserpine is the frequent occurrence of diarrhea with large doses. This may aggravate dehydration, and certainly complicates nursing care.

Head injury. The high incidence of head injuries and subdural hematomas in alcoholic patients is generally recognized. In the management of the alcoholic subject during his acute phase, phenothiazine has the significant advantage that it does not mask the development of an expanding intracranial lesion. The patient may be regularly aroused from his sleep and his neurologic status evaluated. If the patient cannot be aroused, then we should strongly suspect a subdural hematoma.

Drug Addiction

Occasionally the physician will encounter instances of excitation or agitation due to the withdrawal of drugs to which patients have become addicted, or due to excessive use of central nervous system stimulants. Since these syndromes are of comparatively short duration, the use of the phenothiazine compounds in their treatment appears preferable. We have found that doses of 100 to 150 mg. of promazine, orally or intramuscularly every four to six hours, may be necessary to control the symptoms of drug withdrawal. Large doses are preferable and their continued administration every four to six hours maintains the patient in a state of sleep until withdrawal symptoms spontaneously disappear (usually within five to seven days).

In cases of excitation resulting from the excessive use of central nervous system stimulants, a large initial dose of promazine (100 to 150 mg.) is indicated. The frequency and size of subsequent doses should be gauged by the response of the patient.

Psychoses with Agitation

The initial management of disturbed psychotic patients can best be accomplished by resorting to institutional care for diagnosis and beginning of therapy. In many such instances, agitation may be so marked that the patient can be transported to the hospital only if effective sedation is instituted at home. For this purpose promazine is usually effective when given intramuscularly or intravenously in doses of 150 to 200 mg.

There are many types of psychoses, either inherently of brief duration or having short-lived excitatory phases, in which continued confinement to a psychiatric hospital may be avoided. The patient may be managed either in the home or in a general hospital with the aid of subcortical blocking agents. This is frequently the case in senile deterioration with episodic confusion and agitation. In such instances initiation and continuation of treatment may well remain in the hands of the practitioner. Doses of the phenothiazines required may vary from 50 to 300 mg. given orally (when possible) as often as four times a day. The magnitude and frequency of the dose will depend on the patient's response. These drugs, as well as reserpine, may be useful in the prophylactic treatment of nocturnal confusion, so common among the aged population.

Promazine administered parenterally is probably preferable for the management of acute delirium associated with febrile illnesses, or psychotic states occasionally complicating the immediate postoperative period. Fabing has reported that azacyclonol (Frenquel) is also effective in the later condition, although we have been disappointed in its therapeutic efficacy even in large (200 mg.) parenteral doses.

Those psychoses which have no apparent excitatory component and are manifested almost exclusively by depression do not, as a rule, respond well to treatment by the tranquilizing agents. In fact, these drugs might well aggravate the depression in such cases.

Miscellaneous Uses

We have found the phenothiazines to be a useful adjunct for the performance of necessary diagnostic studies in irrational or unmanageable patients. Radiologic observations, lumbar puncture, bronchoscopy, etc., may be done without resistance after the administration of 100 to 150 mg. of promazine or chlorpromazine.

Value of Ataractics in Perspective

It should be emphasized that to date, experience with these drugs has not been adequate to make definite statements concerning their relative effectiveness, particularly with regard to long-term therapy. It would, however, be foolhardy to believe that any one agent would be effective in correcting all of the various types of psychoses and neuroses. This would be tantamount to saying that all diseases of the gastrointestinal tract could be satisfactorily managed by one drug. At the present time the only safe conclusions that can be drawn are those pertaining to the relative value of the various agents in the management of acutely disturbed patients.

It would be rather naive to expect that drug therapy alone would be completely adequate for restoring or maintaining a state of normalcy in the mentally disturbed patient. It has been repeatedly demonstrated that no disease is completely managed by drug therapy alone. Drug therapy in psychiatric disease should be considered merely as an adjunct to other forms of therapy; the social, environmental and interpersonal relationship cannot be ignored. There can be no doubt that the ataractic agents render the patient more accessible to psychotherapeutic procedures; they may serve as a crutch which should be removed if and when normal psychobiologic homeostasis can be achieved.

The effectiveness of these agents serves to support the contention that psychiatric disorders may well result from disturbances in energy utilization or neural transmission, and strengthens the concept of an organic basis for their etiology. The advent of these drugs makes it possible for the physician to manage many of these patients in the home and, when necessary, to have them admitted to general hospitals for diagnostic studies and institution of therapy. This avoids the stigma currently associated with admission of such patients to a psychiatric hospital, and reduces the costs to the patient.

WHAT'S NEW AND USABLE IN THE CHEMICAL TREATMENT OF ABNORMAL BEHAVIOR

John T. Ferguson, M.D.

My work is treating the mentally ill. Not the new admissions at our Traverse City State Hospital, but the chronic regressed patients who, according to all statistics, were beyond the point of no return. It is from our work with these patients that we have collected a large part of the material to be presented today.

What can this mean to you whose field is general practice? Just this: The new methods of chemically reversing advanced, apparently irreversible mental illness are also applicable to the behavior problems you doctors meet in your daily work.

Patients do not arrive at our hospital with fancy psychiatric diagnoses any more than they arrive that way to you family physicians. They all come to all of you and to me for exactly the same reasons—either they cannot live with themselves or they cannot live with others in their communities. But you say these reasons are too vague. What is it, specifically, that brings the mentally ill to the general practitioner—and then to us at the State Hospital?

The simple answer comes out of a study of many complaints leading to admission. It boils down to *behavior*. Behavior of such an abnormal caliber that those closest and dearest to the sick, could not endure it any longer.

All of you are familiar with abnormal behavior of this type—it has existed thousands of years before its description in the learned nomenclature of Bleuler and Sigmund Freud. Many of you have prayed for help that would some day prevent you from having to make another committing statement.

The possible chemical control of abnormal behavior by methods that can be used by the general practitioner—that is our goal. The recent development of what may be called "behavior drugs" gives promise of treatment that will attack and eliminate many of these socio-medical problems in each community. This work has now progressed to a point where it can be passed on for test in the field—by you family doctors.

Our research has progressed until today most of our efforts are concentrated on the investigation and evaluation of new behavior drugs. And, I do mean new, as many of the compounds we are investigating today are numbered, rather than named, and although it may seem odd, many of them are as yet completely unknown to the *Ladies Home Journal* and *Time Magazine*.

This type of research is usually called clinical investigation. However, most of us like to consider ourselves as Medical Test Pilots—the men behind the scene who help to iron the bugs out of the new drugs for the physicians in the front lines. Doing this is not always easy, and the results are not always as successful as we anticipate. It is not easy because after the new drugs have gone through the laboratory and have been tested thoroughly we must analyze the reports, checking closely for activity, safety, side reactions and toxicity. We do this until we find one that has possibilities in our field. Further laboratory tests are then run against known compounds of like action. If the results of this comparative study reveal activity that is better or more specific than those compounds already being used, we file a Food and Drug Administration investigators' form and start testing the drug clinically. As part of our research we work out activity and dosage. Far more important for you doctors, to my way of thinking, are our observations and evaluations of the safety, side reactions, contra-indications and limitations of each compound based upon many months of their use.

As our work progresses, we make reports of that which we have seen. We do this as honestly and simply as we can, in order that the greatest number possible will understand our methods, see how we obtained our results and be able to administer the new drugs with understanding and confidence.

We have prepared such a report for you, a report that we feel will shed some new light on everyday behavior problems, as well as help you in managing them.

None of the present drugs by themselves will control all behavior problems because each drug is rather specific for one type of behavior, and the behavior of an individual is usually a mixture of overactivity and underactivity. This is true of normal as well as abnormal behavior. None of us carries a full head of steam all the time, just as none of us has our fires banked all the time. However, most of us are able to control ourselves and, as a result of this, can live with the stresses and strains that confront us each day.

It is when the response of an individual to the pressures of life is such that he cannot control himself—it is then that we have abnormal behavior. The abnormality may be covered up well, or it may be severe enough to disturb the relatives and neighbors.

I cannot give a one, two, three plan for diagnosing treatable behavior. But I can say that each of you is doing it every day. Take the patient who comes into your office with or without specific objective pathological signs—before you talk to her two minutes you have mentally recorded the fact that she is tense and nervous or that she has the "blues" and is down-in-the-dumps. It is the same method whether the patient be eight or eighty. With but few exceptions, however, the behavior of the patient is mixed in character.

That is, in most patients, regardless of the outward behavior manifestation, there is an element of the opposite present. Let me repeat—*in most patients, regardless of the outward behavior manifestation, there is an element of the opposite behavior present.* I have stressed this mixture of behavior within each patient because a simple understanding of it will greatly increase your success with the new drugs and eliminate many of the difficulties you are now encountering.

To better understand what I mean, and to show you how we worked it out let's go back a couple of years. The first of the new behavior drugs we had were Serpasil and Thorazine—tranquilizers; quieters. Within a few months, the lay magazines were loaded with articles of praise for which they could not coin enough superlatives. I recall one that went so far as to spread a headline across two pages, "Mental Cure Found," or words to that effect. The pressure was great. Medical publications followed the trend with articles of the same caliber. Enthusiasm had no bounds. Let me refresh your memory by quoting from an article:

"Patients showing marked habit deterioration such as soiling, wetting, and destructiveness, become more cleanly, less destructive, and better able to care for themselves; and patients given to outbreaks of violence, with a tendency to assault, become much better adjusted to their environment and their activities are more easily directed into useful channels following treatment."

Fine—except that which I have just read was taken from a 1926 issue of the *American Journal of Psychiatry* and is talking about bromides.

Like the bromides, it was only natural that history should repeat itself. Reserpine and chlorpromazine were soon used to treat everything from falling hair to falling arches. As their use increased, so did the failures and side-reactions. A sour note appeared to overshadow the glowing praise that had heralded these drugs into existence.

When we discounted the failures associated with indiscriminate use, the percentages came up fast but there was still a fly-in-the-ointment. We went fly hunting! With the treatment of our first very overactive group, the results had been excellent, so we treated a less active group. Not so good. They didn't smooth down as well as the first group. The next stratum of the overactive group was even worse. Why? We didn't know, but we looked and checked and then did some thinking. The last group hadn't done as well because they showed more underactive features quicker than the others. It was the same for the second group when compared to the first. From our experience with barbiturates, we know that an analeptic would act as a pick-up. We tried it with caffeine. Only mild success—but we had a lead. Behavior must be mixed. If true—and we could balance these two behavior components within an individual—it is then that we would have our goal—active tranquility. We tried every analeptic we could find. The results were fair, but none was consistent. It was then, well over a year ago, that Ciba permitted us to try two new analeptics. One was good, the other looked most promising. As often happens in our type of research, the first one went sour. But the other one, methylphenidylacetate, which is marketed as Ritalin, more than fulfilled our fondest expectations. It not only relieved the side-reactions of Thorazine and Serpasil—it also increased our improved percentages by creating an awakening toward reality within these patients. It was more than a "picker-upper," it was a true psycho-analeptic.

Realizing this, we lost little time in trying Ritalin by itself on the negative, underactive behavior group. We had excellent results with our first negative group. Ritalin relieved most of their underactive behavior smoothly and without the blood pressure, pulse and appetite changes or the jitters associated with many of the other analeptics we had tried. Then, as with the overactive behavior series, we saw our results fall off as each successive stratum of underactivity was treated. When we added Serpasil and saw our improved percentages increase —it was then that we felt we could produce active tranquility. We hadn't been down the road before, so we traveled cautiously changing doses, watching and recording. As the days turned to weeks, all went well but the months ruined us. Something mysterious was happening to our patients, just as many of you have seen it happen to yours. They just plain weren't doing so well.

Today, fifteen months, 700 patients and eleven drugs later, we feel we have found some of the answers that will help you in the chemical management of behavior problems.

Each of the new behavior drugs has, like digitalis and insulin, specific indications and contraindications. To use them successfully one must know their limitations, their good and their bad points and their clinical course.

The literature, loaded as it is with ambiguous and contradicting statements, makes a true study of each drug impossible. What then are you to do? Concentrate on one analeptic and one tranquilizer. Study them, know them, use them and understand them clinically—separately and combined. They will be enough. Let me show what I mean—

Figure 1 represents behavior problems as they walk through your office door. From the shading, one sees that some are outwardly very overactive, others are quite underactive. Most are near normal.

If only a tranquilizing drug is used, results will be similar to the dark area shown in Figure 2. The most overactive will be helped most. The less the overactivity, the less they will be helped. For a tranquilizing drug, I use Serpasil, because I consider it the least toxic and the safest to use for increased motor activity, aggressiveness, anxiety and tension. It has proven best for me with all overactivity, both mental and physical.

If treatment is confined to an analeptic, results will be similar to the shaded area shown in Figure 3. The more underactivity present, the better are the chances for helping the patient.

For an analeptic drug, I use Ritalin, because within therapeutic limits I have found it to be without side effects. It has proven safest and best for me with underactivity, both mental and physical.

Let's go a step further and consider treatment for both overactive and underactive behavior patients. The overactive patients are treated with Serpasil and the underactive patients with Ritalin. From the clear area in Figure 4, it can be seen that there is still a big segment of behavior that is not being touched.

If you look at this another way, it is then that you see more clearly how this untouched behavior segment has both overactive and underactive components, each of varying intensity. It is definitely mixed (Fig. 5). How do you attack it?

First, you can set up your results as percentages to see how many behavior problems will be responding to Serpasil and how many will be responding to Ritalin, after at least a year. This is quite important because in any practice, the lasting benefits of the future are far more important than are the spectacular cures of today. Roughly, 10 to 15 per cent of all overactive patients on Serpasil alone will be doing fine after a year. About 5 to 10 per cent of under-

From left to right:
Fig. 1, 2, 3

From left to right:
Fig. 4, 5, 6

From left to right:
Fig. 7, 8, 9

active behavior problems will be all right on Ritalin alone after a year. We see, then, that at the end of the year 75 per cent of behavior problems have not been touched—or will be showing changes from their first improvements (Fig. 6). The reason for this is not an accumulation of the medicines within the patient. It is an actual change within the patient. Where this change takes place with Serpasil and Ritalin, I do not know, but I do know that as the behavior of an individual moves toward normal, there is need for less and less medicine. Most of you know what I mean because you have used Serpasil for some of your hypertensive patients—patients whose hypertension was perhaps the clinical manifestation of increased anxiety or tension. Within a week or two, the blood pressure was down several points on maybe a dose of 0.1 to 0.3 mgm. of Serpasil three times daily. The patient felt like a new man. Life was more bearable for him. For the first time in years, he was living. You've heard it—and felt good—until months later when the patient came in depressed or complaining of always being sleepy. I have seen it happen on 0.1 mgm. of Serpasil daily. I have also seen this same patient add 10 mgm. of Ritalin twice daily to his daily 0.1 mgm. of Serpasil and improve to a better mental and physical level than at any time in the past ten years. Therefore, to treat behavior problems properly, each must be treated individually as a mixture of overactive and underactive components.

To illustrate what we mean, in Figure 7 we have not only placed the two behavior components side by side, but we have also shaded the areas to show how, as the underactives awaken toward reality and the overactives "simmer down," each will not only need less and less of their original medicine, but to arrive at an active tranquility they will each need to have the second drug added.

Figure 8 is the same as Figure 7, but with the dosages added. In each section we have used a dosage range, rather than a mandatory figure. We did this to stress the individuality of each patient, as two patients with the same clinical behavior pattern quite often require different dosage levels.

Here approximately 15 per cent of the overactive group have no clinically recordable underactive component. This type of patient will require larger doses of Serpasil than any of the others. This dose range is usually 5 to 15 mgm. of Serpasil per day, although it may have to be raised with a few overactive cases. Results with this overactive group will be faster and smoother if the parenteral Serpasil is used.

A safe rule-of-thumb to follow for parenteral Serpasil is this—"If the patient can be given 7.5 grains of Sodium Amytal then 5 mgm. of Serpasil can be given. If not, then use 2.5 mgm. of Serpasil." Either dose may be repeated every three to six hours, if needed. On the underactive side, there are approximately 10 per cent who will require 60 to 90 mgm. of Ritalin a day. This works best when given 20 to 30 mgm. three times daily.

It is from these two groups—the very overactive and the very underactive—that State Hospitals secure most of their admissions. Proper treatment of this type of patient, therefore, should reduce materially the number of commitments each general practitioner will be forced to make in the future. It is a challenge to good medicine.

In this central group, very few patients will require as much as 1.5 mgm. of Serpasil or as much as 40 mgm. of Ritalin daily. In fact, the 0.1-0.5 mgm. Serpasil and the 10-20 mgm. Ritalin daily dosage will be used more than any other, as most patients will not be too far from normal behavior when first seen.

Using divided doses will give smoother action. We like a three times daily schedule. The medicine may be given before, after, or with the meals. It may be crushed and put in the food or beverage, if necessary.

Although we show the range for the combined use of both drugs, only a small part of treatment will start that way. In most cases, there will be a dominant behavior. If it is underactivity, start with Ritalin. If it is overactivity, start with Serpasil. Then, as the dominant behavior starts to resolve, add small amounts of the second drug. We have found that early addition of small amounts of the second drug—5 mgm. of Ritalin two or three times daily to the patient on Serpasil, or 0.1 to 0.2 mgm. of Serpasil added to the patient on Ritalin—produced better results and is easier on the patient and the doctor than to do nothing until side reactions or bad effects appear. Learning to add the second drug as soon as the original dominant behavior started to resolve caused us more headaches than any other point, yet the facts behind it are so simple I feel guilty whenever I think about it.

Let us consider Figure 9. Behavior is like a teeter-totter. (1) Normal behavior fluctuates, but maintains balance—even though one component may be dominant.

(2) It is when one factor—overactivity or underactivity is clinically manifested—that we have abnormal behavior. It is the inability of the individual to keep in balance that usually brings him to your attention.

If Serpasil is given in amounts sufficient to decrease the overactivity—is it right that this overactivity should reach normal and stop? Of course not. (3) It is like putting a rock on one end of it to stop at center. (4) Unless the dosage is adjusted in proportion to the patient's improvement, it is only right to expect the drug to continue acting on the overactive component until the negative remains clinically.

(5) Now, if we add Ritalin to the point that this new underactivity decreases, we again cannot expect the behavior to reach normal and stop. (6) It will again go on until the original overactivity manifests itself—even though the patient is on the original Serpasil dosage.

(7) From this we see that we could continue adding to each side as they went up and down—we could add until we exceeded therapeutic limits. Remember my headaches—it can be done. I recall one underactive patient during the time I was learning about this—I got her up to 8 mgm. of Serpasil three times daily. That is right—an underactive patient on a dose of 24 mgm. of Serpasil and 90 mgm. of Ritalin each *day*. Today she is doing fine on 0.2 mgm. of Serpasil and 10 mgm. of Ritalin three times daily.

Don't do it the hard way—add the second drug when the patient starts to improve. It will take less drugs—and less time.

(8) After the patient is balanced for a month or two, decrease both drugs in proportion. (9) That is, if he is on 1 mgm. of Serpasil and 20 mgm. of Ritalin three times daily, cut the dose to 0.75 mgm. of Serpasil and 15 mgm. of

Ritalin three times daily. Do this every couple of weeks. (10) In this way, it may be possible to eliminate both drugs. If not, you will arrive at the proper maintenance dose.

The cause of abnormal behavior is not always known to us. Consequently, there will be times when a balanced patient will be temporarily upset. The addition of extra Serpasil or Ritalin for a short time will usually help the patient through these upset periods.

Think of the controlled diabetic patient. If he overeats, he takes more insulin. If he fasts, he cuts his insulin. The same, in relation to the amount of mental strain, is basically true in the treatment of behavior problems. However, the diabetic person cannot do this unless he has had it explained to him. Therefore, for the best results with behavior problems, it behooves the physician to explain to patients, or their relatives, the action of each drug, what the drugs are expected to do and what the patients should report in order that the physician may adjust the drugs properly to reach the desired goal—active tranquility.

Doing this will be easy, and the results will be good with the average behavior problem. However, there is one type of behavior that is being seen more and more each day, which we have been asked to discuss more thoroughly. It is the behavior of senility, the biggest challenge.

In many cases, it is possible to control, ameliorate or even reverse the abnormal behavior of these elderly patients. The method is the same as that which we have already outlined, but since many consider the abnormal behavior manifestations of senility to be irreversible, we feel a report on this new approach to the problem is needed.

Age, length of illness and the usual physical infirmities of this group are not contra-indications to either Serpasil or Ritalin.

No special diagnostic or laboratory techniques are needed, although we have used them in approximately 300 cases. Clinical observations will be the most important criteria for starting doses as well as adjustment.

Those elderly patients showing a predominance of overactivity should be started on Serpasil. A good starting dose is 0.2 mgm. three times daily.

Those elderly patients showing a predominance of negative behavior should be started on Ritalin. A good starting dose is 10 mgm. of Ritalin three times daily.

The elderly patient about whom you are not sure, or who has mixed behavior, may be started on both Serpasil and Ritalin at the same time. A good starting combination is 0.2 mgm. of Serpasil and 10 mgm. of Ritalin three times daily. It is possible—and with a wide margin of safety—to raise these starting doses if you feel the initial behavior warrants such an increase.

The first change may be within two or three days or it may take as long as three weeks to produce it. Checking the patient every day or two for this period will allow regulation of the dose as needed to produce clinical change.

As the clinical behavior pattern of each patient starts to shift toward normal, either the original dose will have to be reduced or the second drug added.

With overactive elderly patients, a reduction in motor activity or aggressiveness, or anxiety and tension is desirable. When this decrease is seen clinically without any evidence of reduced mental activity—it is then best to reduce the

Serpasil gradually before adding Ritalin. If, on the other hand, the reduction includes decreased mental activity—it is then best to add Ritalin. In a few elderly patients, lethargy may be seen before the motor activity or aggressiveness is reduced. When this happens, a small amount of both drugs should be added—the Ritalin to overcome the lethargy and more Serpasil to take care of the motor activity. These cases are rare, but should you have one, remember to work at it with both drugs—or you'll be in for a trip on the bouncing teeter-totter.

The maintenance dose for most overactive elderly patients will be near 0.25 mgm. of Serpasil and 5 mgm. of Ritalin three times daily. About one-fourth of these patients will require either a higher regular dose of Serpasil or an occasional extra dose of Serpasil.

The number of the underactive patients in the senile group will be about one-half or one-third that of the number of overactive patients. I can't tell why, but I can say that a negative, withdrawn, quiet patient loaded with tension, anxiety or resistance should be considered overactive and treated as such. Consequently, a furrowed brow, sweaty hands or refusal to follow normal routines when seen in a patient—regardless of the negative front he tries to assume—should be an indication to start on Serpasil and to treat the patient as an overactive person.

It is usually because of the confusion and disorientation in these negative patients that they resist—they don't understand, so they resort to survival tactics—they fight it—they resist it.

Thus, a negative patient is one who is without tension, anxiety, or resistance. He can be confused or disoriented. Usually, he is one who requires help or prodding to follow daily routines. He follows easily, making few if any decisions for himself.

The Ritalin may produce clinical change in these patients within a couple of days. If there is no change within three or four days, the dose should be raised to 30 mgm. three times daily and if there is no change for three or four days, it is then advisable to add Serpasil which in most cases will produce a change so that the drugs can then be balanced.

The patient who improves his negative clinical pattern without evidence of excess motor activity or aggressiveness, when his behavior moves toward normal, can have the Ritalin gradually reduced. When there is clinical evidence of overactive behavior, along with the mental awakening—it is then that Serpasil should be added to the Ritalin. Most negative patients will be maintained on a dose near 0.2 mgm. of Serpasil and 10 mgm. of Ritalin three times daily. Here again, after the patient has been in balance for a period of time, both drugs can gradually be reduced to find the maintenance dose.

Senile patients will do better and have a smoother life if kept on a maintenance dose. The relatives of these patients usually demonstrate less anxiety if the medicines that helped Grandpa or Grandma are continued.

Speaking of relatives—what can you offer them? What can you tell them the drugs will do for Grandma? You cannot offer them complete rejuvenation for their loved ones. In fact, you can't offer them too much unless they want to help. Why? The drugs by themselves do not have the power to carry the senile patient back—they can produce within the patient the ability to participate—the total improvement will be in almost direct proportion to the help and tender loving care they receive.

If you are sure that the patient will be helped and reassured, and then reassured again as the drugs act to produce a lessening of his confusion and an increase in his orientation—if you are sure—then you can tell those taking care of the patient that he will show a trend toward a more productive, normal activity. There will be an improvement in his ability to co-operate and a new interest in his outlook on life, and himself. He will enjoy himself more, sleep and eat better and take better care of himself. Most important to the relatives—you can tell them he will need less special care and attention—he can be managed without having to be committed to a mental hospital.

How do I know you can say these things? I know because I've seen them happen. Not just once, but many times. Today almost one-half of my committed senile patients could go home, if they had a home to which to go.

I do not know how many of your elderly patients with behavior problems will end up in an institution, but I do know that by early detection and treatment of their abnormal behavior you will reduce the number and make this a much better world in which to grow old.

DRUGS RECENTLY INTRODUCED IN THE TREATMENT OF PSYCHIATRIC DISORDERS

Irvin M. Cohen, M.D.

A variety of new pharmacologic agents useful in the management and treatment of functional disorders have become commercially available in the United States within the past three years. Their introduction has been met by an almost unparalleled reception, a response which has emphasized the growing need for practical drug therapy of symptoms of psychologic origin. Three types of drugs compose these recent advances in neuropharmacologic research: (1) the tranquilizers, (2) the euphoriants, and (3) the nonbarbiturate hypnotics. The tranquilizers are fundamentally sedatives in the sense that they are designed to relieve tension and reduce psychomotor activity. Their uniqueness lies in their ability to do so without disturbing intellectual function. The euphoriants and nonbarbiturate hypnotics are lesser but nonetheless important developments, their significance being in the advantages they offer over existing preparations and their wider clinical applicability.

The ultimate position which they will occupy in therapeutics remains to be determined. Early overenthusiasm is being replaced by the more realistic appraisal that they are mainly of value in symptomatic control, and that cures are rare, if not fortuitous. Unpredictability of therapeutic response and occurrence of objectionable side effects and complications are major defects in the products presently available. Another undesirable feature is the cost, which may become economically burdensome to the patient.

Space does not permit detailed discussion of each of the new drugs. This paper is therefore intended as a brief review of those in widest use, and as a guide to the practicing physician.

TRANQUILIZERS

To utilize the tranquilizers most effectively, a clear understanding of certain facts and therapeutic principles is required:

1. Improvement is not related to diagnosis, but to the presence or absence of certain clinical features in the illness.
2. Dosage is determined entirely on the basis of therapeutic response and must be adjusted to the requirements of the individual case.
3. The margin of safety is great. Fatal termination following overdosage is almost unknown.
4. The patient in tranquilizer-induced sleep can always be awakened. If the patient cannot be awakened, an untoward reaction has occurred, the nature

of which must be ascertained immediately.
5. Side effects are common but usually disappear during treatment.
6. Habituation is rare. Addiction does not occur.

Chlorpromazine (Thorazine.)—Chlorpromazine, a chlorinated derivative of phenothiazine, was synthesized in France in 1950 and was widely used in Europe for two years prior to its introduction in this country in May, 1954. Its spectrum includes psychiatric illness of all classifications, but it is most effective if there is evidence of (1) agitation, (2) anxiety, or (3) aggression, irrespective of the diagnostic entity in which the manifestation may appear. Improvement ranges from mere reduction of intensity of symptoms to apparently complete resolution of illness. Results have been poor in withdrawn or hypochondriacal patients, or when there is secondary gain from symptoms in the form of familial sympathy or overindulgence. Chlorpromazine appears to be capable of worsening depressions and perhaps even mobilizing incipient cases and should not be used in such cases except temporarily to reduce agitation.

The required dosage is highly variable and must be determined strictly on the basis of clinical response. It is believed that many failures with chlorpromazine can be attributed to inadequate dosage. In my experience effective oral dosage for most neurotics is in the range of 200 to 600 mg. daily, whereas psychotic patients have generally required 400 to 800 mg. daily. As much as 3,200 mg. daily have been given without untoward effects.

There has been much discussion of the toxicity of chlorpromazine. The consensus seems to be that although it produces many undesirable side effects and occasionally serious complications, it is in most cases a relatively safe drug which can be utilized without undue risk. With several exceptions, side effects are due to physiologic action on various levels of the nervous system; they are usually temporary and rarely require termination of treatment. One or more can be expected to occur, the most frequent being drowsiness, weakness, nasal stuffiness, and orthostatic hypotensive symptoms. Precipitous fall in blood pressure may occur, particularly after intramuscular injection. If the patient remains responsive and there are no other signs of shock, no special treatment is needed. Should vascular collapse occur, norepinephrine should be used since chlorpromazine may reverse the action of epinephrine. Special precautions should be taken with the aged, to whom intramuscular injections should not be given except when unusual indication exists. It is now generally believed that complications referable to the skin, liver, and hemopoietic system are idiosyncratic phenomena which occur in patients sensitive to this drug. Numerous studies have been devoted to chlorpromazine-induced jaundice. The process has been found to be a reversible reaction which spares the parenchyma and confines itself to temporary occlusion of the biliary canaliculi. Since patients not developing jaundice show no disturbance in bile secretion or hepatocellular function, chlorpromazine probably does not involve the liver except in the presence of sensitivity. The misconception exists that large dosages or prolonged administration increases the risk of liver damage; actually, the incidence, which is approximately 1.5 per cent, is unrelated to these factors. Dermatologic complications usually appear after two weeks of administration, generally resolve quickly, and not only may disappear without interruption of treatment but ordinarily do not recur on subsequent administration. Parkinsonism may occur, particularly when daily dosage exceeds 600 mg.; resolution is usually rapid when dosage is reduced. The rarest complication, agranulocytosis, which occurs most frequently in females and during the sixth week of administration, demands prompt detection and immediate treatment by antibiotics and corticotropin.

Reserpine.—Sedation produced by reserpine is qualitatively similar to that of chlorpromazine, although it does not usually induce sleep except when given parenterally or in large oral dosages. However, the two drugs differ in many respects. Chlorpromazine lowers blood pressure by a combination of peripheral sympatholytic and adrenolytic effects; reserpine, by reducing central sympathetic activity. Chlorpromazine produces tachycardia (compensatory to orthostatic hypotension), hypochlorhydria, and constipation; reserpine, bradycardia, hyperchlorhydria, and increased peristalsis.

Therapeutic effects of reserpine resemble those of chlorpromazine in that it also reduces anxiety and calms psychomotor excitement. Clinical indications are roughly identical, and comparison studies reveal results to be approximately equivalent. Rapid effect can be obtained from both drugs by parenteral administration, although it is my impression that chlorpromazine is the more potent in controlling hyperactive psychotics. Oral reserpine acts slowly, sometimes requiring several weeks for maximum results, and it is wise to warn the patient of this. When rapid relief is needed or desirable, chlorpromazine is preferable. When time is not a factor, choice between these two drugs rests on individual preference and consideration of risks involved. I have found chlorpromazine to be of greater value in patients who complained of "nervousness," vague feelings of unrest, and similar indicators of free-floating anxiety. Patients who exhibit chronic low grade but partially disabling tension states seem to derive more benefit from reserpine, particularly when headaches are the presenting complaint.

Daily dosage for neurotic patients is 0.5 to 5.0 mg. daily. In the management of severely agitated or assaultive patients a combined intramuscular-oral regimen is indicated. Injections of 2.5 to 5.0 mg. in conjunction with oral doses of 1.0 mg. twice daily are given in the early phase, injections gradually being replaced by increasing oral doses usually to a level of 4.0 mg. daily or higher if necessary. Combined chlorpromazine-reserpine therapy recently has been suggested, but whether the effect is synergistic or additive is debatable.

Reserpine has fewer side effects than chlorpromazine though they tend to be more subjectively distressing. The most frequent are nasal stuffiness, weakness and fatigue, and loose stools. No grave complications have been described. The most common complication is Parkinsonism, which is reversible and usually resolves on reduction of dosage or temporary discontinuance of medication. Reserpine may induce depressions, and it is my growing impression that such depressions are more difficult to treat than the usual psychogenic depressions.

Meprobamate (Equanil, Miltown).—Meprobamate is chemically a derivative of mephenesin, exerting similar but more intense sedative and muscular relaxing properties. It appears to be of considerable value in anxiety and tension states and allied psychosomatic conditions. Relief is usually negligible if features indicative of anxiety are absent or if anxiety is of psychotic proportions. Psychosomatic manifestations in which it has proved useful include tension headaches caused by sustained contraction of the muscles of the scalp and neck, low back pain due to muscle tension, pylorospasm, and recurrent blushing.

The dose is 400 mg. three to four times daily. In some cases tolerance develops rapidly and doubling of the dosage may be required. In others improvement may allow halving. Side effects consist mainly of drowsiness and weakness in the early course of treatment and occasionally gastric discomfort. In contrast to the phenothiazine derivatives and reserpine, it has no significant effect on the autonomic nervous system so that side effects of this type are generally absent. Meprobamate is not entirely free of complications. Allergic skin reactions may occur, and in my series an anaphylactoid reaction occurred one and one-half hours after an initial dose of 400 mg. The reaction persisted for 96 hours and consisted of an initial stage of shock followed by prolonged hypotension, fever, and generalized skin eruption. Adkins has described 1 death occurring after a first dose of Equanil. Postmortem examination revealed nonspecific changes.

Promazine (Sparine).—Promazine is a modified form of chlorpromazine. Milligram for milligram it is less potent than chlorpromazine, but when used in sufficient quantity can produce similar calming action on the acutely disturbed patient. Its comparable efficacy in the less dramatic indications has not yet been established. The side effects of promazine appear to be less intense and perhaps fewer than those of chlorpromazine. There is considerably less effect on blood pressure. Precipitous drops in pressure are unusual, even after intravenous administration. Postural hypotension is not uncommon, however. Claims that promazine is free from complications must be discounted as premature. In this regard it should be discounted as premature. In this regard it should be remembered that jaundice due to chlorpromazine was not described until it had been in use for more than two years.

The indications for promazine are essentially similar to those of chlorpromazine, that is, as symptomatic control in the anxious, agitated, or aggressive patient. Since it has limited hypotensive effect, promazine may be injected intravenously, a valuable advantage under certain conditions. The initial intravenous dose is 50 to 150 mg. depending on the degree of excitation. In general, these doses are sufficient, but if the desired calming effect is not apparent within 5 to 10 minutes, additional doses up to a total of 300 mg. may be given. The oral or intramusclar dose is 25 to 200 mg. at four to six hour intervals, depending upon the response of the patient. To reduce the possibility of potentiation of alcohol, the initial dose in the acutely inebriated patient should not exceed 50 mg.

Hydroxyzine (Atarax).—Hydroxyzine is a recently imported Belgian drug. There is yet a paucity of reports in the American literature describing its effects, but extensive clinical trials in Europe and Mexico have shown it to be particularly useful as short term therapy in temporary conditions of emotional stress. It appears from these studies that hydroxyzine is indicated in those cases in which mild barbiturates ordinarily would be prescribed, the advantage of hydroxyzine being that mental acuity is not disturbed. Whether its tension relieving capacity surpasses that of the barbiturates has not been definitely determined, although one group, in describing good results in the treatment of neurogenic skin eruptions, found it superior to phenobarbital.

The therapeutic dose of hydroxyzine is well beyond its toxic dose. Effects generally can be noted within 20 to 60 minutes after administration although in a few cases therapeutic results may not become apparent for several days. Most adults require 25 mg. twice to four times daily. In the control of psychologic symptoms in children, such as hyperactivity, nightmares, and sleeplessness, 5 to 15 mg. once or twice per day in the form of syrup or suppository is suggested by the manufacturer. One of the chief recommendations of hydroxyzine is the relative absence of side effects and the fact that there have been no indications of impairment of hemopoietic, liver, or renal functions. Drowsiness, which usually disappears after the first two or three days of therapy, is the most frequent side effect. Dryness of the oropharynx, rhinorrhea, increased peristalsis, and headache also may occur.

Azacyclonol (Frenquel).—Azacyclonol is a drug about which there has been considerable controversy. It has been reported to abolish hallucinations in a variety of syndromes, including acute and chronic schizophrenia, acute and chronic alcoholic hallucinosis, senile hallucinatory states, and postoperative confusion. Psychiatrists differ widely in their evaluation of azacyclonol, some describing dramatic results, other believing that it has no appreciable activity. Azacyclonol has been subjected to limited clinical trial at the University of Texas Medical Branch Hospitals. Although no definitive conclusions regarding its efficacy have been reached yet, the results to date have not been impressive. The suggested dose is 20 mg. orally three times a day. Azacyclonol apparently has no side effects, and many times the suggested dose can be given without untoward clinical or laboratory reaction.

Euphoriants

Pipradol (Meratran).—Pharmacologic agents which effectively alleviate feelings of depression and fatigue have been available for some time in the form of the sympathomimetic amines, particularly those of the amphetamine series. However, these drugs have certain undesirable properties which often limit their clinical application. They frequently induce anorexia, feelings of uncontrollable restlessness, insomnia, and occasionally cardiovascular pressor reactions. Pipradol is a new antidepressant drug that apparently does not stimulate the sympathetic nervous system to any appreciable extent and only rarely affects appetite.

Very satisfactory results in the treatment of depressions have been described. Our results at the University of Texas Medical Branch have not been as encouraging. We have obtained symptomatic benefit in some cases in which depressive symptoms and complaints of lack of energy were prominent, but in my experience its greatest value has been a counteractive of drowsiness and fatigue induced by chlorpromazine and reserpine.

Low toxicity provides a wide margin of safety, and the dose may be freely adjusted according to individual requirement. As an alerting agent, 1 to 2 mg.

three times a day is ordinarily effective. Larger doses are usually required for relief of depressive symptoms. In mild and moderate depressions the average dose is 3 to 5 mg. three times daily. More severe degrees of depression may respond to higher doses, but in my experience they eventually must be treated by other methods. Unpleasant side reactions such as tension, restlessness, and emotional lability may appear at any dosage level but are most common in the range of 12 to 15 mg. per day. Some difficulty in falling asleep may occur if the drug is taken too close to bedtime, but protracted insomnia is unusual.

Methyl-Phenidylacetate Hydrochloride (Ritalin).—Methyl-phenidylacetate hydrochloride is a mild cerebral stimulant of the order of pipradol. Its therapeutic indications are similar although it is my impression that methyl-phenidylacetate hydrochloride is slightly more effective than pipradol in depressions and has less tendency to produce emotional lability. Neither drug should be given to anxious or agitated patients since either may intensify these symptoms. Tranquilizer-induced drowsiness can be counteracted by 10 mg. twice or three times daily. Depressive symptoms usually require twice this amount or more.

Nonbarbiturate Hypnotics

Older nonbarbiturate hypnotics such as bromides, chloral hydrate, and paraldehyde are effective somnifacients but possess certain undesirable properties. Bromides, in particular, are dangerous because of the high incidence of intoxication. They have been largely replaced by a variety of derivatives of barbituric acid, which, although very versatile and extremely useful, are themselves not entirely satisfactory. They frequently cause hangover, are capable of respiratory depression, and often induce an initial stage of excitement, especially in the aged.

A new group of hypnotics in which these effects are reportedly absent have been introduced under various trade names, including Dormison (Schering), Placidyl (Abbott), Valmid (Lilly), Noludar (Hoffman-La Roche), and Doriden (Ciba). They have no common chemical origin but all are characterized by short, rapid action, quick excretion, and low toxicity. They are thus most useful in patients who have difficulty in falling asleep. Although reports indicate that in sufficient dose some may equal barbiturates in producing night-long hypnosis, it is probable that the long acting barbiturates are more reliable in patients who have frequent nocturnal awakening. The relatively low potency of these drugs also limits their use in highly disturbed patients in whom deep, prolonged narcosis is needed. No deleterious effects on the liver, kidneys, or blood have been reported. The absence of side effects and a wide margin of safety recommend them for use in elderly patients, who are notoriously sensitive to sedatives. The comparative value of these drugs has not been definitely established, but it appears that they are useful additions to the battery of sedative-hypnotics now available.

Summary

A series of pharmacologic agents with varied effects on mental functioning have recently been introduced. The actions, indications, therapeutic results,

66 *The New Chemotherapy in Mental Illness*

dosage, and clinical toxicity of these tranquilizers, euphoriants, and hypnotics are briefly discussed. Although the ultimate position of these particular drugs remains to be determined, their development represents a significant advance in the management and treatment of psychogenic symptoms.

EVALUATION OF THE THERAPEUTIC EFFECTS OF DRUGS IN PSYCHIATRIC PATIENTS

Lincoln D. Clark, M.D.

Introduction

The introduction of the phenothiazine derivatives, chlorpromazine (Thorazine) and promazine (Sparine); the rauwolfia alkaloids; and more recently such drugs as phenyl-piperidylacetate ester (Ritalin), pipradol (Meratran), azocyclonol (Frenquel) and meprobamate (Miltown, Equanil) has aroused much enthusiasm for pharmacological treatment of psychiatric illness. It can be reasonably expected that during the next few years many drugs with "ataractic," "psychotropic," or other alleged therapeutic properties will become available for clinical trial.

Such trials, depending upon the judgment and skill with which they are carried out, can have various results. Ideally, within the limitations of the descriptive methods currently available, they should offer an accurate account of the behavioral and therapeutic effects of a drug. However, they can and frequently do lead to publication of inaccurate or false results. This gives rise to the almost predictable sequence which in recent years has followed the introduction of drugs of unusual interest or promise. It consists of initial overenthusiasm, usually based upon a small number of preliminary, optimistic reports; this is followed by disenchantment as subsequent, more systematic studies fail to verify initial claims; eventually an accurate picture of the usefulness and limitations of the drug evolves. Meanwhile, there is a long period of false expectations, wasted therapeutic and investigational time, and disillusionment to both patient and physician. This sequence is already evident in the psychiatric field under discussion and presumably will become more conspicuous as the number of available drugs multiplies.

Evaluation of the psychological and behavioral effects of drugs involves one of the key problems in psychiatry, i.e., the creation of reliable methods for observing and recording phenomena which are intrinsically difficult to estimate or even define. However, assuming that methods of reasonable reliability for observing such events can be devised, one must then design the study to ensure confidence that the critical variable, the drug, and not a variety of other possible variables, is the determining factor in the observed change. These intervening variables of drug evaluation are numerous and in many instances subtle and difficult to detect.

Many fine contributions on method and experimental design for drug evaluation are available in the literature. Unfortunately, this information and implied recommendations have not had as much influence upon investigational practices as one would hope. It has also not been as readily accessible, in summarized form, as it might be to the busy physician or psychiatrist who, in the final analysis, must critically review available data on therapeutic effects to decide upon the most useful agent.

It is the purpose of this paper to summarize a number of the more frequently used methods of drug evaluation, with comments on their relative value and to review possible sources of error in their use. An effort has been made to organize the material in a readily accessible, schematic form. Many comments will be self-evident to the reader in terms of common sense and his basic knowledge of scientific method.

GENERAL COMMENTS

The kinds of data with which we are concerned consist of the following: (1) verbal accounts by the subject as to his state of mind, given either spontaneously or in response to inquiry; (2) verbal and behavioral response of the subject to standardized verbal or symbolic stimuli (e.g., psychometric tests) or to structured performance problems or social situations; (3) inferences by observers about the significance or verbalizations and behavior, particularly as evidence of degree of mental disturbance; (4) observations of the routine behavior of the subjects in terms of capacity for self-care, work performance, interpersonal relationships, and social problem solving, and inferences therefrom as regards degree of mental disturbance.

Conclusions as to therapeutic effects must therefore depend upon communicational data and observations of individual and interpersonal behavior. These will always represent a complex resultant of several factors. They consist of the neurophysiological effects of the given drug (and concomitant representation in awareness), of their effects in turn upon the functioning personality in all its perceptive, integrative, and executive aspects and rich individuality, and finally of the physical and interpersonal environment insofar as it facilitates or limits expression of this altered mental state. These are invariable parameters conditioning the type of behavior with which we are concerned as psychiatric observers. Such parameters of personality and environment are of course not relevant in the case of drugs which in adequate dosage would predictably produce, for example, general anesthesia or convulsive seizures in all individuals. They are of considerable importance, however, for drugs affecting behavior in its conscious, adaptive aspects, as in treating psychotic patients.

It is obviously important for investigators to define standards of "therapeutic" response or "improvement." Such standards have both quantitative and qualitative aspects. Statements that patients showed "no improvement," "slight improvement," or were "much improved" have little meaning unless information is given about the criteria of improvement used and the means by which these were rated. These standards would be met in elementary form, for example, if an indication of mental illness such as hallucinations were reported as present or absent on the basis of specified observations. With more elaborate methods such as rating scales, the specific items of behavior sampled can be numerically rated at appropriate intervals and the significance of the changes in the ratings evaluated by statistical means.

There is another reason for specifying the nature of the improvement obtained in mental patients. It is well known that patients can remain grossly psychotic and yet become passively cooperative, less overactive and destructive, or more docile. These changes can be achieved by intensive activity programs or a variety of other means. Such improvement may be more important to the custodian than the patient. On the other hand, evidence of resolution of the psychotic process, reconstitution of non-psychotic defenses, or significant degrees of social re-integration would represent improvement of very different significance.

SOURCES OF ERROR AND THEIR CONTROL

A. *In the Observers*

(a) Regardless of their conscious good intentions or intellectual honesty, investigators are subject to bias when observing patients treated with a drug from which therapeutic or other psychological effects are anticipated. There is wide latitude for selective attention or inattention to the many facets of behavior available to our inexact methods of observation. The choice of events observed and recorded and the repression of others may be subtly affected by the investigator's unconscious needs for achievement. Other observers or raters, depending upon their feelings toward the principal investigator, may unconsciously please or, more rarely, displease him by their observations on the treated patients. These are only a few of the many possible sources of bias. They can be controlled only by use of a design which "blinds" observers or raters as regards the drug-treated subjects. This may be difficult to achieve. Raters may expend much effort to overcome the "blinding" because of their pride in uncovering drug effects, or resolve their curiosity about such effects by extracurricular study of available periodicals. The investigator may be quite unaware of these activities.

This becomes more of a problem if the drug being studied has been previously reported or if the drug-treated subjects can be readily identified among the placebo controls by the occurrence of conspicuous subjective or side effects. An inert placebo may be unsatisfactory under these circumstances; it may be preferable to use a known drug which mimics these effects.

(b) There is another less apparent source of error. As an interviewer or rater sees patients on repeated occasions over an extended period, making comparisons between present and past behavior, he may note more evidence of self-help, social skill, rewarding interpersonal behavior, etc., and describe them as improvement. Actually, it may turn out that these features were previously present but not observed. In large institutions with limited staff there is a tendency to think of patients as stereotypes, or perhaps caricatures, with certain conspicuous features of the individual determining one's way of thinking of him. This may markedly condition the initial behavioral ratings. Introduction of a drug study into such a setting intensifies observation and focus upon individual behavior. Increasing awareness of the details or resourcefulness of a patient's ward adjustment may be recorded as improvement. This source of error can only be controlled by the use of an adequate baseline control period during which ratings or observations become stabilized.

(c) Whether one is using standardized interview or behavioral rating scale methods, certain preliminary steps are important. The observers should be trained in the method employed. Their reliability or standard error on successive ratings at adequate intervals of time should be determined. Multiple, independent raters or interviewers are desirable and inter-rater comparisons on the same subjects should be carried out. Markedly deviant raters should be withdrawn. Such raters or interviewers may be found, for example, to be reacting with halo effect to some facet of the patient's behavior to which they are personally sensitive.

B. In the Patients

(a) "Spontaneous" variations in the course of the psychiatric illness and "spontaneous" improvement may be very appreciable sources of error, particularly in evaluation of the treatment of patients with acute schizophrenia or affective psychoses. The longer the duration of the drug therapy, the more of a problem such errors become. An adequate number of cases must be treated and the results compared with a comparably managed control group. Some of the difficulty can be avoided by drug trials on chronic, stabilized psychotic patients.

(b) The number of cases to be used for drug-tested and control groups and the choice of methods by which they are selected are critical decisions in a drug study. The statistical and other considerations involved in this problem cannot be discussed in this paper. It is obvious that treated and control groups should be as comparable as possible. If matched groups are used, the prognostic or other criteria used for matching should be specified.

(c) It is well known that individuals may differ widely in sensitivity to equal amounts of the same drug. This fact should be considered in a drug study. The results from treating a group of patients with a standard dose may be quite different from those obtained when dosage has been pushed to some level of "tolerance," "toxicity," or other individualized end point. The body weight of the patient also affects dosage response. The effects of a given amount of drug will be obviously different when given to a hundred pound person as opposed to one who may weigh twice as much. Reporting dosages as mgm./kgm. would help in this regard.

(d) Intervening variables may affect patient behavior during a drug study as follows:

(1) A new medication, especially if acccompanied by enthusiasm and optimism on the part of the staff, may in itself have beneficial effects upon behavior. However, these suggestive effects are generally limited in extent and short in duration. They can be controlled by a placebo group and adequate length of drug trial. The patients of course should be "blind" as to the nature or anticipated effects of the drug being given.

(2) Failure to hold the ward environment constant, both physically and in terms of personnel, may introduce intervening variables. These include

changes in activity programs as well as addition or withdrawal of personnel or changes in their quality. The introduction of rehabilitation efforts in the course of a drug study, as improvement makes these more feasible, will of course exaggerate apparent drug effects.

(3) Significant improvement in therapeutic climate may be a side effect of the introduction of a drug study. This is particularly true of "back wards" or other settings which have previously been therapeutically inactive, or where available therapeutic methods have not achieved significant gains for long periods. There may be increased interest and enthusiasm on the part of the physicians and improved morale and motivation among nurses and aides. These attitudinal changes may be reflected in more active participation and interpersonal exchange with patients and an assumption that there is greater potential for rehabilitation than before. Of course, such potential may have previously existed. If there is a "blind" control group, it may share these effects and move behaviorally closer to the drug group to the extent of their influence.

(4) Another, less apparent, intervening variable can arise from the drug-induced or "spontaneous" improvement of several patients involved in a drug study on a ward. If such improvement is appreciable, especially if it brings increased social integration, these patients can significantly increase the availability of rewarding social contacts or otherwise stimulate the non-responders to the drug as well as the control group. The "atmosphere" of the ward becomes generally better. This sequence would not be undesirable from a therapeutic standpoint. From an investigational standpoint, however, it can lead to overestimation of drug effects by stimulation of non-responders and underestimation by improving the functioning level of the control group.

Methods of Drug Study: Their Advantages and Limitations

A. Interview Methods

These methods depend primarily upon introspective reports from the patient, but specific aspects of such information can be elicited by inquiry and additional information inferred from the subject's behavior in the interview situation. Many refinements have been made in such methods to control sources of error in both subject and observer. These refinements include:

(1) Double-blind techniques to conceal the nature of the drug given and its anticipated effects from both patient and interviewer.

(2) Use of an adequate number of subjects and controls to minimize individual differences. Controls should receive an appropriate placebo.

(3) The use of standardized interviews in order that the observations may be more precisely repeated by the same interviewers or confirmed by others.

(4) The use of multiple, independent interviewers for each subject in order to control rater bias and differences.

(5) Methods for carrying out systematic, more objective analysis of the interview content.

(6) Introduction of periods of drug and placebo administration, by "doubleblind" methods, into a prolonged series of structured interviews such as are involved in psychoanalytic therapy. The observer-therapist has in this

instance a rich knowledge of personality dynamics which may modify drug effects. Only a very limited number of cases can be studied by this intensive, longitudinal method. At the conclusion of the study, an effort is made to correlate data from the therapist's day-to-day notes with the intervals of drug or placebo administration.

With suitable controls and refinements, as outlined above, these basic methods of clinical psychiatry can afford valuable and extensive information about the psychological and therapeutic effects of drugs. The data can be more precise in terms of the psychic mechanisms and interplay of personality forces involved in a drug effect than those obtained by the rating scale methods discussed below. In pilot studies of a new drug, interview methods can be useful to obtain an impression of the aspects of personality function affected by the drug. These can become leads for the choice of appropriate rating scales or other more systematic observational methods.

However, if high standards of reliability and control are required, these methods can become remarkably cumbersome and laborious. The number of skilled interviewers available is frequently small. Moreover, the interview situation samples only a limited portion of the patient's total behavior. One may miss significant changes which occur during the non-observed portion of the patient's day. In the case of psychotic patients, especially if they are regressed or withdrawn, interviews may be grossly inadequate samples of their behavior.

B. Evaluation of Drug Effects by Use of Psychological Tests

Psychological testing represents essentially a structured interview during which standardized tests involving psychomotor performance are given or standardized verbal or symbolic stimuli are presented to elicit thought processes or projective responses. They have many of the same advantages and disadvantages as interview methods. In general, they have limited value for evaluating the therapeutic effects of drugs in mental illness. Some tests, those measuring psychomotor performance, have good reliability and can be repeated, but they give very limited information. Others, such as the projective tests, afford more extensive psychological information but do not hold up well on repetition and are subject to the same interpretational bias and need for double-blind control as interview techniques.

C. Evaluation of Drug Effects by Use of Behavioral Rating Scales

These methods are extensively used at present. A variety of behavioral rating scales are available or similar scales can be devised for the problem at hand by routine methods of scale design. It is obviously important that the items in the scale correspond to behavior which is presumed to be sensitive to drug-induced change. The necessity of rater training and determination of rater and inter-rater reliability have already been discussed. It is desirable to have multiple, independent raters who sample a reasonably wide range of the patient's daily activity. Improvement as manifested by ratings should have statistical significance when compared with baseline or control ratings.

Rating scale methods make it possible to employ ancillary ward or hospital personnel and to study large groups of patients. They can be well-controlled if the intervening variables are considered and they give rough quantitative results. However, the behavioral information obtained is limited to the items rated. Some aspects of drug-induced behavioral change may be missed by exclusion from the scales. They give limited information by which one can predict a drug response in an individual case.

D. Evaluation of Drug Effects by Sociometric Methods

These methods have been used only to a limited extent for the study of drug effects. They consist essentially of various techniques for carrying out systematic observations on personal and interpersonal behavior in the ward or other setting. Verbal and non-verbal exchanges between patients and patients and staff are recorded. Intervening variables and other sources of error must be controlled and intervals of adequate duration sampled at comparable intervals. Although more difficult to quantitate, such methods can be remarkably sensitive in disclosing the effects of drugs on social integration, problem solving, and other important aspects of interpersonal dynamics which are, of course, critical areas of disability for the psychotic patient.

FINAL COMMENTS

As was noted in the introductory section, pharmacological treatment of psychiatric illness is a rapidly expanding and promising field. It is likely that an increasing variety of drugs will become available for therapeutic trial. The use of adequate observational methods and an experimental design which controls intervening variables has been described as a necessary condition to ensure accurate drug evaluation. The harm which can accrue from publication of inaccurate or misleading conclusions about therapeutic effects has been emphasized. A critical appraisal of some methods of drug evaluation and sources of error in their use has been made. It is hoped that this information will be of value to physicians and psychiatrists who must make decisions about the validity of therapeutic trials reported to them. In turn, it behooves those reporting drug investigations to describe methods, design, controls, subjects, and circumstances of the study in such a way that critical appraisal of the results and comparison with the results of other studies become possible.

NEW DRUG THERAPIES IN PSYCHIATRY

F. A. Freyhan, M.D., Patricia Turner, M.D., and Rita Stenzler, M.D.

When, at the end of 1953, European psychiatry reported with growing interest about new pharmacological agents which made possible major changes in therapeutic management, we decided to organize our clinical work in a manner which would favor an intensive investigational program with pharmacological therapies. As one of the first American psychiatric hospitals to use chlorpromazine as a major psychiatric therapy, we were able to contribute our experiences to the development of therapeutic methods, assess the range of clinical effectiveness and start a carefully planned follow-up study. One advantage of our early start has been the accumulation of a vast complex of clinical data which enables us to carry out comparative studies with various new drugs which may eventually surpass the therapeutic benefits of those now at our disposal. Our main interest here concerns the two drugs which had the greatest impact on psychiatry. The already momentous literature on chlorpromazine and reserpine attests to their clinical and experimental prominence. It is the purpose of this paper to bring a condensed summary of our clinical experiences.

For the sake of brevity, we will focus attention on the following unique and specific actions of chlorpromazine and reserpine. Both drugs, though chemically different, effect mesencephalic and diencephalic systems in a manner which causes changes in autonomic functions and inhibits psychomotor activity. On the autonomic level, we find changes in blood pressure, body temperature, metabolism and sleep patterns, to name but a few. In the sphere of psychomotor behavior, we observe a decrease of drive, impulsivity and affective tension. Since neither drug affects the cortex, there is no sedation in the ordinary sense. Intellectual functions are not impaired and consciousness remains intact. It is evident then that we are dealing with highly specific actions which differ fundamentally from other drugs previously used for psychiatric purposes.

A comparison with insulin will demonstrate the fallacy of generalization as implied in the popular term "tranquilizer." In the case of diabetes, insulin will normalize the blood sugar level and reduce hyperglycemia. If, in another case, the blood sugar is normal to begin with, insulin by the very same physiological action will lower it to what now becomes an abnormal hypoglycemic level. While the pharmacological action of insulin is the same in both instances, the clinical effect has changed from desirable to undesirable. The same principle applies to the so called tranquilizing drugs. In the case of a disturbed, tense, restless or agitated patient, the inhibitory effect on psychomotor activity expresses itself as calmness, lassitude and emotional harmonization. This is a favorable response to the therapeutic agent. Patients, on the other hand, who are depressed, apathetic, hypochondriacally fatigued and worried frequently show already manifestations of psychomotor retardation. The use of "tranquilizers" here enhances or provokes depression and reduces still further feelings of energy and vitality. The resulting therapeutic failure does not stem from the drug but from misapplication.

We place great emphasis on the specificity of both drugs' action in order to show the need for meaningful therapeutic criteria. Psychopathological states which express themselves symptomatically through a common path of hypermotility, abnormal drive, increased emotional tension and impulsivity, are most apt to benefit regardless of the nature or etiology of the disorders. Conversely, clinical states with depression, apathy and emotional withdrawal require a different therapeutic approach, specifically electroconvulsive therapy (E.C.T.) in as far as depressive states are concerned.

Our evaluations of therapeutic responses are bound to be realistic. We do not depend so much on the completion of rating scales as on personal daily observations and follow-up studies. We are favored in this endeavor by the close, continuous contact with patients and their families which results from being the only psychiatric hospital for an entire state.

Chlorpromazine

Chlorpromazine, i.e. Thorazine, has emerged as the most potent therapeutic agent thus far at our disposal. Our comments are based on experiences with 623 patients who had completed treatment before June 1, 1956. Thorazine has been primarily responsible for successful changes in therapeutic management. All those restrictive measures were discontinued which had been necessitated by the disturbing aspects of mental illness: noise, destructiveness and aggressive behavior. The traditional practices of hydrotherapy, isolation, restraints, maintenance E.C.T. and administration of sensorium clouding drugs became obsolete as soon as Thorazine was found to be a potent replacement which could be administered on a maintenance basis for indefinite periods.

At no time did we combine Thorazine therapy with other somatic therapies (E.C.T., insulin, sedatives). Administration of the drug was started intramuscularly in the majority of cases and changed to the oral route by the end of the first week. In general, total daily doses started with 200 mg. and were increased up to 800 mg. The majority of patients responded to daily doses of 400-800 mg. Others required up to 2100 mg. a day.

The question of safety and toxicity has passed through various stages. The complexity of the drug's action and the high degree of individual variation in responsivity require close supervision and caution. While it is true that severe, even fatal, complications occur, it is also apparent that many reactions initially believed to be toxic in nature should be considered as physiological effects of an agent which influences a network of vital cerebral and cellular mechanisms. The number of criteria for interruption of therapy has steadily decreased although it should be stressed that the diagnostic facilities of the hospital permit continuation of therapy which would be risky in an out patient setting. Allergic skin reactions occurred in 63 patients (10.1 per cent). If extensive, they were sufficiently disturbing to necessitate interruption of medication. In most cases, however, addition of antihistaminic drugs sufficed to bring about prompt improvement. Teldrin spansules proved most effective because of the uninterrupted antihistaminic action. There was no incidence of contact dermatitis among nurses or attendants. Desensitization appeared to develop with regularity since patients remained free from allergic disturbances after medication was resumed. 14 patients (2.2 per cent) developed jaundice. With the exception of 1 case, recovery was uneventful within 2 to 3 weeks. One female patient, age 52, developed a severe hepatic disorder with evidence of persistent biliary obstruction, high blood cholesterol and alkaline phosphatase. Transfer to a medical service became necessary since striking changes in lipid metabolism continued for many months. In case of jaundice, treatment was always terminated and never reinstituted. Recent investigations by Shay indicate that jaundice is a drug sensitivity reaction which can be predicted by the use of serum alkaline phosphatase determination as screening tests during the administration of the drug. An abnormal elevation soon after the start indicates a warning signal. If medication is stopped until the phosphatase value returns to a normal level, desensitization takes place in most cases which permits safe continuation of treatment. Our own studies with this screening technique are still in the beginning stage, but there is hope that jaundice will cease to be a serious obstacle.

There were 30 cases (4.8 per cent) with a variety of toxic reactions. These included generalized edema, vomiting, diarrhea, high fever, a grand mal seizure in a nonepileptic person and a case of marked abdominal distension with evidence of beginning paralytic ileus. Termination of treatment resulted invariably in prompt recovery. Two agitated senile patients died during treatment. While death could not be directly attributed to the medication in view of the pathological findings, there was clinical evidence that poor drug tolerance causing cardiovascular collapse contributed to the fatal outcome.

Parkinsonism characterized by rigidity, tremors, loss of associated movements, facial fixity, difficulties in swallowing and mastication and occasional other symptoms developed in 69 patients (11.1 per cent). We want to stress the fact that subtle manifestations of extrapyramidal involvement occur more frequently and should be regarded as normal drug effects upon the subcortical motor system. Our observations strongly suggest that both chlorpromazine and reserpine inhibit psychomotor activity in a manner which changes the functional balance of the extrapyramidal system causing symptoms which, if more pronounced, assume the characteristics of the Parkinsonian syndrome. Our observations clearly indicate that individual disposition plays a decisive part since the severity of this drug-induced Parkinsonism does not depend on duration of treatment or the quantity of the drug administered. Detailed data will be the subject of another publication.

Duration of treatment depended on the nature of the disorder as well as on the individualized therapeutic goal. Table 1 gives a collective survey of the duration.

TABLE 1 (DURATION OF TREATMENT)

	No.	Per Cent
Up to 30 days	240	38.5
31 to 60 days	200	32.1
61 to 90 days	94	15.1
More than 90 days	89	14.3
Total	623	

Table 2 presents an analysis of the therapeutic results in relation to the disorders. It should be noted that the affective psychoses are divided into two groups, one exclusively for manic psychoses, the other for depressions, especially of the involutionary type. "Anxiety states" applies exclusively to psychoneurotic patients.

The following principles of evaluation were applied. A specific therapeutic goal was formulated in each case in terms of target symptoms. The complete disappearance of these symptoms was rated "very good," partial elimination "good," lack of improvement "unsatisfactory" and aggravation of symptoms "worse." The social degree of improvement depends essentially on the magnitude of the target symptoms in the total clinical picture. The elimination of syndromes of disturbed psychomotility, for example in acute manic psychoses, in agitated involutional and disturbed catatonic states or in acute toxic brain syndromes can well mean total clinical improvement. By contrast, the unchanged paranoid ideation of a schizophrenic still interferes with a good social result although the treatment has been quite effective in terminating hostile-aggressive behavior. A thorough discussion of the therapeutic implications will be presented in another publication. In a summarizing fashion, the following conclusions seem justified:

(1) There is a high correlation between therapeutic effectiveness and psychopathological states characterized by hypermotility syndromes. This is also indicated by the favorable response encountered in cases of agitated depressions in contrast to the total failures observed in neurotic and psychotic depressions.

(2) As a major therapy, if critically selected, it is as effective as, and in some respects superior to other somatic therapies which were previously considered as treatments of choice. The psychological advantages inherent in this therapeutic approach have greatly influenced and improved the social climate of the hospital.

(3) There is at present no evidence that the immediate therapeutic results will change the long-term prognostic patterns of the functional psychoses.

230 patients (36.9 percent) are now at home. This global figure as such is of no particular relevancy. It should be stated, however, that the majority of these patients would previously have received other somatic therapies in order to recover. Indefinite maintenance therapy enables certain patients to leave the hospital and to resume their normal activities. Since this offers new clinical and social aspects of therapeutic management, we instituted last February a home care program which now includes 60 patients. The purpose of this

program is to determine what methods are most adequate and safe in the use of maintenance therapy as a means of keeping suitable patients compensated.

TABLE 2 (RESULTS OF TREATMENT)

	Schizophrenia Per Cent	Manic Psychoses Per Cent	Other Affective Psychoses Per Cent	Anxiety States Per Cent	Organic Syndromes Per Cent	Drug or Alcohol Addiction Per Cent	Personality Disturb. Per Cent
Very Good	26.2	50.0	23.6	29.6	21.6	52.5	37.5
Good	51.9	31.0	44.4	44.5	47.1	40.0	31.3
Unsatisfactory	21.9	19.0	29.2	22.2	28.4	5.0	31.2
Worse	0.0	0.0	2.8	2.8	2.9	2.5	0.0
Total No. of Cases	324	42	72	27	102	40	16

RESERPINE

Reserpine, i.e. Serpasil, influences the same psychopathological syndromes in a grossly similar fashion. Much of what has already been said about the therapeutic criteria in reference to Thorazine applies to Serpasil. Distinctive differences exist, however, which require special consideration. Our series comprises 164 patients who had completed treatment before June 1, 1956. In general, Serpasil proved to be less dependable in the treatment of acutely psychotic patients. Therapeutic results were less satisfactory. The greatest effectiveness was noticed in the control of chronic disturbed patients, especially in the geriatric group.

Courses began as a rule with simultaneous administration of intramuscular and oral medication. Injections were continued for 2 or 3 weeks or longer if the result was unsatisfactory. The average dose varied between 5 to 10 mgm. intramuscularly (2 to 5 mg. orally). The doses were lower for senile and higher for manic patients reaching in a few cases a maximum of 30 mg. a day.

There was no incidence of allergic dermatitis. The absence of liver dysfunctions offers obvious advantages. This is, however, somewhat offset by the higher frequency of toxic reactions. 17 patients (10.4 per cent) developed a variety of complications which necessitated termination. These included cardio-vascular crises and collapse, edema of the ankles and face, persistent diarrhea, severe weakness, lethargy and a peculiar breathing difficulty characterized by loud, labored breathing apparently due to spastic contractions in the upper respiratory space. Two senile patients died in a sudden state of circulatory collapse. While the causes of death could be attributed to pathological findings, the unexpected suddenness seemed due to the contributory effects of the medication. One patient, not included in this series (medication was given for non-psychiatric reasons) died of a massive gastro-intestinal hemorrhage caused by a duodenal ulcer which had not been diagnosed prior to autopsy. Finally, one patient died of sudden respiratory arrest associated with the development of extreme Parkinsonian rigidity.

28 patients (17.1 per cent) developed Parkinsonism. Basically, the Parkinsonian syndrome follows the same pattern as described with Thorazine. While the action of reserpine involves the subcortical motor system in a clinically

similar fashion, certain differences can be observed which are significant. In the first place, the incidence of Serpasil-Parkinsonism is higher. Secondly, drooling which is rarely seen with Thorazine occurs frequently. Lastly, many patients complain of an "inner unrest" and feel unable to relax or sit still. This restlessness which resembles "kinesia paradoxa" as described in the literature on paralysis agitans and encephalitis, interferes with the therapeutic progress, especially when complicated by insomnia. On the whole, Parkinsonism, if not too severe, does not justify interruption, since the addition of anti-Parkinsonian drugs suffices to control tremors and rigidity.

Table 3 provides the data on duration of treatment. The fairly large group continuing for 3 and more months includes 10 schizophrenic and 19 patients with chronic brain syndromes.

TABLE 3 (DURATION OF TREATMENT)

	No.	Per Cent
Up to 30 days	52	31.7
31 to 60 days	52	31.7
61 to 90 days	26	15.9
More than 90 days	34	20.7
Total	164	

Table 4 presents the therapeutic results, arranged on the same principle as in reference to Thorazine.

The interpretation of the results should not be on comparative basis with Thorazine. The Serpasil series is smaller and differs in the proportional representation of the various disorders. Results with the manic psychoses were mediocre as half of the cases showed no improvement at all while only one reacted very favorably. Other authors have advocated the addition of sedatives; however, we abstained from such combinations in order to explore the full range of therapeutic potency on the drug's own merits. The results in schizophrenia cannot

TABLE 4 (RESULTS OF TREATMENT)

	Schizophrenia	Manic Psychoses	Other Affective Psychoses	Anxiety States	Organic Syndromes	Drug or Alcohol Addiction	Personality Disturb.
	Per Cent	Per Cent	Per Cent	Per Cent	Per Cent	Per Cent	Per Cent
Very Good	7.4	8.3	25.0	0.0	6.8	50.0	0.0
Good	44.1	41.7	41.7	20.0	54.2	25.0	25.0
Unsatisfactory	48.5	50.0	33.3	80.0	39.0	25.0	75.0
Worse	—	—	—	—	—	—	—
Total No. of Cases	68	12	12	5	59	4	4

be fully understood without a detailed breakdown. We were most impressed with the favorable responses of chronic cases with long records of disturbed anl unsocial behavior. These patients, if kept on medication for several months, emerged from their primitive existence of isolation and showed ability for social participation. Senile patients and those with chronic arteriosclerotic brain syndromes reacted quite favorably. Some of these patients are notoriously difficult because of noisiness, aimless physical activities and paranoid outbursts. Serpasil reduces the overactivity and facilitates more harmonious group behavior. Special caution must be taken with regard to dosage since geriatric patients are more prone to have hypotensive crises, to suffer from dizziness and drowsiness. Ritalin seems effective in counteracting these effects without exerting an influence on mood or psychic tempo.

In conclusion:
(1) The range of clinical effectiveness includes all psychopathological states with hypermotility syndromes. The mode of therapeutic effectiveness is gradual and cumulative rather than immediate. This renders the drug less useful in the treatment of acute psychotic states.
(2) Therapeutic advantages over other somatic forms of treatment can be observed in chronic schizophrenic and geriatric disorders.
(3) There is no evidence of a therapeutic influence on ultimate prognostic patterns of the functional psychoses.

MERATRAN AND FRENQUEL

Many psychopathological states require pharmacological therapies because of psychokinetic retardation, depressive dysphoria and behavioral apathy. We wish to state categorically that electro-convulsive therapy remains unchallenged as the only effective therapy for depressive psychoses. A pharmacological therapy for depressions does not exist as yet. Stimulants, primarily the drugs of the amphetamine group, have long proved their value as supportive measures in the treatment of depressive fatigue and emotional energy deficits.

Meratran was introduced as a new central stimulant which differs from sympathico-mimetic drugs in that it does not cause cardio-vascular pressor reactions, dilated pupils or sweating. Preliminary reports indicated its usefulness in the treatment of depressions as well as in schizophrenic states characterized by apathy. We treated 31 patients of which 22 were schizophrenics. These patients were chosen because of apathy, blocking and total lack of initiative. The non-schizophrenic patients displayed depressive moods with mild retardation. Dosage levels varied between 2.5 and 40 mg. daily, with an average of 10 mg. a day. Duration of treatment was from 5 to 60 days, averaging 2 to 3 weeks.

Anorexia occurred frequently. Treatment of 6 patients had to be discontinued because of nausea and severe loss of appetite. Several patients became activated but complained of jitteriness and anxiety. Two patients previously unproductive and lethargic became delusional. Of the 22 schizophrenic patients, five reacted favorably showing decrease of blocking and apathy, while 6 remained unchanged or developed undesirable reactions. Three of the depressed patients improved, 6 remained unchanged. While these results are inconclusive because of the smallness of the series, they do not suggest that Meratran has therapeutic advantages over the amphetamines. On the psychological side, there was little appreciable change in mood. Motor activation alone did not suffice to implement an improvement in feeling or attitude. Physically, anorexia frequently complicated the therapeutic progress. Further studies are needed to gain a better understanding of the drug's potentialities.

Frenquel, despite its structural resemblance to Meratran, was found to have opposite effects on laboratory animals. Far from acting as a stimulant, it diminishes spontaneous activity. Moreover, it blocks the hallucinogenic effects of mescaline and LSD-25. A number of investigators advocated its clinical use in the treatment of disturbed patients, especially those with hallucinatory states. Available reports differ widely. In some, intravenous administration is stated to be effective in relieving patients of their psychotic symptoms within a few hours. In others, the observers failed to notice any effects whatsoever, beneficial or toxic, regardless of length of treatment. Our own observations are limited to 8 patients. These patients were carefully selected on the basis of vivid hallucinatory disturbances associated with schizophrenia in 6, with acute alcoholic brain syndromes in 2 patients. Medication was started with repeated intravenous injections, totalling 100 to 180 mg. the first day. Oral medication was substituted on the second day and maintained for the duration of treatment which varied from 13 to 55 days. Dosage levels averaged 100 to 200 mg. daily with 800 mg. as daily maximum. In one case with alcoholic hallucinosis, all symptoms disappeared within 48 hours. In all other cases hallucinations, even during and immediately following intravenous injections, remained equally vivid. The drug appears to be quite harmless since even large doses did not produce any observable toxic symptoms. With the exception of the one alcoholic case, there was no evidence of therapeutic effects. While these results can hardly be called encouraging, further studies are in progress which will be concerned with a variety of toxic brain syndromes. The experimental evidence seems to suggest that toxic rather than schizophrenic hallucinations can be modified with this drug.

Prospects

A new science of psychopharmacology has come into existence. Drugs which produce model psychoses offer new insights into cerebral processes. Model psychoses in turn become the experimental testing ground for new therapeutic agents. Advances in the biological sciences contribute on a growing scale to the evolution of concepts on normal and abnormal behavior. What does this offer to clinical psychiatry?

The unsatisfactory overall results in the treatment of mental disorders, only too strongly in evidence in the biometrical statistics, demands that we are alert and receptive to new ideas and ever ready to modify therapeutic approaches. Psychiatric therapies are composites of somatic, psychological and social methods. Any attempt to single out one and exclude others has resulted in therapeutic failures. The introduction of new drug therapies, when seen in the context of this perspective, is not a matter of unsound optimism versus hostile skepticism. What is called for is an imaginative program of research and therapeutic integration. Not so much the fact that we now possess new drugs as the hope that this is only the beginning of therapeutic progress in psychiatry appears to us encouraging.

PROGRESS IN PSYCHIATRIC THERAPIES

Paul H. Hoch, M.D.
Commissioner, Department of Mental Hygiene, State of New York

This presentation gives a general view of the present status of psychiatric therapies. It is designed to be informative, but by no means authoritative, since many therapeutic attempts and practices have perforce been omitted. I shall first discuss somatic therapies and then the problems of psychotherapy.

No conspicuous progress has been made in insulin therapy. Variations of the technique have been introduced, but none is superior to that evolved during the past years. The use of insulin therapy has decreased progressively in recent years, probably because it is expensive and time-consuming, and needs a great number of personnel. Its declining use is interesting, considering that it is held by many to be superior to electroshock treatment in many cases of schizophrenia. Insulin and electroshock are most effective in the early phase of illness, when a considerable number of patients are helped. Unfortunately many do not retain this improvement. In a 5-year follow-up the difference between shock-treated patients and nonshock-treated patients is only slightly in favor of the former.

In electroshock treatment the development indicates experimentation with different currents, for instance unidirectional pulsating currents instead of alternating ones. It is claimed that this form of electroshock therapy is less damaging to the brain tissue because less severe electroencephalographic alterations are observed. It is also claimed that this form is less apt to produce memory impairment and confusion. Some of these claims are substantiated by some investigators. Other investigators, however, remain skeptical because no convincing evidence, based on well-conducted studies with controls, has been brought forward to prove its superiority. Some feel that, even though convulsions from unidirectional current do not produce as much alteration in brain function as those induced by alternating current, they are not as intense and therefore therapeutically less effective.

There is a general tendency to experiment with treatments less drastic than convulsions or insulin coma. Among those are electrical stimulation, photic stimulation, CO_2, subconvulsive metrazol, and subcoma insulin treatments. None of these treatments has been able to supplant electroshock; their value in psychiatric therapy is highly controversial, or they are considered entirely valueless. More research in these fields would be of great interest in clarifying the situation, especially in defining the value of electrical stimulation of certain parts of the brain as compared with the massive diffuse application of electrical current.

In addition to such procedures applied outside of the skull, there has been experimentation in implanting electrodes in the brain, especially in the septal area, and applying mild electrical stimulation through these electrodes. Therapeutic claims are made for this procedure in connection with schizophrenia and intractable pain. These experiments are based on controversial theoretical grounds. It has not been convincingly demonstrated that emotional regulation is localized in certain parts of the frontal lobe; it is known, however, that the subcortical gray has as much or more to do with it than the frontal lobe. The procedure of implanting electrodes would be justified from a clinical if not from a research point of view, if the results were far better than those with other methods of treatments. This is not apparent, however, according to available reports. The cumbersomeness of the procedure and the possible mortality rate also mitigate against its widespread use. Nevertheless, investigations of stimulation of the subcortical gray should continue to disclose more about therapeutic possibilities which do not concentrate on the cortex but on those parts of the brain where emotional and vegetative regulation is initiated.

Progress has been made in electroshock therapy by the introduction of drugs to soften convulsions. Curare and the newer drugs—tubocurare, anectine, and others—are used. The newer drugs are safer than curare, but probably still not safe enough to become a standard part of electroshock treatment. These drugs, however, in all probability will in the future become safe enough to permit electroshock therapy without any great danger of fracture. Further research in this field is indicated.

In the past few years various prognostic tests have been introduced based on the response of the nervous system to adrenaline, mecholyl, or atropine, and other drugs. These tests supposedly give reliable information as to the outcome of shock therapies or psychosurgery. They are important research tools, but their clinical use still remains very controversial.

Re-examination of the role of the vegetative nervous system in emotional disorders should be a major therapeutic research aim. New blocking agents, new stimulating techniques, and new neurophysiological registration methods will enable us to do a more refined study on different level functions of the vegetative nervous system.

A great deal of experimentation and investigation has been done in the last few years to determine which operation is therapeutically most suitable in specific types of mental cases. There are many publications on indications for psychosurgery, on how brain function relates to psychic functioning, and on how mental disorder is affected by surgery. Today there is a tendency to use different operations for cases of long-standing, markedly disorganized schizophrenics and for chronic neurotics, or well-preserved schizophrenics. In the former group classical lobotomy is still used; in the latter the trend is to use smaller operations, such as topectomy, cortical undercutting, lower quadrant lobotomy, medial lobotomy, etc. The personality damage is apparently less than with larger operations. The main complications are still the occurrence of epileptic seizures in about 5-20% of the cases. The therapeutic results are much better with these modified surgical procedures in chronic neurotics, pseudoneurotic schizophrenics, and well preserved schizophrenics than the results with lobotomy in chronic, deteriorated schizophrenics. Nevertheless, for the latter group classical lobotomy is preferable to the smaller operations.

More intensive research is indicated to find a more reliable way to assess indications for psychosurgery and to predict its outcome. Investigations in this field have demonstrated that the frontal lobe does not contain emotional "centers" which can be localized. How much one cuts seems to be more important than where one cuts. The quantitative relationship between the amount of brain substance rendered inoperative in relation to mental symptomatology will have to be investigated further. Interest is shifting from the frontal lobe to the connections of the frontal lobe with the thalamus and the hypothalamic areas. Most likely further experimentation with a stereotaxic approach will try to find out which fiber connections are the most important ones in transmitting emotional impulses. Should these fiber connections become better known, it will be possible to use smaller and more exact operative procedures than are in use today. The refinement of the operations would reduce the possibility of personality damage. In the opinion of many investigators this possibility is still present, even though the serious personality impairments due to the operation are not based on the operation alone, but on the influence of the organic brain damage on a schizophrenic process. Procaine infiltration of the frontal lobe is also now used for prognostic and therapeutic purposes. It is too early to tell whether or not this method works, and it is not clear whether repeated injections of procaine in the brain produce organic damage.

There has recently been a great deal of activity in the biochemical and pharmacological approach in psychiatry. An increasing number of chemical compounds are offered which influence mental symptomatology to varying degrees. Their value in psychiatry is still not properly assessed because they have been used for a comparatively short time. The reaction of psychiatrists to the value of these drugs is characterized by controversial opinions. Some have made very enthusiastic reports in the lay and professional press about the use of some of these drugs. Others feel that we are dealing here with nothing but sedatives of a different chemical structure than those already in use. As is so often the case, the truth most probably lies midway between these opposite views. New compounds such as *Rauwolfia serpentina* and chlorpromazine are very effective in certain psychiatric conditions, for example, in controlling excitement states, reducing or eliminating confusional states, and in many instances in clamping down on tension and anxiety manifestations. In many cases, after the elimination of the excitement the underlying disorder still remains. The action of these drugs is fairly universal in excitement states, but much less so in anxiety and tension states. In some patients the response is good, and their anxieties are eliminated; in others, the drugs do not produce any amelioration of the symptomatology. Likewise, some agitated depressions respond, but many depressions do not. It is not yet known why some persons respond and others do not. The drugs are quite effective in acute schizophrenic episodes, especially if tension, anxiety, hallucinations, and delusions are present. In such cases these drugs are rapidly replacing electroshock treatment. On the other hand, in chronic schizophrenia these drugs in many instances are not effective even though some patients do show improvement. Claims are made in the European literature that after the use of these drugs for a few weeks the patients are cured and their psychosis or neuroses disappear. Most likely this is true only for a few selected patients. The majority are relieved of anxiety while they are taking the drugs, but the symptoms return if their use is discontinued. It should also be stated that these drugs have disagreeable side actions, partly physical and partly mental, which will prevent their use for quite a number of individuals for whom they would otherwise be effective.

One of the new drugs, Thorazine, is of interest because seemingly it affects certain parts of the brain that have something to do with motor control and with emotional and vegetative regulation. This drug seemingly affects the reticular substance. In high doses it produces Parkinsonian syndromes, in smaller doses it reduces motor activity and also emotional overcharge in excitement, tension, and anxiety states. A better understanding of the way Thorazine works and the location of its action would contribute to a better understanding of neurophysiological changes linked to emotional and vegetative alterations. It is also of interest that psychoses experimentally produced by mescaline and LSD25 can be counteracted by Thorazine and other substances like sodium amytal, Desoxyn, and several others. These counteracting agents are not specific; many different chemical compounds have the same effect. But if a compound like Thorazine is able to clamp down on the funtion of the reticular substance as an activator of the cortex, the occurrence of certain psychotic manifestations can be prevented.

We believe there are indications that in the next few wears pharmacological psychiatry will play a very great role. Various compounds will be offered to reduce anxiety, others to alter mood states. This will enrich our therapeutic armamentarium, especially in conjunction with psychotherapy. It is obvious that if some of these chemical therapies are successful, psychotherapy will have to be adapted to them, and modifications will have to be made in psychotherapeutic technique. If it is possible to reduce an individual's anxiety or to increase his ego strength with drugs, the psychotherapeutic procedure with such an individual will be different than it has been in the past.

There is great need for a better scientific evaluation of the effectiveness of psychiatric therapies for the mentally ill. Lack of such evaluations constitutes a handicap which limits progress in treatment, and makes it difficult for psychiatrists to work with a confident sense of direction. The literature presents considerable data which may be interpreted clinically as being for or against the effectiveness of certain therapies, but very often, even after a long time, no firm conclusions have been reached. Moreover, some of the methodology or standards under which such evaluations are made are open to criticism. There are very few follow-up studies, and those that have been made are often inadequate, not only quantitatively in that too few patients are followed, but also qualitatively in that the supposedly improved patients are not seen by psychiatrists, but are reached only by questionnaires. We also lack a comprehensive methodology of evaluating improvement in a patient. Criteria of improvement are judged by different psychiatrists in different ways, because there is no agreement as to criteria. For example, one psychiatrists judges a patient's improvement on social adjustment, another on sexual adjustment, and a third on insight. Some use descriptive manifestations, others special psychodynamic formulations which vary with the different psychodynamic schools. Some are satisfied if the patient returns to the premorbid level of adjustment, others would expect a complete reconstruction before they would call the patient recovered.

The lack of evaluation of therapy is specially conspicuous in the realm of psychotherapies. The efficacy of many of these therapies rests on belief, not on scientific evidence. There have been very few systematic attempts to evaluate claims concerning psychotherapy. In fact, there is virtually no precedent for studying effects of psychotherapy in any form of mental disturbance by a control design. The opinion is often expressed that no form of psychotherapy can ever be evaluated by a control design because of the irreducible differences between patients and therapists, the multifactorial and intangible nature of the therapeutic process, etc. Just because of these doubts experiments in evaluation of psychotherapy are urgently needed. Should it be demonstrated that evaluation of psychotherapy is possible, then the very important next step will have to be taken, namely, a comparative evaluation of different forms of psychotherapy. What kind of patient needs what kind of psychotherapy, which one will benefit most from a certain form of psychotherapy are unsolved issues. Conclusions about short psychotherapy versus prolonged psychotherapy, symptomatic psychotherapy versus reconstructive psychotherapy are based on subjective clinical impressions, not on scientific evaluation.

Some progress, however, has been made. The American Psychoanalytic Association is interested in follow-up of patients under treatment, and also in organizing projects to evaluate therapies. Some such evaluative projects could be organized in such a way as to cross-validate a number of tests and assessment procedures, diagnostic and prognostic. No tests or rating scales or even clinical judgments of staffs have ever been systematically validated for a long-range follow-up of patients. We have very little information on the predictive value of ratings and clinical judgments. Some of the intended projects would permit us to validate judgments of clinical staffs against the judgment of an outside evaluating agency, assess rating scales against clinical appraisal, assess the reliability and validity of psychological tests in comparison with clinical judgments and rating scales, validate prognoses based on either clinical judgments or tests and rating scales. Such studies are, of course, difficult to organize and they are expensive. However, we hope that they will be attempted. They will have a very great effect on the theory and application of psychiatric therapies.

Progress has been made in defining group therapy more sharply. Many different forms are still used, and for this reason it is very difficult to assess and compare success and failure with this form of therapy. Interaction in a group situation, transference, and countertransference between the members of the group and the therapist have been studied rather intensively in the last few years. Studies of this kind will give us a better understanding of group psychology which in the past has been patterned very much on individual psychology. It is apparent that in the group situation psychic manifestations occur which are different from individual psychic interactions and should be differentiated from them. For instance, the paranoid behavior of an individual and the paranoid behavior of a whole group, even though they show similarities, differ in many essentials.

Indications for group therapy have also been studied. It has been assumed that group therapy is applicable when a large number of cases have to be treated and no individual therapy is available, when individual therapy is not successful, and finally when the patient's impairment of functioning is essentially in a social situation. It is obvious that indications for group therapy versus individual therapy will have to be studied in more detail. The controversial issue of whether group therapy is as effective as individual therapy will have to be resolved. This is an issue about which a great many psychiatrists have doubts. It is already apparent that we cannot say that one or the other of these therapies should be used; we must decide what kind of patient, in what constellation, would benefit more from group or from individual therapy, or from the application of both simultaneously. The application of group and individual therapy in different phases of a patient's treatment probably would be the most satisfactory solution, or group therapy after individual therapy, to clarify the patient's ability to handle social situations in a group setting. The use of group therapy, especially in child psychiatry, merits special attention. Many papers on group therapy indicate a tendency toward elasticity in approach. This elasticity, however, should not go so far as to permit a chaotic application, without goal, of any technique a therapist may think of.

In the last few years progress has been made in the application of psychotherapy and psychoanalysis. It has become apparent that the same treatment technique cannot be applied in all psychiatric conditions and that it is not possible to apply the same treatment with only slight modifications in markedly divergent disorders. It has been found that many of the older descriptive diagnostic designations, although not accurate in every respect, nevertheless indicated syndromes with different reaction potentials to therapy. Today special treatment techniques are evolved for schizophrenics, psychopaths, paranoid reactions, various personality disorders, alcoholism, and a number of other conditions. The differences are most conspicuous in the treatment applied essentially in the neuroses and in the treatment of schizophrenics. In the latter patients psychotherapy which utilizes analytic principles as to interpretation and motivation is more active, more ego-supportive, and more environment-manipulative than is customary in the neuroses. In connection with these treatment modifications, it has become obvious that the function of the ego must be studied; even though progress has been made in its delineation and on its function, we are still very far from being able to understand how the ego integrates and regulates the different psychic forces. Further investigations of the function of the ego in relation to therapeutic manipulation will be of paramount importance. It should be emphasized that there is an increased tendency to incorporate "common-sense" therapeutic measures into the treatment of many psychiatric conditions, especially in the special conditions mentioned above. Such measures have been used in a non-codified form for a long time. Now they can be integrated and refined in connection with psychodynamic observations made on such patients.

The integration of different therapeutic measures in a special condition, for instance, alcoholism, into a composite treatment has yielded much better results than were formerly obtained. Many alcoholics today receive individual or group psychotherapy. In addition they are linked to Alcoholics Anonymous with its very powerful social group forces, and they also use Antabuse to prevent drinking on a psycho-chemical level. The present treatment of alcoholism shows how the different facets in psychiatry—the somatic, the psychological, and the social—can be used simultaneously to control a condition which probably would not yield comparably good results if treated alone by one or another of these methods.

The progress made in the last few years in the field of psychotherapy may be summarized in the following 12 points. It is not feasible to discuss these points in detail; they are presented only in very broad outline.

1. It is increasingly recognized that theory and practice in psychotherapy or psychoanalysis are not identical. This recognition has resulted in a tendency to objectify the therapeutic process with recorded interviews and observations of the therapist at work, in order to find out how psychotherapy looks in action in distinction to what the therapist thinks is going on during the session.

2. A search is being made for a common denominator in the different psychotherapies. Further research in this area is strongly indicated. Different schools have very divergent theories about the functioning of the human psyche; nevertheless they claim the same therapeutic results. If it should be demonstrated that one of the psychodynamic systems is superior to others, we would be able to discard the less effective ones. If, however, it should be shown that all these different theoretical systems are similar in therapeutic action, then we would know that the theoretical constructions are not as important as some unknown common denominator in therapy. This common denominator may be the skill, experience, and emotional attributes of the therapist rather than the framework within which he works. It is also possible, however, that forces which are not yet elucidated are operating in psychotherapy.

3. Psychotherapy, regardless of its specific theoretical foundation, has become more comprehensive in a sense that the different facets of psychic functionings are given consideration in therapy. It has become apparent that the conflict is not as important in the neuroses as the inability or ability to handle it. Originally in psychoanalysis the instinctual forces of the id were emphasized; later on, the ego. The conscious behavior of the individual, as well as his unconscious, is fully appraised today. Besides the sex drive, the power drive is investigated. The dynamics take into consideration the individual's social goals, his past adjustment as much as his present adjustment. Both the organismic dynamics and the social dynamics are given consideration.

4. An increasing amount of investigation is being done on transference and countertransference, and their roles in psychoanalysis and psychotherapy. In this field progress will be made if, in addition to the emotional relationship under investigation, the ability of two interacting persons to communicate is better understood.

5. The assets of the patient are taken into consideration to a much greater degree than in the past, when the main investigation concentrated on the liabilities.

6. There is a much greater awareness than in the past of the limitations

of psychotherapy and psychoanalysis. Two resultant trends are discernible. On the one hand, there is a tendency not to accept statements that the patient is noncooperative or schizophrenic or constitutionally inferior to other patients in his ability to participate in psychotherapy, but to try to evolve treatments suitable for patients whose resistance is comparably much more marked and much more deeply rooted. On the other hand, it is recognized that in many patients somatic therapy will have to be used to cut through depressions, panic, and other emotional states which prevent the patient's fruitful cooperation in psychotherapy. The therapeutic goals are also more realistic, in not expecting a complete reconstruction of every patient, and in accepting more modest therapeutic goals.

7. Insight is not stressed as much as formerly. It is recognized that insight into conflicts, although it can be conveyed verbally and even emotionally, does not necessarily mean an improvement in the patient in respect to handling of the conflicts.

8. A more reverent attitude than in the past is evident about the forces that operate in a psychotherapeutic cure. What these forces are is admittedly often unclear, even when dynamically every facet of the case is apparently explained.

9. There is greater awareness of the social environment and its fostering or retarding effects on psychotherapy.

10. It is increasingly realized that etiology and motivation are not the same. Motives of a patient's behavior in action can be investigated and satisfactorily explained, but this explanation does not necessarily mean that the etiology of the disorder is then clear.

11. A constant re-examination is being made of fundamental theoretical concepts as they pertain to therapy. This should lead to clarification of old concepts—relegating some to the realm of psychiatric archeology, and making the theoretical structure on which psychotherapy is based clearer, simpler, and more comprehensible.

12. The gap between psychoanalysis and psychotherapy is closing even though the relation between the two is still a very controversial question. Some psychoanalysts emphasize the chasm between psychotherapy and psychoanalysis and others stress the common operational background and technique.

In the field of psychosomatic medicine, intensive research is going on in many places. It is an established fact that emotional factors play an important role in a primary or in a contributory way in many organic disorders. It is not clearly known, however, in which disorders the emotional participation is secondary and in which the emotional factor is paramount or primary. It would be important to differentiate the disorders of the second group more carefully from those of the first. Even though it is basically correct that emotional components are present in any disease, this concept carries the intrinsic danger of diluting the application of psychosomatic tenets to such an extent that some of the specific observations which have been made in a special group of disorders will be lost. However, the contributions of psychiatry to general medicine should not be minimized. These contributions are growing and are already influencing some of our concepts on etiology, organismic behavior, and adaptation which formerly did not give consideration to the emotional factors.

Some of the therapeutic research in this field is preoccupied with psychodynamic formulations and in much of this work we can clearly see that there is very little relationship *per se* between the dynamic constellation and the physiological function. The meaning of the symptoms remains purely psychologic, although the effect of the stimulation or tension is physiologic. If we study the tension production and discharge of the organism we find that we are dealing with physiological phenomena which relate only in general terms to the subjective meaningful experiences of the organism. This part of the research is usually preoccupied with studying physiological deviations based on emotional changes such as anger, anxiety, and hate. Linkages to the more subtle psychodynamic elaborations, however, are usually difficult to make. Therefore, research still continues on parallel lines and will so continue until a new methodology is evolved which will make it possible to demonstrate essentially where the junction is accomplished between these two mechanisms, the symbolic motivational one and the physiological one. One of the great difficulties here is that we do not have adequate measurements for emotions. The quantity of an emotion and its discharge toward the periphery is very important in producing clinical symptoms. Many of the psychosomatic disorders do not become manifest until the emotional charge reaches a certain quantity.

From a therapeutic point of view, many problems will have to be examined. To mention a few: Why is a particular organ selected in a psychosomatic condition? What happens if the vegetative nervous system stimulation of an organ system is blocked? Will this person now develop another psychosomatic sickness or another form of neurosis, or will he remain cured? Re-examination of the contention that certain emotional conflicts or psychodynamic constellations are specific in affecting a certain organ system is imperative. Many investigators have grave doubt that such correlations exist in a clear cut way.

In many individuals shifts occur from one region of the body's functional system to another. These shifts occur under the pressure of psychic events and are seemingly random displacements. But, if the results of recent investigations are confirmed, it appears that they follow well-defined courses. For instance, shifts from muscle to skin or other secretory activity manifest themselves more frequently when muscle action is able to be activated and then undergoes inhibition and weeping takes its place as a means of discharging tension.

The alternation between psychotic manifestations and psychosomatic symptoms is also of great interest. It has to be stated, however, that many patients have psychotic manifestations and psychosomatic symptoms simultaneously and that this group is most likely larger than the group in which the psychosomatic symptoms alternate with the psychotic ones.

Psychiatry, during its development, has stressed different aspects of the functions of the individual. It started with the investigation of the pathology of the nervous system and the internal milieu of the organism, and later on moved on to investigate the external milieu, the social and cultural influences, as determinants of human behavior. In the future our aim should be better to integrate these two aspects of psychic functioning in order to evolve a more comprehensive and more effective therapy.

A COMPARATIVE STUDY OF VARIOUS ATARACTIC DRUGS

Paul E. Feldman, M.D.

Director of Research and Education, Topeka State Hospital, Topeka, Kansas

Current literature seems to be divided into those articles that aver that the new tranquilizing drugs are of value in the treatment of psychiatric disorders and those that assert that the present claims are unjustified and unfounded.

Kline, Hoch, Winkelman, Goldman, Kinross-Wright, Ayd, and many others have written extensively about the value of ataraxics, all of them finding these drugs to be of considerable value in the treatment of psychiatric disorders; the precise degree of "success" shows variation with perhaps one reporter enjoying greater success with one drug than with another.

The other aspect of the controversy is well represented by the experiences of Sabshin and Ramot, who conclude that the drugs are of little value. Certainly, if the attitude reflected in their paper were present in the authors during the trial period, it might account for their failure with the drugs. I reported a similar phenomenon in "hostile" investigators. Some writers have implied that the drugs are of value only when the total treatment program was inadequate or nonexistent. Sabshin and Ramot imply that enthusiastic reports "emanated, primarily, from institutions with the greatest need for immediate results."

Bross has pointed out, "the 'missing' of advantageous new treatments may be just as serious in medical experimentation as the error of claiming non-existent advantages for a treatment."

The great mass of evidence to date supports the contention that the ataractics are of some value. This, however, leaves little room for complacency until such a time as the efficacy, specificity, and mode of operation of these drugs are clarified.

This study may have value over and above comparative studies of drugs that compile the results of separate investigators who have worked in dissimilar settings, inasmuch as a number of uncontrolled variables are eliminated by using the same clinical observers and similar patients. Also, the unique size of our staff permitted the use of large numbers of patients without encumbering any one physician with the burden and shortcomings of studying drug responses in large numbers of cases.

Our study extending over 2 years has involved 1,450 drug trials on 1,238 patients. No trials have been included in which medication was administered for less than two months. Table 1 indicates the size of the study and the number of staff men who contributed their time and effort in evaluation of these patients. All reports were rendered by staff psychiatrists or residents in training in psychiatry, and though these physicians may have utilized information received from other disciplines in their evaluations, their final conclusions were, for the most part, based upon their own individual observations.

Each contributing physician studied approximately 10 patients on any one drug. The limited individual case-load permitted them to know their patients most thoroughly and they were in an excellent position to detect any changes. The use of large numbers of observers was intentional in order to obtain a more sober perspective of the value of these drugs and to avoid a biased report.

TABLE 1

Drug	Number of patients in study	Number of staff members participating
Thorazine	763	49
Pacatal	110	15
Frenquel	56	10
Thorazine combined with reserpine	276	34
Serpasil	245	35

Method

Criteria

The method consists essentially of the clinical rating of 24 aspects of behavior on a 4-point scale and the conversion of these ratings into an over-all rating utilizing a 6-point scale. For purposes of this comparative study, ratings of "moderate," "moderate to marked," and "marked" improvement were considered significant positive changes. Ratings of "no improvement," "slight,"

TABLE 2
COMPARABILITY OF TEST GROUPS UPON THE BASIS OF CHRONICITY OF ILLNESS

Percentage of patients

Duration of illness (Years)	Thorazine	Pacatal	Frenquel	Thorazine combined with reserpine	Serpasil
0-1	4.1	—	3.6	4.0	5.1
1-2	6.3	—	3.6	4.0	2.5
2-5	22.4	15.5	14.3	14.3	9.4
5-10-	19.0	10.4	21.4	10.3	13.7
Over 10	48.2	74.1	57.1	67.4	69.4
Over 5	67.2	84.5	78.5	77.7	83.1
Over 2	89.6	100.0	92.8	92.0	92.5

and "slight to moderate" improvement were considered negative results. The inclusion of "slight to moderate" improvement under significant change would have made our results appear more startling but would not alter our general conclusions.

Clinical Material

Table 2 indicates the extent of chronicity of illness of the patient groups. Upon the basis of duration of illness as the prognostic factor, the Thorazine group appears in the best light and the Pacatal group in the poorest, but, even in the former, 89.6% of the patients had been mentally ill in excess of 2 years.

Table 3 indicates a close correlation in the diagnostic composition of the groups, other than for the Frenquel group in which the schizophrenic segment was greater. Upon the whole, based upon diagnostic categories, no group would appear to have a significant prognostic advantage over any other.

Drugs

Five varieties of medication were studied during this evaluation: Thorazine (chlorpromazine HCI), Pacatal (N-methylpiperdyl-3-methylphenothiazine), Frenquel (alpha-4-piperidyl diphenyl carbinol HCI), Serpasil (reserpine), (Chlorpromazine HCI [100 mg.]—reserpine [1 mg.]/tablet).

Medications were provided in both tablet and ampule form and all routes of administration were utilized with the preponderance of patients receiving oral medication. When a quick response was desired, the intramuscular route was employed.

TABLE 3
COMPARABILITY OF TEST GROUPS UPON THE BASIS OF SIMILARITY OF DIAGNOSTIC COMPOSITION

Percentage of patients

Diagnostic category	Thorazine	Pacatal	Frenquel	Thorazine combined with reserpine	Serpasil
Schizophrenia	79.3	70.9	92.9	77.5	80.5
Chr. brain syndromes	11.3	14.5	7.1	9.0	8.1
Mental deficiency	2.1	3.6	—	4.5	2.4
Manic-depressive reaction	3.4	3.6	—	4.5	5.7
Involutional reaction	2.1	—	—	2.5	0.8
Psychoneurotic reaction	1.1	7.3	—	2.0	0.8
Psychopathic personality	—	—	—	—	0.8
Children*	0.7	—	—	—	—

*Behavior disorders and childhood schizophrenia.

TABLE 4
IMPROVEMENT BY DIAGNOSTIC CATEGORIES

Percentage of patients improved

Diagnostic category	Thorazine	Pacatal	Frenquel	Thorazine combined with reserpine	Serpasil
Schizophrenia	65.4	42.9	27.0	50.0	39.4
Chr. brain syndromes	58.1	25.0	*	45.0	10.0
Mental deficiency	50.0	*	—	40.0	66.6
Manic-depressive reaction	69.2	*	—	45.0	10.0
Involutional reaction	75.0	—	—	33.3	*
Psychoneurotic reaction	75.0	25.0	—	50.0	*

* Number of patients too small to be significant.

Results

Improvement

Table 4 indicates the relative effectiveness of the various drugs tested. Results ranged from 10% effectiveness of Serpasil in the treatment of chronic brain syndromes to 75% effectiveness of Thorazine in the treatment of involutional psychotic reactions.

Table 5 indicates the changes in the various evaluative criteria upon which the over-all evaluation was based. None of the drugs consistently altered the entire gamut of behavior, with some drugs being more effective than others on some aspects of behavior. Thorazine appears to be outstandingly superior to the other drugs tested in respect to general therapeutic efficacy. A similar conclusion was reached at the International Colloquium on Chlorpromazine and Neuroleptic Medications in Psychiatric Treatment held in Paris, October 1955. Kurland pooling the results of various investigators studying chlorpromazine and reserpine also found Thorazine superior, but Kovitz *et al.* found reserpine "slightly superior" to Thorazine.

In our study, a combination of Thorazine and reserpine appears to be the second most effective drug. In the amelioration of combativeness, self-mutilatory trends, and compulsivity, Thoraserpine appears to have a slight advantage

TABLE 5
INDIVIDUAL RESPONSES OF EVALUATIVE CRITERIA
Percent improved

Criteria	Thorazine	Pacatal	Frenquel	Thorazine combined with reserpine	Serpasil
Dress	48.3	18.4	4.3	15.6	16.8
Orientation	30.0	8.0	0	15.4	6.0
Memory	29.5	6.2	0	18.7	5.2
Delusions	48.0	4.5	4.0	23.6	13.6
Hallucinations	58.0	20.0	10.5	24.2	12.5
Negativism	57.3	27.0	36.4	45.1	25.7
Hyperactivity	72.5	31.3	21.4	55.7	38.0
Hostility	67.1	33.3	25.0	54.4	31.9
Combativeness	70.3	30.6	28.6	75.8	34.7
Bizarre mannerisms	55.1	12.0	11.1	33.3	14.4
Appropriateness of conversation	49.0	25.0	9.1	46.0	15.5
Realistic planning	30.7	15.8	20.0	21.7	2.3
Amicability	55.6	22.2	5.9	42.1	27.0
Sociability	43.9	23.5	0	34.4	20.9
Accessibility	53.3	29.3	4.5	43.6	18.5
Participation in adjunctive therapy	42.6	24.2	11.8	40.3	14.7
Appetite	52.1	27.7	0	33.3	17.7
Sleep	55.4	33.3	0	32.2	20.0
Tension	70.6	34.3	0	42.1	23.7
Self-mutilation	42.9	20.0	0	54.5	11.1
Judgment	23.8	5.0	0	12.1	1.0
Insight	12.3	5.3	0	10.9	1.0
Affect	33.3	11.5	5.3	30.0	5.0
Compulsivity	33.3	6.3	0	35.7	18.4

over the other drugs. Barsa and Kline concluded that "combined reserpine-chlorpromazine therapy seems to have certain advantages over therapy with reserpine alone."

Pacatal, Frenquel, and Serpasil also produce significant changes, but not of the magnitude of Thorazine. In view of the manufacturer's claims of a high degree of specificity of Frenquel for hallucinations, our results in this respect (10.5% effective) were most disappointing. For such aspects of the evaluations as "insight" or "judgment," none of the drugs appeared to be significantly efficacious.

TABLE 6
RELATIVE EFFICACY OF VARIOUS DOSAGE LEVELS

	Dosage	Percent of patients significantly improved
Serpasil	1 mg./day	40.0
	2 mg./day	47.4
	3 mg./day	22.2
	4 mg./day	40.0
	6 mg./day	45.8
	8 mg./day	33.3
	10 mg./day	33.3
	12* mg./day	12.5
Thorazine combined with reserpine	1 tab./day	33.3
	2 tab./day	48.7
	3 tab./day	40.0
	4 tab./day	70.6
	6 tab./day	55.5
	8* tab./day	40.0
Frenquel	60 mg./day	0.0
	80 mg./day	100.0
	120 mg./day	28.6
	180 mg./day	100.0
	240* mg./day	0.0
Pacatal	100 mg./day	16.7
	150 mg./day	38.5
	200 mg./day	33.3
	300 mg./day	45.0
	400 mg./day	40.0
	500* mg./day	25.0
Thorazine	100 mg./day	38.1
	150 mg./day	62.9
	200 mg./day	73.5
	250 mg./day	75.0
	300 mg./day	64.3
	400 mg./day	62.9
	450 mg./day	64.7
	600 mg./day	82.7
	800 mg./day	58.0
	1,000* mg./day	72.2

* And over

Dosages

Other than for the most minimal of doses, all medications were equally effective throughout the gamut of their individual dosages. (Table 6). Within the limits of error imposed by the structure of our study, the higher dosages did not manifest any superiority, therapeutically, over the moderate dosages. Serpasil appears slightly more effective in its lower ranges, Thorazine combined with reserpine in daily dosages of 200:2-600:6, Pacatal in dosages of 300-400 mg./day; and Thorazine from 150 mg./day upward.

Efficacy

Therapeutic efficacy based upon chronicity of illness follows the pattern of being more effective in early, acute cases, but therapeutic responses were elicited at all stages of chronicity. Thorazine most consistently appears effective at all stages of chronicity.

TABLE 7
RESULTS BASED UPON CHRONICITY OF ILLNESS
Percentage of patients improved

Chronicity (Years)	Thorazine	Pacatal	Frenquel	Thorazine combined with reserpine	Serpasil
0-1	76.9	—	0.0	100.0	25.0
1-2	80.0	—	0.0	40.0	66.6
2-5	66.2	33.3	50.0	44.4	54.5
5-10	70.0	33.3	33.3	69.2	37.5
Over 10	61.7	34.9	18.8	28.8	32.1

TABLE 8
INCIDENCE OF SIDE-EFFECTS
Percentage of patients

	Thorazine	Pacatal	Frenquel	Thorazine combined with reserpine	Serpasil
Drowsiness	19.2	26.2	—	58.0	21.1
Parkinsonism	6.6	1.5	—	23.2	4.1
Allergy	4.2	1.5	—	2.9	0.9
Dizziness	3.4	29.2	—	12.0	1.6
Hypotension	3.4	7.7	—	7.2	1.6
Depression	1.8	1.5	—	7.2	0.8
Jaundice	1.6	1.8	—	0.7	—
Blood changes	1.6	—	—	—	—
G.I. symptoms	2.1	9.2	—	6.5	0.8
Turbulence	1.8	3.0	10.7	—	6.5
Dryness of mouth	3.8	.4.5	—	—	—
Blurred vision	0.5	12.3	—	—	—
Edema	0.8	—	—	4.3	—
Salivation	0.6	—	—	11.6	—
Incontinence	0.6	—	—	11.6	—
Weakness	1.3	—	—	2.2	—
Lactation	0.5	—	—	0.7	—
Slurred speech	—	6.0	—	—	—
Amenorrhea	0.5	—	—	—	—
Seizures	1.1	—	—	—	—

Side-Effects

A substantial number of side-effects were produced with all drugs except Frenquel, in which turbulence was the only side-effect noted. Rinaldi *et al.* also noted an absence of side-effects with Frenquel.

Of the more serious side-effects (Parkinsonian, jaundice, and blood changes), Thorazine combined with reserpine and Thorazine showed the highest incidence (Table 8). Lemere treating 88 patients with chlorpromazine-reserpine found a lowering of the incidence of side-effects and concluded that "some of the side-reactions are cancelled out." Eiber had a similar experience with a smaller series of patients.

Comparative Responses

A substantial number of our patients have received independent trials with more than one drug. In between trials, these patients have been without medication so that they had an opportunity to revert to their pretrial state before a new medication was introduced. Table 9 indicates comparative responses of these patients.

It appears that all the drugs are capable of eliciting a response—in individual cases—over and above that elicited with a previous drug. Our findings are at variance with the experience of Bennett *et al.* who found "usually, where one drug was found ineffective, so was the other." On the other hand, Rinaldi *et al.* found reserpine helped the largest number of patients. They confirm our experience that "in no instance were all patients helped by any one drug."

TABLE 9
COMPARATIVE RESPONSES

Thorazine patients changed to a combination of thorazine and reserpine

No.	%	Net change in response	
9	12.7	−2	
12	16.0	−1	29.6% less improvement
17	23.9	0	
8	11.3	+1	
6	8.5	+2	
11	15.5	+3	46.5% greater improvement
4	5.6	+4	
4	5.6	+5	
Total 81	100		

Serpasil patients changed to a combination of Thorazine and reserpine

No.	%	Net change in response	
4	11.4	−2	
3	8.6	−1	20.0% less improvement
10	28.6	0	
1	2.8	+1	
9	25.7	+2	
6	17.1	+3	51.3% greater improvement
2	5.7	+4	
Total 35	100		

Thorazine patients changed to Frenquel

3	10.0	−4	
2	6.7	−3	79.7% less improvement
10	33.3	−2	
9	30.0	−1	
2	6.7	0	
4	13.4	+1	13.4% greater improvement
Total 30	100		

Serpasil patients changed to Frenquel

5	38.5	−2	61.6% less improvement
3	23.1	−1	
3	23.1	0	
2	15.3	+1	15.3% greater improvement
Total 13	100		

Thorazine patients changed to Pacatal

1	2.7	−4	
6	16.2	−3	55.9% less improvement
5	13.5	−2	
5	13.5	−1	
8	21.6	0	
5	13.5	+1	32.5% greater improvement
7	19.0	+3	
Total 37	100		

Serpasil patients changed to Pacatal

2	7.7	−2	30.8% less improvement
6	23.1	−1	
11	42.3	0	
4	15.4	+1	26.8% greater improvement
3	11.4	+2	
Total 26	100		

SUMMARY AND CONCLUSIONS

1. Clinical evaluations have been made upon 1,450 trials with chlorpromazine, a combination of Thorazine and reserpine, Frenquel, Pacatal, and Serpasil.

2. The patient material utilized for this study consisted of a very chronic, inpatient population of a state hospital with a very high percentage of schizophrenic reactions.

3. All 5 compounds tested appear to be of benefit in some respect, but not to the same degree.

4. Thorazine appears to be the most generally effective, and Frenquel the least.

5. All drugs appear most effective in the treatment of early cases and least effective in the very chronic.

6. High dosages of drugs do not appear to provide any benefit over and above the benefit derived from moderate dosage.

7. The incidence of side-effects is highest with Thorazine and Thorazine combined with reserpine and lowest with Frenquel.

8. Combined Thorazine-reserpine therapy does not follow the prediction that the good effects of each drug would be potentiated and the ill effects merely additive. Thorazine-reserpine produces a prohibitively high incidence of serious untoward effects.

9. Patients who do not respond to one drug may respond to another. Patients who respond moderately to one drug may respond maximally to another.

10. No single diagnostic category seems to respond outstandingly to any one drug.

11. Hyperactivity, combativeness and tension respond best to ataraxics. The response of insight, affect, judgment, and realistic planning is disappointing.

12. Our results support the concept that ataractic drugs are of value in the treatment of psychiatric disorders.

SOME OBSERVATIONS ON THE USE OF TRANQUILIZING DRUGS

Thomas S. Szasz, M.D.

The widespread acceptance and use of the so-called tranquilizing drugs constitutes one of the most noteworthy events in the recent history of psychiatry. This development is being hailed in many quarters as the beginning of a new era in psychiatry and "mental health." Even when these drugs are not claimed to "cure" the patient, it is asserted that their use makes him more amenable to other forms of "therapy," either within the hospital or outside. The purpose of this essay is not to evaluate the effects of these drugs on behavior. We accept as a premise (without, however, necessarily subscribing to it) that the pharmacological agents under consideration (chlorpromazine, reserpine, etc.) do indeed bring about the behavioral changes currently ascribed to them. What I wish to comment on, rather, is the *social fact* that these drugs are used. This event itself can rightly be made the subject of scientific inquiry. Indeed, such an inquiry would seem to be desirable to counterbalance and complement an otherwise one-sided enthusiasm and optimism about this novel aspect of psychiatry. No detailed exposition of the sociopsychological aspects of psychopharmacology as therapy will be attempted here. I shall confine myself to sketching briefly some of the considerations which arise in connection with a contemplation of this subject. These may be conveniently organized around the following three questions: 1. What do we, as physicians and psychiatrists, do when we prescribe these drugs? 2. Whom do we treat? 3. Is what we do right (just)?

Some—or perhaps many—will undoubtedly disagree with my suggestions about how best to answer these questions. Be that as it may, I think all will, or should, agree that raising such questions, and thinking about them, is the duty of all thoughtful men faced with measures of such far-reaching medical and social implications.

Does Psychiatry Deal with "Mental Illness"?

Modern psychiatric thought is influenced by and reflects chiefly two sources of knowledge. One of these is medicine, including its basic sciences, such as chemistry, physics, biology, and pharmacology; the other source is sociology, psychology, anthropology, philosophy, semantics, and other disciplines dealing with experience, symbolism, and behavior. Some schools of psychiatric thought lean more heavily on one, and some on the other, of these two metaphorical "parents" of psychiatry (e. g., psychosurgery and psychotherapy and their respective theories). Still others try to combine what they consider the best features of both (e. g., psychoanalysis, "neuropsychiatry," etc.). The result is that there exists a much greater "hodgepodge" of methods and concepts in psychiatry than in most other branches of medicine.

Conceptually, the use of tranquilizing drugs rests on the medical model of "disease." In this context we deal with two principal notions, namely, "disease" and "symptom" (or "sign"). Thus, pneumonia is a disease; chest pain, cough, fever, and leukocytosis are its symptoms and signs. Similarly, we hear speculations about whether the drugs in question "cure mental illness" or whether they only control its "symptoms." Most investigators claim no more than symptomatic control. The abolition of anxiety, tension, restlessness, and combative behavior are thus regarded as analogous to the control of pain, discomfort, and excessive fever by acetylsalicylic acid in an infectious illness. The implication of all this, of course, is that, while we do not yet have penicillin which will *cure the disease,* we might achieve such a result by dint of perseverance, and thus "cure mental illness." If, by the way of comparison, I may be permitted to cite a somewhat inelegant example of this sort of program, I would recall a slogan which was popular in the early days of Nazi Germany. It was: "Today we conquer Germany—tomorrow the whole world." In medicine, first we are satisfied with mastering (controlling) symptoms; later we hope we shall be able to do the same with the disease. The history of bacteriology and the control of infectious diseases shows that this can be done. In view of this, what possible objection can there be to an analogous pharmacological approach to "mental illness"?

The objection, of course, is a familiar one and consists of the possibility that the things which we now call "mental illnesses" are not "diseases" at all. In other words, suppose that the model of "disease-and-symptom" does not apply to the phenomena under study. If such should prove to be the case, we would, at best, be wasting our time, and, at worst, be damaging our patients and society.

This is not the place to consider the evidence for or against the view which regards psychiatric disorder as "mental illness." While it is popular nowadays to speak of "mental illness," many psychiatric investigators have found that the psychological and social approach to behavioral phenomena greatly limits the relevance and value of this conceptual model. A moment's reflection will show that our present custom of considering everything (and human behavior does encompass almost everything) to which a physician addresses himself as "disease" is no more rational and useful than considering all sorts of diverse happenings in terms of economic, political, or religious concepts. Similarly, we persist in calling all that transpires between physician and patient "treatment," no matter how disparate these phenomena might be, and even disregarding whether or not the "treatment" helps the patient. Szasz and Hollender have called attention to three major categories within the broad concept of "disease." They noted that each different concept of "disease" carries with it its particular view of "treatment" and "cure." Moreover, historical and scientific change often leads to changing concepts of "disease." For example, what in one era was regarded as "disease" became the "symptom" of the next scientific epoch, and so on. Not long ago, fever was an "illness," and its disappearance was "cure." Today tuberculosis, malaria, and typhoid are still widely regarded as "diseases." At the same time, we are also at ease with another view of these disorders, according to which they are "symptoms" of certain social (economic, public health, etc.) conditions. These examples are trivial and are cited only to remind us that "disease" is not an impersonal, objectively given "entity"—which "exists" in nature and waits for man's discovery of it—but, rather, that it is a concept which we *make* as we go along in the exploration of our experiences.

PHILOSOPHICAL PROBLEMS RAISED BY USE OF TRANQUILIZING DRUGS

Let us turn our attention now to the three questions mentioned at the beginning of this essay. I shall briefly indicate the generally accepted, that is, official or "scientific," answer to each of the questions. These will be supplemented by some considerations which are recommended as further, perhaps more appropriate, "explanations" for the phenomena at hand.

1. What do we, as physicians and psychiatrists, do when we prescribe tranquilizing drugs? The commonly accepted answers include the following: We treat the patient's "symptoms," such as tension, agitation, and combativeness, which are manifestations of his "mental illness." We make the patient more tractable and therefore more amenable to hospital management or auxiliary "therapy" as an outpatient. We relieve the acutely disturbing manifestations of a behavioral disturbance, and this might lead to a readjustment of the whole person ("cure").

2. Whom do we treat? This question might sound trivial but it is not. It is inherent in the foregoing comments that we treat the "patient." Yet it is equally obvious, and often explicitly stated, that these drugs make the disturbed hospitalized patient more manageable (i.e., less disturbing to ward personnel and other patients). Accordingly, we also treat the hospital staff and patients other than those who receive the drug.

3. Is this form of treatment justifiable, or, in other words, is it right? Obviously, the answer must be yes; otherwise, it would not be generally accepted practice. This is the normative concept of "right" as used in jurisprudence in a democratic society. Yet we know that patterns of behavior—whether pertaining to medical practice or to political conduct—generally approved at one time may be looked upon in quite another light at a later time. This alone commands caution against the ready equation of statistical frequency with "rightfulness."

Now we turn to the objections to the foregoing "explanations" and the consideration of other possibilities. The following comments rest, of course, on the assumption that so-called psychiatric disorders do not lend themselves to fruitful analysis and management in terms of the medical model of "disease-and-symptom." For our present purposes we prefer to regard them in sociologic terms as deviant forms of behavior, and in psychologic terms as "conflicts" and attempted "solutions" of conflicts. While it may be objected that the psychosocial aspects of mental retardation, senile psychoses, psychoses with metabolic or endocrine disease, and many other types of "psychiatric disorder" do (or may) lend themselves to fruitful understanding and treatment in terms of the traditional medical model, the possibility still remains that the majority of the so-called "functional psychoses" will have to be approached differently. Be that as it may, I wish to make explicit that this essay rests on the latter assumption but it does not imply that all "psychiatric disorders" (now so called) can be relevantly dealt with in terms of "conflicts."

Is it not possible that the use of these drugs represents a modern version of the "furor therapeuticus"—a traditional "occupational disease" of the physician? The last several decades have brought us, in rapid succession, various forms of "shock treatments," psychosurgery, and, lastly, the tranquilizing drugs. All have in common the fact that they provide socially sanctioned patterns of medical action and thus help the physician to do something when he is faced with a psychiatric problem. (It is not implied in this context that these methods are not helpful but that psychotherapy is!)

The answers to the second question ("Whom do we treat?") might be implemented as follows: We treat ourselves. This possibility must—I submit—be considered in all forms of treatment. Furthermore, we treat the patient's environment, in the widest sense of this word (family, hospital staff, other patients, society at large, etc.). This claim is supported by the "fact" commonly agreed upon, that the chief alterations in the patient produced by these drugs pertain to making his behavior more socially acceptable. These drugs, in essence, function as chemical strait jackets. The restraint of patients who annoy society is, of course, a time-honored procedure. What is significant in this context, however, is the possible confusion of motives, actions, and results. In other words, when a "disturbed" patient is forcibly restrained, it is clear that this serves the protection of those about him and of the community at large. It may or may not be also "helpful," in the long run, to the patient himself. When a similar effect is accomplished by chemical means, it is much easier to mistake the process for "treatment," the primary aim of which is to "help the patient."

The foregoing considerations lead directly into our third question ("Is it right to treat patients this way?"). The more we consider the complexity of this matter, the more dubious it becomes whether or not this mode of treatment is justifiable. To me, it seems hardly right to emphasize that these drugs "help the patient," inasmuch as it is more apparent that they help others (e. g., like the segregation and confinement of patients with leprosy).

Deviance and Rebellion in "Mental Illness"

The foregoing words of caution imply criticism. Criticism is rarely welcome and is often particularly resented when the critic has, so to speak, nothing better to offer than that which he criticizes. This all too human reaction to criticism has probably played a role in stimulating the advocates of psychotherapy to claim more for this mode of influencing people than can be readily substantiated. While I am personally impressed by the role of psychological and social forces in human relationship, I definitely want to avoid casting this essay into the framework of physiological versus psychological forms of therapy in psychiatry. It seems to me that words of caution and criticism—when appropriate—must stand on their own feet. The suggestion of better alternatives is desirable but is really another matter altogether. (No one expects a drama critic to write a better play than the one on which he comments. Similarly, the inadequacy of a scientific hypothesis may be demonstrated without necessarily suggesting a better one. Why should it be otherwise in the case of therapeutic techniques?)

With this premise in mind, I shall sketch briefly a conceptual model of psychiatric disorders which is different than the one which has been criticized. This model is not novel, since it is held by many psychiatrists. It will be restated here—perhaps greatly oversimplified—not in order to acquaint any one with this aspect of psychiatric theory but only as background information to substantiate and clarify the doubts which have been raised about the use of tranquilizing drugs.

Most so-called psychiatric conditions, such as schizophrenia, depression, alcoholism, and so forth, show us the individual in conflict either with specific individuals or with society as a whole. It is fundamental to our understanding of problems of mental health that, on the whole (sociologically speaking), compliant behavior tends to be viewed as normal and deviant behavior as abnormal. In all "mental illness" (we use this word, without subscribing to its misleading connotations, only for ease of communication) the patient vacillates between compliance with and defiance of parental—and later social—commands and expectations. Often this problem leaves society relatively uninvolved, especially when the person experiences the wishes to submit or rebel primarily in relation to his own inner images of his parents and their substitutes. In patients with schizophrenic and other disturbances—who make up the population of mental hospitals and who are the potential candidates for tranquilizing drug therapy—we invariably see the individual in some degree of overt (social) conflict with those about him. The so-called "disturbed" patient may or may not be "disturbed" in terms of his own feelings. The term reflects more accurately the fact that he disturbs others. This, among other things, is what we mean by deviant behavior.

An analogy may be drawn to the model of an infectious disease. We view such a disorder as a sort of battle between the organism, on the one hand, and the microbes, on the other. The microbe is an "enemy" (within); here we lean on the metaphor of nations engaged in warfare. Similarly, we might picture "mental illness" as revolving around the theme of a battle between the patient's own sense of identity, on the one hand, and those whom he feels thwart his needs and endanger his survival. The original adversaries are usually his parents. Later others in authority may take this role, as, for example, physicians, or often "society" as a whole. Assuming that such a battle is indeed what happens, and that what we call "mental illness" is a manifestation of it, what alternatives for interference in this process are open to us? Again, with due allowances for oversimplification, the following three basic modes of action present themselves: 1. To interfere as little as possible in the patient's life and let him "work out" the conflicts as he sees fit. The minimum interference ("treatment") would have to include making sure that the patient does not seriously injure himself or any one else, (e. g., humane confinement). 2. To concentrate on separating the "combatants." This takes place when patients are forcibly restricted to institutions and are otherwise segregated from society. This casts society into the aggressive and damaging role in which it has already been conceived by the patient. It makes the "working out" of the conflict more difficult. As a rule, this arrangement leads to the permanent defeat of the patient and the victory of the forces of society (at a certain price to the latter, which it is willing, however, to pay). 3. Lastly, to employ sanctions against the patient in an effort to make him conform to the demands of society (parents). Shock therapy, lobotomy—and other measures collectively, and with good reason, called the "drastic therapies"—might be viewed as doing just this. The use of tranquilizing drugs belongs in this category.[2] In a similar context, Meerloo aptly spoke of "medication into submission."

By approaching the problem of "mental illness" in terms of a conflict between the patient and other people (or, broadly, society), we are better able to clarify certain questions about whether the tranquilizing drugs constitute good therapy and whether their use is morally justifiable. In most medical situations the patient does not present the physician with the dilemma of helping him and hurting society, or vice versa. Apparently, in some psychiatric situations he does just this. Physicians have been proud, and justly so, that they have eliminated, to a very large extent, the element of moral judgment from their daily work. If a patient has a broken bone, the physician will set it whether he be sinner or saint. Unfortunately, however useful this model of the physician's role may have been in the past, it appears that we must now modify it or give it up in psychiatry.

Accordingly, physicians will have to clarify the effects of their ministrations in behavioral disorders. They will have to be clearer than heretofore about whether they help the patient or others. Are they agents and representatives of the best interests of the patient, his relatives, the hospital, or society? What if these interests clash?

Without belaboring these issues further, it is clear, in summary, that (if our hypothesis is correct) the best interests of the patient necessitate the maximal recognition of his right for self-determination, growth, and the working out of conflicts. On the contrary, the greatest (immediate) protection of society may conceivably lie in the use of severely repressive measures against deviant citizens, whatever the cause of their behavior.

Yet it must be noted here that it is held by many that possibilities for defiance of authority and deviances from social norms—within certain clearly set limits—must remain open to the individual as a prerequisite for his "mental health," as well as for the well-being of a free, democratic, heterogeneous society. Thus, excessive sanctions against individuals manifesting deviant behavior might effectively protect society for a short period; its danger, for the long run, is that the protective measures themselves might bring about a trans-

---

[2] In this essay I have aimed only at an analysis of the use of tranquilizing drugs in situations which are formally recognized as "psychiatric." Accordingly, the observations and inferences presented either do not apply or apply only partially to the widespread prescription of these substances in general medical practice.

formation of the social structure such as was not desired by those who advocate the protective measures in question. Which "treatment" is justifiable and which is not will depend on the position which we take about these and similar questions. In any event, what is ethically "wrong" is to use a mode of "treatment" which benefits others than the patient and claim that it is for his welfare. It is in this connection that I see the gravest dangers in the use of tranquilizing drugs, and, for that matter, also of certain other forms of psychiatric treatment, including psychotherapy. In other words, when patients had to be restrained by the use of force—for example, by a strait jacket—it was difficult for those in charge of their care to convince themselves that they were acting altogether on behalf of the patient. The use of drugs (and of psychotherapy) removes the safeguards inherent in the guilt feelings of the therapist. Restraint by chemical means does not make us guilty; herein lies the danger to the patient.

Summary

The purpose of this essay is to inquire into, and call attention to, some sociopsychological aspects of the current vogue of using tranquilizing drugs in psychiatric disorders.

The use of these drugs rests on the premise that psychiatry deals with "mental illness" and that such illness presents a problem essentially analogous to that encountered in medicine (and particularly in infectious disease). There is evidence to suggest that this "medical" model of behavioral disturbance is inadequate and misleading. If such disturbances do not constitute "diseases" which manifest themselves in certain "signs" and "symptoms," then measures based on this concept are likely to be faulty, and probably harmful to patient, physician, or society.

A brief analysis of this problem is organized around the following three questions: 1. What do we, as physicians and psychiatrists, do when we prescribe tranquilizing drugs? 2. Whom do we treat? 3. Is this form of treatment justifiable? The generally accepted answers to each of these questions are summarized. They are followed by suggestions for additional possible "answers," the most important of which are (1) that the use of these drugs may represent a new "symptom" of the ancient occupational disease of physicians known as "furor therapeuticus"; (2) that we treat ourselves and the patient's social environment, and (3) that whether we hold the treatment to be justifiable or not will depend on what position we take vis-a-vis the patient's conflict with other persons and society.

In conclusion, the role and significance of defiance of authority and of deviance from social norms in "mental illness" (and in all modes of human life, for that matter) are briefly mentioned. These considerations are emphasized in an effort to substantiate the legitimacy, and possible value, of taking a position of caution and criticism with respect to the widespread use of tranquilizing drugs in medical and psychiatric practice.

A REVIEW OF THE NEWER DRUG THERAPIES IN PSYCHIATRY

Vernon Kinross-Wright, M.D.,
Department of Psychiatry, Baylor University College of Medicine,
Houston, Texas

Reference to the psychiatric literature of the past year leaves one in no doubt that the chemotherapy of mental diseases has come of age. The use of drugs in psychiatry is hardly new; scarcely a year having passed by in the last two decades without the introduction of some chemical designed to relieve mental symptoms. What then is so striking about our present interest in drugs? It is, that in the first instance in the space of two or three years there have been published in excess of two thousand articles on chlorpromazine and reserpine; and in the second, that considerable uniformity of opinion about these drugs is expressed by members of a specialty noted chiefly for its disagreements.

No one of the newer drugs approaches the therapia magna. Some of them, however, do appear to represent major advances in the management of disturbed patients, in the relief of unpleasant symptoms and perhaps in some cases, in the actual resolution of illness. Some of them bid to catalyse new approaches to the understanding of cerebral function.

It is not intended that this paper shall provide an exhaustive review of the recent advances in psychiatric chemotherapy. The subject is still too complex and controversial. The successful introduction of chlorpromazine and reserpine has given a tremendous impetus to the chemical treatment of mental illness. Scarcely a week goes by without a new compound or a variant of an established one being submitted for investigation. As a result, the situation is rapidly becoming so chaotic that even a specialist in the field grows befuddled. Methods of communication in psychiatry have always been poor. We do not have the background of experimental methodology enjoyed by other branches of medicine and our training has rarely included much pharmacology or biochemistry. We are largely dependent on the pharmaceutical houses for our information and it is to their credit that they have not taken advantage of us. Even they do not feel completely secure, for the correlation between the effects of drugs upon the behavior of experimental animals and that of our patients is not as great as we would like.

The author will now draw largely upon his own experiences with them in commenting upon some of the new drug therapies.

Chlorpromazine was the first of the so-called "tranquilizing" drugs to become popular, though some of its chemical relatives now being investigated (phenergan, parsidol) had been utilized before for different purposes. Chlorpromazine owed its introduction into psychiatry to the fact that it potentiated barbiturates, a phenomenon now recognized to be inconstant in man. In the space of three years it has become one of the most widely used drugs in medical practice. Broadly speaking, it is used in psychiatry in three ways. Firstly as a mild sedative for the multitude of patients with neuroses, psychosomatic disorders and situational reactions. Secondly a chemical restraint for the disturbed and excited psychotic. Thirdly in more intensive dosage it is given in an attempt to abolish psychotic symptoms. The literature suggests many other indications for chlorpromazine too, but most of these can be fitted into one of the three categories above. Some facts are clear about the drug. It is not a euphoriant. It does not appear to have the addictive qualities of the barbiturates and withdrawal symptoms are unknown. The sedative and hypotensive effects are only rarely absent. The margin of safety is extremely great. Good effects have been reported with doses of 15 mg. to 4500 mg. per day. Chlorpromazine has a spectrum of biological activity paralleled by few other drugs, and hence has many side effects. This activity appears to be shared by many phenothiazine derivatives in varying degrees and we may confidently expect to see relatives of chlorpromazine put to therapeutic use in the future.

Reports on the therapeutic efficacy of chlorpromazine are sharply divergent. On the one side there is talk of reducing the schizophrenic population in the state hospitals by 25% or more; on the other, statements that good results are meager and transitory. The bulk of opinion, however, tends to suggest that chlorpromazine is an excellent inhibitor of overactivity and mental confusion. Excellent because it is effective, does not impair consciousness, increases appetite, and is simple to administer.

There is no doubt that it is effective in allaying anxiety and reducing tension in the neuroses. European findings in regard to the obsessive-compulsive states have not been found generally true in this country, however. Behavioral disturbances in children have responded well, often dramatically. It is worth mentioning that children tolerate chlorpromazine very well. While most workers view the drug as a symptomatic treatment or as an aid to psychotherapy and other measures, a number of workers including the author, believe that intensive treatment with large doses actually modifies or interrupts the course of some types of schizophrenia. Following the period of intensive dosage an indefinite period of maintenance on a smaller dose is commonly necessary. It seems that in these cases the individual's capacity to react psychotically is inhibited even though his inability to deal with his life situation may persist. Indeed in experiments with monkeys designed to produce chlorpromazine Parkinsonism, the author has found that immature animals show very little response to the drug aside from sedation and lessened drive.

The various lines of research about the action of chlorpromazine upon the central nervous system will not be discussed. Alteration of function of the reticular system and hypothalamus has been demonstrated in animals, and in one human fatality pathological changes were present in these areas.

The complications of chlorpromazine therapy have been exhaustively dealt with in the literature. At this same meeting last year, the author presented his ideas upon this subject. It is important to distinguish between complications such as jaundice, dermatitis and agranulocytosis, and concomitants of the actual therapeutic action of the drug such as hypotension, lethargy, hormonal changes and Parkinsonism. The incidence of jaundice varies from .1 to 3% in different parts of the country. It is possible that the higher figure contains cases of jaundice unrelated to the drug. Jaundice and agranulocytosis are presumably the same sorts of idiosyncratic response seen with other drugs such as thiouracil and methyltestosterone. They are not related to dosage—in fact, seem to occur more frequently with minimal dosage. The only positive sign of overdosage with chlorpromazine known to the author is a toxic-confusional state.

A clear understanding of the side-effects of the newer drugs is very essential to the practising physician. These drugs bring about drastic changes in the function of both central and peripheral nervous system in addition to the idiosyncratic responses. For this reason they require careful prescription. It is scarcely justifiable to relieve a mild tension state or stomach upset at the expense of several months of jaundice.

In summary, chlorpromazine is a drug with a wide range of safety but with widespread effects upon the organism. It is often effective in relieving anxiety. It is the most useful inhibitor of psychomotor excitement yet discovered. In larger doses it may block the manifestations of schizophrenia. Depressive illnesses are not usually helped by the drug though the author has secured good results in these cases with energetic administration. In some instances, chlorpromazine may precipitate depression. Indiscriminate usage of chlorpromazine may be attended by unjustified morbidity.

Reserpine was introduced in this country shortly after chlorpromazine. It is a drug of ancient lineage, being an alkaloid isolated from the Rauwolfia root used as a sedative in the East for centuries. Despite the fact that it bears no discernible chemical relationship to chlorpromazine its effects on abnormal behaviour are generally similar. It, too, is a sedative and an inhibitor of psychomotor excitement without significant effect upon the brain cortex. While differences in the effect of the two drugs upon the reticular system have been demonstrated, both produce Parkinsonism. Reserpine occasionally causes convulsions which is in keeping with animal experiments. Chlorpromazine lowers convulsive threshold in some individuals while raising it in others. In animals the latter drug is an anti-convulsant.

Reserpine, in the author's experience, has a rather unpredictable onset of action. Oral medication frequently does not produce effects in the patients until several days have elapsed. This is sometimes true with intramuscular injection. Sedation with reserpine is not so marked as a rule as with chlorpromazine, though ambulatory patients on roughly equivalent doses of the two drugs often complain more about the lassitude associated with reserpine. The hypotensive response to reserpine is milder and more prolonged. Patients rarely complain of dizziness. Reserpine has not been implicated in the production of jaundice, and idiosyncratic responses (dermatitis, edema) are less frequent. In large doses Parkinsonism is a very frequent occurrence with reserpine (about 50% in the author's cases). Both drugs have a tendency to increase or produce depressions sporadically especially in neurotic and hypertensive patients. With reserpine, however, the depression may be severe, necessitating hospitalization and electroshock. The author has seen three such cases.

There is as yet a paucity of reports examining the relative merits of the two drugs. It is the author's impression that the majority of psychiatrists active in the field favor chlorpromazine over reserpine for psychotic patients. The author now rarely uses reserpine in this type of patient because of unpredictability of onset of effect, liability to depression or increased tension, and relative lack of effect upon basic psychotic behavioural patterns. In the neuroses and in children's behavioural disorders there is apparently little difference between the two agents, though the author again favors chlorpromazine for its more positive action.

Combinations of the drugs have been tried. Better results in psychotic patients with fewer doses of either drug and fewer side effects have been noted. The author has secured good results in a number of manic and schizophrenic patients resistant to either drug given singly. However, side effects were increased. The value of a combination of two novel and inadequately evaluated compounds must be largely speculative at this time.

From among a large number of compounds studied for analeptic properties two have been selected for clinical use because of the low toxicity. Meratran and Ritalin have essentially similar action and comparable to that of amphetamine. Chemically they are both piperidine derivatives. Both are central stimulants with a less vigorous action than that of the amphetamines. Neither is said to be accompanied by overactivity of the sympathetic nervous system. In the author's series of patients this has been generally true though occasional patients have developed autonomic symptoms. Neither drug causes anorexia. They share an anti-depressant action though in the author's experience this has only been consistent and substantial with depression resulting from reserpine or chlorpromazine. Results in reactive and endogenous depressions have been fair but not superior to those obtainable with amphetamine. Both have a tendency to increase anxiety where it is already present, sometimes to an alarming degree. This is probably an unavoidable property of any stimulant drug. However, in a few instances the drugs have had a paradoxical calming effect in anxious patients. Meratran is reported as being effective in the treatment of certain tics. Given intravenously by the author it has induced a conspicuous though temporary reduction of drug-induced Parkinsonian symptoms.

It may be concluded that both Meratran and Ritalin possess the desirable effects of amphetamine with fewer side effects. In addition, Meratran may have a more specific effect upon certain conditions associated with muscular hypertonus.

Frenquel, the next drug to be discussed, is remarkable in that its empirical formula is the same as Meratran. It differs in that the piperidyl ring is substituted at the 4 position instead of the 2. In experimental animals it tends to antagonize the action of Meratran, i.e., it is a tranquilizing drug. In normal human subjects in substantial doses the drug is without discernible pharmacological effect. Fabing, however, has demonstrated that it readily inhibits the development of psychotic response to Lysergic acid diethylamide or reverses the response once it has occurred. On the basis of these experiments Frenquel has been used in the treatment of a wide variety of psychiatric conditions. There has been a wide divergence of opinion among investigators about its usefulness. Some have claimed excellent results with deliria and acute schizophrenia; others using small doses over longer periods have secured results in more chronic psychoses. The author has obtained poor results with all schizophrenics though admittedly has not given the drug over long periods. He has obtained results comparable to those achieved with chlorpromazine in some cases of toxic-confusional psychoses. The compound appears to be without side effects. Judgment must be withheld at this time.

The last drug to be reviewed is Meprobamate, otherwise known as Miltown or Equanil. Meprobamate is chemically related to Myanesin and has generally similar properties. It has, however, a longer duration of action, is less toxic and produces greater muscular relaxation and has some anti-convulsant action. While it has been described as a "tranquillizer" it has quite different effects from reserpine and chlorpromazine, and is without significant effect on the autonomic nervous system. In two published studies good results were noted in a variety of patients—mostly in the neurotic category. The author in a double-blind controlled study with 30 mixed neurotic patients has been unable to detect any significant improvement attributable to Meprobamate. It must be said, however, that several patients with symptoms of occipital tension and low back pain have responded to the drug very satisfactorily. A number of severely agitated psychotic depressions responded to Meprobamate in large doses by a lessening of agitation though the depressive affect was unaltered. Side effects include mild dermatitis and excessive sleepiness.

It would be premature to draw conclusions, but the author's present opinion is that Meprobamate has the same order of effect on psychiatric patients that barbiturates do with the addition of a more specific muscle relaxation. It should be useful in conditions associated with much muscular tension.

The science of predictably influencing human behaviour by the use of drugs influencing the central nervous system is making great strides. Experimentally we can produce and abolish psychoses at will. The substances discussed above are but the early forerunners of a whole host of compounds. The need for effective screening techniques, standardization of terminology and improved communication among psychiatrists is urgent.

We must not expect too much of these drugs for human behaviour is more than a biochemical process. Let us not, however, underestimate either their power to do good—and harm if given without due care.

Part Two

CLINICAL EXPERIENCE:

(A) IN PSYCHIATRIC DISEASE

USE OF THE TRANQUILIZING PROPERTIES OF RESERPINE

J. Campbell Howard, Jr., M.D., and Frank J. Vinci, M.D.

Pharmacology

The essential pharmacologic effects of reserpine (Serpasil), isolated and identified by the Ciba team of Mueller, Schlittler, and Bein, consist of two main properties: (a) the ability to decrease sympathetic nervous system activity and (b) the ability to tranquilize.

A characteristic of emotional turmoil is an overplay of the sympathetic nervous system, often causing tachycardia, pallor, clamminess, increase in blood pressure, and other similar symptoms. The same mechanism by which reserpine reduces blood pressure can alleviate these effects of hyperexcitement. With the decrease in adrenergic outflow, there may result a parasympathetic predominance that can account for some of the side effects of the drug such as cardiac slowing and increased bowel activity. Actually, some of these so-called side effects together with the sedative properties can be put to good use. These will be considered later.

The tranquilizing action of reserpine, allaying irritability and irritation, unlike that of the barbiturates or other hypnotics is not achieved by cortical depression. As a matter of fact, according to Rinaldi and Himwich, "reserpine produces an alert electroencephalographic pattern" whereas the "barbiturates induce a pattern of sleep." Thus, to explain this action, we must look further. "The chief central mechanisms through which emotional behavior is mediated are known to be located in the hypothalamus." From various studies it appears that the hypothalamus is involved. Schneider *et al.* have shown that the sham rage of a decerebrate cat can be controlled by reserpine.

Clinical Uses

Being accustomed to the general rule of specific medications for specific conditions, the broad indications for reserpine may make it sound somewhat like the famous old "patent remedy." However, the wide gamut of uses is not so far fetched as it may appear on first impression. There are very few illnesses that do not require emotional adjustment, and therefore, as will be shown, its wide prescription is logical.

Neuropsychiatric Application. True Psychoses. In view of the vast amount of studies reported in the literature concerning the role of reserpine in the treatment of disturbed psychotics, mental deficiency, and behaviour problems, the subject is only listed and will not be considered in detail.

PSYCHONEUROSIS. In this group of disorders, such as anxiety reactions, hysteria, or phobic reactions, the patient overreacts to various stimuli. Reserpine tones the reactions down, insulating the patient from his environment. This can be illustrated by the remarks of one of Wilkins' female patients: " 'I am not less ambitious, I'm not less aggressive, I'm not less effective. I just don't seem to *have* to do the things I used to. Before, I felt I had no control over myself. I *had* to do things. Now I don't care, I don't even notice things. Dust doesn't annoy me. Before, I knew it wasn't important, but I had to clean it up. Now I let it go for two weeks, and it doesn't bother me.'" A further practical use in this connection is in the patient with globus hystericus.

Clinical evidence indicates that reserpine should not be used in depression or depressive states except in those patients who are perhaps on the way out of a depression or withdrawal state, reaching the point where they are making some restitutive change. At this time their anxiety can be controlled so that they can devote more of their emotional drive to overcoming conflicts.

Dosage: The psychotic group requires large doses, usually starting with 5 mg. parenterally and increasing up to 10 mg. or more if necessary. Generally, 3 to 5 mg. is given at the same time by mouth, and after one to three weeks, oral medication alone (5 to 15 mg.) may be enough. For the neurotic, 0.1 to 1 mg./day will generally be sufficient.

These dosage recommendations do not constitute a hard and fast rule. The dose should be individualized according to the patient's response. Once maximum therapeutic effects are reached, as a general rule, the amount of medication should be reduced to the minimum that will maintain the desired effects.

Psychosomatic Medicine. Under this heading will be considered the conditions in which emotional tension may cause or aggravate physical symptoms, the control of which will usually lead to greater or more rapid improvement or better adjustment to the disability.

CARDIOVASCULAR SYSTEM DISORDERS. Hypertension: In the treatment of hypertension, besides its ability to reduce blood pressure by its effect on the sympathetic governing center, the sedative properties afford a means of helping the patient to worry less over his diagnosis, his business, or other problems that tend to aggravate or perpetuate hypertension.

Post-Coronary Occlusion: Anxiety, depression, and tachycardia are all frequent findings after a myocardial infarction. The use of reserpine causes the patient to relax, helping him to accept the disability, and also reduces the heart rate to a more normal pace. Angina pectoris might also be included under this category. Slowing of the cardiac rate allows more time for coronary filling. Decreasing the anxiety may also help lessen the attacks.

Rhythmic Disturbances: A common side effect of reserpine is cardiac slowing, due to a depression of the sympathetic nervous system and a resultant parasympathetic predominance exerted over the vagus pathways. Attacks of paroxysmal auricular tachycardia so frequently seen in high-strung persons can sometimes be prevented by the drug, but it has no place in the treatment of an acute attack. The anxieties caused by premature auricular and ventricular contractions may be lessened by the patient being made less conscious of them or by a reduction in their occurrence.

Neurocirculatory Asthenia: The so-called soldier's heart or man with the soiled shirt (from putting his hand over his heart) can be helped by both actions of reserpine.

Dosage: In these cardiovascular disorders, 0.1 to 1 mg./day has usually been sufficient. Once full benefits have been achieved, the dosage should be reduced to a lower maintenance level. Frequently 0.1 mg./day is enough even for the hypertensive.

FUNCTIONAL GASTROINTESTINAL DISORDERS. Functional gastrointestinal upsets, mucous and ulcerative colitis, are all closely tied to emotional disturbances and in many instances are caused by them. Reserpine's tranquilizing action has been found to be very helpful in preventing or decreasing the frequency and severity of these attacks. In spite of the fact that reserpine, due to vagal predominance, will increase gastric volume, acidity, and intestinal motility, apparently the sedative effect can more than offset these side effects in some instances. In other words, in many of these patients the psychic factors must play a major role. Antacid and anticholinergic medication such as oxyphenomium bromide (antrenyl) should be given together with reserpine, particularly during its use in functional upper gastrointestinal lesions.

DERMATOLOGIC CONDITIONS. There is no question that psychogenic factors greatly influence the progress of many skin diseases as well as causing them. Rein and Goodman, Genest *et al.*, and others have reported reserpine to be helpful in a variety of disorders such as chronic eczema, lichen planus, hyperhidrosis, neurodermatitis, urticaria, and some cases of psoriasis. It should not be considered specific therapy but an adjuvant, although where nervous factors are the prime cause, perhaps reserpine alone may clear up the lesions. Because it may take several weeks for the full effects of the drug to be obtained, immediate results cannot be expected. However, even after three or four days of treatment, pruritis may be dramatically relieved. Why it should be so helpful when itching is present is difficult to explain.

OBSTETRICS AND GYNECOLOGY. Reserpine may be helpful in all of the following conditions: premenstrual tension, dysmenorrhea, menopausal syndrome, frigidity, and nymphomania. For premenstrual tension and dysmenorrhea, reserpine should be taken for 10 days before the expected menses; for menopausal symptoms, continuously. Whatever the cause, the theories being numerous, there is little question about there being a state of tension in the premenstrual syndrome. In the menopause, there are anxieties and fears and in many patients a hyperreactive vascular system, all of which can be aided by reserpine.

Even though frigidity is the direct opposite of nymphomania, according to Greenblatt, reserpine is effective in either case. This can be explained in the following manner. The sexual response of the human female is tempered and influenced by many factors: psychogenic, anatomic, physiologic, and state of health. Whereas most men are in a constant state of frenzy, women, for the most part, demonstrate either a passive acceptance or a passive resistance. Few of them have that positive drive known as "libido." The frigid female does not enjoy marital relations because of latent or patent hostility for the "stronger sex" and refusal to accept a subordinate position. Her frigidity is, in fact, a form of pugnaciousness. With the administration of reserpine to 5 frigid women, libido per se as a positive force was not noticeably increased, but receptivity was so improved in 2 of them that they willingly accepted their mates. On the other hand, in 2 women with such nymphomaniacal tendencies as to prove disturbing to their husbands and to themselves, the sedating action of reserpine proved of decided advantage in lessening the constant urge. Reduction in the tension states causing these conditions brought the patients' responses to a more acceptable level.

WEIGHT GAINING. There is a general tendency for some patients on reserpine to gain weight. This actually can be put to good use. Many people without specific disease, characterized by Shakespeare's "lean and hungry look," as well as those with illness such as tuberculosis are emotionally high strung to a degree that it either affects their eating habits or makes them burn off what they eat. Calming the individual and reducing the expenditure of nervous energy allows him to relax, take time to eat, eat more, and not burn up calories so fast. For the tuberculous patient, in addition to helping him gain weight, reserpine can help him adjust to his disability.

Although no studies have been carried out, the sedative properties might help the overweight bulimic individual, who eats and eats because of emotional problems, lose weight by lessening his tensions and therefore his dependence on oral gratification.

HEADACHES. According to Barrett and Hansel, reserpine is effective in vascular types of headaches regardless of the basic mechanism involved. It is especially useful in the histaminic type, which is the most common of the vascular headaches. Friedman also reported that it has value in tension headache, particularly of the hypertensive variety, but has little effect on migraine. Of course, the use is prophylactic and the drug is not for acute cases.

BRONCHIAL ASTHMA. Pharmacologically, a sympathetic stimulation, as with the administration of epinephrine, to relax the constricted bronchioles is the general rule in treating the acute asthmatic attack, not the use of a sympathetic depressant such as reserpine. However, all who have had anything to do with asthmatics are cognizant of the role that emotional disorders play in triggering an asthmatic attack. Segal and Attinger reported that of 56 chronic bronchial asthmatics, 4 had less dyspnea and 22 were not as jittery or disturbed. Acute attacks were less severe and less prolonged and could be more easily relieved with standard measures.

Dosage: For all the above-listed conditions, a range of from 0.1 to 1.0 or 2.0 mg. of reserpine has been employed. Generally, once the full effects have been obtained, the dose can and should be reduced to a lower maintenance level. Because reserpine requires at least two to four days to begin to work, and up to four or more weeks to produce full effects, it makes no difference whether the total daily dose is given once a day or is divided—results are the same either way. The dosage for the remainder of the indications will be discussed under the specific use, as different amounts are required in these instances.

PEDIATRIC USE. High-strung, tense children and those with behavior disorders can be relieved by the tranquilizing action of reserpine. Since children tolerate the drug well, even fairly large doses (up to 5 mg./day or more) can be employed. The more disturbed the child, the larger should be the dose. Talbot reported that 29 per cent of 32 infants, 6 weeks to 1 year old, who were hyperactive, irritable, and had bizarre sleeping patterns were helped. On doses of 0.1 to 0.3 mg./day, there was complete remission of irritable behavior in 19 cases.

Enuresis in 16 of 17 children responded without other medication or fluid restriction. The single failure was found to have a duplication of one ureter. The average dose was 0.75 mg./day.

GERIATRIC USE. Both the so-called normal geriatric patient and the senile psychotic can be helped. In the former group, Ayd reported that on reserpine the geriatric patient adjusted better to his situation, both at home and in nursing homes, and could remain there instead of entering a psychiatric institution. Sainz, in a study of 750 ambulatory and hospitalized elderly psychotics, found considerable improvement in behavior and a lessening of quarrelsomeness, apprehension, and negativism. The dosage should be individualized depending on the severity of the symptoms and the response.

ALCOHOLISM. The unsatisfactory management of the acute alcoholic, particularly of his excitement, tremors, and hallucinations, with hypnotics such as paraldehyde is well known. For adequate sedation, the patient must be knocked out and he may develop pneumonia and urinary infections, become a nursing problem, and may become addicted to the hypnotic. Neuer, Avol and Vogel, Greenfield, and others, studying the tranquilizing properties of reserpine, found that such patients could be quickly brought under control, some within as few as nine hours and all within 48 hours. On an average, patients were symptom free in 24 hours. To obtain more rapid effects, one or two 2.5 to 5 mg. doses were given parenterally about three hours apart. A repeat parenteral dose was given the second and third day, if necessary; otherwise, 0.5 to 1 mg. of reserpine per day was given by mouth. Patients quieted down but were not forced to be bedridden as a result of heavy sedation. Greenfield treated 28 patients with a milder variety on an outpatient ambulatory basis, starting them with a parenteral dose of 2.5 mg. Later in his work he found that the addition of 10 mg. of oxyphenomium bromide three times a day by mouth was helpful in settling intestinal upset associated with the alcoholism. The dosage should be individualized for each patient and the drug used cautiously in patients on Antabuse or with cardiovascular problems. The blood pressure reduction may be greater in the latter groups. Several investigators have alluded to the possibility of long term therapy with reserpine by mouth, helping to lessen the emotional problems that lead to drinking and thereby aiding in rehabilitation. This would have to be combined with an adequate medical and Alcoholics Anonymous program. West, at the American Psychiatric Association Meeting in May 1955, reported success in 25, improvement in 7, and failure in 8 persons under such a program begun in January 1953, but to prove its value further, more extensive trials are needed.

HEAD INJURIES. The use of opiates and hypnotics in acute head injuries or post-craniotomies is not advisable because of the masking of vital signs such as pupillary size and respiratory rate by these drugs. Lambros and Steelman have both reported that when reserpine was used, vital signs were not masked and patients were not restless and could help themselves. Lambros also found that abnormal neurologic signs and symptoms regressed more rapidly and headache was negligible. "Ten patients with acute closed type of head injuries were given Serpasil 1 to 2 cc. (2.5 to 5 mg.) every 2 to 3 hours intramuscularly. No patients who were in shock were treated with Serpasil."

CONVULSIVE DISORDERS. Lambros and Barsa and Kline found the tranquilizing effect of reserpine helpful, not so much as a preventative, but more in terms of sedation and of aiding the patient to adjust to the difficulty. From 0.5 to 1.5 mg. of reserpine was given.

SIDE EFFECTS

Before giving any drug, one should have a knowledge of what it can do, how it works, and what side effects may occur. If it is recalled that reserpine decreases sympathetic nervous system tone, allowing parasympathetic predominance, many of the so-called side effects that are actually normal physiologic responses can be easily remembered, such as, nasal stuffiness, nausea, increased intestinal activity, cardiac slowing, and reduction in blood pressure (usually not below normal). Lethargy or tiredness can be explained on the basis of the tranquilizing action. Generally, most of these symptoms subside as therapy is continued. If they are bothersome, however, "side effects may be adequately controlled by reduction of dosage or by the addition of other drugs: lethargy—Ritalin; nasal stuffiness—antihistamines; jitters—lower dosage; nausea—Antrenyl." The development of a Parkinson-like syndrome or of the agitated behavior

TABLE I
Side Effects and Their Management

Side effect	Management
Nasal stuffiness	Topical vasoconstrictors such as naphazoline
	Antihistamines orally or topically such as tripelennamine
	Methyl-phenidylacetate may also help
Bradycardia	Usually not sufficient to be troublesome; lower dosage
Hypotension	Usually not a problem—bed rest and, if severe, *l*-arterenol
Gastrointestinal complaints	
Nausea or vomiting	Anticholinergics such as oxyphenomium bromide and antacids
Diarrhea	Reduce dosage—usually subsides without treatment
Lassitude and drowsiness	Methyl-phenidylacetate, 5 to 10 mg. 3 times a day; reduce dosage
Depression—usually preceded by agitation, insomnia, also a history of depressive tendency	Stop medication and methyl-phenidylacetate may be given
Side effects seen during psychiatric use—high dosage	
Turbulence and agitation (Kline turbulent phase)	Glutethimide, 0.5 to 1 Gm., may quiet patient (Barsa and Kline feel this is an important phase of therapy); some reduce dosage
Parkinson-like syndrome	Reduce dosage
Convulsive episodes	In psychotic patients occasionally they may occur during early weeks of therapy; handle on individual basis

TABLE II
General Indications and Dose Range

Indications	Daily dosage range
1. True psychoses	2.5 to 5 mg. intramuscularly plus 1 mg. twice a day orally
2. Psychoneurosis	0.25 to 1 mg. orally
3. Cardiovascular disorders	
a. Hypertension	0.5 to 1 mg. orally
b. Post-coronary occlusion	0.1 to 1 mg. orally
c. Rhythm disturbances	0.1 to 1 mg. orally
d. Neurocirculatory asthenia	0.1 to 1 mg. orally
4. Functional gastrointestinal disorders	0.1 to 0.5 mg. orally plus oxyphenomium bromide, 10 mg. 4 times a day
5. Dermatologic conditions	0.25 to 0.5 mg. orally
6. Obstetrics and gynecology	
a. Premenstrual tension	0.25 to 1 mg. orally
b. Dysmenorrhea	0.25 to 1 mg. orally
c. Menopausal syndrome	0.25 to 1 mg. orally
d. Frigidity and nymphomania	0.25 to 1 mg. orally
7. Weight gaining	0.1 to 1 mg. orally
8. Headaches	0.25 to 1 mg. orally
9. Bronchial asthma	0.25 to 1 mg. orally plus antiasthmatic therapy
10. Pediatrics	
a. Hyperkinetic children	0.2 to 5 mg. orally
infants	0.1 to 0.3 mg. orally
b. Enuresis	0.25 to 1.5 mg. orally
11. Geriatrics	
a. Normal geriatrics	0.25 to 1 mg. orally
b. Senile psychoses	3 to 5 mg. orally
12. Alcoholism	
a. Acute phase	2.5 to 5 mg. parenterally repeated in 3 hours if necessary
b. Chronic phase	0.5 to 1 mg. orally. The addition of oxyphenomium bromide, 10 mg. 3 times a day, is helpful in settling intestinal upset associated with alcoholism
13. Head injuries	2.5 to 5 mg. intramuscularly every 3 hours
14. Convulsive disorders	0.5 to 1.5 mg. orally

that is described by Kline as the turbulent phase of reserpine therapy is an effect that occurs on higher psychiatric dosage, such as 10 to 15 mg./day or more, when reserpine is given by the parenteral route and not when employed for the above conditions.

The most serious reaction that may occur is the onset of a depressive syndrome, as reported by Freis and others. In patients whose level of activity is lowered at the start of therapy, or who have a history of a depressive tendency, the drug should be used with caution, if at all. If one is to employ reserpine, low dosage should be used and an analeptic drug such as methyl-phenidylacetate hydrochloride may be given concomitantly. Ayd, Ferguson, and others have found that the latter counteracts the lethargy associated with reserpine therapy.

In several cases of reserpine-induced depression, Ferguson reported that "administration of phenidylate to these patients appeared to overcome the depression and clear the drowsiness sufficiently to permit an awakening-to-reality and some physician-patient contact." Ayd has not found this to be true. Further study will be necessary before the exact influence of Ritalin in reserpine-induced depression can be determined.

The development of insomnia, agitation (except in psychotics), or symptoms of mental depression, which are to be differentiated from lethargy or tiredness, calls for watchfulness on the part of the physician. The dose of reserpine should be reduced or discontinued. Some of the patients showing these signs have gone on to develop a depressive reaction.

Summary

1. The essential pharmacologic actions of reserpine, namely, the tranquilizing effect and reduction of sympathetic reactivity and parasympathetic nervous system predominance, are reviewed.
2. The uses of the tranquilizing effect in hypertension, post-coronary occlusion, rhythmic disturbances, neurocirculatory asthenia, true psychoses, psychoneurosis, functional gastrointestinal disorders, dermatologic conditions, obstetrics and gynecology, weight gaining, headaches, bronchial asthma, pediatrics, geriatrics, alcoholism, and head injuries are discussed.
3. The dosage recommendations for the above conditions are given.
4. Side effects, their significance, and their management are reviewed.

THE USE OF RESERPINE IN AN ACUTE PSYCHIATRIC TREATMENT SETTING

Garfield Tourney, M.D., Detroit,
Emil M. Isberg, M.D., Miami, Florida,
and Jacques S. Gottlieb, M.D., Detroit

Increasing attention is being given to the utilization of reserpine in the management and treatment of psychiatric disorders. This most potent single alkaloid derivative of the Indian plant Rauwolfia serpentina has been reported to be of value in the therapeutic approach to acute and chronic schizophrenia, depressed states, anxiety symptoms, agitation, obsessive thinking, disturbed behavior patterns associated with mental deficiency, toxic states, and chronic organic brain syndromes. The description of such applicability in this heterogeneous group of disorders merits repeated observation and study before conclusions concerning the efficacy of reserpine can be made. In this brief communication, experiences with the use of the drug under the conditions of an acute psychiatric treatment center will be described.

The Patient Population

In the acute psychiatric treatment setting patients are hospitalized because of relatively acute psychiatric disorders, or acute exacerbations of more chronic psychiatric illnesses. The majority of such cases are of acute or chronic schizophrenia, but a number of depressions, severe psychoneuroses, psychophysiologic disorders, character neuroses, and toxic and organic disorders are seen. The majority of the patients were initially treated as inpatients, but for others hospitalization was not definitely indicated or could be forestalled with treatment on an outpatient basis. Many of the patients were initially treated with reserpine after hospitalization, others in conjunction with psychotherapy or electrotherapy; but the greatest number were placed on the reserpine treatment after the failure of psychotherapeutic or somatic techniques. In those patients to whom the reserpine was given in conjunction with other therapies, an attempt was made to evaluate solely the effects of the reserpine in this study. All hospitalized patients participated in recreational and occupational therapy programs during the therapy with reserpine. No control series of patients was used in this study, and in the development of techniques for the administration of the drug no consistent dosage and method of application were used. Because of this, it must be admitted that the results of this study are largely impressionistic, but they do lead to certain definite conclusions regarding the therapeutic value of reserpine and the need for further investigation.

Method of Administration and Dosage

Patients with moderate to marked excitement and increased psychomotor activity were placed initially on relatively high doses of reserpine, usually 7 mg. or more of the drug per day. Usually 5 to 10 mg. of the drug was administered intramuscularly and supplemental oral medication given if the patient was cooperative. No more than 13 mg. of the drug was administered in any one day. This high dosage of the medication would be maintained until there was a reduction in the psychomotor excitement and other features of the disturbed symptomatology, or the appearance of moderate to severe toxic symptoms. The dose would then be gradually reduced, and the patient switched to the oral preparation of the drug, at a level for the maintenance of the improved state of the patient. This reduction could usually be begun in five to seven days and a maintenance level reached in approximately two weeks. If there was no remarkable change in the patient's symptoms in 7 to 14 days, the drug was often discontinued, and other accepted therapeutic methods were utilized to cope with the patient's difficulties. Patients who had previous therapy with failure were treated with reserpine in the same manner if the severity of their excitement and disturbed behavior was moderate to marked. Because of the nature of the hospital setting, patients could not be kept for prolonged studies while being treated with an experimental drug, and it is realized that many patients may have been inadequately treated because of this. However, it was thought that if the drug had any specific action on mental illness, this effect should begin to be apparent within the period of 7 to 14 days.

Patients suffering with mild to moderate overactivity and agitation, moderate to severe anxiety, bizarre thinking, and depressive symptoms were placed on moderate doses of reserpine, that is, 4 to 6 mg. per day. This was usually given orally, but on occasion was administered by the parenteral route.

Finally, those patients with mild psychomotor disturbances, symptoms of mild to moderate anxiety and depression, or bizarre thinking without associated agitation were given the drug in low dosage, that is, 1 to 3 mg. per day. Some patients have been treated for only short periods of time, and others have been followed on the medication for over six months. The continuation of therapy largely depended on the therapeutic results and the complications from treatment.

Complications of Reserpine

A number of side-effects of the drug have been reported. These include hypotension, bradycardia, fatigue, listlessness, somnolence, diarrhea, Parkinsonian syndrome, and others. In this study, the commonest complications evident were hypotension, weakness and fatigue, dizziness, nasal congestion, and drowsiness. A Parkinsonian syndrome developed in the treatment of seven cases. Four patients, all suffering from chronic undifferentiated schizophrenia, described a state of added apprehension over a feared loss of control of their impulse life and were resistant to further treatment with the drug. This reaction occurred after the ingestion of a relatively small amount of the drug, 3 to 6 mg., and cleared after therapy was discontinued. Two patients had allergic

TABLE 1.—*Complications of Reserpine*

	No. of Cases	Hypotension	Nasal Congestion	Flushing of Face	Weakness and Fatigue	Dizziness	Drowsiness	Parkinsonian Syndrome	Hypothermia	Depression	Loss of Control	Allergy	Diarrhea	Treatment Discontinued Because of Complications
High dosage (7 mg. or more)*														
2 wk. or less	21	15	5	1	8	4	4	2	0?	0	1	0	1	4
2-4 wk	8	6	2	0	2	1	1	2	1	0	0	0	0	0
1-2 mo	2	0	0	0	1	0	0	0	0	0	0	0	0	0
2-4 mo	2	1	0	0	2	1	0	0	0	0	0	0	0	0
4 mo. or more	5	3	3	1	4	2	4	1	0	1	0	0	0	0
Moderate dosage (4-6 mg.)*														
2 wk. or less	10	5	1	0	1	0	0	1	0	0	0	0	0	0
2-4 wk	6	3	1	0	2	0	1	0	0	1	0	0	0	0
1-2 mo	2	0	0	0	1	0	1	1	1	0	0	0	0	0
2-4 mo	2	1	0	0	0	0	0	0	0	0	0	0	0	0
4 mo. or more	0	0	0	0	0	0	0	0	0	0	0	0	0	0
Low dosage (1-3 mg.)														
2 wk. or less	10	1	2	2	3	1	1	0	1	0	1	2	1	5
2-4 wk	9	0	1	0	3	0	1	0	0	0	1	0	0	0
1-2 mo	10	0	2	0	0	0	3	0	0	0	0	0	1	0
2-4 mo	11	0	5	0	3	0	0	0	0	0	0	0	0	0
4 mo. or more	3	0	1	1	2	0	0	0	0	0	1	0	0	0
Totals	101	35	23	5	32	9	16	7	3?	2	4	2	3	9

* High and moderate dosages were usually maintained for less than two weeks, and then the dosage level was adjusted to a minimum for control of symptoms, this frequently being 3 mg. per day, but varying from 1 to 6 mg. a day.

responses after receiving only 2 mg. of the drug. In the first, there were erythema, edema, and intense itching of the palms and the soles, and in the second, a typical asthmatic attack. These reactions ceased after discontinuing the drug, but they were reproduced by a second administration of reserpine. Side-reactions were somewhat more noticeable in patients receiving a high dose of the drug, but no marked difference was evident. In two patients symptoms of a retarded depression occurred. Therapy was discontinued in nine cases because of the appearance of the complications. At first, we noted more alarm when complications occurred, and probably had a tendency to discontinue the drug too early, without reducing the dose initially to see whether the complications could be avoided by this procedure. The complications occurring and their relation to the dose of the drug are summarized in Table 1.

Results of Treatment

The drug was found to be of value as a tranquilizing agent, reducing agitation and overactivity, improving patient's responses to interpersonal stimuli, decreasing concern over and reducing the expression of delusions and hallucinations, alleviating anxiety and obsessive concern, and managing delirium. Essentially no effect was noted on depressive symptoms. In fact, several of the psychotically depressed had an intensification of their depression during the therapy.

Of the 58 schizophrenic patients studied, 27 showed no change, 11 demonstrated an improved hospital adjustment but required further hospitalization, 11 improved enough to be maintained outside the hospital, although many florid signs of schizophrenia remained (slight improvement), and 9 patients made a moderate recovery (moderate improvement) and were able to return to many of the responsibilities of work, home, and family. However, of the 20 discharged patients, 5 relapsed and required further treatment and hospitalization. Three of these patients relapsed while on the medication. The drug was effective only in the control of the secondary schizophrenic symptoms, such as agitation, restlessness, delusions, and hallucinations, and was found to produce no alteration in the primary symptoms of the disorder, mainly, the affective and associative disturbances characteristic of the illness. This amelioration of symptoms improves ward morale and fosters better personnel-patient relationships. Patients begin to socialize, and for the first time are able to verbalize

TABLE 2.—Results of Therapy with Reserpine

	No. of Patients	No Clinical Response	Improved Hospital Management	Slight Improvement— Dischargeable If Hospitalized	Moderate Improvement	Marked Improvement	Relapse Under Treatment	Treatment Discontinued Because of Complications
Schizophrenia								
Paranoid type, acute	12	4	1	2	5	0	2	1
Paranoid type, chronic	27	11	7	6	3	0	3	0
Catatonic type, acute	5	2	1	1	1	0	0	2
Simple type	1	1	0	0	0	0	0	0
Schizoaffective type	4	3	0	1	0	0	1	0
Chronic undifferentiated	7	5	1	1	0	0	0	3
Childhood type	1	0	1	0	0	0	0	0
Mental deficiency with psychosis	2	0	2	0	0	0	0	0
Psychoneurotic anxiety and related symptoms	22	8	1	12	1	0	?	2
Obsessive-compulsive neurosis	2	0	0	2	0	0	0	0
Alcoholic addiction	3	3	0	0	0	0	0	0
Involutional depression	4	3	1	0	0	0	0	1
Psychotic depressive reaction	1	1	0	0	0	0	0	0
Psychophysiologic headache	3	0	0	0	3	0	0	0
Acute brain syndrome	4	0	0	0	3	1	0	0
Chronic brain syndrome	3	0	1	0	2	0	0	0
Total	101	41	16	25	18	1	6?	9

some of their emotional difficulties in therapeutic interviews. Therefore, reserpine appears to be a valuable adjunct to supportive and psychotherapeutic programs.

Anxiety and related neurotic symptoms were relieved somewhat in the psychoneuroses and personality disorders, but there appeared to be no effect on the basic over-all psychoneurotic problem, and hence psychotherapy was necessary. The neurotic symptoms also frequently returned after two to four weeks of therapy, although the medication was continued. Obsessive preoccupation was markedly reduced in the two patients studied. The chronic anxieties and tensions of the alcoholic patients studied were not alleviated by the medication.

In the few cases of delirium and organic agitated states studied there was moderate improvement. The drug will probably be of great help in the management of the agitated senile and arteriosclerotic states.

Results of treatment with reserpine are summarized in Table 2.

Summary and Conclusions

One hundred one cases treated with reserpine were studied in the setting of an acute psychiatric treatment hospital.

The dosage and treatment technique were modified according to the clinical state of the patient. Patients severely disturbed with moderate to marked psychomotor activity were treated with high doses of reserpine (7 to 13 mg. per day), usually for 7 to 14 days. Those with mild to moderate overactivity or severe anxiety were placed on moderate doses of the drug (4 to 6 mg. per day). Patients with less severe symptoms than those in the above categories were treated with low doses of the drug (1 to 3 mg. per day). Modification of dosage was made according to the patient's clinical response and complicating side-effects of the drug.

Common complications of the reserpine therapy were hypotension, weakness and fatigue, dizziness, nasal congestion, and drowsiness. Other side-effects noted, of less frequency, were the Parkinsonian syndrome, feeling of loss of control, diarrhea, depression, and allergic responses.

The drug appears to be of definite value in the management and treatment of schizophrenia. Secondary symptoms of the illness are reduced or removed, but the primary process is still in evidence. However, this improvement fosters interpersonal contacts of a social and psychotherapeutic nature. Where previously a state of pessimism existed among ward personnel and physicians toward the schizophrenic patients, with reserpine, interests and enthusiasm for their treatment develop, which, in turn, undoubtedly play a very important role in the recovery of the patients.

Slight alleviation of anxiety and related neurotic symptoms occurs with reserpine, but this is frequently a transitory response, and the drug appears not to be a substitute for psychotherapeutic measures.

The drug has value in the alleviation and control of the disturbed behavior and other symptoms of acute and chronic brain syndromes.

This preliminary study indicates the need for more careful and controlled evaluation of the therapeutic efficacy of reserpine.

USE OF RESERPINE IN CHRONIC NON-DISTURBED PSYCHOTICS

James Boudwin, M.D.,
Veterans Administration Hospital, American Lake, Washington,

and Nathan S. Kline, M.D.,
Director, Research Facility, Rockland State Hospital, Orangeburg, N. Y.; Department of Psychiatry, College of Physicians and Surgeons, Columbia University, New York, N. Y.

A NUMBER of studies have presented convincing evidence that reserpine has brought about marked improvement in chronically disturbed psychotic patients. No systematic studies have been reported exclusively on hospitalized patients who were *not* markedly or moderately disturbed. The impression has arisen that disturbed patients do better than non-disturbed. To determine whether this was correct, 100 patients were selected from a chronic non-disturbed female ward and given a full course of reserpine treatment. The patients covered a multitude of diagnoses (as indicated in Table I), and age range was from 18 to 67 (see Table II for breakdown). The patients had been institutionalized up to 35 years (Table III) and present hospitalization was from less than 1 to over 23 years (see Table IV for breakdown).

It was felt that this study would also present an occasion to evaluate the effects of an analeptic drug, in this case desoxyephedrine, used in combination with reserpine. There were three purposes in administering the desoxyephedrine: first, we wished to test the hypothesis, still held by some, that reserpine acts beneficially because it is an "ordinary" sedative. The action of the desoxyephedrine would tend to counteract the reserpine if such were the case, and this sub-group would thus have poorer responses than those on reserpine alone; second, we felt it necessary to test the opposite hypothesis, i.e. whether patients receiving the two drugs showed therapeutically better results in terms of discharge rates from the hospital in comparison with those on reserpine alone; and third, we desired to determine whether desoxyephedrine relieved any of the lethargy, sleepiness, or other side effects which are fairly frequent in reserpine treatment. It was also of particular interest to determine the effect of desoxyephedrine on the side effects in view of the fact that two drugs, glutethimide (Doriden) and benztropine methanesulfonate (Cogentin) have been found useful for this purpose.

Subjects

Twelve of the original 100 patients were dropped during the course of the study for a variety of reasons. This included four transferred to other buildings, two discontinued at the absolute insistence of relatives, one who refused oral medication, and three patients in whom the general physical condition was poor before treatment and side effects during treatment were severe. Two pa-

TABLE I: Final Improvement Relative to Diagnosis

	Marked	Moderate	Slight	None	Total
Schizophrenia					
Paranoid	6	7	12	4	29
Catatonic	1	3	17	1	22
Hebephrenic	1	1	14	2	18
Mixed and Other	2	3	3	0	8
Sub-total	10	14	46	7	77
Manic-depressive mixed	1	—	—	1	2
Involutional paranoid	2	—	2	—	4
Other					
Primary behavior disorder	1	—	—	—	1
Alcoholism	1	—	—	—	1
Psychosis with cerebral embolism	—	1	—	—	1
Psychosis with epidemic encephalitis	—	—	1	—	1
Psychoneurosis, mixed	—	—	1	—	1
Total	15	15	50	8	88

tients manifested extremely severe cardio-vascular episodes while on treatment. It is still an open question as to whether reserpine either precipitated or contributed to these conditions. One of the cases terminated in death, but unfortunately autopsy permission was refused. The presumptive diagnosis was

TABLE II: Final Improvement Relative to Age

	Marked	Moderate	Slight	None	Total
10-19	1	0	1	0	2
20-29	1	3	6	1	11
30-39	7	5	19	3	34
40-49	2	6	11	4	23
50-59	3	1	5	2	11
60 +	1	1	4	1	7
Total	15	16	46	11	88

arteriosclerotic heart disease. The other patient had cardiac dilatation from which she is now completely recovered; she is also improved psychiatrically.

MEDICATION

The remaining 88 patients received 3 mg. of reserpine daily for the entire course of treatment. Almost all the patients received the oral medication for a full 15 weeks. The intramuscular medication was administered as follows: 5 mg. daily for the first 10 days, followed by 10 mg. daily for the next 14 days, and then 5 mg. for the next 14 days. There were some minor variations from this procedure of administration since, if side effects became too disturbing, the dosage was reduced. On the other hand, dosage was not reduced until

TABLE III: FINAL IMPROVEMENT RELATIVE TO LENGTH OF TIME SINCE FIRST HOSPITALIZATION

	Marked	Moderate	Slight	None	Total
Under 2 years	3	1	4	1	9
2 to 4 years	6	2	5	—	13
4 to 10 years	3	5	14	—	22
10 years or more	3	7	27	7	44
Total	15	15	50	8	88

the full course of treatment had been given even if the patient showed marked improvement.

The desoxyephedrine was given in doses of 5 mg. twice a day for the first 10 days, and was then increased to 10 mg. twice a day for the next 14 days. At the end of this period, one-third of the patients were continued on 10 mg. twice a day, a second third of the patients were reduced to 5 mg. twice a day, and the remaining third of the patients were discontinued entirely from the desoxyephedrine. This regime was maintained until the end of the test period.

EXPERIMENTAL DESIGN

The group of 100 patients were all started on combined reserpine and desoxyephedrine. A group of patients on this ward receiving reserpine alone in conjunction with a different project were used as controls during this period. At the end of 24 days, there remained 90 patients. These were divided into 3 groups of 30 each to test the effects of high, low, and no desoxyephedrine in conjunction with the reserpine.

SIDE EFFECTS

Desoxyephedrine reduced extra-pyramidal symptoms such as drooling, tremulousness, and many of the subjective complaints such as feeling of stiffness of muscles or joints. The general impression gained was that although these were less frequent and severe than with reserpine alone, the reduction was not as dramatic as seen with benztropine methanesulfonate or glutethimide. One distinct improvement was that the patients on desoxyephedrine, during

TABLE IV: Improvement Relative to Duration of Present Hospitalization

Duration of Hospitalization	Disturbed (150 patients) Markedly improved	Total	Non-Disturbed (88 patients) Markedly improved	Total
Under 1 year	9 (69%)	13	2 (40%)	5
1 to 3 years	14 (38%)	37	7 (27%)	26
3 to 5 years	5 (17%)	29	3 (30%)	10
More than 5 years	4 (6%)	71	3 (6%)	47
Average	21%		17%	

the period when they were on intramuscular reserpine, showed markedly less somnolence and lethargy, and were found less frequently stretched out or sleeping on benches or floor. After the intramuscular reserpine was withdrawn, there appeared to be no difference in reaction to oral reserpine between patients who were on high doses of desoxyephedrine, those on moderate doses, and those on none. The indication is, therefore, that the desoxyephedrine may be a useful adjunct of therapy during the period of administration of intramuscular reserpine, but it is probably not of significant help when the patient is on the oral dose alone.[1]

Therapeutic Results

The therapeutic response of the patient was not related to the administration of desoxyephedrine. Four of the patients on the high doses of desoxyephedrine and five of those receiving no desoxyephedrine during the maintenance period showed marked improvement, whereas six of the patients on low doses of desoxyephedrine showed this same degree of improvement. This, of course, pertains only to the reactions during the oral phase, since all of the patients received desoxyephedrine during the intramuscular phase.

In reviewing the results in respect to improvement of these non-disturbed patients as a group, ratings are used similar to those in earlier publications by our group. "Marked improvement" means ready for discharge, or discharged; "moderate," "slight," and "no change" are also used as previously indicated. In presenting the degree of improvement, it should be borne in mind that these patients were selected from a building housing 614 such females. The 48 most disturbed patients in the building had already been placed on a chlorpromazine-reserpine comparison project; another eight patients had been treated clinically, and are therefore not included in this study. The 100 patients selected originally for this project were chosen because they appeared on clinical grounds to be those with the best prognosis

---

[1] In ambulatory neurotic patients treated in private practice, the desoxyephedrine appears more effective. Whether this is due to differences of reaction related to diagnosis or to the lower doses of reserpine (0.1 to 4.0 mg.) has not been determined. There is evidence that lighter doses of desoxyephedrine may be more effective.

in this continued-care building. It is therefore cautioned that the results obtained on this group might not be obtained if 100 patients were selected at random from this same building.

Therapeutic Lag

Of the 88 patients, eight showed no change, 34 slight improvement, 38 moderate improvement, and eight marked improvement when evaluated during the final week of therapy. As we have noted elsewhere, there is not infrequently a therapeutic lag, i.e., patients who have shown only moderate improvement while on treatment will continue to progress after medication has been withdrawn. This is particularly true in the group of patients who, at the termination of therapy, appear to be apathetic, disinterested, and somewhat withdrawn from social participation. As the weeks pass, these patients become "reactivated," and not infrequently this continues until the patient is deemed well enough to leave the hospital. One month after the termination of active drug medication, the entire group was again carefully evaluated. One of the eight patients who had markedly improved had relapsed at the end of eight days (see Table V). Eight patients who were deemed only moderately im-

TABLE V: Changes in Improvement Relative to Disturbance at End of Medication and One Month Post-Medication

	Marked	Moderate	Slight	None	Total
Rarely disturbed					
Last week of treatment	5	19	15	4	43
1 month later					
Relapsed	1 →	4 →	0	0	—
Improved	— ←	5	1	0	—
Occasionally disturbed					
Last week of treatment	3	11	15	3	32
1 month later					
Relapsed	0	6 →	0	0	—
Improved	—	0	0	0	—
Semi-disturbed					
Last week of treatment	0	8	4	1	13
1 month later					
Relapsed	0	5 →	0	0	—
Improved	— ←	2	0	0	—
Total					
Last week of treatment	8	38	34	8	88
1 month later	15	17	48	8	88

proved at the end of the reserpine treatment continued to progress to such an extent that they were judged markedly improved and were approved for convalescent status. This brought to a total of 15 the number of patients approved for discharge from the hospital.

Age

As in previous studies, the therapeutic response was not significantly related to age. There is some tendency for patients in the 30-39 year age group to show a more favorable response than in some of the other groups. However, on a percentage basis those in the 10-19 and the 50-59 year groups did even better, so that the impression that age is an extraneous factor continues.

Diagnosis

The few organic cases did not do so well as the group average. Also, as in the disturbed patients, the paranoid and mixed schizophrenics did better than the hebephrenic and catatonic. The favorable response of some of the manic-depressives and involutionals are encouraging, but because of small numbers they cannot be said to be more than suggestive.

Duration Since First Hospitalization

As had been anticipated, the longer the time since initial hospitalization, the poorer the prognosis. However, almost 7% of the patients hospitalized over 10 years ago were markedly improved.

Length of Present Hospitalization

In a completely consistent manner, the shorter the duration of the present hospitalization, the better the prognosis. Since three years is generally regarded as a cutting point, it is significant that between 10% and 11% of the patients hospitalized this long were markedly improved.

Over-all Results

In summary, 17% of this group were markedly improved, contrasted with a group of 150 actuely disturbed patients where 21.3% were markedly improved. Since duration of hospitalization is a major factor in prognosis, the groups should be contrasted in each sub-group.

When it is considered that the patients on the non-disturbed ward were felt to have the best prognosis, whereas those on the disturbed ward were chosen because of management problems, it is probable that with comparable selection the differences might have been even more marked.

Conclusions

In respect to the questions raised in the opening paragraphs: 1) The addition of desoxyephedrine does not reduce the effectiveness of reserpine, 2) nor does it increase the therapeutic activity, and 3) it has usefulness in the management of subjective side effects, lethargy, and somnolence, particularly in the early stage of treatment when intramuscular reserpine is being used.

The results seem to bear out the general impression that disturbed patients have a somewhat more favorable prognosis (21% markedly improved) than the non-disturbed (17% markedly improved).

These patients were selected as having the best prognosis of those available in this building. In all, however, approximately 90% of the patients in each of the categories showed at least some noticeable degree of improvement.

In the month following treatment, one of the "rarely disturbed" relapsed, but five others improved from "moderate" to "marked," and one from "slight" to "marked." The other most notable shift was that whereas none of the semidisturbed had improved immediately following treatment, two of 13 became markedly improved.

Evaluation of results must be by categories graded according to duration of hospitalization, since prognosis is directly related to this factor. Age can be ignored as a bearing variable and diagnosis is of secondary importance. Organic cases, including lobotomies, as a rule do not do so well as other types of patients. Among the schizophrenics, the paranoid and mixed types have the best prognosis.

Discussion

Now that experience has been obtained with both disturbed and non-disturbed chronic patients, some estimate can be made of the probable effect[2] on the total mental hospital population. Both groups (disturbed and non-disturbed) have shown up to seven percent improvement, even among the chronic patients. Allowing for some relapse, it appears that a minimum of five percent of the chronic mental hospital population of the country could be discharged if adequately treated with reserpine and/or chlorpromazine in conjunction with adequate clinical care. In the future, there is the likelihood of new pharmaceutical products which may advance this percentage still farther.

Summary

1. A group of 88 chronic non-disturbed patients were treated with reserpine. The results were significant (91% improved, of whom 17% were improved enough for release). The number of discharges, however, is less than for the disturbed patients (21% released). This is also generally true when duration of hospitalization is equated for the two groups.

2. The addition of desoxyephedrine to the regimen reduced subjective side effects and kept the patients from extremes of lethargy during the intramuscular phase of treatment. In the later phases of treatment, a control group on reserpine alone did as well as the two test groups who were on reserpine plus low or high doses of desoxyephedrine.

3. Desoxyephedrine did not nullify the effects of reserpine treatment, which would indicate that the "active principle" is not primarily a sedative one in the usual sense. On the other hand, although it helped with side effects, it did not agitate the patients in a manner that improved their prognosis.

4. The present study calls attention to a most important factor—the

---

[2] The responsibility for these estimates are those of N. S. K. alone.

therapeutic lag. Eight of the 15 patients eventually ready for discharge did not begin their most marked improvement until after the drug had been withdrawn. There is evidence that this was more than a continuation of prior improvement.

OBSERVATIONS DURING THE TREATMENT OF 175 PSYCHOTIC PATIENTS WITH RESERPINE

By Rudolf B. Freund, M.D.

In October 1954, reserpine therapy was started at Utica (N. Y.) State Hospital. Since that time, 175 male patients, suffering from all types of the major psychoses, have been treated. The indications for treatment were based on signs and symptoms rather than diagnoses. Disturbed behavior and destructiveness, motor hyperactivity or catatonic stupor, un-co-operativeness, and paranoid attitude were the absolute indications. Included, were a few extraordinary morbid conditions, such as Huntington's chorea, multiple sclerosis, mental deficiency and physical conditions due to trauma, in which attitude and behavior justified treatment under relative indications. Statistical evaluation still appears inappropriate because the figures in the different groups are too small, and the observation period is too short. The method of treatment, developed by trial and error, coincides fundamentally with the one described and recommended widely in the literature, principally by N. S. Kline, and his coworkers. The three stages observed in the course of treatment with reserpine generally, as described by Barsa and Kline, can be confirmed as occurring only in patients who do not suffer from an organic involvement or who have not been subjected previously to extensive courses of physical treatment.

All of the side effects, already described by others, can be confirmed and could be eliminated either by temporary reduction of the doses or by short temporary interruption of the course of application from three to six days.

The impression was gained that different brands of reserpine had possibly a different incidence of untoward side effects, an observation difficult to understand if one assumes that one deals with a pure, homogeneous alkaloid. However, similar observations, depending on the technics of the different manufacturers, occurring in specific fractions of digitalis will be remembered. If this observation should be confirmed, a rigid standard of pharmacologic testing and manufacturing may become necessary.

When the course of treatment was temporarily interrupted, it was usually observed that a new impulse was added to the effect of the drug. It was the writer's impression that the response to the treatment was enhanced thereby and that improvement occurred more suddenly. If this observation, made in individual cases, continues to be valid, it may prove that a phase-treatment (treatment in phases) with short intermissions is a preferred method for certain cases.

It is agreed upon by all authors engaged in pharmacological research as well as in clinical observation of the effect of reserpine (and also of chlorpromazine) that, for the first time, drugs are under investigation which touch off reactions in psychotic patients not observed previously with drugs or any other method of treatment. The physiological work of Cannon and Ranson, of Penfield and especially W. R. Hess, conducted independently from consideration of the reserpine effect, and the *ad hoc* studies of the research teams of Ciba and Squibb have laid down the fundamentals for speculations as to how reserpine might interact in the complex mechanism which determines the functioning of the emotional and affectual spheres. Should the neurophysiologic research which is going on at the present time prove that a precisely defined chemical agent acts directly on specific structures in the hypothalamic area, then a complete reorientation will occur in the conception of the psychiatric disorders now called functional.

The observation of Barsa and Kline, that the patients who respond favorably to reserpine treatment usually pass through three successive stages of behavorial and emotional changes, seems to be fundamental. Patients first enter a sedative phase, from which they go into the turbulent stage, during which specific psychotic manifestations and secondary symptoms, such as hallucinations and anxiety, become more pronounced. This second phase is especially important, because it reveals more frankly underlying or hidden psychotic material, the knowledge and understanding of which opens the future path to the indispensable psychotherapy. During this stage, possible suicidal trends might become extremely active and require close supervision. Entering the third, the integrative phase, the patient is accessible to and requires psychotherapy, which will help essentially to bring the reserpine treatment to a success. One must emphasize that the reserpine treatment *per se* does not heal a mental illness, but may enable us to apply psychotherapy successfully.

During reserpine treatment, specific actions of the drug could be observed:

One, seen in a few outstanding cases of manic-depressive psychoses of the manic type, could be called a "normotonic action," to indicate that the drug can change the psychodynamic "tone." Psychodynamic tone may be considered to be the specific state of mind of an individual as it appeared to observers in his individual setting prior to his break with reality.

A patient (A. M.), 74 years of age, had his first admission to Utica State Hospital in 1909 and his fourth (present) admission in 1947. He was diagnosed as manic-depressive, manic type, and is the prototype of a manic patient. This patient has destroyed, over the years, more state property and has been involved in more fights than any other individual patient in the hospital. He was full of mischief, obscenity and profanity and expressed them happily in an extraordinarily noisy and aggressive way, being in full contact and oriented at all times. In his overactivity and appearance, in the absence of somatic symptoms or signs appropriate for his chronological age, he gave the impression of a man in the late 50's until he was started on reserpine treatment in October 1954. He went through all the three stages; and, six weeks after the start of the treatment, he was a different person. He had been, as just described, a typical manic and is now a quiet, very co-operative, well-behaved, clean man appearing and acting his chronological age. The "normotonic" transformation has occurred. He asked to be transferred to a ward where he would not hear other patients' profane or obscene language, of which he now complained. He wanted to stay where it was quiet, and where a man of his age could quietly spend his evening of life. This patient is today comfortable and uncomplaining, lives on an old men's ward and receives a maintenance dose of 0.1 mg. reserpine daily. This case may serve as a typical example for five similar cases of manic-depressive psychosis, manic type, of long standing in whom the normotonic action was observed. Two of these patients, for whom adequate arrangements could be made, have left the hospital on convalescent care status and are adjusting well on a normotonic level.

In schizophrenic patients, especially those with catatonic or paranoid symptomatology, mainly those whose illness are of not too long duration and who have had no, or not more than one, course of physical treatment, the action of reserpine appears to be different. It is like the breakdown of the glass wall behind which the schizophrenics live their own lives unconcerned about the outside world, haunted by their fantasies and dreams or happy with their autisms. As soon as they enter the "integrative stage" with reserpine, they become eager to establish contact again with the world they escaped after clashing with major or minor problems. There is no such pouring-out of information as was seen during the war when elicited by amytal or pentothal, in the acute breakdowns. The reaction is rather eagerness for companionship, the craving of the immature or early-arrested personality to re-establish interpersonal relationship. It resembles a "healthy" attitude, a "fresh-air-breathing" mood, which is both expressed and shown. It seems like a waking-up after a hibernating sleep when these patients want to stretch their limbs, and want to put to work the resting energies that they are suddenly aware of. In the history of this hospital, so many patients have never before volunteered for work and physical activities. They look forward to, and ask for, interviews; they behave congenially toward the personnel and toward other more unfortunate patients for whom they show an unusual sympathy. One could call this action of the treatment the cathartic one in order to emphasize the change from the foggy-turbulent condition in which the schizophrenic patient lives.

Still another effect of reserpine, which is not necessarily essential for its psychiatric use, but which seems to be significant for the circulatory system, can be observed clinically. The remarkable absence, or rarity, of undesirable accidents caused by sudden hypotension seems to be the result of an effect of the drug on the diastolic, rather than on the systolic, blood pressure, with the establishment of a pulse pressure more beneficial to the circulatory functioning than in the latter case. Rauwolfia serpentina apparently shares this faculty with another species of the same Apocynaceae family, the Nerium oleander, from which is derived an excellent drug, oleandrin, which, in the absence of more familiar drugs, gained special significance and appreciation during the last world war. Being more accessible than Rauwolfia serpentina, the Nerium oleander might help to lead to new sources of drugs which contain the reserpine principle.

After the introduction of reserpine treatment, electric shock and insulin treatment could be eliminated entirely from the author's service. So far, they have not been missed, even in a service of 900 patients with an average monthly transfer rate of 21 patients from the admission service. There seems to be, however, no contraindication—in the future course of development of the drug treatment—to the interpolation, in selected cases, of single symptomatic shock treatments.

A major problem arose soon after the initiation of reserpine therapy when, on a single ward, a whole group of disturbed patients, simultaneously started on the treatment, changed uniformly in a very short time. The "old hands" among the attendants became bewildered at the unusual change of "mood climate" on the ward. They became suspicious and soon—when the turbulent phase set in—an attitude one might call relief prevailed. They said: "You see, we were right. We have seen that before, it was only the sedation!" The writer started weekly conferences at that time with the entire personnel, in the beginning giving formal informative lectures. These were soon changed to informal round table conferences; and the writer believes today that these are indispensable. A new spirit developed, and a previously unknown, congenial, teamwork atmosphere spread. The nurses and attendants felt suddenly that their observations and detailed information about changes occurring in patients had become an essential and integrative basis for the continuation of a therapeutic program which could change an "institution" into a "hospital."

The personnel of the social service department and those of the occupational and recreational therapy departments requested individual and specific briefings on the new developments which reflected on their particular activities and relations with the patients. An entirely new and enthusiastic spirit swept through the hospital, penetrating into each branch, including the administrative and business offices. An enormous amount of additional work and planning was necessary. It was not always easy to satisfy the demands for the new drug, and problems of supply and demand still arise today, with a reorientation of budgeting. It reminds one of the logistic work of staff officers during World War II (when new weapons suddenly outmoded great supplies and made new provisions imperative). In a great centralized system like the state mental hospitals, such sudden changes involved a great amount of work and planning which can only be done successfully if there is enthusiasm.

The main burden of work on the hospital level must be carried by the ward personnel, if this new approach to the treatment of mental diseases is to become completely successful. Valuable information is gained from the nurses and the attendants during the routine informal conferences. A competition began in the writer's service among the wards as to which had more patients on treatment and as to who could give the most pertinent information about treatment conditions. While previously, a worker did not care too much about which ward he might be stationed on, or about how often changes were necessary, an identification with a specific ward could now be noticed, and pride would be expressed about results and changes in the ward atmosphere. The ward personnel of the previous "disturbed" ward—where the program started—resented this "disturbed" classification and asked to be called the "active treatment group" because, "It discriminates against our ward and frightens or annoys our patients and their visitors." The ward physicians have learned to know the nurses and attendants from entirely different angles; and the beneficiaries of the mutual better understanding and appreciation are—again—the patients. It seems true that a new classification and organization of the wards will become necessary. The big unwieldy wards of 80 and more patients, where patients have been assembled according to their need of supervision are becoming more and more inconvenient. Smaller units are urgently required, where one can let patients live according to their stages of treatment. This program would have more in mind than formerly the purpose of rehabilitation and the specific interests and abilities of patients and ward personnel. On this reorientation in the set-up of the mental hospital will depend to a great extent the success or failure of the new treatment.

Rehabilitation rather than plain occupation must gain greater importance in the occupational therapy program. The integrated patients themselves come forward with suggestions, and many are eager to perfect their hobbies into adaptable occupations for the time when they are ready to leave. This may involve re-evaluating the worth of recreational activities. One cannot help observing that these may take too much time in the day's routine. Recreational activities may have to be integrated as privileges, as relaxing measures after a good week's rehabilitating work.

Of course there have been failures in treatment. The writer believes that patients who have previously had several courses of physical therapy or have undergone lobotomy without success do not go successfully through the three reserpine stages. There were others for whom the writer's indication of reserpine treatment was wrong and who later responded better to chlorpromazine. Experiences with mental defectives and with epileptic patients are still not very encouraging. However, the observation period is too short and the number of treated cases in these groups too small for adequate judgment. As of now, the opinion of the personnel is divided with regard to these groups. Much still has to be learned in regard to proper indications and in regard to dosage, to bring the new treatment to full success.

Three major factors appear to the writer to be of a foremost importance in paving the way for successful reserpine treatment in mental hospitals: (1) creating a harmonious therapeutic team, closely knit and uniformly trained and inspired, comprising all branches and levels of personnel; (2) following up the slightest signs of arising initiative in patients and guiding it into rehabilitating activities: (3) providing more time for direct psychotherapeutic activities by the psychiatrists, by relieving them of the growing burden of clerical work (performed more cheaply, more efficiently and quickly, by administrative assistants taken from the clerical secretarial ranks).

Summary

One hundred seventy-five patients have been treated with reserpine in Utica State Hospital since October 1954. Indications for treatment were not based on diagnosis, but on signs and symptoms. Disturbed behavior and destructiveness, motor hyperactivity, catatonic stupor, unmanageability and un-co-operative behavior were the absolute indications. Only a few extraordinary conditions, such as Huntington's chorea, multiple sclerosis, mental deficiency and physical traumatic condition were considered justifiable as relative indications for treatment.

Statistical evaluation appears inappropriate because the numbers in the different groups are too small and the observation period too short. Clinical and other personal observations, however, are:

1. A specific action of reserpine seems to occur in the regulation of the psychodynamic tone of patients with manic-depressive psychosis. This partial action may be called the "normotonic" effect and may be considered a static function.

2. Another partial function of reserpine appears to occur in some schizophrenic patients. This function lies in a different category and can possibly be called the activating function—in contrast to the static effect—because the schizophrenic patients are activated, after going through a turbulent phase, to step out of their own world of unreality into the moving world of contacts, interpersonal communication and initiative. One might call this the cathartic function, thinking of catharsis in the analytical interpretation.

3. Another effect of reserpine can be observed, not necessarily an essential one for its psychiatric use, but one significant for the circulatory system. The remarkable absence or rarity of undesirable side effects like orthostatic hypotension, fainting or similar circulatory accidents, seems to be the result of an affect on the diastolic rather than on the systolic pressure, depending on an action on peripheral resistance. This establishes a pulse pressure more beneficial to circulatory functioning than in the alternative case. This effect of Rauwolfia serpentina may be called a normotensive action, comparative to the action observed in other cardio-circulatory drugs deriving from the Apocynaceae family.

4. Electric shock and insulin coma treatment can be eliminated entirely. They have not been missed so far in a service of over 900 patients, with an average monthly transfer rate of about 21 patients from the admission service.

5. Efforts toward reorientation of nurses and attendants become indispensable. These require the special attention and activity of the physicians. Regular conferences with informative lectures and informal round table talks have become a regular routine. A new and closer contact between physicians and ward personnel and also a stronger contact with the other branches of therapeutic activities have been established. An entirely new spirit of enthusiasm and psychotherapeutic approach has resulted.

6. On the administrative level of our hospital system, a different attitude will have to prevail in order to carry to success the many new problems following the introduction of reserpine. Selection of personnel will have to take into account the fact that persons will be needed who are able and willing to work with—rather than merely watch over—the patients. Occupational therapy must extend into a rehabilitation program with adequate diversified facilities. Recreational activities will have to be integrated as relaxing measures after a full week of rehabilitation work. Recreational activities should again become a privilege, instead of being a substitute for the kind of meaningful work that guides a patient toward normal extrahospital life.

7. The old large wards will have to be split up into smaller units. They

should be filled with patients according to their stages of improvement and rehabilitation, and of their mutual personal relations. Small wards will serve better the needs of the patients for the establishing of interpersonal relationships.

8. Reserpine treatment is unsuccessful in patients who have had previous courses of physical therapy or who have undergone lobotomy without success. It seems to have only individual effect in selected cases of epileptics or mental defectives. Only tranquillizing results were obtained in organic cases.

Acknowledgment

Supervisor, nurses and attendants deserve the special thankful appreciation of the writer. Only their co-operation, understanding and untiring willingness to undertake additional work and responsibilities carried the reserpine program to a success. It is not possible to name every member of the team, who shared equally in the work, but the writer wishes to express his special thanks to Messrs. J. McHugo, T. Murphy, H. Blakely, L. Darmody and J. Higgins, as representatives.

RESERPINE IN THE TREATMENT OF PATIENTS WITH CHRONIC MENTAL DISEASE: A CONTROLLED STUDY

Lawrence Koltonow, M.D.

The chronically ill mental patient who requires close supervision but is still not badly deteriorated constitutes a growing problem in state mental institutions. In view of the many optimistic reports, the present study was undertaken to determine the value of oral reserpine in these patients. We began without a preconceived plan or goal.

The study was performed on a ward of patients requiring close supervision in view of histories of dangerous or potentially-dangerous acts. All were considered to be security risks, and only rarely was a patient moved to a more comfortable or a more deteriorated ward.

Of a total of 82 patients, 79.5 per cent had been hospitalized for from two to eight years; 22.5 per cent, over six years. Three-quarters had a diagnosis of schizophrenia, and two-thirds of these were paranoid type. Only a few were well enough to receive recreational therapy, and few were visited or taken out of the hospital for visits.

Procedure

Behavior during successive periods on varying doses of drugs was carefully noted. The hospital pharmacist arbitrarily separated the patients into two groups, one of which received placebo tablets during the entire period of study. Although differences between drug and placebos soon became obvious due to drug effects, the attendants were not informed which was which. Medication was given each morning after breakfast, and the dosage altered for all patients simultaneously.

The patient's charts were all reviewed before the study was started. All the patients were interviewed before instituting treatment, frequently during treatment, and at the end of treatment. The impressions of the physician and attendant were noted at each interview. At the end of treatment, the daily ward and nurses reports were examined and evaluated as to recorded changes on the ward and on an individual basis. In general, the observations were twofold: one, specific patient behavior, and two, general ward behavior.

The dose was raised and lowered as follows: 2 mg. for 1½ weeks; 3 mg. for 2 weeks; 4 mg. for 5 weeks; 5 mg. for 6 weeks; 4 mg. for 1 week; 3 mg. for 1 week; 2 mg. for 1 week; 1 mg. for 5½ weeks. There were a few breaks in the consistent administration of the drug. A group of patients which developed clinical Parkinsonism were placed on placebo, later were given the drug again. Also, two known epileptics were given reduced dosage. One patient of the 82 refused the medication for a short time. One patient became very disturbed and had to be transferred to a seclusion ward, removing him from the study.

RESULTS

We observed somewhat the same sequence of responses that has been reported previously, that is, sedative stage, turbulent stage and stage of integration.

At about the third to fourth week while on 3 mg. a day, the patients were noticed to be "more forceful" in expressing themselves. There were many challenges for fights, but fewer fights than normal.

At the seventh week, on 4 mg. a day, we had a period where the food consumption doubled on the ward. The patients gained weight very rapidly. There were more fights, but of less intensity. Near the eighth to ninth weeks, their weights generally started to revert to normal although the drug was not decreased.

At the ninth to tenth week, on 5 mg. a day, we first noticed clinical Parkinsonism in *five* patients, with typical mask-like fascies and cogwheel rigidity. The medications for these men were changed to placebo, and all their symptoms soon disappeared. Later, more men showed the same symptoms, but they were continued on the drug. As the dosage was lowered, their symptoms also disappeared. The original five men were again placed on reserpine after their Parkinsonism disappeared, and again they developed the same symptoms. However, as the drug dose was lowered and eventually stopped, their symptoms also disappeared.

About the eleventh or twelfth week, still on 5 mg. a day, we were especially aware of increasing sociability on the patients' part. The patients who had not talked with the ward doctor or attendant in years would engage in conversation. Fights now decreased in number. After 5 weeks on 5 mg., we began decreasing the dosage rather rapidly. The ward became more restless and noisy. Some patients who were improved seemed not to be affected by the decrease in dosage, some required maintenance of 1 to 3 mg. a day to prevent regression.

After five and a half months, the experiment was stopped completely. There were signs that the ward would revert to pre-control behavior. The most improved men were moved off and given jobs. Some patients who showed signs of improvement, as noted above, were restarted on the medication.

The general feeling was that the drug made the ward quieter and the patients much easier to handle.

Patients were divided into three major groups: improved, no change, or worse. The improved were qualified as Grade I, II, and III. Grade I improvement meant that the patient showed only minimal improvement such as being less combative or resistive or quieter. Grade III meant that the patients were well enough to be given a job and possibly transferred from the ward. Grade II was somewhat in between, that is, they showed marked improvement but were not well enough to hold a job.

Of the 41 patients who received reserpine, 24 showed improvement (58%), 16 showed no change, 1 was worse. Of the 24 showing improvement, 11 of these showed Grade I, 6 showed Grade II, 7 showed Grade III. Of those on placebo, 2 showed improvement, 35 showed no change, and 2 were worse. Of the 2 showing improvement, one was Grade I, one was Grade III.

A breakdown into diagnoses showed that of the 32 schizophrenics receiving reserpine, 19 showed some improvement. Eight of these were Grade I, 6 were Grade II, and 5 were Grade III. A majority of the schizophrenics were paranoid type. A breakdown into types of schizophrenia and improvement showed that 50 per cent of the paranoid schizophrenics were improved. Three out of three (100%) catatonics were improved, 4 out of 4 (100%) simple schizophrenics were improved, and 3 out of 4 (75%) hebephrenics were improved. Five of the patients on the drug were diagnosed as mentally deficient with psychosis. Three of these showed improvement.

One of the remarkable differences noted was that of weight change during therapy. The patients gained weight, some very rapidly, while the dosage was increased and later lost weight with continuation of drug. The average weight gain of those on reserpine was 10.6 pounds as contrasted to 3.2 pounds for those on placebo.

The average age of those showing improvement was 38.4 years, the remaining patients average 47.8 years.

Side Effects

The most pronounced side effects were flushing, agitation, stiffness of legs, swelling of the face, aching of the legs and tremor. Of those on reserpine, 27 per cent complained of walking difficulty due to stiffness of the leg while 14 per cent complained of aching of the legs. It might be speculated that these were premonitory symptoms of clinical Parkinsonism. All the side effects disappeared when the drug was stopped or markedly decreased.

Interpretation

We feel that the results showed that in a group of mentally ill patients who require constant close supervision, reserpine produced significant behavioral improvement as contrasted to placebo. Of the 41 patients on the drug, 58 per cent improved; 17 per cent improved enough to be able to be transferred off the ward and given responsible work assignment. In view of the above statistics we might speculate as to areas where the drug would be of value. First is that the ward would be easier to supervise and therefore produce more efficient attendant care. Secondly, patients who otherwise seem to show no hope might respond enough to work or even be discharged from the hospital.

The gain in weight, we believe, is significant and might be a prognostic aid in evaluating the effect of reserpine.

We would like to comment on what can be called a "therapeutic paradox." When we asked the attendant to evaluate the progress of the patient, he often stated the patient was worse. When asked why, it was reported that the patient became disobedient, more restless, more talkative, and more of a nuisance. From the attendant standpoint, the patient was worse. However, we saw, as the study continued, that these were the first signs of improvement. It was as if the shell of schizophrenic autism and withdrawal was being weakened and the patient was re-entering the world of reality. He no longer would sit quietly in a chair most of the day, but would reach out for more human contacts. This often led to fights as we noted in the study. For example, one patient paced back and forth almost continuously and, for a time, was difficult to control on the ward. Later he was improved enough to be transferred to a very comfortable ward and is now holding a job. The first signs of improvement and therapeutic effect often make ward management and attendant work more demanding.

Certainly, the attendants should be oriented as to this phase so that they will not be disturbed. During our study, it became evident that the success or failure depended to a good measure on the complete cooperation of the attendants.

Summary

The results of a five and a half month control study on the use of oral reserpine in a close supervision ward show the drug to be definitely pharmacologically active and effective in influencing patient behavior. Ward behavior was quieter and more easily managed. Some patients improved enough to be transferred to more comfortable wards and were given work assignments. In view of the above findings, the possibility of routine administration to all chronically ill patients could be considered.

RESERPINE IN HOSPITALIZED PSYCHOTICS: A CONTROLLED STUDY ON CHRONICALLY DISTURBED WOMEN

Arthur Lemon Arnold, M.D., and Harry Freeman, M.D.

A voluminous literature has accumulated on the efficacy of reserpine in mental disorders, particularly in psychoses accompanied by uncontrolled behavior. As yet few reports have included double-blind controls with a published breakdown of the specific areas of clinical change. Hollister found the dosage to be the most influential factor in a series of studies using varied doses, with the results expressed in terms of hospital adjustment. Hoffman and Konchegul, Campden-Main and Wegielski, and, more recently, Sommerness, Forster, and Cowden reported similar studies.

The present study was intended primarily to determine an effective dosage of reserpine in chronic disturbed schizophrenic women, using a double-blind technique, for comparison with the effect of administering placebos and of giving no medication at all.

It was hypothesized that in adequate dosage reserpine will effect tranquilization of chronically disturbed psychotic women. In order to test this, it was necessary (1) to control the effects of suggestion on the patients, nurses, and physicians; (2) to control the reflection of general improvement in the ward environment on the patients in the study; and (3) to record accurately many details of behavior.

Present Investigation

Experimental Design.—On the ward in which are treated the women who are the most disturbed (in terms of difficulty of hospital management—combative, destructive, denuditive, smearing, self-mutilative), those who were in psychotherapy or who were receiving electroshock therapy, who had had frontal lobotomies, or who consistently refused oral medications were excluded from the study but were retained on the ward. It was felt that results with lobotomized patients might not be applicable to patients whose brains were anatomically intact. Of more than 90 patients, all but 28 were thus excluded, and these 28 were studied (by the project observer, A. A.) for three weeks, after which ratings on a modified Malamud-Sands Worcester Rating Scale were made of their behavior. Observations were thus systematically recorded for (1) neatness of appearances, (2) level of motor activity, (3) expressivity

TABLE 1.—*Means and Ranges of Variables Used in Matching Patients for Reserpine, Placebo, and Nontreated Groups*

Variables	Reserpine		Placebo		Nontreated Group	
	Mean	Range	Mean	Range	Mean	Range
Age	44.6	23-66	52.2	34-67	44.3	29-58
Years in hospital	13.9	2-44	16.1	7-42	14.6	2-32
Baseline behavior score	50.0	17-73	50.5	27-75	44.3	28-69

of face and gesture, (4) flexibility of responses, (5) control of hostility, (6) socialization (with disruptiveness and inaccessibility as extremes), (7) control of attention, (8) amount of speech, (9) level of mood, (10) quality and (11) demonstrability of feelings, (12) accuracy of perception, (13) logicality of thought, (14) defensive position (with omnipotence and nihilism as extremes), and (15) accuracy of self-evaluation. These 28 patients were then assigned (by the project administrator, H. F.) to one of three groups matched as to age, length of time since first hospitalization, and severity of disorder, as indicated by the base line rating scores. From Table 1 it may be seen that the matching was done rather accurately. One group of 10 patients was assigned to receive reserpine tablets; the second group of 10 was designated to receive identical placebos, and the third group of 8 was to receive no medication. The group to which any patient belonged was not known to the observer. For the duration of the study, no other therapy was given.

Method. At intervals of approximately two weeks the observer recorded a behavior rating of each patient, in the scoring of which a numerical increase indicates greater abnormality. The reserpine dosage (all oral) was controlled by the administrator and was known only to him, the dose being the same for all patients in the reserpine group. At the start, 1.5 mg. of reserpine was given daily, and this was increased at 5 weeks to 3.0 mg., at 7 weeks to 5.0 mg., and at 9½ weeks to 8.0 mg., at which level it was continued for 13 weeks, when (in the 22nd week of medication) the reserpine was discontinued.

Since the patients included in the study constituted less than a third of the ward population, and neither the nature of the medication nor a breakdown of the group was known to ward personnel, an atmosphere of pervasive and contagious enthusiasm, full of expectation of dramatic improvement, did not arise. The ward was not redecorated, and new, stimulating activities were not introduced into the ward routine. This was admittedly a stringent setting, but, as far as possible, factors related to "wonder drug" enthusiasm were avoided in an effort to measure drug effect alone as far as practicable.

Untoward Effects. Several such effects in patients in the reserpine group caused some difficulty later in the assessment of the data. In the 11th week one patient, aged 66, developed sufficient orthostatic hypotension that she was transferred to the geriatric medical service by the ward physician, and reserpine was discontinued. Another patient, aged 55, developed mild congestive heart failure with moderate ankle edema at the conclusion of the study

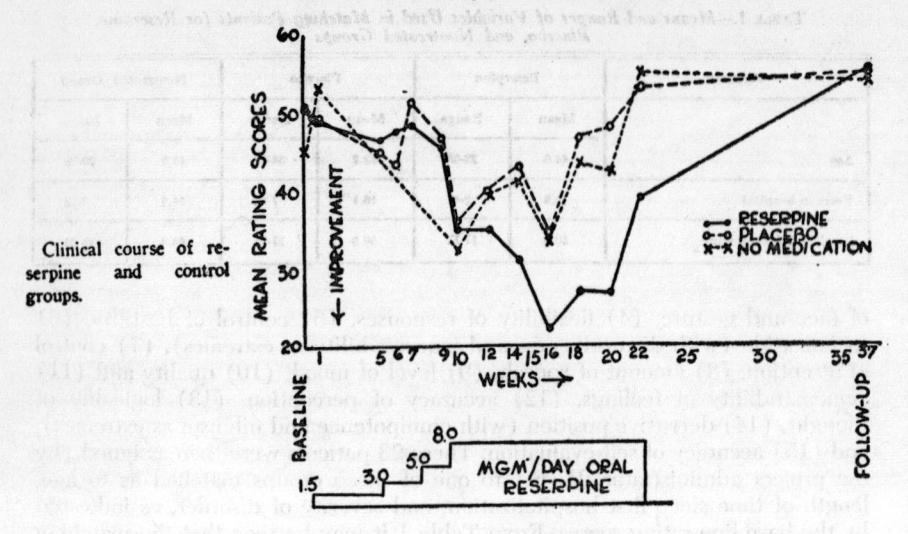

Clinical course of reserpine and control groups.

TABLE 2.—*Significance of Changes in Ratings for Individual Items in Rating Scale fo Reserpine Patients Between a Four-Week Period on 3.0 and 5.0 Mg. Dosage and a Five-Week Period on 8.0 Mg. Dosage, and for the Placebo Patients Between the Same Periods; and Significance of Comparisons of the Changes in the Two Groups for Each Item*

Item	Reserpine (N=7) Change	P Value	Placebo (N=10) Change	P Value	Reserpine vs. Placebo P Value
Neatness of appearance	24	...	−12	...	
Level of motor activity	33	...	10	...	
Expressivity of face and gesture	29*	0.05	20	...	
Flexibility of responses	47*	0.02	23	...	
Control of hostility	50*	0.02	37	0.02	
Socialization	48*	0.02	1	...	0.05†
Control of attention	33	...	−6	...	
Amount of speech	25*	0.05	−5	...	
Level of mood	45*	0.02	30	...	
Quality of feelings	35*	0.5	38	...	
Demonstrability of feelings	40*	0.05	40	0.02	
Accuracy of perceptions	42	...	35	...	
Logicality of thought	−1	...	−30	...	
Defensive position	41*	0.05	43*	0.01	
Accuracy of self-evaluation	−3	...	−81	0.01‡	

* Differences within reserpine and within placebo group are statistically significant by Wilcoxon's test for paired replicates.
† Differences between corresponding values in reserpine and placebo groups are statistically significant by the Mann-Whitney u test.
‡ Significantly worse to the 0.01 level of confidence.

and required bed rest for a week to regain cardiac compensation; a similar situation has been reported by Perera. A third patient, aged 57, frequently inactive, developed sudden signs of bowel obstruction and died just before going to surgery, in the 17th week of the study; autopsy findings did not rule out fecal impaction. Another patient, originally assigned to the reserpine group, refused all medication from the start and was transferred by the administrator to the control group which received no medication. Only one expected side-effect occurred, in which case a 29-year-old patient in the reserpine group developed Parkinsonian tremors at the conclusion of the study, but this was mild and was not present a week after the medication period.

Results. There was no significant difference between the mean of the group receiving placebos and the mean of the group receiving no medication. Further, there were no significant differences between the means of these two control groups and that of the reserpine group until after the 10th week, when the reserpine dose had been increased to 8.0 mg. daily. It should be noted that only the divergent trends between the groups, rather than the absolute levels of the ratings, are pertinent, since the latter fluctuated over the period of the study, and it can be seen that whatever factors were operating affected all three groups. The mean rating scores of the placebo and nontreated groups were in the direction of improvement on 8.0 mg. daily and continued as a trend for 10 weeks, but in the final 2 weeks of medication this divergence decreased (Figure). When the follow-up observations were recorded 15 weeks after medication was discontinued, the mean score of all groups had returned to the base line level.

Statistical Analysis (Table 2). Those who received reserpine showed significant improvement in socialization, control of hostility, flexibility of responses, level of mood, expressivity of face and gesture, amount of speech, quality and demonstrability of feelings, and defensive position. Those who received placebos improved significantly in defensive position, control of hostility, and demonstrability of feelings; they worsened significantly in accuracy of self-evaluation (perhaps only relatively, reflecting increased familiarity with the patient). As a whole, all rating items considered, the reserpine group showed improvement greater than that of the placebo group, and this was statistically significant to the 0.05 level of confidence. The only aspect of behavior, however, showing improvement in the reserpine group which was significantly greater than that shown by the placebo group (by an extremely conservative statistical test) was socialization; five reserpine-treated patients showed remarkable improvement in this respect.

Illustrative Responses. Certain individual responses are illustrative of the effects noted above. Patient 1, age 30, denuditive, smearing, and apathetic, had been hospitalized six and one-half years and had had electroshock treatments during her first year in the hospital. Her base line rating score was among the worst in the reserpine group. After about two weeks on 8.0 mg. daily she was dressed, attentive, and able to communicate verbally. Improvement in this regard continued, reaching a peak 4 weeks later, but declined thereafter until, after 12 weeks on the same dosage, she was bizarre in her dress, deluded, and hallucinated, and was again unable to communicate her thoughts clearly. At the follow-up, less than four months after reserpine was discontinued, she was essentially the same as at the beginning of the study.

Another patient in the reserpine group, Patient 9, age 23, hospitalized seven years, was hallucinated and grimacing, combative, and explosive in her reactions at the start, and showed an unsteady, but marked, improvement in her control of assaultive and destructive behavior, with appropriate and pleasant expression and clarity of thought, after having received 8.0 mg. of reserpine daily for two weeks. She was even able to help serve meals to bed patients in an adjacent ward. After 12 weeks on this dosage, however, she was again so out of control that she enucleated her own eye.

A patient in the placebo group, Case 13, age 47, hospitalized over 10 years, was intensely preoccupied, pacing restlessly, constantly picking at her skin, and virtually uncommunicative. While there were slight fluctuations in her ability to respond meaningfully, her condition remained essentially unchanged throughout. Another placebo patient, Case 15, age 49, hospitalized over 20 years, was explosive, noisy, and socially disruptive, and had received without benefit pentylenetetrazol U.S.P. (Metrazol) convulsive therapy, hydrotherapy, and electroshock therapy. Near the end of the study she became calmer and was under adequate control nearly all the time except while dining in the cafeteria; there was no reversion to the initial abnormal level at the time of follow-up.

One of the patients who received neither reserpine nor placebos, Case 28, age 37, hospitalized over 10 years, with no satisfactory response to two courses of electroshock therapy, was hallucinating, silly, and bizarre in dress when the study began. By the 16th week she was still quite dependent and her expression was awkwardly exaggerated, but she was calm and more controlled. Eight weeks later, however, she again showed considerable scattering and was silly and aloof.

Summary

The data obtained may be summarized as follows:

1. No difference between the reserpine group and the placebo group appeared in the 28 chronically disturbed psychotic women until 8.0 mg. of reserpine was administered daily.

2. The placebo group did not differ from the group who were given no pills.

3. On the basis of an analysis of the scores on the individual items of a psychiatric rating scale, reserpine in adequate dosage (compared with a placebo) was found to produce statistically significant improvement in socialization; no other items showed improvement which was within the 0.05 level of confidence.

4. Great variation in amount and duration of improvement occurred, so that no patients were well enough to be discharged and all who had improved relapsed partially while receiving the same amount of reserpine, suggesting an escape from the medication effect.

5. Fifteen weeks after medication was discontinued, the mean rating scores of all three groups had returned to the base line level of abnormality.

BEHAVIORAL CHANGES OF CHRONIC SCHIZOPHRENICS IN RESPONSE TO RESERPINE

Roy E. McDonald, M.D., Robert B. Ellsworth, Ph.D., and Jane Eniss, R.N.

Purpose of Study

This study has to do with the action of reserpine on the behavior of chronic schizophrenics. It is reported because of the experimental design employed, despite the risk of repeating the conclusions of many similar studies. The study was designed with the thought that only one major variable (reserpine) was desirable, i.e., that the validity of results should not be lessened by the fact that either the raters who evaluated the behavior change of the patients or the patients themselves had any information concerning the identity of the drug group. For this reason, a double-blind design was used, with adequate experimental and control groups.

Procedure

A ward of 27 chronic schizophrenics, average hospitalization nine years, was selected for study, because as judged both by the estimate of their situation and by testing devices there had been no appreciable change in their behavior in over three to six months. No organic or scheduled psychotherapy had been conducted with this group for over a year; there was a stable ward, personnel, and activity environment. Thirteen patients for the drug and fourteen patients for the placebo group were selected by the toss of a coin on the basis of seating arrangement in the dining room. All four patients at each table received the same medication. Three milligrams of reserpine or a like amount of placebo was placed daily in the coffee or fruit juice by the nurse. She was the only one who knew the identity of the groups, and she did not participate in rating the patients' behavior.

The drug was administered over a 73-day period. The amount accepted by the subjects was from 65% to 100% of that offered, and 80% of the patients accepted at least 85% of their medication.

Behavioral rating scales were devised to cover the patient's behavior in everyday occupational and correctional (exercise) therapy. A previously reported scale, the Hospital Adjustment Scale, was used to evaluate the ward behavior of each patient. The O. T. and C. T. scales were devised to measure possible behavioral improvement in these areas. The usual item analysis and scale-construction methods were used in developing these scales, with an adequate period of training for each rater.

Drug Toxicity

Most evidences of drug toxicity were transient and minimal, having to do with nausea, anorexia, and diarrhea. One patient steadily lost 20 lb. in weight. One patient developed unilateral arm clonus, which disappeared upon withdrawal of the drug; no evidence of organicity was noted in a full neurological study.

Results

Table 1 presents the record of significant changes in the patient's behavior for each patient who participated in the study. It is to be emphasized that only definite behavior changes are recorded under the H. A. S., O. T., and C. T. (columns 1, 2, and 3 respectively). Calculation of behavioral changes on the rating scales was completed before anyone knew the identity of the pa-

TABLE 1.—*Significant Changes in Patients' Behavior*

	Experimental Group					Control Group			
Patient No.	H. A. S.	O. T.	C. T.	Evaluation	Patient No.	H. A. S.	O. T.	C. T.	Evaluation
1	+	..	..	....	14	..	..	..	....
2	..	..	..	(+)	15	..	..	..	....
3	+	+	..	(+)	16	..	..	+	....
4	..	+	+	(+)	17	..	..	+	....
5	+	..	+	(+)	18	..	..	..	....
6	..	..	..	....	19	+	..	..	....
7	..	+	..	....	20	..	..	..	....
8	..	..	..	....	21	..	..	..	(+)
9	..	..	+	....	22	..	+	..	(+)
10	+	+	+	(+)	23	..	..	..	.
11	..	..	..	....	24	+	..	..	....
12	..	..	..	....	25	..	+	..	.
13	.	+	+	....	26	..	..	..	....
	4/13	5/12	5/12	(5/13)	27				
						2/14	1/13	3/13	(2/14)

tients in the experimental (drug) group. The following procedure was used to determine whether or not a definite change had occurred:

1. The same rater rated the same patient each month throughout the study.
2. A base-line score was established for each patient at the beginning of the study, and it was assumed that any change in score from this base line could indicate error on the part of the rater and/or improvement-regression in the patient's behavior.
3. A standard error was, therefore, established for each rater, so that a decision could be made as to whether or not a change in score represented a significant change in the patient's behavior (Table 1).

A plus (+) is recorded for a patient only if the difference in his score at the end of the study and his base-line score is greater than the rater's standard error. Two patients in the control group (21 and 24) and two patients in the experimental group (3 and 8) did not attend O. T. or C. T. activities and were not rated in these areas.

At the end of the study, the entire staff was asked to evaluate (last column) each patient's possible behavioral change. The staff members were asked to report "a change that hits you between the eyes, not one that you have to look for."

If at least 90% of the statements favored a change for the better, and there was no more than one dissenting vote among the 22 people present, a patient received a plus (+) in the "Evaluation" column. This was used as a "check" on the three behavioral scales which were used in actually determining whether or not a patient had improved.

Table 1 indicates that slightly more patients "improved" in the experimental group than in the control group, if any change in any area is accepted as "improvement." If, however, incidences of "improvement" are calculated for those patients changing in two or more areas, then the difference between the two groups is greater. By the exact method of calculation, the difference between the two groups is at the 0.03 level of significance (Table 2).

An additional significant finding was that there were more incidents of change occurring in the experimental group than in the control group. With

TABLE 2.—*Number of Patients Who Improved in Two or More Areas in Experimental and Control Groups*

	Experimental (Drug)	Control (Nondrug)
Improved	5	0
No change	8	14

$P = 0.03$.

TABLE 3.—*Number of Incidents of Improvement in the Experimental and Control Groups*

	Experimental (Drug)	Control (Nondrug)
Improved	14	6
No change	21	32

x^2 5.36 >0.02 level.

the x^2 test of the total "incidents of change" in C. T., O. T., and H. A. S. (ward), the experimental group differed from the control group at a 0.02 level of significance (Table 3). No significant correlations occurred among the three scales: hence the x^2 test was used here.

Improvement for the most part was gradual, significant improvement on the rating scales occurring by the second month. One patient appeared to have obtained results only after four to five months of therapy.

GENERAL IMPRESSIONS

In terms of informally observed improvement, the patients in the experimental group could not be selected from those in the control group by anyone's guessing and identification of these groups. The ward was nonetheless noted to be "quieter" and the patients more "tractable." The nurse reported: "Prior to the institution of reserpine, patients seemed restless . . . there were frequent altercations . . . in general a rather tense, tight atmosphere. After . . . six to eight weeks the ward seemed . . . quieter . . . fewer altercations . . . Patients seemed more relaxed. . . more aware of each other. . . began asking for more to do."

The testing devices measured such areas as Cooperation, Contact Span, Participation, Interest, Concentration, Alertness, and Accessibility. Consistently improved ratings in those patients who were favorably influenced by the drug were seen only on those items which measured Accessibility and Contact Span.[1]

An independent study, involving a more exact method of analyzing the changes which occurred as a result of the drug, is currently under analysis. A variation of a method reported by Osgood and Suci was applied to the patient population. Two main results were obtained: (1) A factor analysis of 20 rationally derived scales, on which all the patients had been rated, revealed four independent factors; (2) a combination of pattern and cluster analysis showed that at least five distinct subgroups in this particular patient population were extracted, as defined by the different scores on the four factors. The first tentative results indicated that those patients who "improved" under the drug showed the greatest change on the factor preliminarily labeled "capacity." That is, those who improved moved in the direction of a higher capacity rating. Moreover, those patients with a high initial capacity rating seemed to be the least affected by the drug. This analysis is not yet complete and will be reported at a later time. It would appear, however, that capacity encompasses both the accessibility and the contact span areas of the other rating scales.

COMMENT

It would appear that the administration of reserpine to chronic schizophrenics alters their behavior, as judged from the testing devices employed. That reserpine was the only consistent major variable in the study would strengthen this conclusion and make observed changes attributable to the drug alone. Especially is this likely to be true if, before any patient is accepted as changing, he must change in at least two different areas. If he changes in only one area, one cannot eliminate the possibility that he had changed as a result of the incidents specific to that one area. If he changed in two or more areas, it was felt that a definite over-all change had probably occurred in the patient, independent of what may have happened in one specific area.

It should be emphasized that reported changes are major ones and do not have to do with subtle changes or their interpretation, as in an interview-type study. Since, at the conclusion of the experiment, no one was able to assess

---

[1] A later cluster analysis revealed that the items in these two rationally labeled areas were actually highly interrelated.

better than by chance who was given the drug, the tidiness of the double-blind design in drug research was preserved. The importance of the double-blind structure was additionally illustrated by what happened to the ratings of patients once their identity became known. Thirty days after the end of the study proper, patient identity having been divulged to the raters, 100% of the experimental group was rated as significantly improved on one of the scales.

That the change induced was gradual, and in no instance (save one) dramatic, was illustrated by the fact that the identity of the drug group remained unknown. Yet the overall changes in those "improved" patients were real and significant. From the point of view of the ward personnel, definite overall quieting was noted, and, on the rating scales, there was seemingly consistent improvement in the areas of Contact Span and Accessibility.

This study is in agreement with a growing number of other studies and supports the conclusion that reserpine is a valuable adjunct in psychiatric therapy for some chronically hospitalized schizophrenics. However, the results appear to be somewhat more conservative than those reported in less carefully controlled studies, although there has been little opportunity to compare these results with those for studies using similar groups and experimental designs. It is hoped that as more drugs become available for psychiatric use, experimental designs such as that used in this study will be used early in their evaluation.

Summary and Conclusions

The double-blind design was successfully employed in the evaluation of the effect of reserpine on the behavior of lengthily hospitalized chronic schizophrenics.

Reserpine in a dose of 3 mg.[2] appears to have a salutary effect on the behavior of some of this population when evaluated by the testing devices described.

Seeming improvement was noted primarily in the areas of Accessibility and Contact Span.

Major toxicity did not occur.

---

[2] In five patients who did not respond to the initial dose, the drug was given in the amount of 8 mg. At the end of 31 dosage days no improvement was noted and one patient exhibited Parkinsonism.

RESERPINE (SERPASIL) IN THE MANAGEMENT OF THE MENTALLY ILL

Robert H. Noce, M.D., David B. Williams, M.D., and Walter Rapaport, M.D.

In our preliminary report, we reported on 74 mentally ill and 15 mentally retarded patients who received reserpine for periods as long as seven months in duration. The oral dosage averaged 2 mg. daily, and the parenteral dose was 1 to 10 mg. Eighty per cent of the patients manifested improvement that was due to the alkaloid. Many regressed patients became alert and sociable, while the hyperactive, noisy, assaultive group became tranquil. The use of restraints, seclusion, and electroconvulsive therapy decreased by at least 80% after the inception of this treatment. Many patients no longer revealed psychotic symptoms, and it was possible to place on indefinite leave of absence or discharge status many patients whose prognosis had been regarded previously as hopeless. The patients selected for treatment in this project were only those who had a poor prognosis. They were the so-called back ward patients who had been mentally ill for many years. Most of them were schizophrenics. The same criteria were used for the selection of the 15 mentally retarded patients treated. They were the most difficult patients to manage from the standpoint of ward care and training, having I. Q.'s varying from 2 to 34. Because most of the mentally retarded patients of Modesto State Hospital are in the low intelligence-quotient diagnostic categories, we requested that future studies in the mentally retarded with all I. Q. ranges be conducted in institutions whose facilities are devoted entirely to the care and treatment of the mentally retarded. At the present time, several institutions are conducting further research with reserpine in the treatment of the mentally retarded. Therefore, since the completion of the preliminary report, our efforts in the study have been devoted exclusively to the treatment of the mentally ill.

SELECTION OF PATIENTS

In the present study, 247 patients, consisting of 30 male and 217 female, practically all psychotic, were treated with reserpine for periods ranging up to 12 months. The majority of these patients, 165 in number, are classified as schizophrenics of the following types: paranoid, 73 patients; catatonic, 49; hebephrenic, 16; mixed, 16; chronic undifferentiated, 4; simple, 3; schizoaffective, 3; acute undifferentiated, 1. The remainder of patients selected came from a wide variety of diagnostic categories (see table). We decided to evaluate the effectiveness of reserpine in the treatment of recent mental illness of much shorter duration as well as to continue to treat many chronically ill patients. The age range of patients treated was from 15 to 80 years, the average age being 44 years.

RESULTS

Inasmuch as orally given reserpine is a slow-acting drug, immediate results may not be observed. The majority of patients revealed some improvement within a week or two with parenteral medication. In a significant number of patients, if improvement is at all possible it will be noticed within a period of two months; however, many regressed patients may require six months' treatment in order to manifest maximum improvement. In hyperactive, noisy, combative patients and in the regressed, seclusive types treated with parenterally given reserpine, partial alleviation of their symptoms was observed within one or two hours, as well as increased alertness and more interest in environment.

The following criteria were utilized in determining improvement: 1. Slightly improved. Depressed, withdrawn patients show some improvement in mood and exhibit more interest in their environment and ward activities. They cooperate better in feeding, dressing, and bathing themselves, as well as maintaining toilet habits. Violent, agitated patients have 25% to 50% less need for sedation, restraint, electroconvulsive therapy, and seclusion and may participate in rehabilitation therapy. 2. Moderately improved. Patients exhibit infrequent episodes of unsociable behavior. They are able to care for themselves except possibly during these episodes. At least 75% less restraint, shock, and sedation are required, and the patients participate in rehabilitation therapy. 3. Markedly improved. Patients require no sedation, hydrotherapy, electroconvulsive therapy, restraint, or seclusion. They become sociable, agreeable, and always take part in rehabilitation therapy. They exhibit no episodes of verbal or physical abusiveness and care for themselves completely. If hallucinations and delusions are present, patients do not react thereto. They may be in remission.

In some patients who showed cyclic periods of hyperactivity, combativeness, and/or raucous behavior these cycles were eliminated. In other patients the psychotic episodes decreased in duration and severity. Some patients experienced a partial or complete remission. Hallucinations or delusions were observed no longer; or, if these disabling symptoms persisted, the patients manifested a healthy indifference to them. Some paranoid schizophrenics, as well as other types of psychotic patients, have revealed these remissions. Schizophrenic patients appear to respond more favorably to reserpine than patients in other diagnostic categories; however, the number of patients in these other categories is small, and no conclusions can be formulated. The paranoid and catatonic schizophrenics revealed a more favorable response to therapy than other types.

We have observed that, in the majority of patients, reserpine improved appetite. Thus it produced physical as well as mental improvement. Significant weight gains were observed in 75%. This favorable influence on barostatic mechanism was utilized in treating the soma as well as the psyche in our patients, who usually manifested some degree of physical debilitation as well as mental symptoms. Because a state of paraympathetic dominance is induced by reserpine, constipation is alleviated. As a general rule, those patients without evidence of organic brain damage revealed a more satisfactory response to reserpine than those with pathological cerebral changes. However, remarkable improvement in the socialization of some psychotic patients with brain damage has been noted. In some patients, inhibitions were decreased, thus enabling them to verbalize and "act out" their feelings. This ventilation and "acting out" facilitated psychotherapy. Reserpine has caused many patients to be aware of their psychosis and to become dissatisfied with it, resulting in a motivation to improve themselves mentally and physically. For example, a paranoid schizophrenic who was hostile and aggressive was given reserpine treatment. After a few months' treatment she asked the ward nurse, "How can I improve my mental condition? I want to be on a ward where there are more social activities so that I can help myself to get well enough to leave the hospital."

Dosage and Side-Effects

Reserpine, 5 mg. given intravenously or intramuscularly, was administered daily or every two days for 5 to 10 days. The dosage was varied from 2.5 mg. to 10 mg. On the first or second day of treatment, oral therapy with reserpine was started, 1 mg. twice daily. After the first week, oral dosage was increased or decreased according to the patient's response. In elderly patients with severe arteriosclerosis and/or hypertension these doses were decreased by one-half. This prevents syncope and hypotensive episodes in elderly patients. If the medicament was well tolerated, the dosage was increased slowly for optimal effect. Patients receiving reserpine required diligent observation and constant adjustment of dosage to their changing clinical conditions. At times, slight increases in dosage caused more effective response. On the other hand, decreasing the dosage resulted in more alertness in some patients. The optimum dose is that which produces maximum therapeutic response with minimal psychomotor retardation.

If further acute psychotic episodes occur during therapy, it is preferable to treat the patient more intensively by the use of parenteral as well as oral medication. When these acute exacerbations have subsided, treatment is confined to the oral method of administration. We wish to emphasize that sufficient dosage of reserpine over a long period of time may produce a far more satisfactory therapeutic response than smaller doses administered for a short period of time. The latter method of treatment may produce little or no improvement in the patient.

The side-effects were minimal. Patients were able to maintain an ambulatory status while taking reserpine. Many of them participated in industrial therapy throughout the hospital. Parenteral administration of 5 mg. or more causes dermal vasodilatation, manifested by flushing of the skin, hyperemia of the conjunctivas, and shivering within an hour after administration in some patients. They may experience transient nausea and lassitude for a period of 12 to 24 hours. Increased dreams, polydypsia, polyuria, and diarrhea have been observed. In other patients, no symptoms except lassitude may be evident. Some individuals manifest no undesirable symptoms whatsoever. After the expiration of 24 hours, a significant number of patients experience marked subjective improvement, and it is not unusual for them to make such statements as, "I feel better than I have felt for a long time," or, "I feel as frisky as a colt!" Sometimes slight vertigo is experienced, but this is not of an incapacitating nature. Although hypotension, with blood pressure as low as 80/50 mm. Hg and cardiac rates as low as 60, has been observed in some patients, it has been asymptomatic, except for the salutary, tranquillizing effect. The hypotension and bradycardia respond well to ephedrine sulfate, 3/8 grain (25 mg.) once or twice daily, orally or intramuscularly, if an elevation in blood pressure is desired.

OTHER TREATMENT

Electroconvulsive Therapy.—Fifty-six patients, or 22.7%, received electroconvulsive therapy in conjunction with reserpine. The glissando technique was employed, utilizing Dale and Medcraft units. This combination therapy was employed for the following reasons: 1. Patients taking reserpine were distributed all over the hospital in various wards and therefore were under the care of numerous psychiatrists, some of whom preferred to use electroconvulsive therapy. 2. Some patients did not reveal optimal therapeutic improvement with reserpine alone, but showed marked improvement with the combination of reserpine and electroconvulsive therapy. This applies especially to deteriorated patients. 3. Patients who were depressed and suicidal were administered combination therapy because, obviously, our goal was to eliminate the suicidal ideation and attempts as quickly as possible.

The administration of electroconvulsive therapy is facilitated by reserpine because anxiety, tension, fear reactions, negativism, resistiveness, and combativeness are eliminated or decreased considerably. Many patients had received well over 100 electroconvulsive treatments without improvement prior to receiving reserpine. When reserpine therapy was instituted, in many cases it was possible to discontinue electroconvulsive therapy because of the marked improvement in patients' conditions. Thus it is evident that many patients were refractory to electroconvulsive therapy but did respond to reserpine alone. Hyperactive patients revealed normal motor activity, noisy patients became much more sedate in their verbalizations, and seclusive, withdrawn patients became more alert, extroverted, and cheerful in their demeanor. Since the inception of this study, electroconvulsive therapy for patients receiving reserpine has been decreased by 75%. It was possible to administer a smaller number of treatments because of the potentiating effect of reserpine on electroconvulsive therapy. In no instance was any undesirable effect observed in employing the combination of electroconvulsive therapy and reserpine. No apnea or respiratory or circulatory impairment was noted, revealing that this combination therapy is a safe procedure. Reserpine lowers the convulsive threshold. We have observed that satisfactory grand mal convulsions were produced with lower voltages and shorter durations of time.

Barbiturates.—A small number of patients were given supplementary treatments with barbiturates. Most of them did not improve in their mental condition; in fact, some of them became more disturbed, necessitating elimination of the barbiturate. However, a few patients did improve more with the combination of reserpine and barbiturates than with reserpine alone, indicating that reserpine potentiates the effects of barbiturates in some patients. Reserpine has proved to be efficacious in the treatment of many agitated and hyperactive senile patients who had been treated with barbiturates with unsatisfactory results. Their symptoms were alleviated considerably, and they were able to develop some degree of insight into their mental conditions. In arteriosclerotic patients, confusion and disorientation were alleviated partially or completely.

Natural History

We have observed that reserpine facilitates the care of disturbed medical patients and is especially useful in the treatment of hyperactive postoperative patients. We are cognizant of the natural history of many diagnostic categories that are characterized by remissions and relapses. Therefore, some patients who were receiving treatment with reserpine may have been approaching, and would have manifested, a remission without any treatment. By the same token, any patient receiving electroconvulsive therapy, insulin therapy, or psychotherapy may be near a remission so that, when this remission occurs, the treatment is regarded often as the sole causative factor in the patient's improvement. This common denominator in many mental illnesses, namely, the natural history of the disease, is germane to all methods of therapy in psychiatry and is no more important in reserpine treatment than in other methods of treatment. Reserpine alleviates agitation, anxiety, and tension in both psychotics and neurotics, regardless of pretreatment blood pressure. Antisocial, negativistic patients are able to think in a more clear manner.

Interdisciplinary Program

In conjunction with reserpine, it is desirable to conduct a "total push" program. In this program the efforts of workers in all disciplines, namely, psychiatrists, psychologists, social-service workers, rehabilitation therapists, and nurses, are combined in a team approach under the leadership of the psychiatrist. This unified effort is a more effective therapeutic approach than the effort of workers in one discipline only. Also, wholesome social and environmental factors are provided in this therapy, which allows the patient maximum freedom of activity. Pianos, television sets, planters on walls, pictures, and drapes can and should be placed on wards for disturbed patients after reserpine treatment has been instituted. Patients enjoy music, and they take pride in homelike decorations as they become more aware of and more interested in their environment. Our female "security" wards have lost their austere appearances and resemble college dormitories at the present time.

The patients' improvement must be explained and interpreted to relatives, with the hope that they will supervise them on indefinite leave of absence. For example, a regressed 65-year-old schizophrenic, who had been hospitalized for 16 years and who had not been visited by relatives for a long time, improved greatly with reserpine therapy, regaining her contact with reality. She wrote to her relatives, asking them to visit her. They were disinterested and did not visit. Consequently, the patient became depressed. Although she improved greatly with reserpine therapy, she is still somewhat depressed because she is aware of the rejection by her spouse and other relatives; however, we will find a placement for her in a family-care home.

REPORT OF CASES

CASE 1.—29-year-old married white woman was admitted to Modesto State Hospital on April 26, 1954. She spoke in a vociferous and irrelevant manner, grimaced, and struck her head on the walls. The diagnosis was schizophrenic reaction, catatonic type. The history revealed that she had received six months' intensive treatment, including insulin and electroconvulsive therapy, in another hospital three years previously. Upon admission, the patient received an electroconvulsive treatment. This was ineffective, for she resumed her bizarre, hyperactive behavior 10 minutes later. Reserpine, 5 mg., was administered intravenously on April 26, 27, 28, and 29, simultaneously with 1 mg. by mouth daily. Within an hour after the initial injection she became quiet and cooperative. Subsequently, she revealed normal mental and physical activity and was able to receive psychotherapy. She was relaxed, had undisturbed sleep, and developed a voracious appetite. Four days after admission she performed bookkeeping work at the hospital. She was discharged on May 7, 1954, taking reserpine orally, 0.5 mg. twice a day. One month later the dosage was reduced to 0.5 mg. once a day. As an outpatient, she received psychotherapy one hour each week for one month.

At the present time, she is taking 0.5 mg. of reserpine orally daily and continues to make an excellent adjustment. She cares for her three children, cooks, and performs housework. She is calm in temperament, not being irritated by small daily annoyances that had previously disturbed her. Her husband observed that she is stable and alert mentally, more so than ever in the past.

CASE 2.—A 33-year-old married white woman was admitted to Modesto State Hospital on Aug. 14, 1953, with a history of confused and delusional behavior for three days. She was hyperactive and combative. The diagnosis was schizophrenic reaction, catatonic type. She had a history of trauma from the psychodynamic aspect. At the age of 16 she attempted suicide. She was an overt homosexual and behavior problem in high school. She married a man much older than herself, and the marriage was unsuccessful. From Aug. 27, 1952, to Feb. 8, 1954, she received 139 electroconvulsive treatments, hydrotherapy, sedation, seclusion, and restraint, but remained combative and destructive. Treatment with reserpine was initiated on Jan. 21, 1954, at 1 mg. twice a day. It was necessary also to administer intravenous medication on a few occasions because she was mildly disturbed. Within a month, significant improvement was noted. She became quieter and more cooperative, making it possible to eliminate sedation and restraint. Since March, 1954, she had been friendly and sociable, and she was assigned to work in the laundry because she requested it. She enjoyed her work, participated in occupational therapy activities, and attended movies. In July, 1954, she went on indefinite leave of absence. She received four psychotherapeutic interviews as an outpatient and continues to make excellent adjustment, performing her household duties and caring for her children. The present oral dosage is 2 mg. of reserpine daily.

CASE 3.—A 55-year-old married white woman was admitted to Patton State Hospital on Jan. 30, 1937, as mentally ill. She was fearful that strange men might assault her and was apprehended in front of the Y. W. C. A. barefooted and in an highly excited condition. The diagnosis was psychosis with syphilitic meningoencephalitis. The blood and spinal fluid serologic tests were positive, and the colloidal gold curve was 4432100000. The physical examination was essentially normal. The neurological examination revealed hyperactive patellar reflexes and fine tremors of the tongue. While at Patton, the patient attempted to kill a psychiatric technician and attempted suicide by cutting her own throat. She received the customary antisyphilis treatments. She was transferred to Modesto State Hospital on Feb. 19, 1948, with the symptoms of combativeness, assaultiveness, and hyperactivity. She spent most of her time in seclusion and failed to respond to electroconvulsive therapy, sedation, and hydrotherapy. She was placed on a regimen of orally given reserpine on March 12, 1954, receiving 2 mg. daily, as well as several intravenous and intramuscular injections of 5 and 10 mg. She has improved to such an extent that she is now working in the sewing room and is quiet and cooperative. She has received no additional somatic therapy for the past six months. Her present medication is 1 mg. three times a day.

COMMENT

Reserpine reduces considerably the need for electroconvulsive therapy, sedation, restraint, seclusion, and hydrotherapy. It is desirable to employ this more conservative method of treatment prior to attempting more radical somatic treatment. Reserpine enables psychiatrists to treat larger numbers of patients because this treatment, which can be administered by nursing personnel, requires less time and energy than other somatic therapies. More important, larger numbers of patients are made amenable to psychotherapy. In regressed patients who have been psychotic for many years, six months' therapy with reserpine may be required to produce maximum improvement. It is recommended that patients who have not responded in a satisfactory manner to electroconvulsive therapy, insulin shock therapy, and prefrontal lobotomy, be treated for a period of two to six months with oral and/or parenteral reserpine, depending upon the patient's therapeutic requirements. The authors, as well as other investigators, have noted that in a significant number of cases it has been possible to eliminate these more radical therapeutic procedures by the use of reserpine. Because reserpine accelerates and increases insight formation, it is possible to decrease the number, and the duration, of psychotherapeutic interviews in a significant number of cases. Reserpine has been an effective therapeutic adjunct in this institution and should prove to be a valuable addition to the present therapeutic armamentarium both in institutional psychiatry and in private psychiatric practice.

Reserpine has facilitated nursing care in 85% of our patients. A large percentage of patients are not as untidy and destructive after reserpine treatment. A significant number of them lose these symptoms and are motivated to socialize and participate in industrial and recreational therapies. The time and energy devoted previously by nursing personnel to custodial duties and in assisting with electroconvulsive therapy is expended at present on therapeutic measures that are rehabilitative in nature. Reserpine has caused many patients to be aware of their psychosis and to become dissatisfied with it, resulting in a motivation to improve themselves mentally and physically. The transportation of psychotic patients and their movements to other states, countries, or hospitals can be facilitated by reserpine treatment.

The majority of patients in this study were schizophrenics (165). The most favorable responses were observed in the paranoid and catatonic types. Thirty per cent of the paranoid type and 45% of the catatonic type improved markedly. During this study, 6.48% of the patients were discharged from the hospital and 21.46% left the hospital on indefinite leave of absence. The total percentage of patients in this study who left the hospital in indefinite leave of absence or discharge is 27.9%. Thirty-six per cent of the patients in this study revealed marked improvement; 28%, moderate improvement; 20%, slight improvement; and 15%, no improvement. Of the patients who have left the hospital, 8.5% received reserpine at home, the oral dosage ranging from 0.5 mg. to 2 mg. daily.

Medicine has been passing through an era of radical somatic treatment of the mentally ill, and we hope that a period is approaching in which more conservative methods of treatment will be favored, one of which is chemical therapy. This period of chemical treatment of the mentally ill is in its infancy, and we believe that more specific drugs will be discovered in the future that will make it possible to treat specific symptoms or diagnostic categories.

Summary and Conclusions

Reserpine seems to be most effective in the treatment of schizophrenia; therefore, this alkaloid is a valuable adjunct in the state hospital, where a high percentage of the population is schizophrenic; however, we have completed only 12 months' study of this particular chemical treatment of the mentally ill. Further research in reference to chemical and physiological disturbances of the cerebrum in mental disorders should provide enlightening information about the effectiveness of reserpine and other chemical therapies. Many of these studies are being conducted by various investigators throughout the country at this time, and we are looking forward to their reports. The use of reserpine should result in annual savings to taxpayers by virtue of its decreasing admissions as well as making possible many leaves of absence and discharges. Many chronic mentally ill patients who were regarded as having a hopeless prognosis have gone, and others will continue to go, on indefinite leave of absence from the hospital.

EFFECT OF RESERPINE AND OPEN-WARD PRIVILEGES ON CHRONIC SCHIZOPHRENICS

Allen S. Penman, Ph.D., and Thomas E. Dredge, M.D.

Reserpine has been described as having a calming or tranquilizing effect on subjects and as exerting its hypotensive and sedative effects through action on the hypothalamus. Plummer stated that probably the most likely region at which reserpine could produce changes in autonomic balance would be "an area of the central nervous system, such as the hypothalamus, where autonomic nervous functions are integrated ... All observed effects of reserpine, including sedation, reduced emotional response, peripheral autonomic alterations, and circulatory changes, are explicable on the basis of an alteration of sympathetic-parasympathetic balance by partial suppression of sympathetic predominance at the hypothalamic level." Adler reported in his study that there is a reduction in hyperactivity, assaultiveness, apprehension, anxiety, and depression. Although he noted that patients varied in response to the drug, there was an obvious decrease in anxiety. Similar improvement was noted by Barsa, who selected patients on the basis of their excited, hyperactive, assaultive, or destructive behavior, regardless of diagnosis, age, duration of illness, or previous treatment. Noce found that the use of the drug reduced considerably the need for electroconvulsive therapy, sedation, restraint, seclusion, and hydrotherapy, and that 30% of paranoid schizophrenics and 45% of catatonic schizophrenics improved markedly. Tyhurst described similar results in his study and suggested that the drug seemed mainly to reduce the emotional disturbance and concern associated with abnormal mental content.

A more recent study, and one with the use of control groups, was carried out by Sommerness and associates, who selected 90 of their most highly disturbed chronic mentally ill male patients and divided them into three groups of 30 each. Thirty were given reserpine (Rau-Sed); 30 were given an identical-appearing placebo, and 30 received no medication. Their conclusions were that reserpine in oral doses of 1 mg. b.i.d. did not effect a behavioral improvement as measured by the L-M Fergus Falls Rating Scale; that it effected a lowering of blood pressure and a slight weight gain, and that the greater attention to the patients inherent in taking blood pressures and weights and increasing the interest of ward personnel resulted in behavioral improvement of all three groups under study.

With the exception of the aforementioned investigation, there appear to be no studies in the literature in which adequate control groups were used in experimenting with the use of reserpine with chronic schizophrenic patients. It has been pointed out by Wolf and Pinsky that patients have shown both psychological and physiological changes when given placebos, and it was felt by us that the effect of the drug must be evaluated with comparable control groups who are to be given placebos or no medication. It is possible that the changes in patients as a result of receiving placebos are due to suggestion, increased attention, and changes in ward routine.

Hypotheses

In general, the studies of the effect of reserpine have indicated a marked reduction in anxiety, hyperactivity, assaultiveness, depression, apprehension, and concern associated with abnormal mental content, and in some instances remission of all symptoms associated with the patient's illness. We set out to evaluate these reported effects of reserpine in a controlled study and, in addition, to observe the effect of granting open-ward privileges to patients who have been on a locked ward for considerable periods of time. The latter was done with the hope of reducing some of the administrative problems of a closed ward, providing added incentive to the patients, and making more open-ward beds available in the hospital. It was also felt that the use of reserpine would result in some patients' making a good open-ward adjustment, whereas previously they had been unable to do so. With these general statements in mind, we tested the following specific hypotheses:

1. Reserpine has a tranquilizing effect on patients which will result in behavioral improvement beyond that which can be attributed to suggestion, increased attention, or changes in ward routine.

2. Open-ward privileges will motivate the patients to change their behavior in an acceptable direction, and will result in increased socialization.

3. Patients receiving reserpine will conform to open-ward rules and regulations, and make a more adequate adjustment to open-ward privileges than patients receiving placebos or no medication at all.

Experimental Procedure and Population

Since the experiment was designed to measure two variables, the effect of placing the patients on open-ward status and the effect of reserpine, it was necessary to select the group from one ward and to include patients who were not known elopers. The Chief of Professional Services and the ward physician of one of the Continued Treatment Service wards interviewed all of the 164 patients in the building to determine by means of a brief screening method which patients could be considered as possible candidates for open-ward privileges. The only criteria for selection were whether the patient could understand the rules and regulations of open-ward status and whether he would promise that he would obey such rules if given these privileges. This screening process resulted in a group of 123 patients who were considered eligible for the research project. From this original group the experimenters eliminated all patients except those with well-established diagnoses of schizophrenic reaction. Any patient who carried a multiple diagnosis or had an accompanying diagnosis of an organic condition was rejected as a candidate for the program, even though his primary diagnosis was schizophrenic reaction.

In order to test the hypotheses and have adequate control of the experimental variables, it was decided that a minimum of 80 patients was needed, to allow for 16 patients in each of the five experimental groups. When the final group of 80 patients was selected, they were distributed at random within the experimental groups. However, since the patients varied considerably in age and length of hospitalization, it was decided to match the groups as much as possible with respect to these two variables. After the original random distribution, some changing was done to control age and length of hospitalization by placing an equal number of older patients in each of the groups. When this was done, it was found that the mean length of hospitalization for each group was approximately the same without any further changing of the patients in any group. The mean age of the groups ranged from 39.8 to 42.7 years, and the mean length of hospitalization ranged from 9.3 to 12.5 years.

The groups were then identified by letters A through E, only the experimenters having knowledge of which groups were receiving reserpine. This was felt to be necessary so that if any medical problems arose it would be easy to check immediately to see whether the patient was actually receiving the drug. Since the experimenters did not rate any of the patients, it was not felt that this knowledge would bias the evaluation of the effectiveness of the treatment. The following is the identification of the groups and the treatment of each. The groups will be identified by these letters throughout the rest of this paper: (*a*) Group A, reserpine and open ward; (*b*) Group B, placebo and open ward; (*c*) Group C, reserpine and closed ward; (*d*) Group D, no medication and closed ward, (*e*) Group E, no medication and open ward.

The entire project covered a period of six months, which was divided into the following three phases: a two-month preexperimental phase, a three-month experimental phase, and a one-month follow-up period. The preexperimental and follow-up phases were established for the purpose of pre- and postexperimental testing and evaluation of the patients, which will be taken up in more detail later. During the entire six months no changes were made in ward routine, assignments of patients to various activities, transfer to other wards, or ward personnel.

Following the preexperimental period of eight weeks, the patients in the open-ward groups were given full open-ward privileges, and the groups on drugs were started on oral doses of 4 mg. daily. The placebo group was given identical-appearing tablets in the same amount. This procedure was continued for 30 days, at which time the dosage was increased to 8 mg. orally on a daily basis for an additional 60 days.

Methods of Evaluation

From the beginning of the preexperimental phase until the end of the follow-up period, each of the patients was rated weekly by three psychiatric aides on the L-M Fergus Falls Behavior Rating Scale, weekly blood pressures were taken, and weight was recorded once a month. By this means a base line was established for behavior, weight, and blood pressures before treatment began, and could be followed during the rest of the experiment.

The Minnesota Multiphasic Personality Inventory (MMPI) was administered to each patient during the preexperimental period, and this test was repeated during the follow-up phase.

In recording the behavior ratings for each patient, the mean of the three raters for each item on the scale was used. The mean of all of the patients' scores for each particular behavior item of the scale was then recorded as the group score for comparison among groups. This allowed for a comparison among groups on each of the various kinds of behavior rated, as well as among groups on their over-all behavior.

The statistical tools used were analysis of variance and significance of differences between related means.

Before discussing results, it will be noted that the total number of patients in the analysis of the experimental data do not total the original 80 patients. A few of the patients eloped or wandered around the hospital grounds, disregarding their assignments or not reporting to the ward according to schedule, and were then placed on a closed section; a few of the patients had to be taken from the closed-ward groups and placed on the open section in place of the elopers because the number of closed-ward beds was limited; a few patients were inadvertently shifted to different assignments in the Department of Physical Medicine and Rehabilitation; one elderly patient died of causes unrelated to the experiment, and a few patients became physically ill during the experiment and were dropped from the groups when they were transferred to the general medical ward. For any of the above reasons, or similar ones, these patients were eliminated from the experiment to rule out uncontrolled variables.

In Group A there were three elopements, and one patient became physically ill; in Group B there were two elopements; in Group C six patients were transferred out of the ward; in Group D five patients were transferred, and in Group E there were three elopements and one death. The total number of patients, then, eliminated from the experiment was 21, and this included 8 elopers, 1 who became physically ill, 11 who were transferred, and 1 death. Elopers included not only patients who left the hospital grounds, but also patients who consistently violated the regulations of open-ward privileges, such as not reporting to assignments or not reporting to their wards or meals at prescribed times. Of the original 16 patients in each group, the final number was 12 for Group A, 14 for Group B, 10 for Group C, 11 for Group D, and 12 for Group E, the total being 59 patients. The behavior ratings for these 59 patients were used for comparison among groups on the L-M Fergus Falls Behavior Rating Scale.

The comparison among groups with respect to pre- and postexperimental MMPI profiles necessarily included only those patients in each group who completed the MMPI both times it was administered, and was further limited to those included in the final 59 patients. For the Groups A through E, the numbers, respectively, are 6, 10, 7, 0, and 9, for a total of 32 patients. Of the original 80 patients who were given the MMPI, the respective numbers are 14, 11, 12, 6, and 12, for a total of 55 patients completing the MMPI. Of the 59 patients remaining in the experiment, 40 had completed the MMPI the first time, but there were 4 in Group A, 2 in Group D, and 2 in Group E who would not complete it the second time it was given. One patient in Group B and two patients in Group D finished the MMPI the second time, even though they did not complete it the first time.

RESULTS

1. *Systolic Blood Pressure.*—As can be noted from Figure 1, both drug groups showed a reliable reduction in systolic blood pressure, with the placebo group remaining relatively unchanged.

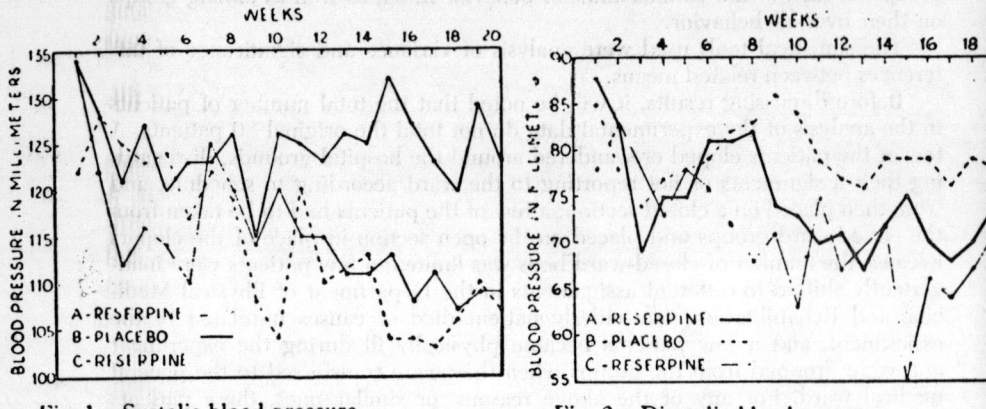

Fig. 1.—Systolic blood pressure.

Fig. 2.—Diastolic blood pressure.

2. *Diastolic Blood Pressure.*—It can be noted from Figure 2 that there was a reduction in diastolic blood pressure in both the drug groups, with the placebo group again remaining relatively unchanged.

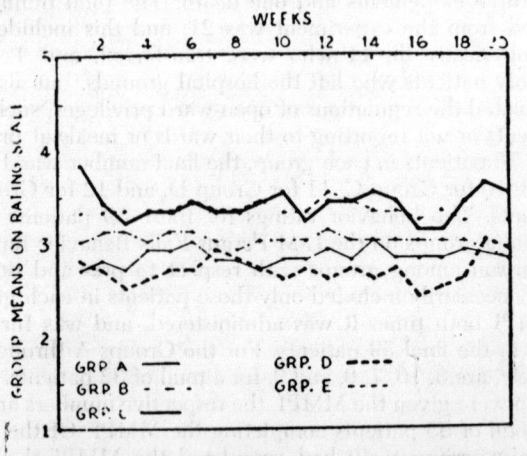

Fig. 3.—Weekly group means on L-M Fergus Falls Behavior Rating Scales.

3. *Weight.*—The two drug groups gained an average of 4 lb., whereas the placebo group showed an average loss of 3 lb.

4. *Behavior.*—There was no significant change in over-all behavior found in any of the five groups studied as measured by the L-M Fergus Falls Be-

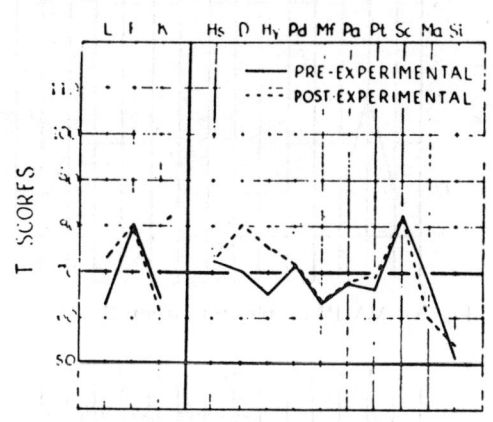

Fig. 4.—MMPI profiles for Group A.

havior Rating Scale. As can be noted from Figure 3, there is no consistent difference among groups, nor is there any trend toward behavioral improvement perceived in any group that could be attributed to drugs, suggestion, increased attention, or changes in ward routine.

5. *MMPI Profiles.*—As can be seen on Figures 4, 5, 6, and 7, there were no significant differences found, with one exception, on any of the scales on the MMPI for the groups studied when the pre- and postexperimental profiles were compared. The one exception is a significant increase on the *Hy* score for Group A (reserpine plus open-ward privileges).

6. *Social Adjustment.*—Open-ward privileges did not result in increased socialization. No significant improvement was found on the scales measuring responses to other patients, psychiatric aides, nurses, doctors, social workers, and psychologists.

7. *Conformity.*—Patients receiving reserpine did not conform better than the placebo and no-medication groups to open-ward rules and regulations. Conformity was measured by the number of elopements and by the number of patients who consistently violated the rules of open-ward privileges by such behavior as not reporting to assignments or to their wards or meals at prescribed times. The number of patients falling in this category was eight, and included three in the reserpine group, two in the placebo group, and three in the no-medication group.

8. *Completion of MMPI.*—With respect to the patients who for one reason or another did not complete the MMPI the first time it was administered, it was not found that reserpine resulted in these patients taking it the second time it was given.

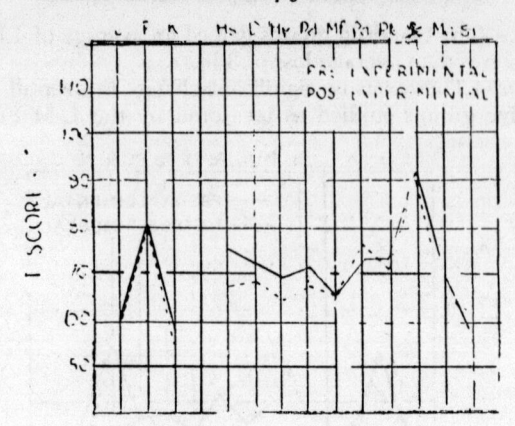

Fig. 5—MMPI profiles for Group B

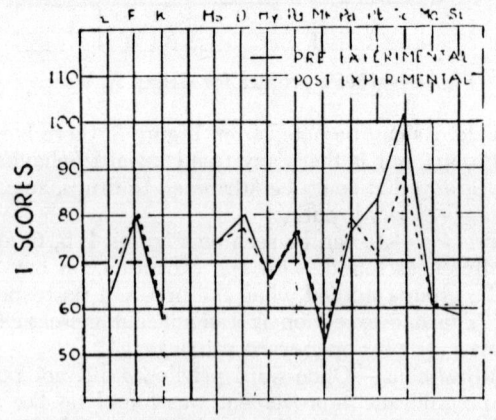

Fig. 6—MMPI profiles for Group C

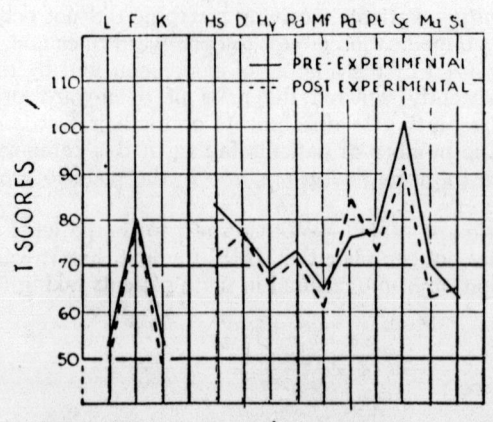

Fig. 7.—MMPI profiles for Group E.

Comment

The finding that the use of reserpine resulted in a reliable reduction of both systolic and diastolic blood pressure is consistent with the findings of other investigators. In addition, as was found in another study, reserpine tended to bring about a slight gain in weight, while the placebo group showed a slight loss in weight. We can offer no explanation to explain this loss of weight with placebo tablets.

The negative results with respect to improvement either behaviorally or as measured by the MMPI may be due to several factors. First, 8 mg. orally per day may not be an effective dosage for chronic schizophrenic patients. Second, reserpine may not have a generalized therapeutic effect on such chronically disturbed patients. Third, the administration of the drug may not have been continued over a sufficient time to obtain positive results. As to the amount of the drug given to the patients, it compared very favorably with the dose given by other experimenters who have reported positive results, and in many cases was considerably more than has been given by others.

As part of the original design, we planned to administer the drug for a period of 90 days. As a result of surveying the literature for previously reported studies of the use of reserpine, it seemed reasonable to assume that positive changes in behavior, if they were to occur, would begin to manifest themselves within this period of time. We also decided to check results at the end of the 90-day period, and, if some improved behavior was observed, to continue the drug for a longer period. Since no changes were noted, it is our opinion that three months on the drug was a sufficient test of its effectiveness. We feel that reserpine given at random to chronic schizophrenics is of little effectiveness, and that further research should be directed toward the development of a set of criteria to be used for the selection of patients who might profit from such treatment.

Although other studies have indicated that increased attention, changes in ward routine, and suggestion have resulted in improvement of behavior, this was not found in this study. We feel that such factors were kept to a minimum in this study, since ward activities were unchanged and all of the patients were already assigned to various activities that kept them busy during the day. The number of ward personnel was not increased, and they were instructed not to show any increased attention to the patients or to comment on the purpose of the drugs.

No harmful side-effects were noticed with the use of reserpine, except in one patient who developed a Parkinson-like syndrome. This disappeared upon discontinuance of the drug.

As has been pointed out, not all the patients completed the MMPI; so it was not possible to compare the MMPI profiles of all the patients in each of the groups. Failure to complete the MMPI was attributed to several things, including negativism and hostility, confusion, and inability to understand directions; a few patients were mute and would not attempt to answer or look at any of the cards, and a few sat in front of the MMPI boxes apparently hallucinating constantly. Some of these patients spent as long as three days on the test without completing it; so further attempts at testing were discontinued. The only change in the MMPI profiles which was significant at the 0.05 level was an increase on the *Hy* scale for Group A, and this finding might be expected to occur by chance when the total number of comparisons made is considered.

The granting of open-ward privileges to chronic schizophrenic patients who have been on a locked ward for a number of years did not seem to have any positive effect on their behavior. It did not result in increased socialization or improved interpersonal relationships, and it did not seem to serve as a reward or as an incentive to change their behavior in a more socially acceptable direction. Patients who were not reporting to their assignments or to the ward at prescribed times were warned about the possible loss of their privileges, but this did not seem to be effective in changing their behavior. As mentioned previously, patients in open-ward groups who violated the rules and regulations of open-ward privileges were returned to locked sections and were dropped from the experiment. However, weekly ratings of them were continued, and these ratings did not indicate any negative change in behavior as a result of the loss of open-ward privileges. This raises the question as to whether being placed on an open ward is very meaningful and rewarding to patients similar to those used in this experiment. It suggests that awarding of open-ward privileges is insufficient to produce improved behavior, and that such a change in ward status should be utilized in conjunction with a total-push type of program, which can usually be more effectively used with open-ward patients.

One of the most interesting results of the experiment is the discovery that even with such a crude screening method as was used in this study potential elopers could be reduced to a minimum. Of the total number of eight listed as "elopers," only three actually left the hospital grounds. One of these was picked up by hospital personnel; one called the hospital from a nearby railroad depot to ask to be returned to the hospital, and one went to his home. The parents of this patient called the hospital to report his arrival and to request that they be allowed to keep him with them. This finding would suggest that many of the other patients in the hospital who have been on locked wards for many years could be placed on open wards, or that many of the locked wards could be changed to open ones. At the present time 45% of the patients in this hospital are on open wards, and it is planned to increase this percentage despite the findings of this study that open-ward privileges per se are not sufficient to produce desired changes in chronic schizophrenics. There are several reasons for this planned change. First, there would be a lessening of some of the administrative problems on the ward. An obvious example is the reduction of time spent by the psychiatric aides in transporting patients to the various activities in other sections of the hospital. Second, it would make available to the patients many activities which are therapeutic but which are not available to closed-ward patients because of the number of personnel that would be required for supervision. This applied especially to the many recreation activities that are conducted on the hospital grounds. Third, the opening of the ward for this study resulted in greatly increased morale of the personnel members on the ward. They no longer felt that they were working on one of the "hopeless" or "back" wards in the hospital, or that nobody was paying any attention to what was going on in their building. Fourth, it would mean a gain in the number of open-ward beds in the hospital and would reduce some of the "waiting time" of patients on closed wards until open-ward beds were available.

Summary

Eighty chronic schizophrenic patients on a closed ward were divided into five groups of 16 patients each. One group was given reserpine and open-ward privileges; one group was given open-ward privileges without medication; one group was given open-ward privileges and placebo; one group remained on a locked section and was given reserpine, and one group remained on the locked section without medication. The drug groups were given 4 mg. orally each day for 30 days, and this was increased to 8 mg. orally per day for the next 60 days. The placebo group was given identical-appearing placebos in the same amount. All groups were studied for eight weeks prior to and for four weeks subsequent to this period of 90 days. Weekly ratings of behavior were made throughout the entire six months, and the Minnesota Multiphasic Personality Inventory was given before and after the three-month period of medication. Measurements were made of blood pressure and weight at regular intervals.

Conclusions

1. Reserpine in oral doses of 8 mg. per day did not result in improvement, as measured by rating scales and by the MMPI, in chronic schizophrenic patients.
2. Patients receiving reserpine did not adjust better on the open ward than patients receiving no medication, as measured by conformity to the rules of the ward and the number of elopements.
3. Awarding of open-ward privileges did not result in improved interpersonal relationships or behavioral improvement.
4. Reserpine did effect a lowering of blood pressure.
5. Reserpine resulted in a slight weight gain.

SHORT-TERM TREATMENT OF PSYCHIATRIC PATIENTS WITH RESERPINE

Stephen B. Payn, M.D., and Fred V. Rockwell, M.D.

The purpose of this study was to evaluate the short-term therapeutic usefulness of reserpine. The patients were treated during a relatively short observation period in the Psychiatric Institute of Grasslands Hospital.

Between October, 1954, and August, 1955, reserpine was given to 100 patients. We confined our study to patients in whom any favorable effect of the drug was likely to be dramatic and unmistakable and could not easily be confused with the spontaneous improvement as a result of the hospitalization. For this reason, too, we usually observed the patient for several days and gave the reserpine only if no spontaneous improvement took place. Our method of evaluating the results differed from that of most investigators insofar as we evaluated each individual patient by daily observation and frequent psychiatric interviews.

Method

In our earlier patients the initial dose of reserpine was 3 to 5 mg. given in one dose intramuscularly, orally, or occasionally intravenously. Thereafter the patient received 1 or 2 mg. or reserpine by mouth once a day. When oral medication was refused, it was given intramuscularly. Later in our study the daily dose from the first day on consisted of 5 to 15 mg. intramuscularly with or without 2 to 6 mg. by mouth. The blood pressure was taken every day immediately before and one hour, two hours, three hours, and six hours after the medication. The nurses kept daily records of the individual patient's behavior and of the number of hours that the patient slept every night. In addition, the patient was seen in psychiatric interviews every few days.

As mentioned before, the medication was usually given after an observation period of a few days when no spontaneous improvement occurred. Occasionally, however, in severely disturbed patients treatment with reserpine was started within a few hours after admission.

General Effect

The first effect of the drug usually appeared about thirty minutes to three hours after the injection and consisted of generalized flushing, chilliness, and tremulousness lasting several hours. These symptoms were rarely seen when the drug was taken by mouth. On the other hand, they did not appear much sooner after intravenous injection than after intramuscular administration. This was also observed by Kline, who therefore believes that some metabolic change has to occur before the drug can become active. Hafkenschiel and Sellers suggest that this change is a conversion of the reserpine into a yohimbine-like substance.

The first effect of the reserpine on the mental condition was a sedative one and sometimes occurred dramatically within a few hours but was usually not apparent until the third or fourth day of treatment. Tension and anxiety were reduced. The patients were less agitated and less assaultive. Their appetite improved, and they were able to sleep better.

It is remarkable that this improvement usually occurred without any change in the mental content. Patients with delusions, for instance, continued to have their delusions but were no longer frightened by them.

After about a week some of our patients showed an aggravation of their original symptoms. They became tense, excited, and assaultive and had delusions and hallucinations. This phase lasted from an hour to several days, but when the medication was continued, the patients improved again.

These observations confirm the description given by Barsa and Kline, who divide the effect of treatment with reserpine into three phases, the sedative phase, the turbulent phase, and the integrative phase.

SIDE-EFFECTS

Only few side-effects were noted. Their occurrence was in no way related to the therapeutic efficacy of the drug. The most common side-effects were those mentioned before: chilliness, generalized flushing, and tremulousness, which appeared from thirty minutes to three hours after parenteral administration and subsided after several hours. As part of the flush reaction several patients had a marked injection of the conjunctival vessels. Some patients had stuffiness of the nose; some had soft stools or gastric discomfort. Drowsiness was not infrequent, and an occasional patient complained of generalized muscle aching. The symptoms usually subsided spontaneously or with symptomatic treatment, but in some cases the dose had to be reduced. Since our patients received the drug for short periods only, they never developed any Parkinsonism, which many authors describe as a common side-effect after prolonged administration.

EFFECT ON THE BLOOD PRESSURE

For the purpose of this study the patients were divided into three groups on the basis of the blood pressure, with the same criteria as those used by Kline:

1. "Normal" blood pressure, between 100 and 149 mm. Hg systolic or between 60 and 99 diastolic pressure.
2. Low blood pressure, anything below that.
3. High blood pressure, anything above that.

The effect of reserpine on the blood pressure was not always consistent. In some cases there was a transient rise a few hours after administration of the drug. In others the blood pressure fell abruptly within an hour or two after the drug was taken but rose again to its original level during the next twelve to twenty-four hours and then fluctuated in an irregular fashion either around the original level or at a lower level. The response often varied from day to day in the same patient with the blood pressure falling one day and remaining unchanged another day. The fall occurred in some patients within two hours and in others after several days. It involved either the systolic pressure alone or both the systolic and diastolic pressure. In our series there were no cases with lowering of the diastolic pressure alone.

Since spontaneous fluctuations of the blood pressure had to be taken into account, the pressure was considered lowered only if there was a drop of at least 25 mm. Hg in the normotensive group and 35 mm. in the hypertensive group.

Of 78 patients with normal blood pressure, 20 responded to reserpine with lowering of the blood pressure, 35 showed no blood pressure change, and 23 had transient lowering with spontaneous return to the original level.

Of 19 patients with hypertension, seven had a blood pressure fall, two had no change, and ten had only transient lowering.

Our series had three patients with low blood pressure. Two of them showed no blood pressure change, while in the third patient an alarming fall in systolic and diastolic pressure occurred.

CASE 1.—The patient, a thirty-eight-year-old woman with far-advanced, active pulmonary tuberculosis, was admitted to the Psychiatric Division because of auditory and visual hallucinations and paranoid ideas resulting in refusal to eat. She received an intramuscular injection of 5 mg. of reserpine initially and 1 mg. by mouth the following day. Her blood pressure was 98/68 before the injection. It remained essentially unchanged until the third day when it was 88/58. The reserpine was withheld, but the blood pressure continued to fall and on the sixth day was 70/20. It rose spontaneously to 94/68 the next day. The patient had no complaints which could be attributed to the hypotension, even when the blood pressure was at its lowest level.

What was unusual in this case was the fact that the blood pressure continued to fall even after the drug was stopped.

There were several other patients in whom the blood pressure fell rather sharply, but in most of them it rose again spontaneously, and the reserpine could be continued, as in the following case.

CASE 2.—A twenty-six-year-old male patient with acute undifferentiated schizophrenic reaction received 5 mg. of reserpine intramuscularly. Before the injection his blood pressure had been 110/72. After two hours it was 96/70, and an hour later it had fallen to 88/38. This fall was associated with pain in his head, back, and abdomen and a feeling of heat alternating with chilliness. He improved spontaneously within a few hours. The blood pressure rose to 100/60 and remained at this level with minor fluctuations. The reserpine was continued with 2 mg. by mouth daily for eighteen days.

In other patients it was necessary to withhold the reserpine or to use ephedrine or phenylephrine (Neo-Synephrine), as in the following patient.

CASE 3.— A twenty-nine-year-old woman with acute undifferentiated schizophrenia had a blood pressure of 100/60 before she was started on reserpine, 5 mg. intramuscularly and 1 mg. by mouth every day. There was no essential change in the blood pressure until the fifth day of treatment when it fell to 60/30. The patient received 50 mg. of ephedrine intramuscularly, and the blood pressure rose again. A second drop occurred on the seventh day of treatment, this time to 68/48. When the reserpine was withheld, the blood pressure rose again. At no time did the patient show any symptoms which were due to the fall in the blood pressure.

What was said about this patient applies to most others. It was astonishing that the marked drop in the blood pressure was rarely associated with any symptoms. This may be partly explained by the observations of Hafkenschiel, Sellers, King, and Thorner that reserpine did not decrease cerebral blood flow so that their patients had no complaints which could be attributed to cerebral ischemia.

Effect on the Mental State

Of 100 patients who received reserpine there were 12 with marked improvement, 18 with moderate improvement, and 28 with slight improvement; that is, 58 patients showed some degree of improvement, while 42 did not improve.

By "marked improvement" we mean a very definite change in the patient's behavior, as shown, for instance, when a patient in catatonic stupor begins to talk or loses his waxy flexibility; or when a patient with incoherent speech full of neologisms begins to talk coherently; or when an agitated, hostile patient becomes quiet and friendly. "Marked improvement" does not necessarily mean that the thought content has changed.

Between "marked improvement" and "no improvement," there are degrees which we called "moderate improvement" and "mild improvement." These terms mean here what they generally mean. Any more precise definition tends to obscure the fact that the evaluation of behavior and emotions is bound to be subjective to a certain degree. Suffice it to say that even for "slight improvement" there had to be a definite change, such as ability to sleep without sedation in a patient who previously slept poorly even with sedation. Whenever there was any doubt about the effect of the reserpine, the result was classified as "no improvement."

The number of cases studied is not sufficiently large to permit accurate statistical evaluation of possible correlations between the degree of improvement and such variables as type and duration of illness, age of patient, and blood pressure response. However, the results of this study are presented as factual observations.

The highest rate of improvement was obtained in the schizophrenic reactions (37 out of 50 patients).

Patients under the age of forty had better results than those over forty. Of 54 patients below forty, 38 improved, whereas only 20 out of 46 patients over forty showed improvement.

Patients with illness of less than two years duration responded better than patients whose first psychotic episode dated back more than two years.

A favorable response to reserpine occurred more often when the drug was given in the early stages of an episode.

There was no evidence of correlation between the therapeutic effect of reserpine and the blood pressure response.

On the basis of the total clinical observations, the authors were left with the impression that the best results were obtained in those patients with the most intense emotional reactions, especially tension and anxiety, regardless of diagnosis.

The results of treatment did not always depend on the dose of the drug. While it has been generally established that the reserpine doses used in the earlier clinical trials were too small, the optimal dose has not yet been determined. Our studies have shown that some patients improve with small doses, while others do not respond to much larger doses. We have no explanation for it. But this apparent inconsistency can hardly be surprising when we consider the complexity of the pathologic condition that we are treating. Obviously further studies will be necessary. Our main intention was to see whether reserpine could be of value in the short-term treatment of psychiatric patients. That it is of definite value can be seen from the following two case histories.

CASE 4.—A forty-year-old woman was transferred to the Psychiatric Institute from the surgical service following a breast biopsy. Although the lesion was found to be benign, the patient was depressed and apprehensive and felt the nurses were conspiring against her. She was convinced something terrible was going to be done to her; she had learned of it "through the air." She spoke of vague hallucinatory experiences. She would often burst into tears and insist she had cancer. Her movements were slow, her appetite was poor, and she required sedation at night.

On her fourth day in the Psychiatric Institute she received 5 mg. of reserpine intramuscularly. This was followed by daily oral doses of 1 mg. About six hours after the injection she watched television and smiled occasionally, and that night she slept without sedation. The next day she was more relaxed and outgoing, talked rationally, ate well, and was able to help with the ward work. Two days later, however, she woke up during the night, was very agitated, said she was "tricked into coming here," and the "spirits" were telling her that something was going on. When the nurse gave her some milk, she asked whether a pill was put into it. Although she was still tense the following day, she soon began to relax again, and from then on she continued to improve. She conversed freely with the patients and nurses, laughed and joked with them, and seemed to enjoy their company. The nurses described her as "the life of the ward."

Blood pressure before the first dose of reserpine was 110/80 mm. Hg and remained unchanged. No side-effects were observed. The patient was discharged to her husband on the ninth day of treatment.

CASE 5.—A thirty-seven-year-old, white woman was admitted to the Psychiatric Institute of Grasslands Hospital in catatonic stupor. She was mute and motionless, stared into space, and showed automatic obedience to the point of waxy flexibility. Thirteen hours after her admission, she received 4 mg. of reserpine intravenously. Thirty minutes later her movements were more relaxed, and she went to the toilet spontaneously, while previously it had been necessary to toilet her. One and a half hours after the injection her face was flushed, and she indicated by gestures that her chest and throat were tight. Half an hour later, she also expressed it in words. She still talked little, usually only in response to questions, and she still had waxy flexibility. She ate fairly well and slept with 0.1 Gm. of pentobarbital sodium.

The next day the improvement was remarkable. There was no more automatic obedience. She talked freely and described her feelings in the following manner: "I was afraid of everything...Mostly of people. Everything looks different now. I'd like to take care of my children and husband the best I possibly can . . . Now I realize my husband doesn't bother with other women. He doesn't drink. He is good to me . . . One morning I heard somebody banging and I was afraid and ran away, but of course I couldn't run away from myself."

The improvement continued for four days during which she received 1 mg. of reserpine by mouth every day. On the fifth day she became agitated, paced up and down, then lay down and stared at the ceiling. When spoken to, she said: "I feel like nobody wants me. My husband doesn't want me. They are making fun of me. Doctor, am I a bad person? I am afraid." The reserpine was increased to 2 mg. a day. In the course of the day her anxiety diminished, and she slept well without sedation. The following day she was transferred to the State hospital in good condition.

In both patients one can recognize the sedative phase, the turbulent phase, and the beginning of the integrative phase. We could never observe more than the beginning of the third phase because the patients reached it at a time when they were ready for transfer to the state hospital.

While reserpine does not cure the patients of their psychoses, the drug is more than just a sedative. Its importance lies in the fact that it establishes contact between the patients and the outside world and thereby makes them accessible to psychotherapy. This is dramatically illustrated in the last case.

Not less striking is the effect that the treatment with reserpine has had on the general atmosphere in the wards. A remarkable change has taken place. The wards are quiet. Fewer patients have to be secluded. Tube feedings are rarely necessary. Less sedation is needed. Sedative packs are hardly ever used. To what extent sedative packs and tube feedings have been reduced is shown in Table I, which compares the number of packs and tube feedings during the first six months of reserpine therapy with the figures during the corresponding six-month periods in the four preceding years.

TABLE I.—NUMBER OF SEDATIVE PACKS AND TUBE FEEDINGS IN RELATION TO RESERPINE

	Sedative Packs	Tube Feedings
Without reserpine		
Oct., 1950 to Mar., 1951	432	159
Oct., 1951 to Mar., 1952	709	155
Oct., 1952 to Mar., 1953	453	64
Oct., 1953 to Mar., 1954	621	107
With reserpine		
Oct., 1954 to Mar., 1955	95	12

Summary

Reserpine was subjected to clinical trial in the short-term treatment of 100 psychiatric patients. Fifty-eight patients improved. While a change in the patients' thought content was rarely apparent, the most striking effect of the drug was the relief of tension and anxiety, resulting in improved sleep, reduction of overactivity, and the establishment of contact with the environment. The wards became more quiet, there was less need for sedation, and tube feedings and sedative packs were practically eliminated.

USE OF RESERPINE ON AN ADMISSION SERVICE

Ernest Gosline, M.D.,
Supervising Psychiatrist, Rockland State Hospital, Orangeburg, N. Y.,

and Nathan S. Kline, M.D.,
Director of Research, Rockland State Hospital, Orangeburg, N. Y.

On the female reception service at Rockland State Hospital, Orangeburg, N. Y., during the year 1954 there were a total of 1093 new admissions and another 233 patients returned from convalescent status and family care. The building has a capacity of 440 beds and it is evident that the problems of management in this group of recent admissions, especially since many patients are acutely disturbed and severely psychotic, is a matter of intense practical concern. In a recent paper by Kline and Stanley it was emphasized that in addition "to discharging patients from the mental hospital there is the equally important problem of maintaining those patients who cannot be brought to a point of improvement sufficient for discharge in as comfortable, healthy, and economical manner as possible." It is not an infrequent occurrence that the memory of the traditional management techniques, such as cold packs, restraints, and seclusion, linger as an unpleasant memory in some patients after they have recovered from the acute phases of their illness.

An evaluation of the effects of reserpine was made with a group of 100 patients, recently admitted to the female reception service; they were selected on the basis that they all presented special problems in ward management. The behavior difficulties include excitements, assaultive and self-destructive behavior, hypomanic states, potentially suicidal and homicidal behavior, depression, agitation, feeding problems, post-shock confusional states, and cases requiring marked sedation, restraint, or seclusion because of their mental condition. Patients in whom there was a delay or contraindication to receiving such somatic therapy as electro-convulsive therapy or insulin coma were also included in this group. Some patients in whom the delusional trend was of such a nature that there were marked disturbances in their relationships with society were included. Another group of patients had difficulties in their inter-personal relationships to the extent that they were extremely annoying to other patients and hospital personnel or were disruptive to ward routine.

SELECTION OF SUBJECTS

These first 100 patients to receive reserpine were selected purely because of the management problems involved without regard to age, diagnosis, duration, or severity of illness. The duration of treatment ranged from a total of 8 days to 7 months. Reserpine was given either orally or on a combined oral and parenteral regime. Age ranged from 15 to 72 years (Table I). The majority of patients received reserpine for one month or longer (Table II). The majority of patients were first admissions (Table III) and there was a wide range of diagnostic categories (Table IV).

TABLE I: AGE DISTRIBUTION
(Range—15 years to 72 years)

Age	Number of Patients
15–25	21
26–35	21
36–45	21
46–55	23
Over 55	14
Total	100

TABLE II: LENGTH OF TIME PATIENTS RECEIVED RESERPINE
(Range—8 days to 7 months)

Under one month	12
1–2 months	52
Over 2 months	36
Total	100

TABLE III: NUMBER OF PREVIOUS ADMISSIONS

None	55 patients
1	20
2	14
3 or more	11
Total	100

METHOD OF ADMINISTRATION

Thirty patients were treated with oral reserpine exclusively, and received from .5 mg. to 4.0 mg., with an average dose of from 2 to 3 mg., daily. Another group of 70 patients received a standard combined parenteral and oral dosage regimen. On the first day, patients received only 2.5 mg. reserpine intramuscularly to test for unusual reactions. Thereafter, patients received 5 mg. reserpine parenterally and 1.5 mg. orally. After 8 days, patients were

TABLE IV: Distribution of Diagnoses

Dementia Praecox, Catatonic type	23
Dementia Praecox, Paranoid type	16
Dementia Praecox, Hebephrenic type	3
Dementia Praecox, Mixed or undifferentiated type	15
Dementia Praecox, other types	2
Total Schizophrenia	59
Manic-Depressive Psychosis	10
Involutional Psychosis	11
Psychoneurosis	3
Character and behavior disorders	3
Psychosis with mental deficiency	2
Psychosis with organic or structural change	12
Total	100 patients

placed on a maintenance dose of 2.0 to 3.0 mg. reserpine by mouth. Dosages were modified to meet individual needs. In the light of subsequent experience, we now regard this dosage as inadequate for therapy in many cases, although it was sufficient to modify management problems as detailed below. Currently we are using larger doses for longer periods in an effort to evaluate the full therapeutic potentialities.

Evaluation of Management

In an attempt to formulate some method for scoring the wide variety of management problems on an admission service, the following classification was evolved:

Group I

This group includes patients who are assaultive, elated, hypomanic or severely disturbed in response to their environment or to their own autistic productions. This group includes patients who ordinarily would be placed on emergency electric shock treatment or be transferred to the disturbed section of the hospital.

Group II

This group includes behavior problems other than those stated above, such as severe regression, stupors, catatonia, suicidal tendencies, self-mutilating tendencies, feeding problems, and cases having sudden short-term sporadic outbursts of disturbed behavior.

Group III

Somatic problems. This group includes special disease entities such as Alzheimer's Disease, epilepsy, and one case of psoriasis. It also includes cases of severe cardiovascular disease, cerebral vascular accidents, fractures, and other physical contraindications to electric shock treatment. Patients who have dehydration, emaciation, and severe hypertension were also included in this group.

Group IV

This group includes those patients who are severe sedation problems requiring massive doses of customary sedatives such as barbiturates, hyoscine, paraldehyde, etc.

Group V

This group is composed of those patients having marked difficulties in interpersonal relationships. This includes those patients in whom the mental content, the anxieties, or the delusional trends are of such a nature that they are a source of difficulty to hospital, family, and to other patients, and also to employees who are directly concerned with their management. Included in this group are patients with strong manipulative tendencies, who arouse the hostilities of others, and then step aside when altercations develop.

Many patients were problems in management in only one area; other patients would be considered problems in management in all 5 areas. Also, in some cases, despite improvement in behavior in categories I, II, III, and IV, the problems in inter-personal relationships (Group V) became pressing as the patient regained contact with reality. The patients were evaluated in relation to whether they were mild, moderate, or severe problems in the specific areas prior to their placement on reserpine and also at the termination of their treatment. The specific scoring categories were combined to determine whether a patient had an overall improvement in management.

EVALUATION OF THERAPEUTIC EFFECT

Although the basic purpose of this study has been related to the management problems, it is noteworthy that there were definite changes in the patients' mental condition while they were receiving reserpine. In evaluating changes in mental condition and improvement, the following categories, as derived from the paper by Barsa and Kline, are used: markedly improved—, moderately improved—, slightly improved—, no improvement—, and worse—. "Markedly improved" means ready for discharge, and other categories are graded accordingly.

Of this group of patients studied, 80 patients had been approved for either electro-convulsive therapy and/or insulin therapy prior to being started on reserpine. Also, several patients were placed on reserpine following electroshock therapy because of a severe post-shock confusional state.

RESULTS

Clinical observations on the patients were made by the authors during the course of daily rounds on the female reception service. In addition, observations by attendants and nurses, and frequent discussion with the resident psychiatrists directly responsible for the patients, were considered in the evaluation of the effect of reserpine. Especially helpful were the frequent, constructively critical discussions with Dr. Charlotte Munn, whose experience as head of the female reception service was invaluable in the clinical evaluation of these patients. The general impression of the ward personnel, nurses, supervisors, and even the families was that the patients receiving reserpine showed more interest in their immediate surroundings, were more sociable, entered into more constructive activities, and were more pliant and flexible in adjusting to the hospital environment. There was a marked reduction in the number of mechanical restraints, seclusion orders, and usual sedation. Despite the patient's frequent complaints of weakness and dizziness during the early stages of treatment, there were very few injuries or accidents. Tube-feeding became almost non-existent in this group of patients. Patients receiving reserpine would occasionally request camisole because of their anxiety and fear-producing impulses, and would not resist the application of the restraint, at times even expressing gratitude.

Another favorable change was seen among the poorly nourished patients. They usually had a marked increase in appetite and showed an obvious pleasure in eating, often to the extent of being the center of good-natured comments from other patients and employees. Personal hygiene and appearance were almost uniformly improved, and some of these women expressed concern about their weight gain. Patients who had previously been disruptive to ward routines, sometimes in a most obtrusive manner, responded dramatically.

The following tables attempt to approach the clinical results in a statistical manner, although it must be emphasized the value of such data is dependent upon accurate clinical appraisal by the psychiatrist.

Previous studies by Barsa and Kline had shown no correlation between therapeutic response and age, and therefore no attempt was made to correlate these when no relationship obtruded itself upon inspection of the data. Table V presents an evaluation of the therapeutic response (as contrasted to management response) of the entire group in respect to diagnosis. The response in the "organic" cases was less satisfactory than for most other cate-

TABLE V: IMPROVEMENT RELATIVE TO DIAGNOSIS

	Marked %	Moderate %	Slight %	None %	Worse %	Number of Patients
Schizophrenia	22	42	24	12	0	59
Manic-Depressive	20	20	20	30	10	10
Involutional	9	73	9	9	0	11
Behavior disorders	100	0	0	0	0	2
Psychoneurosis	67	33	0	0	0	3
Psychopathic Personality	0	0	0	100	0	1
Mental Deficiency	0	50	0	0	50	2
Organic Disorders	8	8	25	42	17	12
Average	21%	38%	20%	17%	4%	100

gories. If these are excluded from the population, overall improvement of 86% (rather than 79%) is found, Again, it should be repeated that the dosage and regimen are now deemed to have been less than optimum, so that decidedly *better* results are anticipated with the more adequate therapeutic regimen we have initiated since December 1, 1954.

Table VI indicates the number and percentage of specific types of management problems and the response to reserpine. Although not convenient for inclusion in the table, the excellent results obtained in clearing up post-electroshock confusional states is worth mentioning. The need for emergency electroshock therapy was also practically eliminated. One very unusual result was the alleviation of a case of severe and chronic stuttering. This recurred when medication was discontinued, and has been relieved a second time with return to medication. The table leaves no question of the value of reserpine in the management of patients on an admission service.

Each patient was also scored from +1 to +3 for their degree of cooperativeness in each of the 5 possible groups. The lowest degree of cooperation was +1 and the greatest, +3. The greatest degree of improvement would thus be 2 points. Similarly, the degree of management difficulty was scored from −1 to −3 in each group. The combined score obtained by subtracting the minus rating from the plus gives an overall numerical index of management status of the entire population. This index before and after reserpine provides a quantification of improvement. The greatest possible shift is 4 points, and Table VII details the improvement in management as measured by this score.

The relative merits of the oral vs. the combined oral and parenteral reserpine are also demonstrated in Table VII. It is noted that disturbed patients, Group I, respond better to the combined (oral and i.m.) medication, whereas there does not appear to be so significant a difference in the other groups. The

TABLE VI: Percent of Patients Presenting Problems of Management

Type	Pre-medication	After Reserpine
Group I (assaultive, disturbed)	72	38
Group II (stuporous, suicidal, etc.)	93	48
Group III (somatic problems)	47	35
Group IV (sedation problems)	81	40
Group V (difficult interpersonal relationships)	81	63

Summary: 72% of patients showed definite improvement in at least one area.

combined treatment involves relatively low doses by present standards, and it is possible that under other circumstances greater differences would appear. Also of significance is the high mean combined index for Group V, which may have some correlation with the possible therapeutic effect of the medication. It is evident that this effect should be more fully explored, and work is at present being undertaken in this direction.

Of the 100 patients, 43 had on this or previous admissions had some previ-

TABLE VII: Mean Improvement as Measured by Management Index

	Reserpine Oral	Reserpine Combined	Percent of Patients Improved
Group I	.4	1.4	53
Group II	1.6	1.7	52
Group III	.4	.5	74
Group IV	.8	1.2	49
Group V	1.0	.9	78

Cooperativeness rated 1 to 3
Management difficulty rated 1 to 3

$$\text{Management Index} = \frac{\text{increase in cooperativeness plus decrease in management difficulty}}{\text{number of patients}}$$

ous form of somatic therapy such as electro-convulsive treatment and/or insulin coma. All patients in Table VIII had been recommended for electro-shock and/or insulin by the clinical director, and ordinarily would have received such treatment.

It was felt, in a careful review of the cases in the light of the descriptions of Barsa and Kline, that 10 of the above patients were transferred to the Shock Unit during an unrecognized "turbulent period," and that they might well have been continued on reserpine. Success in supplanting EST and/or insulin was so encouraging that, on an experimental basis, EST has been entirely discontinued on the female admission service, although it may still be prescribed in emergency circumstances (which as yet has not been necessary).

TABLE VIII: Reserpine and Shock Therapy

	Pre-medication—Scheduled for Shock	Reserpine-Treated—Placed on Shock
Number of patients	80	26 *

Summary: In 67½% of patients scheduled for shock it was unnecessary.

* Ten of these patients we now recognize to have been in the "Turbulent phase" and shock may not have been necessary if treatment had been continued.

Some of the more interesting undesirable side effects of reserpine are listed in Table IX. There were no irreversible toxic effects noted in this series, and there were no deaths. A Parkinson's syndrome was present at some time during the course of treatment in about 5% of the patients. The tremulousness, gastro-intestinal disturbances, excessive salivation, edema of extremities and face, and other side effects were also seen. One side effect not previously reported was that some of the patients developed mydriasis, which is interesting in that miosis is reported as occurring in cats. One patient became overtly and aggressively homosexual, despite no previous history in this respect, and another patient developed cardiac decompensation, which may or may not have been related to the reserpine.

TABLE IX: SOME PROBABLE SIDE EFFECTS

	Percent of Patients
Depression *	9
Obesity	6
Suicidal Trends	5
Erotic Dreams	3
Dermatitis	3

* Believed released by rather than caused by reserpine.

DISCUSSION

The statistical results of this frankly clinical study indicate that reserpine is of definite use in the management of these selected patients. Since the majority of them were treated for only 1 to 2 months (Table III), it would be difficult to explain their improvement in management as due to spontaneous remissions unrelated to medication or as a result of adjustment to routine, since other similar patients not on reserpine rarely showed such marked changes. The present dosage was sufficient to achieve definite improvement in the manageability of these patients and some improvement in their mental condition (Table V). It is believed that the results achieved would have been better if the "turbulent phase" (as described by Barsa) had been recognized, and the patients continued on medication through this period. Also, those 12 patients receiving medication less than 1 month did not receive adequate treatment by our present standards. The results of this study serve as a preliminary and pilot test of the usefulness of reserpine on an admission service. The obvious need for controls to validate and confirm these results has led us to do a comparative study. This work will be reported on subsequently. Since December 1, 1954, all patients entering the female reception service who are in need of somatic therapy are being placed exclusively on reserpine, except for patients needing emergency shock therapy. As a control to this group we have very detailed records of the effect of electro-shock therapy and insulin on this same service for the entire previous year. In addition to this control, we are also continuing the male reception service in the usual admission treatment without the use of reserpine (with the cooperation of Dr. Kern and his staff). The result of this investigation now under way should definitively determine the value of reserpine in adequate doses on an admission service.

Although patients receiving reserpine are less difficult to manage, there are some changes which would seem to require a re-orientation of hospital procedures and of personnel using this form of treatment. Following the initial "Sedative Phase," there is frequently increased agitation, anxiety, fear, and increased psychomotor activity ("Turbulent Phase"). Thus, many of the patients who were initially marked by overt, destructive, assaultive, and generally disruptive behavior, after going through the sedative phase are now internally agitated rather than expressing their agitation directly against their environment. This paradoxical shift from problems of management connected with destructive behavior against their environment to internal anxiety and agitation requires that increased attention be paid to the psychological needs and problems, rather than the simple management of the patients. This has resulted in a necessary re-orientation in the attitudes and behavior of the attendants caring for these patients. The patients themselves show a tremendously increased need for contact with ward personnel, including nurses, psychiatrists, attendants, and others. The patients desire more, frequent and longer visits from their families as well. These patients now are not only aware of their internal problems, but have a great urgency to express them in inter-personal relationships which they formerly avoided. In an effort to meet this need, the use of group psychotherapy has been increased; particularly evident is the striking change in their desire for social contact with other members of the group. This has been associated with an increase in the patients' motility, and the desire to also express themselves in motor activities of a more complex and expressive nature than formerly possible. Patients have shown enhanced interest in art therapy and music; a number of patients have started to learn to play the piano or have returned to their former accomplishments, all in an effort to give expression to what is going on internally. Some patients have entered into occupational therapy with renewed energy and interest, and the demands on these auxiliary services have been markedly increased. The patients have also expressed a desire to participate in ward activities, and many of them have helped with ward routines since this formed another type of contact. This is accompanied by increased alertness and awareness of the needs of the ward, so that patients not infrequently volunteer to carry out certain activities, whereas formerly each step had to be supervised.

In the present study, individuals who had organic or structural changes of the central nervous system did not respond to the same extent in seeking outlets for their increased awareness, anxiety, and agitation. In the functional cases, the various channels of expression are freely used; whether central nervous system impairment interferes with this raises an interesting problem. There was also a welling up of other expressive activities ranging from the expression of infantile erotic impulses, such as pleasures in eating and excreting, to more complex and interesting genital awareness as evidenced by dreams as well as overt activity. Some patients actually expressed their feelings of increased eroticism directly, which at times proved a source of embarrassment to the husbands of patients on visiting days and included some rather unexpected erotic maneuvers directed at physicians on the admission service.

Conclusions

1. Reserpine in either oral or combined oral and parenteral forms is of definite usefulness in the management of patients admitted to a reception service in a mental hospital. This usefulness is more apparent in schizophrenias, manic-depressive psychoses, involutional psychoses, and severe psychoneurotic disorders. It has been of less use in patients in whom a definite organic defect is probably the etiological factor related to their psychosis, such as cerebral arteriosclerosis, and other disorders in circulation, senile psychoses, epileptic psychoses, and mental defectives.

2. This preliminary study indicates that a more prolonged and vigorous course of medication, with larger dosages, is a necessity for definitive evaluation of the therapeutic effect of reserpine.

3. Reserpine treatment presents special problems with the more acutely disturbed patients in an admission service. This requires a re-orientation of ward personnel to meet the psychological changes. This re-orientation includes more attention to the psychological needs of these patients, to their anxieties, and to creating situations in which the patients' increased impulses toward expressing their drives and conflicts in action is given full play. This includes such activities as occupational therapy, recreational activities, and opportunities for helping on the ward in various ways.

4. Possible psychodynamic formulations have been suggested from the material presented.

A CONTROLLED STUDY OF RESERPINE ON CHRONICALLY DISTURBED PATIENTS

M. Duane Sommerness, M.D., Rubel J. Lucero, M.A., John S. Hamlon, M.D., J. L. Erickson, M.D., and R. Matthews, R.Ph.

A review of the available literature indicated no adequately controlled experimentation in the use of reserpine with chronically disturbed long-term mental patients.

It has been noted that patients have evidenced remarkable changes, both psychological and physiological, when treated with placebos. Therefore, it was felt that the effect of the drug must be measured simultaneously with that of the placebo. Since experimenters have observed changes in patients due to placebo, it may be possible that changes ascribed to medicines are sometimes due to suggestive effects.

Quite often the intercession of a different routine on chronic wards will lead to the entire ward showing at least temporary improvement behaviorally. It is therefore necessary to include a nontreated control group.

The effect of suggestion must be measured as well as the effect of an intercession of a break in ward routine when one is attempting to evaluate a drug. For these reasons, it was felt that experiments with the drug, placebo, and control groups must be carried out simultaneously in order to obtain reliable scientific results.

Present Study

Isolation of Problem.—It has been stated that reserpine is effective in counteracting anxiety. Any therapeutic regime that purports to reduce anxiety should be at least minimally effective in alleviating the disturbance of the chronic mentally ill. Therefore, it was felt that reserpine should be tested on highly disturbed patients.

Basic Hypothesis.—Reserpine has a calming effect on disturbed patients which results in positive changes in behavior beyond those that could be attributed to suggestion or interference in the usual ward routine or regimen.

Experimental Design.—The 90 most chronically disturbed male patients in the hospital were placed on one ward. They were divided into three groups by a random numbers table. This randomization resulted in essential equality for diagnosis, behavior, weight, and blood pressure.

One group was given 1 mg. b. i. d. of reserpine (Rau-Sed, Squibb) orally. At the time the experiment was begun, available research indicated that this dose was considered optimum by one investigation, while another investigator considered a 1-mg. oral daily dose optimum. The second group was given an identical-appearing placebo under identical conditions. The third group re-

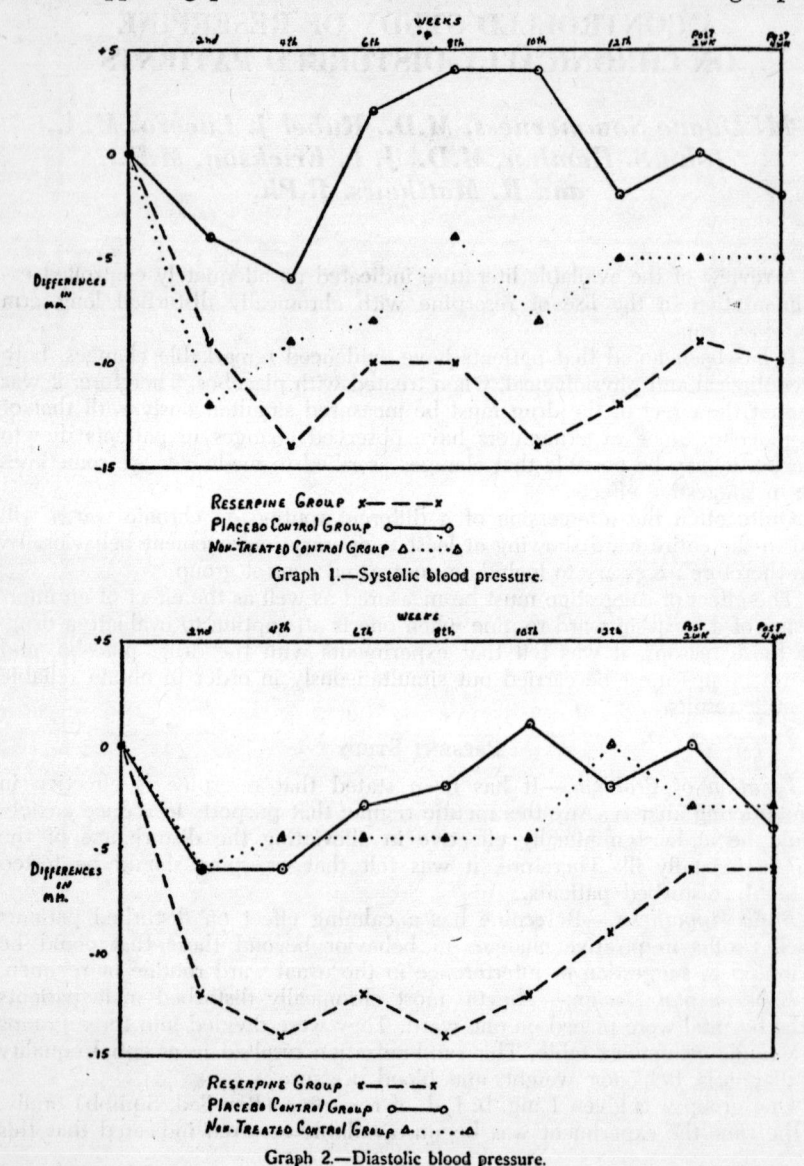

Graph 1.—Systolic blood pressure.

Reserpine Group x― ― ―x
Placebo Control Group o―――o
Non-Treated Control Group △·····△

Graph 2.—Diastolic blood pressure.

Reserpine Group x― ― ―x
Placebo Control Group o―――o
Non-Treated Control Group △·····△

ceived neither reserpine nor placebo but was otherwise under identical conditions.

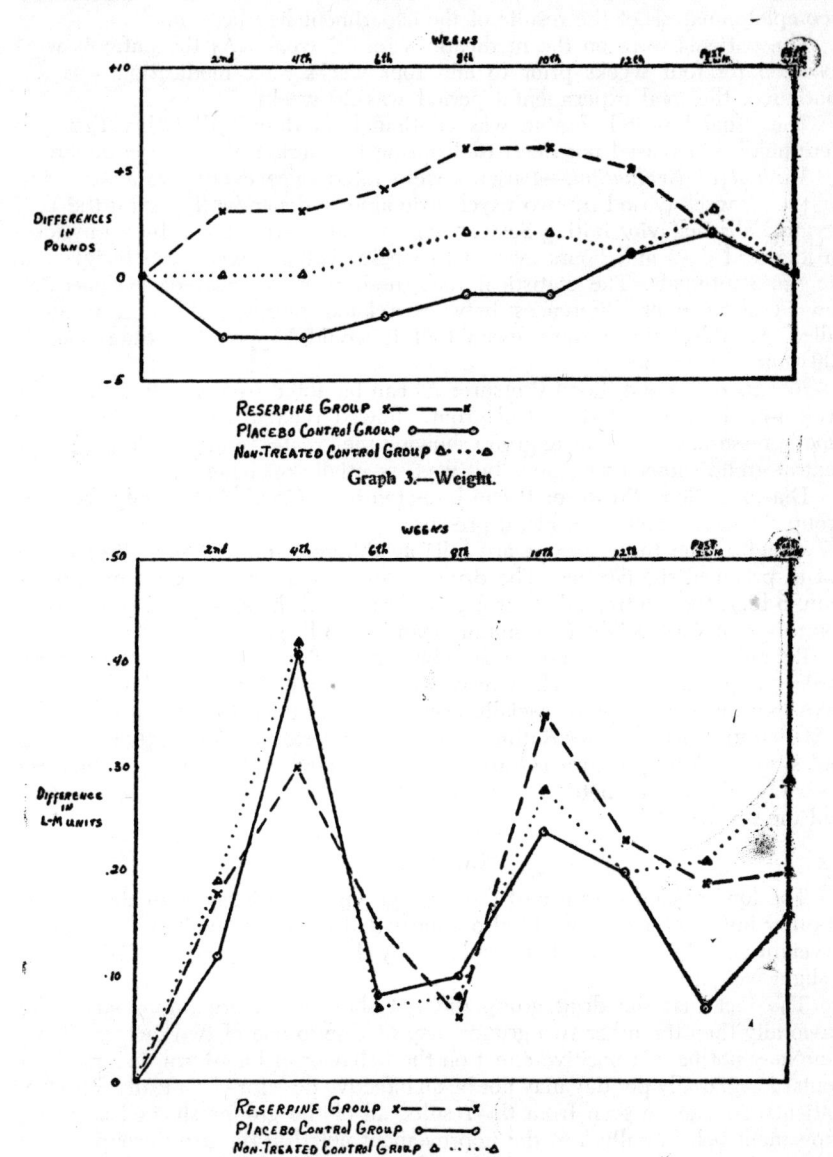

Graph 3.—Weight.

Graph 4.—Behavior average.

The hospital pharmacist alone knew which group received reserpine or placebo. This information was not available to the other experimenters until a complete analysis of the results of the experiment had been made.

The patients were on the medications for 12 weeks. As the patients were observed for four weeks prior to and four weeks after medication was discontinued, the total experimental period was 20 weeks.

The usual hospital routine was continued on the ward. Other therapies were neither increased nor decreased during the period of the experiment.

Method of Evaluation.—Patients were rated once every two weeks during the 20-week period by two psychiatric aides independently, using the L-M Fergus Falls Behavior Rating Scale. Blood pressures were taken by a physician on identical days and hours every two weeks. Patients were also weighed in the same intervals. The statistical tools used were analysis of variance, x^2, and significance of differences between related means. (When a result is called "reliable," the authors mean that it would happen less than once in 100 times by chance.)

Results.—Systolic Blood Pressure: As can be noted from Graph 1, both the drug and the nontreated control group showed reliable reduction in systolic blood pressure, with the drug group showing the greater reduction. The placebo control group showed variations but was essentially unchanged.

Diastolic Blood Pressure: It can be noted from Graph 2 that only the drug group showed reduction in blood pressure.

Weight: The three groups are reliably different, though the difference is not of practical significance. The drug group gained weight (maximum mean gain, 6 lb.); the nontreated control group remained the same, and the placebo control group lost weight (maximum mean loss, 3 lb.).

Behavior: There was no appreciable or consistent difference among the three groups at any time. There was a reliable trend for all of the groups to have improved in terms of socially acceptable behavior (as measured by the L-M Fergus Falls Behavior Rating Scale). It is interesting to note that behavior and systolic blood pressure (Graphs 1 and 4) show cyclic changes which are inversely related (the better the behavior the lower the systolic blood pressure, and the reverse).

COMMENT

The lower blood pressure of the drug group is consistent with the findings of other investigators. It would also appear that reserpine tends to bring about a weight gain. We are unable to explain why the placebo group tended to show a slight weight loss.

The fact that the drug group did not show any more improvement behaviorally than the other two groups may be due to one of two factors: Reserpine may not have a positive effect on the behavior of long-term disturbed patients; 2 mg. orally per day may not be an effective dose for chronically disturbed patients. As can be seen from the results, all of the groups showed some improvement behaviorally, but the improvement noted in the drug group was no greater than the improvement in the other two groups. We have reached the conclusion that having a doctor take blood pressure on patients every two weeks, having the patients weighed regularly, and arousing the interests of the ward personnel seem to account for the favorable behavioral results uniformly obtained in all three groups. Although there was consistent improvement in behavior, it followed a cyclic pattern, lending support to the widely held hypothesis that disturbed behavior in the chronically mentally ill tends to occur in a rhythmic pattern. It is also interesting to note the positive relationship between good behavior and lower systolic blood pressure in this cyclic manner.

Summary and Conclusions

The 90 most highly disturbed male patients with chronic mental illness in a 2000-bed hospital were placed on one ward. Thirty were given 1 mg. of reserpine (Rau-Sed, Squibb) orally b. i. d.; 30 were given an identical-appearing placebo, and 30, no medication, for a period of 12 weeks. They were also studied for four weeks prior to and four weeks subsequent to this period. Measurements were made of behavior, blood pressure, and weight.

Reserpine in oral doses of 1 mg. b. i. d. did not effect a behavioral improvement (as measured by the L-M Fergus Falls Behavior Rating Scale) in chronic disturbed male patients.

Reserpine effected a lowering of blood pressure.

Reserpine effected a slight weight gain.

The greater attention to patients inherent in taking blood pressures and weights and increasing the interest of ward personnel resulted in behavioral improvement in all three groups under study.

IMPROVED BEHAVIOR PATTERNS IN THE HOSPITALIZED MENTALLY ILL WITH RESERPINE AND METHYL-PHENIDYLACETATE

John T. Ferguson, M.D.

This report concerns itself with approximately eight months of the oral administration of a new drug combination (Serpasil and Ritalin) to 225 chronic hospitalized mental patients.

The project was undertaken to evaluate our opinion, derived from treating more than 500 overactive patients with Serpasil and more than 200 underactive patients with Ritalin, that behavior in the chronic mental patient is mixed in character, regardless of the outward manifestation, and should, therefore, respond to a combination of the two drugs more effectively.

Fifteen female wards, often called the "back-wards," with a population of 1,003 were used for the project. From these wards the 225 worst behavior problems were chosen, without regard for diagnoses, time spent in the hospital, or ages of the patients. The project, therefore, included overactive, underactive, and mixed behavior problems.

The group was predominantly schizophrenic, although 19 different classifications were included (Table I).

The length of time each patient had spent in the hospital varied from eight months to better than 52 years, with the average being over 13 years.

The ages of the patients ranged from 23 years to 78 years, and averaged 46 years.

Our preliminary evaluation revealed cardiac abnormalities in 68 of the 225, and 26 of these 68 were on some digitalis preparation. Included in the group were six diabetics, four Parkinsons, three hemiplegics, five seizure patients, and six CNS lues.

Dosage Plan

We used the 0.1 mg. and 1.0 mg. standard, scored Serpasil tablets and the standard 0.2 mg. per teaspoon Serpasil Elixir. For the Ritalin we used the 10 mg. and the 20 mg. scored tablets.

Ward routines allowed a three times daily dosage schedule in which 117 of the 225 received their medicine 30 minutes to one hour before meals, and 66 of the 225 received their medicine 30 minutes to one hour after meals. The remaining 42 of the 225 were quite resistive to medicine, so their tablets were crushed and put in their food or beverage at meal time.

TABLE I: Diagnoses

Schizophrenia		163
Simple	2	
Hebephrenic	41	
Catatonic	55	
Paranoid	38	
Schizoaffective	7	
Acute Undifferentiated	2	
Chronic Undifferentiated	18	
Mental Defective		18
Manic Depressive		15
Chronic Brain Syndrome		18
Syphilis	6	
Arteriosclerosis	5	
Unknown	2	
Senile Brain Disease	3	
Convulsions	2	
Paranoid State		2
Depressive Reaction		4
Anxiety State		2
Antisocial Reaction		2
Involutional Psychotic Reaction		1
Total		225

Our previous experience along with our primary objective—to treat abnormal behavior manifestations—led us to decide on a dosage schedule in proportion to the degree of abnormality present. Consequently, our doses varied considerably. We used from 0.1 mg. of Serpasil t.i.d. up to 20 mg. t.i.d., although we gave three overactive and aggressive patients 20 mg. q.i.d. for several days. Our Ritalin doses ranged from 5 mg. t.i.d. to 30 mg. t.i.d., although we gave several negative patients 50 to 60 mg. t.i.d., with one patient receiving 90 mg.

Of the 225 patients, 134 had a markedly overactive and aggressive behavior pattern; these were started on Serpasil. Seventy-five of the 225 were predominantly negative, and were started on Ritalin. The remaining 16 of the 225 were in the geriatric group and presented a mixed type of behavior, so were started on both Ritalin and Serpasil at the same time.

When the action of the first drug used was such that a change in behavior was noted, then the second drug was added. The combined doses were then adjusted every 24 to 48 hours for each patient as individually needed. This adjustment was usually made so that the Serpasil was increased or decreased by one-half to one-fourth of the previous dosage, while the Ritalin was usually adjusted up or down by 5 or 10 mg. a dose.

However, in changing the Ritalin of previously overactive and aggressive patients and in changing the Serpasil of previously negative patients, it proved best to make minimal changes to avoid a reversal of behavior and the necessity of further readjustment. With this method, the optimal stage was reached quicker and more smoothly.

The combined doses were adjusted for each patient of the group, as described, until such time as we felt that optimal drug action had been reached. Two hundred and one of the 225 reached this stage in less than two months, while 24 of the 225 still required periodic adjustment. Twenty of these 24 were non-psychotics.

During the second month, we ran three experiments for drug activity. In one, we ran a double-blind test on Ritalin. In the second, we substituted Serpasil placebos for Serpasil. In the third, we discontinued both drugs at the same time.

All three experiments proved the drugs to be basically responsible for the improvement in behavior, as reversal to original patterns was evident within four to ten days.

At the end of six months, we discontinued the drugs of the group, and now, after two months, have had to return only 69 of the 225 to their previous dosage.

At no time have we seen any evidence of habituation, although we suspected it in two neurotic patients until we substituted placebos and found their reaction was merely a part of their attention-getting mechanism.

Results in Relation to Behavior

For evaluation of the combined oral use of Serpasil and Ritalin in relation to behavior, we used an 11-category check system and a base profile of behavior for each of the 225 patients. For the check system we covered the following points of behavior (see Table II): (1) Personal Appearance (2) Personal Care (3) Motor Activity (4) Aggressiveness (5) Eating Habits (6) Toilet Habits (7) Night Behavior (8) Socialization (9) Supervision Needed (10) Cooperation in Routine and (11) Rehabilitation.

For the base behavior profile, we used two short essays, covering the 11 points. These were written for us by the attendant-nurses of each ward, one at the start and one for this report.

As our investigation progressed, we found our records were not only giving us an evaluation in relation to over-all behavior but were giving us an evaluation of the medicines in relation to the specific behavior covered by each category. Consequently, we are reporting our observations for each category as if each were a separate study, in the hope that this new approach will help in establishing more specific indications for the combined oral administration of Ritalin and Serpasil (see Tables II and III).

1. *Personal Appearance*

In this category we have recorded a 64.7% improvement in the patients' manner and mode of dress, including care of the hair.

This new interest in appearance has "swamped" our staff beautician with requests for permanents to the degree that she has inaugurated an on-ward beauty program, with patient help, as a part of our Industrial Rehabilitation Program.

TABLE II: CATEGORIZED BEHAVORIAL PATTERNS OF 225 MENTALLY ILL PATIENTS BEFORE TREATMENT WITH RITALIN AND SERPASIL

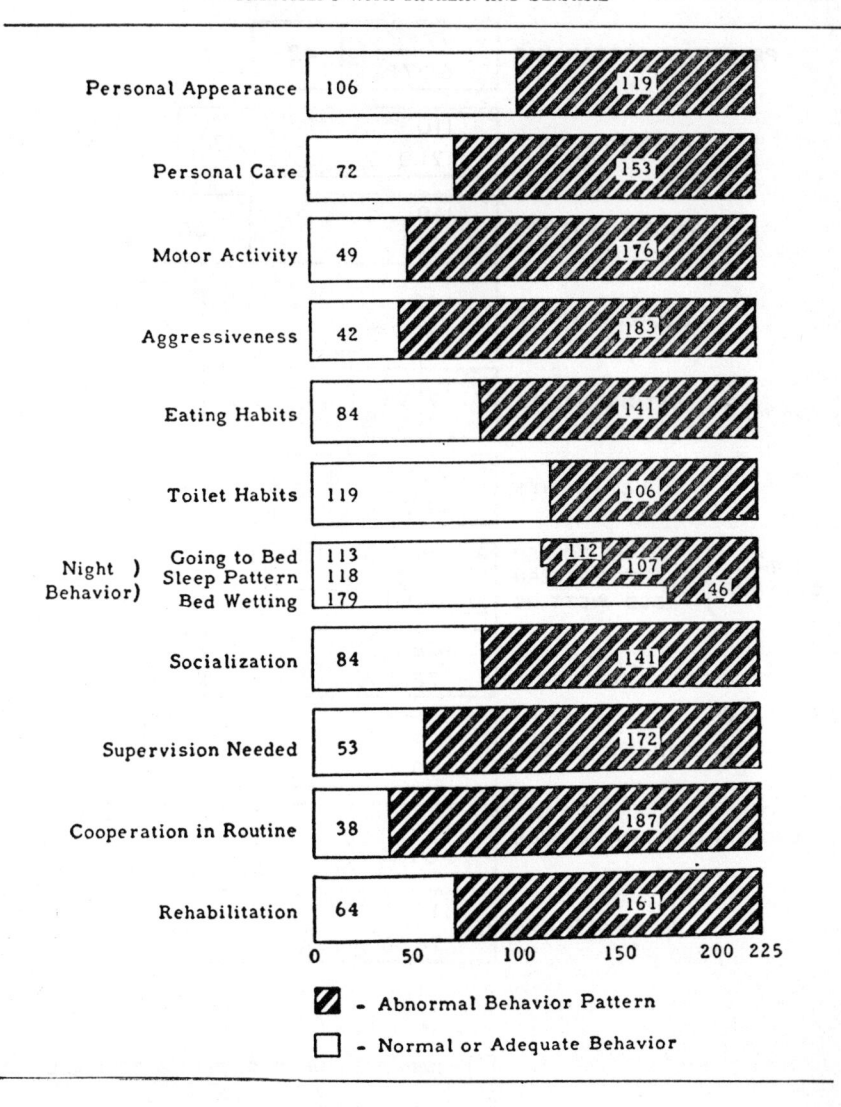

Category	Normal or Adequate	Abnormal
Personal Appearance	106	119
Personal Care	72	153
Motor Activity	49	176
Aggressiveness	42	183
Eating Habits	84	141
Toilet Habits	119	106
Night Behavior — Going to Bed	113	112
Night Behavior — Sleep Pattern	118	107
Night Behavior — Bed Wetting	179	46
Socialization	84	141
Supervision Needed	53	172
Cooperation in Routine	38	187
Rehabilitation	64	161

▨ - Abnormal Behavior Pattern
☐ - Normal or Adequate Behavior

TABLE III: BEHAVIORAL CHANGES AFTER EIGHT MONTHS' THERAPY WITH RITALIN/SERPASIL
(These patients represent the abnormal group shown in Table II.)

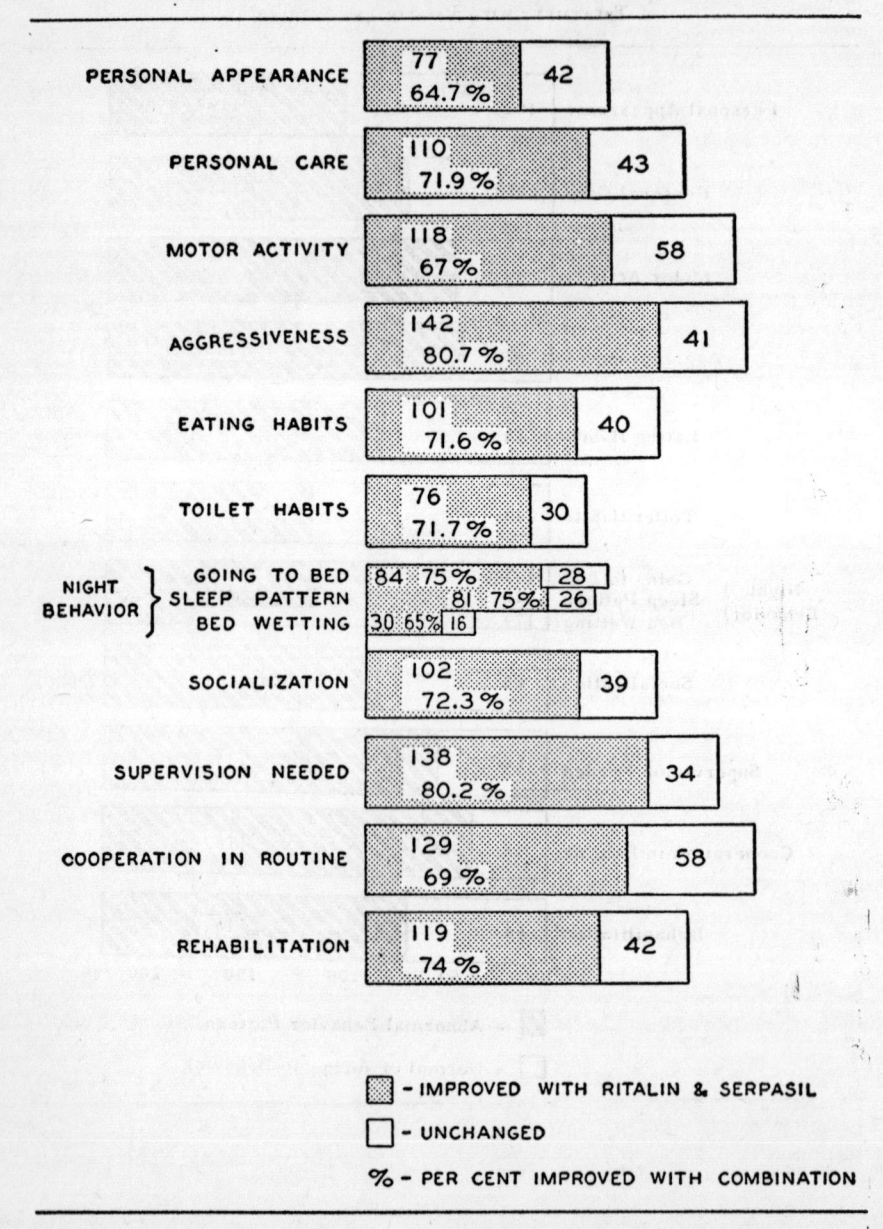

Category	Improved with Ritalin & Serpasil	% Improved	Unchanged
PERSONAL APPEARANCE	77	64.7%	42
PERSONAL CARE	110	71.9%	43
MOTOR ACTIVITY	118	67%	58
AGGRESSIVENESS	142	80.7%	41
EATING HABITS	101	71.6%	40
TOILET HABITS	76	71.7%	30
NIGHT BEHAVIOR — GOING TO BED	84	75%	28
NIGHT BEHAVIOR — SLEEP PATTERN	81	75%	26
NIGHT BEHAVIOR — BED WETTING	30	65%	16
SOCIALIZATION	102	72.3%	39
SUPERVISION NEEDED	138	80.2%	34
COOPERATION IN ROUTINE	129	69%	58
REHABILITATION	119	74%	42

▓ – IMPROVED WITH RITALIN & SERPASIL
☐ – UNCHANGED
% – PER CENT IMPROVED WITH COMBINATION

2. Personal Care

An improvement of 71.9%, along with the over-all interest in personal care created by the medicines, has allowed us to expand our oral hygiene program within the group, even though several of them carry their tooth brushes around their neck.

We have found that improvement in this category is dependent upon and in proportion to the amount of personal retraining the patients can be given as they awake from their dream world or lose their resistance.

3. Motor Activity

We have seen a 67% improvement here, and although the improvement for the underactive groups are, percentage-wise, less than for the overactive groups, we feel the results far surpass our fondest expectations, as nothing so dramatic as that which we have witnessed has ever been done before for these chronic, regressed, negative patients.

4. Aggressiveness

There is an 80.7% improvement in this category, which includes the argumentative, the abusive, the compulsive, the fighter, and the destructive patient, as well as the bashful, the withdrawn, and the hiding patient.

Quite noticeable has been the decrease in the number of arguments, temper outbursts, and fights, to the degree that all the wards are quieter.

Destruction is down over 65% in all phases: furniture, windows, fixtures, mattresses, and clothes. Seclusion is also down in the same proportion. We use no restraints.

5. Eating Habits

In this category we have witnessed a 71.6% improvement in the eating habits of the patients.

The remarkable improvement in the eating habits is considered by our attendant-nurse staff to be the outstanding change that has taken place. Many of the overweight have reduced, while the underweight group have gained. There is also a marked decrease in the spoon-feeders and the feeding problems.

6. Toilet Habits

In this category we found a 71.7% improvement in the toilet habits of the patients while awake.

From our observations, we have found that patients receiving an excess of Serpasil will tend toward soiling and that the adjustment of the Serpasil doses downward to the patients' requirements will stop the soiling.

7. Night Behavior

In this category we have recorded better than 70% improvement in the night behavior of the patients, including the going-to-bed behavior, the sleep pattern, and the bed wetting. There is much less night wandering. The patients can find the toilet easier, and as a result of this we have cut our mattress replacement by better than 70%.

8. *Socialization*

Here we find a 72.3% improvement in the sociability of the patients.

The medicine, by its action, appears to have "awakened" within the patients the ability to participate socially, so that we are having more participation in parties and entertainment.

9. *Supervision Needed*

In this category we have recorded an 80.2% improvement in the nursing time and nursing care the patient needed. Because they are time-consuming, Special Therapies were also included.

A major improvement here is manifested by the fact that we have not given an electroshock treatment to any of the 225 since starting the project, whereas we formerly gave 100 to 125 weekly. This alone has saved us one day a week of a doctor's, a nurse's, and five attendant-nurses' time.

Another improvement is that none of the 225 are now on any form of routine sedation, whereas 82 of the 225 were receiving sedation routinely before starting the project.

10. *Cooperation in Routine*

In this category we note a 69% improvement in the patients' cooperation in routine ward procedures. The patients who were unable to cooperate or were resistive were considered a behavior problem at the start.

The greatest improvement appears to be in those patients that had previously lacked the ability to comprehend or were confused. This improvement appears to coincide with the degree of awakening that is produced, and seems to allow for the re-establishment of former normal reaction patterns, as several have re-entered routine procedures as if they had known how before, at some time.

11. *Rehabilitation*

We have seen a 74% increase in the ability of the patients to enter new situations, along with an increased interest in their environment. This has not only allowed us, but has required us, to broaden our rehabilitation program as the medicines, by themselves, do not have the power to carry the patient alone. They can create within the patient the ability; we must instill the confidence and help establish the security necessary for recovery.

Results in Relation to Physical and Laboratory Tests

Spot tests taken routinely during the eight months have shown no marked change in urinalyses, CBC's, and NPN's from the original values.

Of the 68 cardiac patients, we had two that presented problems not related to the medicine, so that all, including the 26 we kept on their digitalis preparation, have had no ill effects.

Of the six diabetics, all have remained under control.

The four Parkinsons were originally on Artane or Rabellon and Hyoscine. This was discontinued on all four, and at this time they all are improved in their shaking and three of the four have less cogwheel action and walk better.

The three hemiplegics have shown no physical change.

The five seizure patients were taken off their phenobarbital and their Dilantin was reduced. One of the five has had one seizure in the past four months.

All six of the CNS lues are better, although they present a mixed picture. Two of the six talk better, are more understandable, and are much better behaved; two more of the six made no deep changes but are better controlled; the other two of the six have become easier to manage.

Results in Relation to Total Project

At the start the best results were obtained in the schizophrenic group with the hebephrenics and catatonics doing the best and the paranoid type showing the least change. We are now, however, witnessing a reduction of the persecutions and accusations formerly seen in these patients.

The manic-depressive group, because of their completely changing picture, were the hardest to regulate at first. These have now become steady, slightly on the underactive side, but without the great swing.

Most of the senile group have shown a marked clearing of confusion, and, as a result of this, have had good improvement. This group is doing well on a new combined tablet containing 0.25 mg. of Serpasil and 5 mg. of Ritalin given t.i.d.

The mental defectives present a mixed reaction. About one-half of the group have shown improvement compatible with internal change, while the other half have not responded to the drugs other than for control. In fact, most nonpsychotic patients present but little of the deep change seen in the psychotics.

From these observations, we feel that in the true psychotic there has been a definite chemicophysiological change which the Serpasil and Ritalin, by their action, tend to reverse, while in the nonpsychotics this chemicophysiological change has not occurred, so the problem is primarily one of controlling conditioned reflexes and habit patterns.

The basic improvement is such that we feel the age of the patient, time spent in the hospital, or type of ward has no direct bearing on the action of the drugs. However, the degree to which the personnel of the different wards helped the patients as they awakened toward reality was quite noticeable in the patients' total improvement—almost to the point of being in direct proportion.

In fact, the combination has brought new life to our institution, and may be instrumental in changing the hospital from a custodial to a communal treatment center. From a hospital of 3,000 with a waiting list, we are happy to report that we now have over 150 vacancies since inaugurating this and other projects.

TREATMENT OF TWO HUNDRED DISTURBED PSYCHOTICS WITH RESERPINE

Joseph A. Barsa, M.D., and Nathan S. Kline, M.D.

The root of the plant Rauwolfia serpentina Benth., a shrub indigenous to India, was used for centuries in native Indian medicine for the treatment of a wide variety of diseases, including mental disorders. The drug was introduced into the United States for its use in the management of hypertension. In 1952, Muller, Schlittler, and Bein identified a new crystalline alkaloid from the Rauwolfia root. This alkaloid, reserpine, appeared to be the chief active principle of Rauwolfia. In 1954, one of us (N. S. K.) reported on the use of the Rauwolfia whole root and reserpine in the treatment of various psychiatric disorders. The present study is an extension of a study made several months previously, based on the response of 150 chronically disturbed psychotics to reserpine therapy.

SUBJECTS

In a hospital building housing 740 chronically disturbed psychotic female patients, 200 of the most disturbed were selected regardless of diagnosis, age, duration of illness, or previous treatment. They were chosen chiefly for their excited, hyperactive, assaultive, or destructive behavior. Several patients in profound stupor who were severe feeding and management problems were also included. Of the 200 patients selected, 150 had received insulin coma therapy and/or electroconvulsive therapy without lasting benefit. Fifty-five patients were currently receiving maintenance electroconvulsive treatments once or twice a week and had already received from 40 to several hundred individual shock treatments. Fourteen of the patients selected had undergone some form of psychosurgery. The age of the patients selected ranged from 15 to 70. One hundred fifty-nine were given a diagnosis of schizophrenia. The remaining 41 were given the following diagnoses: 7 manic-depressive psychosis, mixed type; 4 involutional psychosis, melancholia; 5 involutional psychosis, paranoid type; 1 involutional psychosis, mixed type; 7 psychosis with mental deficiency; 2 psychosis with cerebral arteriosclerosis; 1 psychosis with cardiorenal disease; 6 epileptic psychosis, epileptic clouded states; 6 epileptic psychosis, deteriorated type; 1 alcoholic psychosis, Korsakoff's type, and 1 psychosis with epidemic encephalitis.

METHOD OF STUDY

In this study 1 mg. tablets of reserpine and 2 cc. ampuls of solution for parenteral use containing 2.5 mg. of reserpine per cubic centimeter were used.

Gradually, in prescribing daily for each patient, one of us (J. A. B.) evolved the following general dosage plan, which could be modified to meet individual requirements. When starting therapy the patient would receive 5 mg. of reserpine intramuscularly and 3 mg. orally each morning. This was continued for 10 days. By this time if the patient was showing a beneficial response (not merely sedation), administration of the oral dose was continued but the intramuscular dose was given every other day for three doses. Then, if the patient's condition still showed evidence of improvement, the intramuscular dose was given every fourth day for two doses, and administration of the daily oral dose was continued. Finally, if the patient's mental state remained favorable, administration of the daily oral dose of 3 mg. was continued, but therapy with the intramuscular dose was discontinued as a regular medication and was given only as a booster dose when the patient became very disturbed. After the first 10 days of oral and intramuscular reserpine therapy, if the patient did not show a beneficial response, administration of the 3 mg. orally and 5 mg. intramuscullarly was continued daily for 6 more days. If there was still no improvement, the oral dose was still given but the intramuscular dose was increased to 10 mg. every other day and 5 mg. on alternate days. This regimen was carried on for eight days. If there was still no improvement, use of the daily oral dose of 3 mg. was continued but the intramuscular dose was raised to 10 mg. daily for five doses. If at the end of this time no improvement was evident in the mental state of the patient, the intramuscular dose was reduced to 5 mg. daily for three doses and then eliminated completely; administration of the daily oral dose of 3 mg. was continued. An oral dose of 3 mg. was found to be the optimal maintenance dose in most of the patients; however, because of side-reactions, the maintenance dose had to be reduced to 2 mg. in six cases and to 1 mg. in two cases. If the patient showed no improvement at any time during the first six weeks, it was found useless to continue therapy. Sometimes a valuable clue as to whether the patient would respond to therapy could be gained in the early days of treatment, when, for a brief period, perhaps only a day, the patient would suddenly shed her symptoms and seem to emerge out of her psychosis. When this was seen it was an indication that the patient would eventually respond to treatment, even though it might not be until many weeks later.

After completing a course of intramuscular injections of reserpine as outlined in the dosage plan above, if the patient showed only a slight beneficial response, it was not found useful to continue the intramuscular injections for a longer period. It was more advantageous to keep the patient on the oral dose for two to three weeks and then to repeat the course of intramuscular injections. There was also evidence to indicate that after two or more months, when a patient had stabilized at a certain level of improvement, it was often possible to raise the degree of improvement by repeating the course of intramuscular injections of reserpine.

All of the patients in this study were started on reserpine therapy at a time when they were disturbed. If they had previously benefited from insulin coma or electroconvulsive therapy, they were given reserpine only after they had shown definite evidence of relapse. The maintenance electroconvulsive therapy was discontinued, and the patients were allowed to become disturbed again before reserpine therapy was instituted. While receiving reserpine the patients were given no other somatic therapy and no other sedative drug, with the exception of anticonvulsant medication in a few epileptic patients. It was found by experience that a minimal course of therapy consisted of at least three consecutive months. To discontinue therapy earlier seriously lessened the patient's chances of achieving a satisfactory result from treatment and increased the possibility of relapse. All of the patients in this study received reserpine from three to nine months, with the following exceptions: one patient died suddenly after one month of therapy (discussed below); therapy was discontinued for seven patients after two months because they had shown no evidence of responding to treatment.

Results

The categories of improvement used in the study are defined as follows: by markedly improved is meant that the patient's mental state and behavior had improved to such an extent that with a normal amount of supervision she would be able to adjust adequately outside of a hospital; by moderately improved is meant that, although the patient was not well enough to live outside of a hospital, her behavior had improved to the extent that she was usually cooperative and was adjusting fairly well to the hospital environment; by slightly

TABLE 1.—*Improvement with Reserpine in Respect to Diagnosis in 150 Cases*

Diagnosis	Markedly Improved	Moderately Improved	Slightly Improved	No Improvement	No. of Cases
Dementia praecox					
Paranoid	4	12	10	3	29
Catatonic	17	27	13	11	68
Hebephrenic	1	8	6	4	19
Mixed	4	4	1	1	10
Dementia praecox, total	26	51	30	19	126
Manic depressive, mixed	1	1	1	..	3
Involutional psychosis, melancholia	1	1	..	1	3
Involutional psychosis, paranoid	..	4	..	..	4
Psychosis with mental deficiency	3	..	..	3	6
Psychosis with cerebral arteriosclerosis	..	..	..	1	1
Psychosis with cardiorenal disease	1	..	..	..	1
Epileptic psychosis, epileptic clouded states	..	1	2	..	3
Epileptic psychosis, deterioration	..	..	1	..	1
Alcoholic psychosis, Korsakoff's	..	1	..	..	1
Primary behavior disorders, simple adult maladjustment	..	..	1	..	1
Total	32	59	35	24	150

improved is meant that the patient was a little easier to manage but still manifested excited, assaultive, or destructive behavior. The evaluation of the patient in regard to degree of improvement was made by the physician in charge (J. A. B.), the supervising nurse of the building, and the nurse or attendant who was in charge of the particular patient's ward.

The results obtained in this study can be compared with those of the first 150 cases reported in another paper. Tables 1 and 2 are an analysis of improvement according to diagnosis, in the first 150 cases and in the total 200 cases. Furthermore, in both studies it was found that age did not seem to exert an appreciable effect on the degree of improvement. It was also found that the longer a patient had remained in the hospital, and the longer she had been ill, the less were her chances of achieving a moderate or marked improvement. In the first study, however, 5.6% of the 71 patients hospitalized continuously for more than five years were markedly improved and 80% showed some degree of improvement. In the present study 100 patients had been in the hospital for

TABLE 2.—*Improvement with Reserpine in Respect to Diagnosis in 200 Cases*

Diagnosis	Markedly Improved	Moderately Improved	Slightly Improved	No Improvement	No. of Cases
Dementia praecox					
Paranoid	9	19	12	3	43
Catatonic	19	30	16	11	76
Hebephrenic	1	11	8	4	24
Mixed	6	5	2	3	16
Dementia praecox, total	35	65	38	21	159
Manic depressive, mixed	2	1	4	..	7
Involutional psychosis, melancholia	2	1	..	1	4
Involutional psychosis, paranoid	..	4	1	..	5
Involutional psychosis, mixed	..	..	1	..	1
Involutional psychosis, total	2	5	2	1	10
Psychosis with mental deficiency	3	..	1	3	7
Psychosis with cerebral arteriosclerosis	1	..	..	1	2
Psychosis with cardiorenal disease	1	..	..	..	1
Epileptic psychosis, epileptic clouded states	..	2	4	..	6
Epileptic psychosis, deterioration	..	2	3	1	6
Epileptic psychosis, total	..	4	7	1	12
Alcoholic psychosis, Korsakoff's	..	1	..	..	1
Psychosis with epidemic encephalitis	..	..	..	1	1
All diagnoses, total	44	76	52	28	200

more than five years; 8% were markedly improved, and 85% showed some improvement. In both studies 92% of the patients showed a degree of improvement as great as or greater than that achieved by electroconvulsive treatments. In only 8% of cases the patient did not show as much improvement from reserpine therapy as from shock therapy. It should be noted that, in the 8% who did better with electroconvulsive therapy, improvement was not maintained for very long after shock treatments were discontinued.

Fourteen patients in our study had previously received some form of psychosurgery. There were two transorbital lobotomies, three topectomies, and nine prefrontal lobotomies. The analysis of the response of these patients to reserpine was as follows: markedly improved, none; moderately improved, three; slightly improved, six; and no improvement, five. It is seen, therefore, that the improvement in this group was not as great as in the others. However, since all of the psychosurgery patients had been mentally ill for many years, this factor, rather than the psychosurgery, may have been the determining element in their failure to respond to reserpine. Several patients who had shown an inadequate response to reserpine alone were started on a course of reserpine combined with a daily oral dose of 25 to 100 mg. of chlorpromazine [10-(y-dimethylaminopropyl)-2-chlorophenothiazine hydrochloride]. The latter drug seemed to potentiate the effects of reserpine. The results were so encouraging that a large series of patients were given the combined reserpine-chlorpromazine therapy.

Clinical Course

In a previous report, one of us (J. A. B.) distinguished three stages in the patient's course of therapy: the sedative period, the turbulent period, and the integrative period. The sedative period begins very soon after the start of therapy and lasts from 3 to 10 days. In this period the drug produces chiefly a sedative effect, the patient becoming quieter, less disturbed, and perhaps rather drowsy. This is followed by the turbulent period, in which the patient's behavior becomes more disturbed and the delusions and hallucinations are often more pronounced. The patient often complains of feeling strange, not like herself, and feeling at times that she has no control over her impulses. Some patients, exerting considerable control prior to therapy, seem to "break wide open" at this time. Tremulousness, restlessness, mounting tension, and anxiety are prominent symptoms. The duration of this period varies from a day to two or three weeks. It must be emphasized that the patient should be treated vigorously with oral and intramuscular administration of reserpine during the early weeks and that the dosage should not be reduced until the patient has passed over the hump of the turbulent period. The successfully treated patient then passes into the integrative period, in which she becomes more cooperative, more friendly, and more interested in her environment. Delusions and hallucinations gradually fade until they seem to disappear. This final period lasts from one to six (or more) months until medication is discontinued because of the satisfactory therapeutic response of the patient. It must be noted that only those patients responding favorably will successfully pass through these stages. Some patients seem either never to progress beyond the sedative period or, if they do pass into the turbulent period, to be unable to achieve enough ego strength to attain the integrative period, and they return to the sedative stage. In such cases the maximum therapeutic effect to be expected is one of sedation.

Side-Reactions

Drowsiness and a sense of fatigue were frequent manifestations during the sedative period. Generalized tremulousness, increased salivation, dizziness, abdominal cramps, diarrhea, nasal stuffiness, edema of the face and feet, frequency of urination, and paresthesias of the extremities were often experienced during the early weeks of therapy, especially during the turbulent period. In an effort to combat these symptoms, which may be very distressing to the patient, various drugs were used, even though as a rule the above symptoms eventually disappeared spontaneously without the need of reducing the dosage of reserpine. Atropine was used with varying success against the tremulousness. Oxyphenonium (antrenyl) bromide, an anticholinergic substance, was very effective with the abdominal symptoms. Phenylephrine (Neo-Synephrine) hydrochloride or ephedrine nose drops were used to alleviate the nasal stuffiness. Amphetamine derivatives were found useful in counteracting the drowsiness and sense of fatigue when they became very severe. Most effective against the tremulousness, the restlessness, and the feelings of tension, which were especially acute during the turbulent period, was benztropine (Cogentin) methanesulfonate, a synthetic anti-Parkinsonism drug with antihistaminic and anticholinergic properties.

Three patients had grand mal convulsive seizures for the first time during their first six weeks of reserpine therapy. Electroencephalograms taken on two of the patients revealed an epileptic pattern. Two topectomy patients also had convulsive seizures for the first time during the first month of therapy. The electroencephalogram of one of these patients was within normal limits, whereas the other was suggestive of a convulsive disorder. One patient who had had a prefrontal lobotomy in 1949, and who in the year preceding treatment had averaged two convulsive seizures a month, had five grand mal convulsive seizures in the first month of therapy. One patient with idiopathic epilepsy who during the previous year had had no more than one grand mal and two petit mal seizures a month had two grand mal and three petit mal seizures during the first month of therapy. One patient who in June, 1953, had developed her first spontaneous convulsive seizures while receiving a course of electroconvulsive therapy, and who since then had no more than one grand mal or one petit mal seizure a month, had four grand mal convulsive seizures during her first month of reserpine therapy. It is important to note that the above-mentioned increased incidence of convulsive seizures did not occur beyond the first six weeks of reserpine therapy, even though therapy with the drug was continued. Another observation was that the psychotic symptoms and disturbed behavior of the epileptic patients included in this study were very resistant to the beneficial effect of reserpine. Whether the drug has specific convulsant properties, or whether the convulsions were due to the disruption of the body's homeostasis in susceptible individuals, cannot be answered at the present time. Increased appetite and gain in weight commonly manifested themselves early in therapy. If, however, after an early increase, appetite later fell off considerably and became poor, this was usually a sign of overdosage of reserpine. Another sign of toxic effect of reserpine was the development of an organic type of mental confusion. This symptom would disappear when the dosage of reserpine was decreased.

Ten patients while receiving therapy developed a typical picture of Parkinsonism. Three of the patients developed the signs after two weeks of therapy, five after four weeks, and two after three months. All were receiving intramuscular injections of reserpine at the time, and six of the patients had been receiving 10 mg. doses for several days. The patients showed a mask-like facies (this had to be distinguished from the drowsy, lethargic facies, due to the sedative effect of the drug), excessive salivation, drooling, rigidity with cogwheel phenomena, a pill rolling tremor, and a slow, shuffling gait with small steps and loss of associated movements. The rigidity in the patients was usually more marked than the tremor. This Parkinsonian picture was made to disappear merely by reducing the dosage of reserpine. In one patient who developed Parkinsonism, the symptoms were made to disappear, then reappear, and again disappear, by changing the dosage of reserpine. The development of Parkinsonism was not an indication to reduce dosage of reserpine unless satisfactory mental response had already been reached.

Three deaths occurred during the nine months of this study. One patient on the fifth day of therapy committed suicide by hanging. One patient, apparently in good physical condition, died suddenly after one month of treatment. Autopsy permission could not be obtained. Another patient, who had previously shown no evidence of diabetes, although there was a family history of this disease, rapidly lapsed into diabetic coma and, despite treatment for the diabetes, died 48 hours later. This patient had received reserpine for three months. Because of this case and the possibility that reserpine might have activated a latent diabetes, thereafter the urine of all patients receiving reserpine was examined every month. No further cases of diabetes were found. It was felt, therefore, that these deaths were not due to the reserpine therapy.

Comment

Hess showed that stimulation of certain nuclei in the supraoptic area of the hypothalamus of the cat produced a peculiar state of quiescence or sleep, associated with miosis, lowering of body temperature, fall of blood pressure, bradycardia, increased intestinal activity, and slowing of respiration. According to the work of Bein, and Bein, Gross, Tripod, and Meier, reserpine acts directly on central autonomic substrates, possibly in the hypothalamus, and that, rather than a stimulation of the parasympathetic centers, it causes a depression of the corresponding central sympathetic functions. Schneider and Earl in a recent paper have further investigated the mode of action of reserpine.

In the present study, it was noticed that in some patients the improvement produced by reserpine did not last long after therapy was completed. Of 41 markedly improved patients whose medication was discontinued, 2 patients showed evidence of relapsing after being without the drug for one week, one patient relapsed after three weeks, another after four weeks, another after five weeks, another after six weeks, two after seven weeks, and one after eight weeks. The remaining 32 patients (78%) have not relapsed, although they have not received reserpine for as long as five months. The patients who relapsed were treated again and brought back to their former state of improvement. In retreating them, even those who relapsed after a week, it was found necessary to start afresh and give them another complete course of therapy. The value of reserpine in the treatment of chronically disturbed patients can be seen in the fact that, since the advent of reserpine therapy in this building of 740 patients, electroconvulsive therapy has been completely eliminated, whereas previously about 150 electroconvulsive treatments were given every week.

Several questions arise regarding the nature and significance of the turbulent period in the course of therapy. This period is indeed a crucial one, for it presents the biggest hurdle in the successful outcome of therapy. Furthermore, during this period the patient becomes most distressed and suffers the greatest anxiety. Some patients seem to fall apart completely at this time. But is this period an essential step in the successful course of therapy? Does it represent the release of anxiety resulting from the breakup of old behavior patterns? Or is this period of increasing tension and anxiety with the consequent upsurge of defense symptoms merely as a side-effect in therapy? It is a psychic side-effect perhaps derived from the various physiological changes in this parasympathetic dominant stage in therapy? Can, therefore, this period be eliminated without jeopardizing the success of therapy? It has been found that benztropine methanesulfonate can remove many of the distressing symptoms of the period and yet not decrease the effectiveness of therapy. Moreover, when reserpine is combined with chlorpromazine the turbulent period is shorter and less intense, but the potency of therapy is not diminished. Thus, it would seem that a continuing search should be made for drugs capable of eliminating the turbulent period and yet not lowering the effectiveness of reserpine.

Conclusions

Reserpine is definitely of value in the treatment of chronically disturbed psychotic patients. Twenty-two per cent of a group of 200 such patients have improved sufficiently to be judged well enough to leave the hospital. Eighty-six per cent of the patients showed some degree of improvement, and 71% did better with reserpine therapy than with electroshock. Although certain toxic effects of reserpine (including Parkinsonism and convulsions) were observed in the treated patients, none of these were permanent; all of them disappeared when the dosage of reserpine was reduced. There is evidence to indicate that in some patients the therapeutic effect of reserpine lasts only as long as the drug is being administered; however, in 78%, improvement has been maintained after medication was discontinued.

HAS CHLORPROMAZINE INAUGURATED A NEW ERA IN MENTAL HOSPITALS?

Winfred Overholser, M.D., Sc.D., L.H.D.
Superintendent, St. Elizabeth's Hospital, Professor of Psychiatry, George Washington University School of Medicine, Washington, D. C.

The use of drugs in the treatment of mental patients is nothing new. In ancient Greece black hellebore was considered such a specific drug that advice to take a trip to Anticyra, where the shrub grew plentifully, became a common expression. The soothing effects of opium have long been known, and this drug was frequently prescribed even a hundred years ago. Later such sedatives as paraldehyde, chloral, and the barbiturates were developed. These various drugs have had their respective vogues, depending upon the prevailing knowledge of pharmacology and on the rationale of their administration. In more recent years, however, there has been considerable reluctance to use sedative drugs because they were looked upon as merely substitutes for mechanical restraint, as something not therapeutic but merely palliative. Furthermore, such drugs as paraldehyde and the barbiturates, if they quieted the disturbed patient, did so at the expense of impairing his consciousness and even of bringing about stupor. Most of the sedatives used hitherto have likewise been at least potentially toxic or addictive, or both. There have been other periods when drugs were but little used, or when other supposed "cures" dominated the scene, only to lose their popularity. In recent years the vogue of psychotherapy has in the minds of some at least obscured the fact that certain physical approaches can aid in the treatment of mental disorders.

Thanks to the ingenuity of French science, something entirely new in the line of sedatives has appeared on the horizon, namely, chlorpromazine. This drug exhibits the unusual quality of bringing about sedation and quiet without substantial impairment of consciousness. It has a wide range of tolerability, is largely non-toxic, and is not addictive. Serious side-effects have been rare, and the effects which have occurred have been almost entirely reversible. Thus, although chlorpromazine is far from being a panacea it is nevertheless a most useful drug which has demonstrated its wide usefulness wherever used. It has been found useful in several fields of medicine, as in the control of hiccough, nausea and vomiting, the reduction of postanesthetic shock, and obstetrics. It is primarily, however, in the practice of psychiatry and especially of hospital psychiatry that I would speak. An example of the widespread use of the drug in the United States is found in the fact that probably as many as four million patients have had it prescribed for them!

The medical literature is full of the reports of the use of chlorpromazine, and it is obviously impossible to summarize these reports here. Much is yet to be learned about the pharmacological action of the drug, about the criteria for its prescription, and about the elimination of side-effects. Differences of opinion have been expressed as to the optimum dosage, as to the duration of the administration of the drug, whether or not maintenance doses should be continued for an indefinite period. A full evaluation must necessarily wait for a longer period of observation of the effects. There is no doubt, however, that many new vistas have been opened and that many changes have already been noted, particularly in hospital psychiatry.

Let us consider first the effects on the patient himself. The opinion seems to be almost unanimous that patients who exhibit psychomotor activity, assaultiveness, hostility, and negativism show a reduction in their motor output with the administration of the drug. They are less restless, are quite ready to sit quietly, are less assaultive and destructive, are orderly and well behaved. Subjectively they exhibit a marked reduction in anxiety. They are clear mentally, in good contact with their surroundings, and are able to discuss their hallucinations and delusions calmly and with a considerable degree of objectivity. Thus many patients who had previously been inaccessible now become amenable to psychotherapy and the other forms of occupation and recreation which are provided for them on the wards. Although in certain cases of agitated depression a certain amount of quieting has been noted, the drug is not recommended for the depressions in general, particularly those without agitation, electroshock still being practically specific here. Shock therapy in general, which has been used in some hospitals for the treatment of catatonic symptoms and overactivity, has been reduced to a vast degree. At St. Elizabeths Hospital, for example, in comparable six-month periods of 1954 and 1955 it was found that the number of patients was reduced from 177 to 13 and the number of treatments from 1168 to 107. Restraints in general have been used very much less and at St. Elizabeths Hospital we have found that the need of seclusions of our disturbed patients has been greatly reduced. Approximately 10 per cent of our patients are receiving tranquillizing drugs, over half of them receiving chlorpromazine and the others receiving reserpine, a combination of the two, or some of the other tranquilizing drugs.

One controlled study of 50 negro women at St. Elizabeths Hospital was reported recently by Drs. S. Tenenblatt and A. Spagno. They found 80 per cent of the patients improved. Here it should be borne in mind that as in many of the other reports it was the patients who were the most disturbed and who had the least good prognoses who were given the drug. The best results were noted in the treatment of the manic-depressive and the schizophrenic psychoses, particularly the catatonic and paranoid types of the latter. Of 50 patients under treatment only 4 required discontinuance of the therapy on account of untoward effects. Many of the patients who responded had been ill for years and were serious ward problems.

There is no question whatever concerning the tranquilizing effect of the drug on disturbed patients, particularly in those suffering from the paranoid type of schizophrenia and the manic phase of manic-depressive psychosis.

What of the effect on the ward as a whole? Briefly, the atmosphere of disturbed wards has been completely revolutionized. Patients now remain clothed, they are quiet, they do not annoy each other, they conform to the conventions, take an interest in their personal appearance, and in the appearance of the ward. Since the patients are more receptive and more co-operative they demand other activities to occupy them during their waking hours. There is thus a far greater need for the development of recreational, occupational, and diversional therapies, of more psychotherapeutic attention to the patients, of greater interest on the part of the nurses and attendants in providing various programs. Far from reducing the number of problems the drug has merely changed them; there are indeed more problems now than there were before, but these all operate to the advantage of the patient and to his greater comfort.

What of the effect on the staff and the personnel? A far greater interest has been developed. The morale has been increased. A hopeful attitude has come about as patients who had been previously troublesome were noted to be co-operative and helpful and to show other signs of improvement. The psychiatrist has been returned to medicine, as has the nurse, not only by the administration of the medication, but by the increased necessity of attention to possible signs of adverse effects. It has been a challenge to the entire medical and ward personnel to increase attention to the patient and to show more interest in bringing about his improvement, while to the psychiatrist there has been offered an opportunity for a better study of psychopathology, since the patient is now able and willing to discuss his problems, whereas before he might have been entirely inaccessible to investigation and help.

What is the effect on the hospital as a whole? We have already mentioned the decrease in the destructiveness and assaultiveness, the wear and tear on the physical plant and on the clothing. What of the statistics? This is something which must wait for a later evaluation. In some hospitals, as in ours for example, the initial study was done on the most disturbed, least hopeful patients. Although greater freedom has been permitted them as a result, this has not been reflected as yet in a substantial increase in the discharge rates. Many patients are, however, out on temporary visit, and if their improvement holds it is quite likely that they will be discharged from visit in the fairly near future. It has been observed in some hospitals, notably at the Rochester (New York) State Hospital, as reported by B. Pollack, that the number of patients returned to the hospital from trial visit has decreased greatly. There is thus a hope that the number of discharges may be increased and that patients may continue at home with or without maintenance doses of the drug, while at the same time it is not at all impossible that the number of first admissions will be reduced by the use of the tranquilizing drugs in the community. Sound statistics are not available at the moment as to the duration of hospitalization. As a matter of fact, too, the rate of discharge is subject to a number of misinterpretations, and is not necessarily a sound criterion of therapeutic success. It seems quite likely that more activity in out-patient departments and community clinics will be called for as a result of the drug.

What of the effects of the drug on the family of the patient? There has been a marked increase in the hopefulness of the families and in their expectation that their loved ones may be returned to them soon. Unfortunately in the case of some of the patients who have been in hospital for a considerable period of time and who have been psychologically "given up" by the families there appears to be now on the part of some of these families a fear that the patient may be released! Sometimes, indeed, this fear borders almost on panic. These cases are of course exceptional. In general it certainly must be said that the attitude of the family has been vastly improved.

Finally, what of the effect on the community? These drugs have again made the mental hospital a medical institution in the minds of the public. Physicians in general practice are more co-operative and more willing to refer patients for hospital or other psychiatric treatment. Some physicians in the community who are not psychiatrists are using chlorpromazine to treat mild cases of mental illness. Legislative bodies have shown a greater interest in the problems of mental illness, now that a positive and easily administered therapy appears to be available, and the interest of various community groups such as churches and other civic groups has been greatly stimulated. Families have not only become more hopeful but more demanding. Very often indeed they are insistent that the drug be administered, whether or not it be medically indicated! It seems not too much to say too that the community is at last developing an attitude of far greater tolerance toward the discharged mental patient, a greater readiness to accept him back into the community and into industry or his other former occupation.

Mention has been made earlier of the fact that there are some complications which are observed from time to time in treatment with chlorpromazine. We have noted, for example, at St. Elizabeths Hospital in one group of negro women that 36 per cent of the group exhibited the presence of colostrum or milk in the breasts. This is a symptom which has not been very frequently noted in the literature; it is, like most of the other symptoms, entirely reversible and quite insignificant. A fairly common complication, especially if the use of the drug is continued over a period, is a Parkinsonian tremor, often decidedly marked. The tremor, however, subsides promptly when the drug is discontinued. The incidence of jaundice appears to be in general moderate only, and in almost all cases apparently completely reversible when the drug is discontinued. The same may be said of the fever, the photosensitivity of the skin and the erythemas which have been sometimes observed. More serious is the incidence of decrease in white cells, sometimes going to a stage of clinical agranulocytosis. Several cases of death from this cause have been reported. In hospital practice it seems clear that the drug should not be prescribed without occasional tests of liver function and blood counts. If fever occurs, this may be a warning signal and calls for special vigilance. Hypotension has been reported, and emotional depression has been noted in certain cases. It should of course be remembered that no drug which has any beneficial effects whatever is without some potential dangers. Most of the side-effects of chlorpromazine are reversible and the only one which causes a threat to life (fortunately relatively rare) is agranulocytosis, as already mentioned.

Any discussion of chlorpromazine should not fail to take notice of another drug of an entirely different source which has closely related effects, namely, reserpine. It is the impression of some of the workers of the field that this acts somewhat better in organic cases such as the arteriosclerotic group than does chlorpromazine. It is perhaps somewhat less effective in women than in men. It is slower in action and somewhat more cumulative in effect. The mental effects of the drug are related, although the action is less dramatic; it has been noted by some observers that there appears to be a synergism between this drug and chlorpromazine, so that combined therapy may be useful. As in the case of chlorpromazine, a reversible Parkinsonism is frequent. The dangers of hypotension are even greater with reserpine than with chlorpromazine and the presence of gastric ulcer is a decided contraindication. A few deaths have been reported from acute edema of the glottis. The incidence of unfavorable side-effects is perhaps somewhat less than with chlorpromazine.

Some of the "Philistines" may object that both of these drugs, that is, chlorpromazine and reserpine, are merely palliative. This is no criticism of a drug, even though it be meant as such. There are many drugs which are valuable although not basically curative. One has only to think of insulin in diabetes, of liver extract in pernicious anemia, of vitamin therapy in certain of the avitaminoses, and so on. It may be said that after all the anesthetics are merely palliative, since they do not cure pain. There is a place for palliatives in the practice of medicine. Most emphatically we have in chlorpromazine and reserpine two drugs which add greatly to the comfort, first of the patient, of his family, and of those about him. Furthermore, by allaying anxiety and reducing motor activity while at the same time maintaining clarity of consciousness, the patient becomes far better able to make human contacts, to accept psychotherapy, and to profit by it. As long ago as 1914 Freud (who after all began his professional life as a pharmacologist) suggested that "all our provisional ideas in psychology will some day be based on an organic substructure." He went on to say, "This makes it possible that special substances and special chemical processes control the operation of sexuality and provide for the continuation of the individual life in the species."

Today much valuable work is being done by pharmacologists in co-operation with psychiatrists. One thinks of the experimental use of mescaline, of lysergic acid, of serotonin, as well as of the "tranquilizing" or "neuroleptic" drugs. More knowledge is needed about their action. Much more work needs to be done in the development of other pharmacologic agents which may be as effective without having the undesirable side-effects which have already been enumerated.

In the light of our knowledge regarding the psychic effect of the new drugs, is it too fantastic to suggest that perhaps some day those psychoses which we now term, for want of a better word, "functional," may be found to be due in part at least to endogenous chemical substances which act on the central nervous system, and even perhaps if that fact should be established, that chemical antagonists may be developed as therapeutic agents?

There have been many swings of the pendulum in psychiatric treatment—the "moral treatment" of Pinel, the bloodletting of Rush, the "focal infection" era, the prolonged sleep and insulin period, the various psychotherapeutic approaches. Now the pendulum seems to have swung again, this time into a pharmacologic era. This era will bring psychiatry closer to the rest of medicine, and will make our patients more amenable to psychotherapy, both individual and group, and to the other adjunctive therapies. It will increase our knowledge of mental functioning, and most important of all, will aid our patients in their restitution to health and to society.

AN EVALUATION OF PROMAZINE HYDROCHLORINE IN PSYCHIATRIC PRACTICE

Stanley Lesse, M.D.
Neurological Institute of the Presbyterian Hospital of New York and the College of Physicians and Surgeons, Columbia University, New York, N. Y.

This paper represents our initial clinical evaluation of a new synthetic phenothiazine derivative in psychiatric practice: promazine hydrochloride, a gamma-dimethylamino-n-propylphenothiazine hydrochloride. Its formula is very similar to those of the other 2 phenothiazine compounds that have been intensively tested in psychiatric patients; namely, phenergen hydrochloride and chlorpromazine hydrochloride. Promazine hydrochloride differs chemically from chlorpromazine hydrochloride only in that the latter has a chlorine atom attached to the phenothiazine nucleus.

Promazine hydrochloride was studied in our search for an ataraxic drug which would be equal or superior to chlorpromazine as a tranquilizer in psychiatric patients, while at the same time having fewer adverse side-effects.

METHODOLOGY

The case material consists of 50 patients, 45 of whom were seen in private practice, and 5 who were clinic outpatients. Thirty-six were women ranging in age from 28 to 75 years, while 14 were males 35 to 72 years of age. As to diagnoses, 22 had schizophrenia, 15 had agitated depressions, 11 had psychoneuroses, and 2 severe, acute organic mental reactions. The duration of illness varied from 20 hours to 21 years, the vast majority being less than 4 months. All patients were treated with promazine hydrochloride for more than 2 weeks. The longest period of treatment has been 4 months. The majority of patients had had therapy with other ataraxic drugs prior to starting on promazine.

Technique of Evaluation of Improvement Level

The technique used in evaluating the level of improvement was the same as that introduced by us in our initial evaluation of the efficacy of chlorpromazine therapy in private practice. It considers and attempts to quantify, as much as possible, both subjective and objective factors. The criteria used stress the patient's adaptation to routine responsibilities of everyday life in addition to the degree of symptomatic improvement. The degree of pride and pleasure obtained from successful performance was considered also. The details of the scheme are as follows:

I. *Performance.*—(A) Vocational Performance—Key: (1) *Excellent*: full-time employment. Functioning efficiently without strain. Great pride and pleasure from attainments. (2) *Good*: full-time employment. Greater effort required than was necessary prior to illness. Moderate pride and pleasure from attainments. (3) *Fair*: working intermittently with considerable difficulties, frequent absences. Faulty performance at times. Lack of pride and pleasure. (A) *Poor*: unable to perform at all. (B) Social Performance (Individual and Group Interpersonal Relationships)—(1) *Excellent*: active and comfortable. High level of pride and pleasure obtained. (2) *Good*: active but with slight to moderate difficulty at times. Limited pleasure capacity. (3) *Fair*: socializes with great difficulty. Readily becomes very anxious. Lack of pride and very limited and infrequent pleasure. (4) *Poor*: seclusiveness or chaotic relations.

II. *Amelioration of Anxiety.*—Anxiety is defined for our purpose here in its broadest aspect. We consider it synonymous with fear whether this fear is generated by unconscious conflict or actual difficulties. We attempted to quantify anxiety according to a 4-point scale after analyzing this psychophysiological phenomenon into several components; namely, (1) motor component, (2) affectual component, (3) verbal component, and (4) autonomic component. Key: (1) *Calm*: no restlessness. Overt expression of fear, when it occurs, is appropriate to the severity of the actual stress. (2) *Slight restlessness*: slight affectual expression of fear, slight pressure of speech. (3) *Marked restlessness*: pacing. Marked overt affectual expression of fear. Often severe pressure of speech. (4) *Panic*.

III. *Amelioration of Initial Symptoms.*—Key: (1) *Excellent*: all symptoms completely gone. (2) *Good*: symptoms markedly reduced in intensity and frequency. Patient able to cope with them. (3) *Fair*: Slight improvement only, with the symptoms continuing to plague patient most of the time and with marked impact. (4) *Poor*: symptoms unchanged.

IV. *Dreams.*—Whenever possible, dreams were sought out and studied in an attempt to gain additional information. Disappearance of nightmares, decrease in the frequency of rage dreams, and an increase in the frequency of pleasant dreams were points that were evaluated.

The final Improvement Rating was indicated on a 4-point scale which took into account all of the factors described above. Key: (1) I. *Excellent*: full-time efficient employment. Active and comfortable in social performance. Marked pride and pleasure from vocational and social performance. (2) II. *Good*: full-time employment but requiring slightly greater effort than usual. Active socially but with slight to moderate difficulties at times. Slight residual anxiety. Symptoms markedly reduced in intensity and frequency. Limited pride and pleasure from performance. (3) III. *Fair*: working but with considerable difficulties. Frequent absences. Socializing with great difficulty. Moderate to marked residual anxiety. Slight improvement in symptoms. Minimal pride and pleasure from performance. (4) IV. *Poor*: unable to perform vocationally or socially. Anxiety level severe and unchanged. Symptoms unchanged. Absence of pride and pleasure from performance.

Of the 50 patients, 44 were too ill to function socially or vocationally, being completely dominated by their symptoms. The other 6 functioned, but only with very great difficulties.

Clinical Evaluation of Promazine Hydrochloride

Improvement.—Of the 50 patients studied 17 (34%) were considered as presenting excellent or good results (Improvement Ratings I or II). The remaining group obtained very slight benefit or none at all. In other words, the drug worked effectively in approximately one-third of the cases, while it had very slight or no effect in the remaining two-thirds.

Factors Affecting Degree of Improvement.—As with chlorpromazine, age, sex, and diagnosis did not significantly affect the improvement ratings. The factor upon which the degree of improvement appears to rest is the degree of overtly manifested anxiety. Promazine hydrochloride was most effective in patients with marked anxiety, particularly those in whom there was a great deal of motor activity as part of the anxiety. Figure 1 illustrates the relationship between the degree of anxiety and the improvement rating. Note that only 1 patient with relatively slight overtly manifested anxiety showed a significant improvement.

It is my impression also that the drug is more effective in acutely ill patients than in those who have been ill for 6 months or more.

Technique of Drug Administration.—Dosages with promazine hydrochloride were similar to those used with chlorpromazine hydrochloride. The initial daily dose ranged from 50 mg. to 600 mg. per day (average 100 mg.). I have given initial daily doses of 400-600 mg. to patients who were on corresponding doses of chlorpromazine and in whom the chlorpromazine had to be discontinued be-

ANXIETY AS A FACTOR EFFECTING DEGREE OF IMPROVEMENT

DEGREE OF ANXIETY	IMPROVEMENT RATINGS				
		I	II	III	IV
	1	0	0	1	4
	2	0	1	4	5
	3	0	12	12	4
	4	2	2	1	2
TOTALS		2	15	18	15

FIG. I.

cause of a severe side-effect. This changeover was made without any observable difficulty. In severely agitated patients the initial daily dosage was as high as 400 mg. per day. I have used promazine intramuscularly in only 4 patients who manifested extreme anxiety, the maximum dose being 400 mg. spread over 24 hours. The intramuscular promazine appears to be far less painful than the parenteral chlorpromazine. It took effect, in the 3 patients in whom it was very efficacious, in from 15 to 30 minutes, which is about the same as I have found with intramuscular chlorpromazine. As yet I have had no experience administering the drug intravenously. The majority of patients report that promazine taken orally begins to take effect in from 45-60 minutes.

The maximum dose of promazine used was 1,000 mg. per day. It is my impression, however, that if the drug does not have very significant benefits by the time 500-600 mg. per day are used, it will be of no use at higher dosages. However, as with chlorpromazine, if the patient shows definite symptoms and signs of improvement before he has received 500-600 mg. per day, the drug should be increased until maximal benefits are obtained. The maximum dosages were maintained for 2 weeks or longer. They were not decreased until there was definite evidence that the patient had maintained a high level of improvement for several weeks.

The medication was a valuable adjunct to either supportive or analytical psychotherapy, but only in those patients who initially were very tense. These patients at the onset were poor candidates for any type of psychotherapy given on an outpatient basis. The amelioration of the marked anxiety enabled many in this group to cooperate in psychotherapy.

Complications of Promazine Therapy.—We have found that over 50% of patients treated with chlorpromazine had adverse side-effects; in 1 of every 8 chlorpromazine was discontinued because of their severity.

We found that promazine had far fewer side-effects than chlorpromazine, and when present, with 3 exceptions, they were very mild and caused no great difficulties. Mild drowsiness or fatigue and dryness of the oral and nasal mucosa were the only symptoms commonly seen. Of the 14 patients complaining of drowsiness only 6 required amphetamines to counteract the symptom. Slight dryness of the oral and nasal tissues was reported by 9 patients. Hypotensive effects of very mild degree were seen in only 3 patients. Mild pruritis was reported by one patient, while mild constipation and bulemia each were reported by 2 patients. Three schizophrenic patients, all of whom had difficulty with reality control when consciousness was even slightly depressed, demonstrated aggravation of their psychoses.

The drug had to be discontinued because of adverse side-effects in 2 patients. Extreme aggravation of a schizophrenic psychosis was the reason in 1 case, while an annoying maculo-papular eruption over the upper extremities was the cause in the other. With this second patient, it should be noted that many unrelated drugs have caused the same problem. We have not seen grippe-like complications, Parkinson-like symptoms, jaundice or leukopenia in patients treated with promazine. Blood counts performed on 25 patients, while they were on the drug, were all normal.

Patients who had had very severe adverse side-effects with chlorpromazine were switched over to promazine. One who had extreme severe rigidity on 3 occasions with chlorpromazine has been effectively treated with promazine without complications. Two patients who developed jaundice on chlorpromazine were immediately transferred to a similar dose of promazine with rapid disappearance of the icterus. Four patients, 22 with severe general dermatitis and 2 with severe grippe-like syndromes, were also switched to equal doses of promazine with rapid disappearance of the adverse side-effects and without any loss of therapeutic effect.

We have noted no clinical evidence of potentiation of the action of barbiturates by promazine.

Discussion

The reports on promazine hydrochloride have dealt mainly with its effects on hospitalized alcoholics. One report also considered its effect on hospitalized opiate addicts and agitated or confused psychotics. The authors were impressed with the tranquilizing effects of the drug in agitated patients. They were also impressed with its antiemetic properties. A few patients were reported as having slight to moderate postural hypotensive reactions. However, since most of the patients in whom this symptom was reported had organic psychotic effects secondary to alcohol one cannot readily determine whether the promazine, the alcohol, or a combination of both was the major cause of a slight drop in blood pressure. The adverse side-effects of this drug, when compared with those reported for chlorpromazine, appear to be relatively very mild and uncommon.

Our series of 50 patients represented the broad clinical spectrum commonly seen in private psychiatric practice. The drug was given only to those who were severely ill, most of whom would have required hospitalization or ambulatory electroshock therapy, if a tranquilizing drug were not available.

The clinical efficacy of the drug was judged by what we consider a strict scheme that is readily applicable to psychiatric patients seen in private practice, in the outpatient clinics, and in patients following discharge from mental institutions. It stresses the patient's abilities of adaptation and performance both socially and vocationally. In addition, the ability to experience pride and pleasure from his performance is a cardinal feature. The degree of amelioration of anxiety and other symptoms is also important.

On the basis of these criteria we found that 1 of every 3 patients treated with promazine showed very significant improvement. As with chlorpromazine, promazine is effective only in those patients who demonstrate marked anxiety, particularly if the motor component is pronounced. For example, if we consider only the 35 patients who evidenced the greatest degree of anxiety prior to therapy, the drug was significantly effective (improvement ratings I and II) in slightly less than one-half of the cases. On the other hand, as we found for chlorpromazine and the other tranquilizers, the medication was not effective in patients manifesting very little overt anxiety. The diagnoses, the patient's age or sex did not have any significant bearing on the results. The drug was most effective in acute illnesses of less than 4 months' duration.

In therapeutic efficacy, therefore, promazine hydrochloride appears, on the basis of this relatively small series, to be equal to chlorpromazine hydrochloride.

Promazine hydrochloride appears to have great advantages over chlorpromazine because the adverse side-effects produced by the drug have, thus far, been minimal as compared with those caused by chlorpromazine. Promazine can be used effectively in patients in whom chlorpromazine must be discontinued because of severe complications.

Summary

1. Fifty psychiatric patients treated with promazine hydrochloride, a new

phenothiazine derivative, are reviewed.

2. The drug was effective in one-third of the patients treated, but only in those who demonstrated marked anxiety.

3. Dosages and methods of administration are considered.

4. Adverse side-effects are mild and relatively uncommon as compared with those produced by chlorpromazine.

5. Promazine appears to be as effective as chlorpromazine as a tranquilizer in psychiatric practice and deserves further study.

A CLINICAL STUDY OF MECHANISMS OF ACTION OF CHLORPROMAZINE

Erwin Lear, M.D., Albert E. Chiron, M.D., and Irving M. Pallin, M.D.

Chlorpromazine, an amine derivative of phenothiazine, was first synthesized in France in 1950. Subsequently, it was used throughout the continent in conjunction with hibernation anesthesia, and, in May, 1954, chlorpromazine was introduced into clinical use in this country as an antiemetic drug. This agent has been shown to possess a wide range of physiological activity because of its action on the central nervous system. It has been used widely in the field of psychiatry; in the treatment of narcotic addiction and alcoholism; in the palliative management of terminal carcinoma; and in various phases of anesthesia, such as premedication, the control of traction reflexes during anesthesia, and the reduction of postoperative nausea, vomiting, and pain.

Potentiation of many drugs commonly employed in anesthesia, such as the narcotics, barbiturates, and ether, was noted when the agents were combined with chlorpromazine. Our interest in this compound was initially based on its use as an adjunct to premedication, thus permitting smaller doses of preoperative narcotics to be given and hence reducing the undesirable side-effects associated with their administration. The use of chlorpromazine in premedication has been challenged, primarily because it causes hypotension that is refractory to the commonly used vasopressors; chlorpromazine has also been reported to reverse the pressor response to epinephrine. The use of chlorpromazine with spinal anesthetics has also been questioned, since both the spinal anesthetic and chlorpromazine may produce hypotension.

Our experience with chlorpromazine as an adjunct to premedication now includes its use in over 3,500 cases; in over 1,450 of these cases the operation was done with the patient under spinal anesthesia. We became interested in the possibility of producing epinephrine reversal in the human under spinal anesthesia with chlorpromazine premedication. We also analyzed our cases in which the operation was done with the patient under spinal anesthesia in an attempt to elucidate the mechanisms of blood-pressure change associated with chlorpromazine premedication when combined with the spinal anesthesia required for given surgical procedures.

EPINEPHRINE REVERSAL

The pressor response to intravenously given epinephrine is reversed in the laboratory animal after injection of chlorpromazine. Foster and his co-workers, using human volunteers, reported epinephrine reversal on the blood vessels of the hand, where vasoconstrictor tone is highest, after intravenous administration of chlorpromazine. The British investigators proposed that the use of epinephrine to correct chlorpromazine-induced hypotension is "useless if not dangerous." A segment of our series of patients receiving chlorpromazine and a spinal anesthetic was then exposed to attempts at the production of epinephrine reversal. None of the patients in the following series received vasopressors prior to or during surgery except for epinephrine, in the amounts noted with each case. The dosage schedule for epinephrine was based on a range of 0.15 to 0.30 mcg. per kilogram of body weight. The drug was given intravenously, either as a drip or, when this became impractical, as an injection directly into the intravenous tubing. There were no instances of sudden significant blood loss in these patients, nor were surgical reflexes encountered that might have altered the study. Most of the patients dozed under the influence of the premedication, although a few received small amounts of intravenously given thiobarbiturates or nitrous oxide.

Figure 1 shows the blood-pressure record of a 21-year-old female who had received chlorpromazine and a spinal anesthetic. Immediately after administration of the spinal anesthetic, the blood pressure fell 30mm. Hg below the preoperative level, and administration of an epinephrine drip containing 0.5 mg. of the drug dissolved in 1 liter of 5% dextrose in water was therefore started.

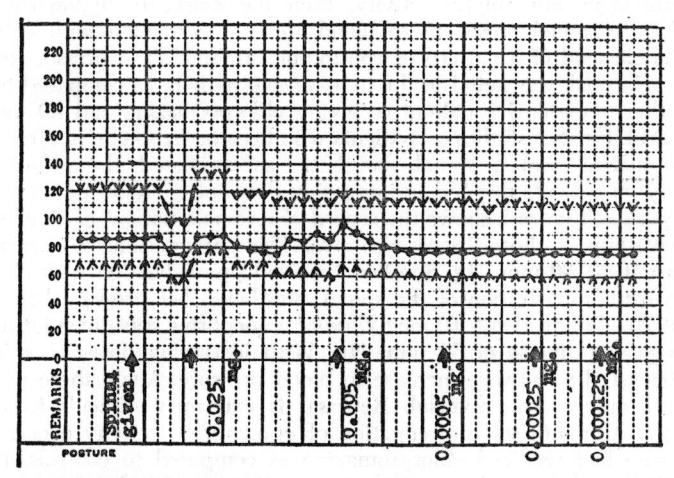

Fig. 1.—Effect on blood pressure of epinephrine drip given to 21-year-old woman under spinal anesthesia who had received chlorpromazine preoperatively.

The patient received 50 ml. of solution, equivalent to a total of 25 mcg. of epinephrine, within the next three to five minutes. The blood pressure showed a peak response of 40 mm. Hg, and, although it began to fall as administration of the drip was discontinued, the base-line pressure became stabilized at a level 20 mm. Hg higher than that immediately after the spinal anesthetic had been given. Epinephrine reversal could not be demonstrated. In an attempt to rule out masking of epinephrine reversal by the dominant pressor response, progressively decreasing doses of epinephrine were given until a dose of 0.125 mcg. was reached. Epinephrine reversal was not demonstrable. The dose range of 0.125 to 10 mcg. was repeated on a number of other patients with no clinical evidence of reversal.

The attenuation of pressor response to epinephrine has also been demonstrated in patients under spinal anesthesia. Three normotensive female patients of the same general age and physical status were studied. One patient received no chlorpromazine and served as a control. The other two received chlorpromazine as a part of their premedication; one of these had a normotensive course, while the other became hypotensive after the administration of a spinal anesthetic. The three patients were given 25 mcg. of epinephrine intravenously. The hypotensive individual showed marked attenuation of pressor response, with a peak pressure increase of only 15 mm. Hg, as contrasted to a 25 mm. Hg rise in the woman given chlorpromazine who remained normotensive and a 30 mm. Hg rise in the control. (We were unable to detect epinephrine reversal in the clinical course of these patients.) After a period of stabilization, 50 mcg. of epinephrine was given to the patients, with an unexpected response from the hypotensive patient. If severity of hypotension be considered the index of chlorpromazine adrenolytic activity, then the markedly hypotensive patient should be extremely resistant to blood-pressure correction with epinephrine, however, instead of a pattern of continuing attenuation, a pressor response of 60 mm. Hg peak was noted in the hypotensive patient, as compared to 40 mm. Hg in the normotensive patient receiving chlorpormazine and 90 mm. Hg in the control. Further studies on patients who became hypotensive after receiving chlorpromazine and a spinal anesthetic substantiated these findings. The hypotensive patients respond to increasing doses of epinephrine with equipressor responses. Figure 2 shows the record of a female patient of similar age and physical status as those discussed above. This patient came to surgery with a pressure of 90/60 mm. Hg. She had received premedication with chlorpromazine. After administration of the spinal anesthetic, her pressure became stabilized at 70/40 mm. Hg. A 10-mcg. dose of epinephrine was given intravenously, with a peak response of 30 mm. Hg. With increasing doses of epinephrine, there occurred a stepwise increase in blood pressure. Again there was no evidence of epinephrine reversal. Reversal is extremely difficult to reproduce clinically. Although some attenuation of epinephrine activity occurred in patients who had received chlorpromazine as compared to controls, there was no significant effect on the equipressor response to epinephrine, and graduated doses of the drug caused stepwise responses in the blood pressure. It has been our clinical experience that the hypotensive patient showed greater response to increasing doses of epinephrine than the normotensive patient who had received chlorpromazine and a spinal anesthetic.

Chlorpromazine in Conjunction with Spinal Anesthesia

Many anesthesiologists have experienced great difficulty in correcting the blood-pressure declines resulting from the combination of premedication with chlorpromazine and spinal anesthesia. Any agent that is to become a routine part of the anesthesiologist's armamentarium should not require that the most potent of vasopressors, with its own inherent dangers, be given to offset side-effects. Consequently, our statistics on the effect of chlorpromazine premedication on blood pressure were reviewed. Variation from patient to patient was studied. Since the level of spinal anesthesia also contributes to alterations in

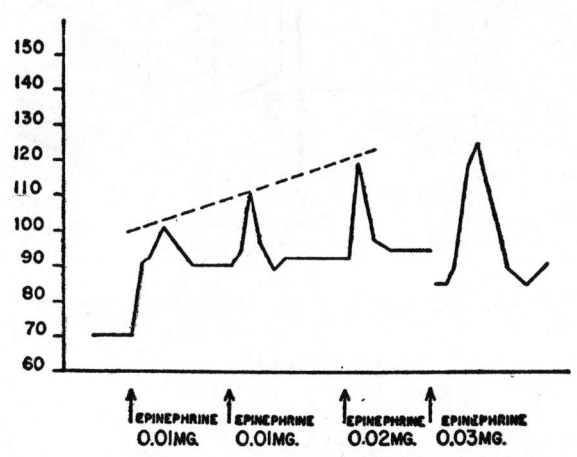

Fig. 2.—Blood-pressure record of patient under spinal anesthesia who had received chlorpromazine preoperatively.

blood pressure, data were reviewed with regard to correlating the level of anesthesia and the blood-pressure changes in patients receiving chlorpromazine. There were 1,450 patients who underwent surgery with chlorpromazine premedication and under spinal anesthesia. Five hundred fifty-one (38%) underwent major gynecologic surgery; 261 underwent abdominal surgery (of these, 59 had intestinal operations; 19, gastrectomy; 128, gallbladder surgery; 19, abdominal-perineal surgery; 13, appendectomy; 19, laparotomy; and 4, sympathectomy); 188 (13%) had hernia repair; 145 (10%) were operated on for hemorrhoids; 203 (14%) underwent major genitourinary surgery; 58 (4%) had orthopedic surgery; and 44 (3%) underwent miscellaneous procedures. The ages of the patients ranged from 14 to 84 years, and patients in all risk categories were included.

Blood Pressure Change After Premedication.—The patients were classified into three general groups on the basis of degree of blood-pressure change after premedication as compared to blood pressure on admission. Patients exhibiting a fall in pressure of 30 mm. Hg or less were placed in group 1, those with a fall of from 31 to 60mm. Hg in group 2, and those with falls of over 60 mm. Hg in group 3. Control patients who received standard premedication fell predominantly into group 1 (92%). By way of contrast, only 80% of the 1,450

228   The New Chemotherapy in Mental Illness

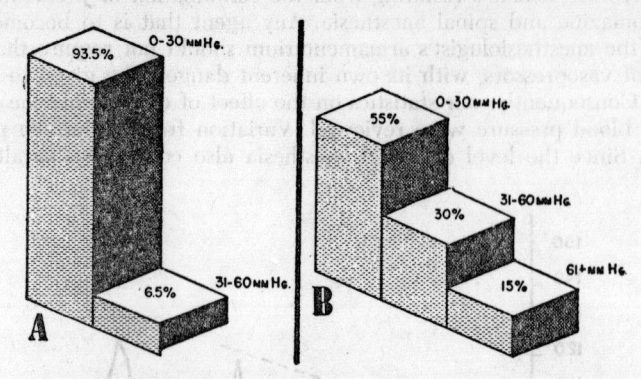

Fig. 3.—Blood-pressure falls of patients, A, with pressures on admission of less than 140/90 mm. Hg and, B, with pressures on admission of 140/90 mm. Hg or greater.

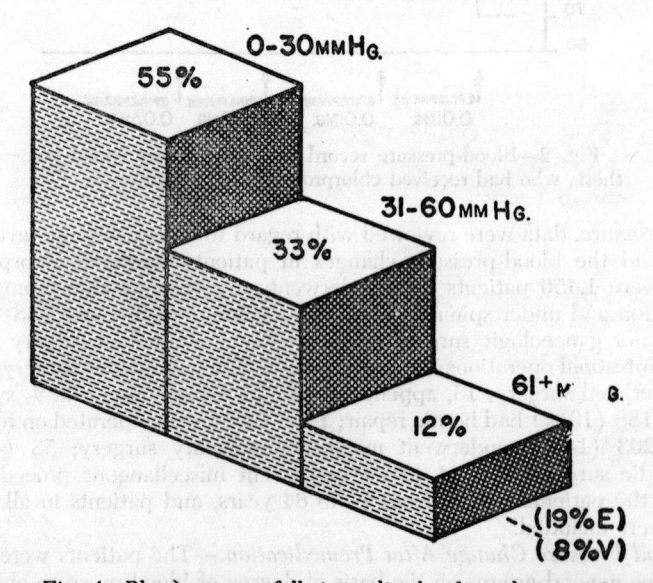

Fig. 4.—Blood-pressure falls immediately after administration of spinal anesthetic as compared to pressure on admission in patients receiving premedication with chlorpromazine and under high spinal anesthesia (T-4) for upper abdominal surgery. 19% E = ephedrine; 8% V = methoxamine (Vasoxyl) hydrochloride.

patients receiving chlorpromazine premedication fell into group 1, while 16.5% fell into group 2 and 3.5% into group 3. These figures would appear to substantiate the observations of numerous investigators that the use of chlorpromazine does increase the incidence of preoperative hypotension. If, however, only those patients receiving chlorpromazine who had pressures on admission of under 140/90 mm. Hg are included in the analysis, the percentage of patients now in group 1 rises to more closely approach the control figures, as will be noted in figure 3. It should be emphasized that all patients with pressures on admission of 140/90 mm. Hg and greater are not necessarily hypertensive; the hypertension in a number of these patients represents a reaction to the stress imposed upon them by the hospital admission. There were 303 patients, or 21% of the 1,450 patients, with blood pressures on admission of 140/90 mm. Hg or greater.

Blood Pressure Change After Administration of Spinal Anesthetic.—There was a marked lowering of blood pressure in all patients in the series after the administration of a spinal anesthetic. In the over-all series, only 53% of the patients were in group 1, with lowering of pressure from that on admission of 0 to 30 mm. Hg, while 31% were in group 2 and 16% in group 3. Of the 303 patients with pressures on admission of 140/90 mm. Hg or greater, 21% were in group 1, 33% in group 2, and 46% in group 3. (See figure 3A).

Level of Spinal Anesthesia.—The blood-pressure change immediately after administration of the spinal anesthetic is related to the level of anesthesia re-

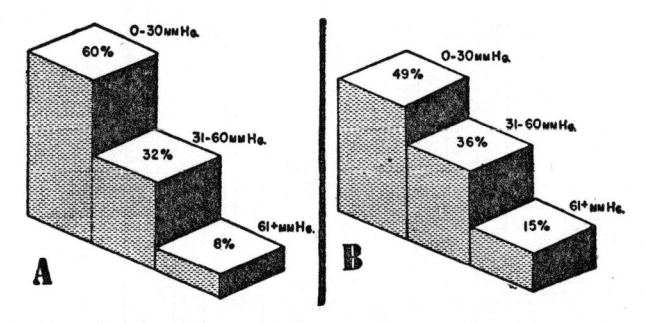

Fig. 5.—Blood-pressure falls immediately after administration of a spinal anesthetic as compared to pressure on admission in patients receiving premedication with chlorpromazine and under low spinal anesthesia (T-8) for lower abdominal surgery by, A, the vaginal approach and, B, the abdominal approach.

quired for a given type of surgery. High levels of anesthesia reduce the area wherein compensatory vasoconstriction normally occurs. In a patient who has received premedication with chlorpromazine, the level of spinal anesthesia plays little active role in the blood-pressure pattern. Figure 4 illustrates the observation that blood-pressure changes in patients under high spinal anesthesia

(T-4) exhibit little difference when compared to those in the over-all series (fig. 3A). Blood-pressure changes in patients under low spinal anesthesia (T-8) (fig. 5), such as is given for major gynecologic surgery, also compare favorably to those in the over-all series (fig. 3A).

The effect of the lithotomy position on blood pressure, as in vaginal plastic surgery, is minimized. Figure 6 shows the record of a 49-year-old female who came to the operating room for repair of a cystocele and rectocele after receiving standard premedication. After administration of the spinal anesthetic, the patient was placed in the lithotomy position and the pressure was permitted to become stable. When the pressure maintained itself for 15 minutes, 12.5 mg. of chlorpromazine was given slowly intravenously. The blood pressure fell sharply 60 mm. Hg below the patient's control level. This dose was repeated at 15-

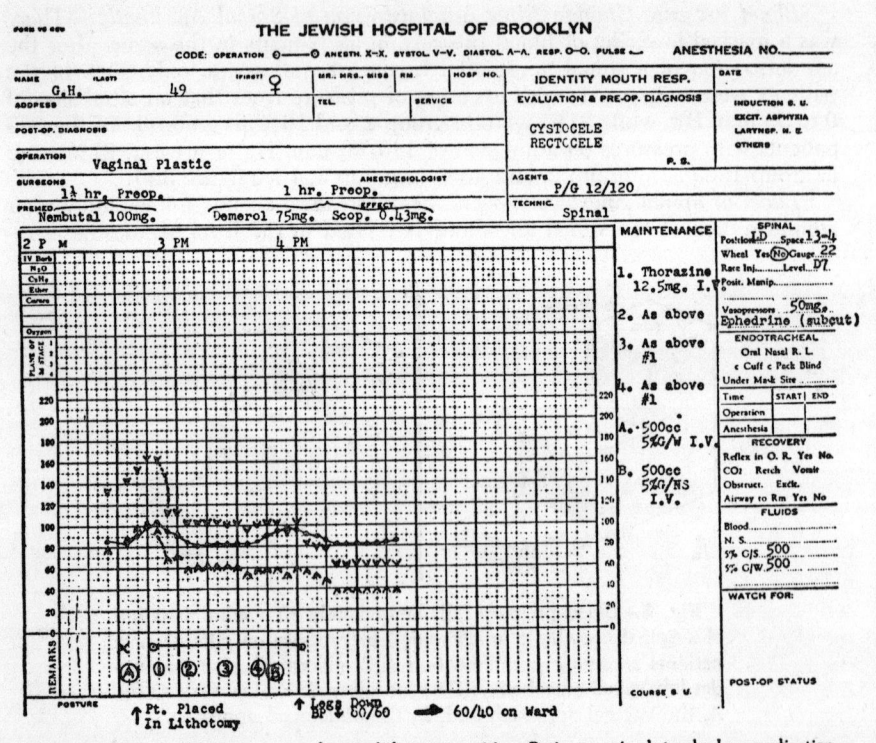

Fig. 6.—Record of patient operated on in lithotomy position. Patient received standard premedication.

minute intervals until a total of 50 mg. of the drug had been given. There was no further drop in blood pressure, however, until the end of the procedure, when the patient's legs were lowered. The hypotension corrected itself approximately three hours post-operatively. Figure 7 shows the record of a patient undergoing a similar procedure, except that the patient received premedication with chlorpromazine. Immediately after administration of a spinal anesthetic, the blood pressure continued to fall, despite the use of the lithotomy position. The blood pressure returned to its preoperative level shortly after the patient was returned to her bed.

Blood Pressure Changes After Use of Vasopressors Before Administration of Spinal Anesthetic.—The commonly used vasopressor agents are of three basic types: myocardial stimulants, cerebral stimulants, and peripheral constrictors. Ephedrine acts directly on the myocardium, increasing cardiac output and hence raising the blood pressure; there is also some degree of arteriolar constriction. Methamphetamine (Desoxyephedrine) hydrochloride is primarily a cerebral stimulant, although it causes some increase in myocardial activity and some peripheral constriction. Methoxamine (Vasoxyl) hydrochloride is a vasopressor with an entirely peripheral effect; the bradycardia often associated with the use of this agent may be of central origin. Figure 8 shows blood-pressure changes after administration of a spinal anesthetic to the entire series of patients receiving chlorpromazine preoperatively, each of whom had received one of three vasopressor agents. These data confirm the observations of many with regard to the ineffectiveness of routine doses of the standard vasopressors. Methoxamine, however, appears more effective in preventing the severe pressure falls (over 60 mm. Hg), as can be seen by contrasting the percentage of patients in group 3 for each of the three pressor agents studied.

COMMENT

The central action of chlorpromazine is apparently responsible for the majority of physiological alterations associated with its use. Early in the course of study of this compound, ganglionic blocking properties were thought to be responsible for the hypotension not infrequently seen. A number of studies have subsequently demonstrated the fact that chlorpromazine was not a true ganglionic blocking agent. Adrenolytic properties have been demonstrated in the laboratory animal. We have noted epinephrine reversal in the laboratory but have been unable to reproduce this phenomenon clinically. Although some degree of peripheral activity contributes to the clinical picture, the central action of this drug is responsible for its wide range of physiological effects. In the series of patients receiving chlorpromazine and a spinal anesthetic, the blood-pressure changes are primarily a result of chlorpromazine administration rather than a function of the level of anesthesia. Vasopressors, regardless of mechanisms, are unable to correct the pressure changes with any degree of constancy. The concomitant use of barbiturates in patients under spinal anesthesia who have received chlorpromazine further aggravates blood-pressure changes and increases the resistance to correction with vasopressors. The additive effect of barbiturates and chlorpromazine is related to the ability of both compounds to depress the hypothalamus and the reticular activating system.

The hypothalamic region of the diencephalon is responsible for the regulation of temperature and the sleep processes. The posterior nuclear group in the hypothalamus, when stimulated experimentally, produces a number of reactions characteristic of sympathetic activity: dilatation of the pupils, sweating, inhibition of intestinal activity, liberation of epinephrine, tachycardia, and a rise in

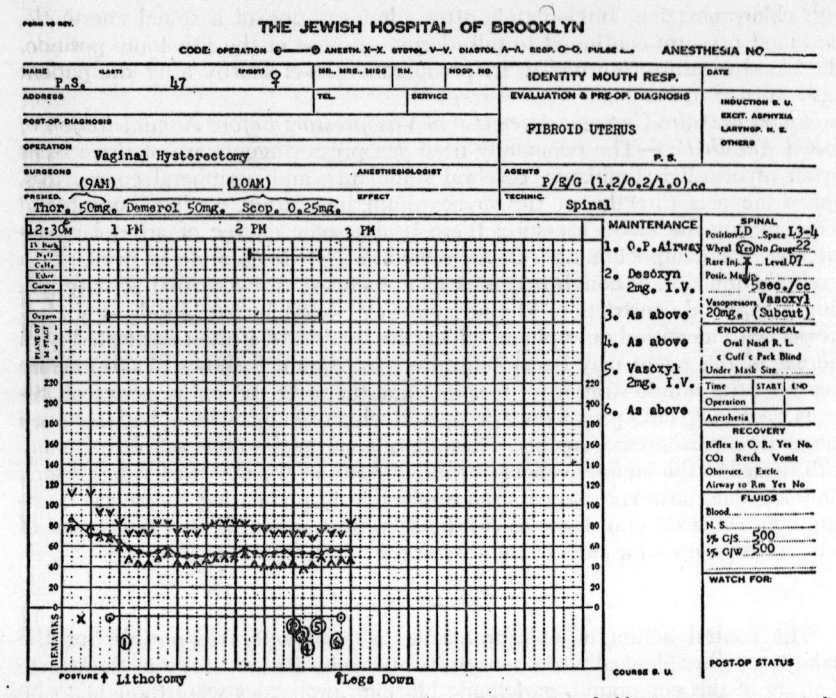

Fig. 7.—Record of patient operated on in lithotomy position. Patient received chlorpromazine preoperatively.

blood pressure. The depression of sympathetic activity, temperature regulation, and the sleep regulatory processes noted with the use of chlorpromazine are the results of a reduction in hypothalamic activity.

With the increasing knowledge of function within the central nervous system, it has become apparent that no one center in the brain entirely controls the activity of a system. Evidence of sympathetic activity can also be elicited from those areas of the prefrontal cortex that are thought to represent cortical projection of the hypothalamus. The thalamus, gyrus fornicatus, and ascending reticular activating system are also related to sympathetic function. The ascending reticular activating system is a multisynaptic medial brainstem structure that receives collateral fibers from the classic ascending sensory pathways. Sensory input to this system must serve a function common to all sensory input, the maintenance of a state of alertness at cortical levels for incoming stimuli. Depression of this system produces marked somnolence in the laboratory animal, with limited response to stimuli (auditory and olfactory), and would appear to be the neurophysiological basis of ether analgesia (Artusio).

Peripheral sympathetic activity and circulating epinephrine also contribute to the maintenance of cortical activity as a function of the stress reaction of an organism. That this occurs by mechanisms other than circulatory has been demonstrated experimentally. Studies implicate the reticular activating system as the cause of the increased cortical activity after rises in the amount of circulating epinephrine. If the brain stem cephalad to the quadrigeminal bodies is severed, with cerebral circulation remaining intact, intravenously given epinephrine does not produce intensification of cortical action potentials. Laboratory animals given chlorpromazine premedication exhibit attenuated responses to intravenously given epinephrine. Depression of the reticular activating system and hypothalamus by chlorpromazine probably accounts for the wide activity range of this compound.

The antishock property of chlorpromazine is related to a combination of central effect and the peripheral manifestations of this effect. Normally, under conditions of stress, the sympathetic nervous system responds with a mass reaction. (See fig. 8). Vasoconstriction and an increased cardiac output are the results of hypothalamic activity on the adrenal medulla, while the adrenal cortex responds to hypothalamic activity by way of neural connections to the anterior hypophysis and the subsequent production of corticotropin (ACTH). The reticular activating system, too, responds to stress by increasing cortical sensitivity to incoming stimuli; its role beyond that of an arousal mechanism is not fully understood at present. Vasomotor activity increases under adrenergic

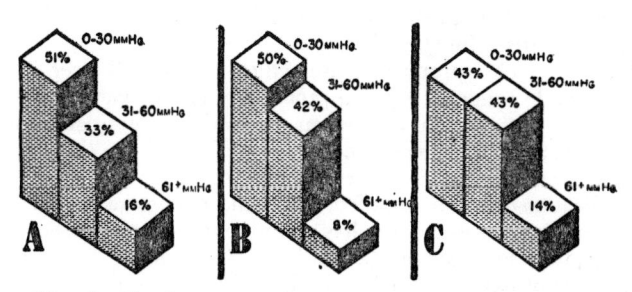

Fig. 8.—Blood-pressure changes after administration of a spinal anesthetic to patients who had received premedication with chlorpromazine and, A, 50 mg. of ephedrine; B, 20 mg. of methoxamine (Vasoxyl) hydrochloride; or, C, 20 mg. of Methamphetamine (Desoxyephedrine) hydrochloride.

influence, with constriction of precapillary sphincters and the consequent shunting of blood to the vital centers (heart and brain) to the exclusion of the remainder of the body. In early shock, renal blood flow, which normally represents about 25% of total circulating volume, falls to approximately 10% or less of its usual amount. There is a 75% reduction in femoral blood in experimental animals exposed to nonhemorrhagic shock. This large reduction in flow occurs before there are any noticeable blood pressure changes, so that the animal can be said to be in the compensatory stage of shock at a time when pulse and blood pressure offer no warning signs of shock per se.

The persistence of vasoconstriction eventually leads to areas of localized ischemia, with the subsequent release of tissue metabolites and breakdown products. The integrity of an anoxic capillary bed is further disturbed by tissue breakdown products, and vasoconstriction yields to dilatation and to increased membrane permeability, with consequent fluid loss. Dilatation of the capillary bed in areas affected by the shunting of blood leads to the formation of large stagnant pools of blood, which further diminishes the already embarrassed circulating volume. Eventually, peripheral failure leads to a central vascular collapse.

With the reduction in sympathetic reaction to stress that occurs with administration of chlorpromazine, renal and splanchnic vascular beds receive a more adequate share of available circulating blood volume; tissue anoxia is reduced, vascular integrity maintained, and fluid loss from altered permeability is absent. This discussion is not meant to infer that a permanent protection from shock exists but rather that there is a prolongation of the temporary state during which corrective therapy can be instituted without exhausting the patient's reserve. In the patient who has received chlorpromazine, the blood pressure responds early to blood loss, and hence blood replacement is begun at a period when blood loss might have been masked by compensatory vasoconstriction without chlorpromazine. Should extensive intravenous therapy fail to return blood pressures to reasonable levels, the addition of conservative amounts of vasopressor will elicit a marked response from a dilated vascular tree of good integrity and adequate functional reserve.

We have used chlorpromazine premedication in well over 3,500 patients undergoing a wide range of surgical procedures and of varying risks and ages. Clinically, these patients do well when exposed to potentially traumatic and hemorrhagic surgery. The incidence of surgical shock in the operating room is less than it was previously. What hypotension does occur under chlorpromazine premedication is safely handled. First, the patient who has received adequate sedation before operation has a reduction in metabolic activity and, therefore, requires less oxygen. Secondly, patients under anesthesia receive a high percentage of oxygen. Finally, the liberal use of intravenous therapy (not vasopressors) tends to restore blood pressure.

Summary

While epinephrine reversal is rather easily reproduced in the laboratory animal, clinically this phenomenon is difficult to produce in the human. Epinephrine continues to cause an equipressor response in patients who have received chlorpromazine. Chlorpromazine premedication is associated with a 20% incidence of hypotension, as compared to a 7 to 8% incidence with standard premedication. If patients are arbitrarily divided into two groups, those with pressures on admission of below 140/90 mm. Hg and of 140/90 and greater, then the response to chlorpromazine in the former group compares favorably to the response noted with standard premedication. The blood-pressure change after administration of a spinal anesthetic in the patient receiving chlorpromazine is more a result of the administration of this agent than a function of the level of anesthesia. Standard vasopressor agents are of little value in correction of pressure change under spinal anesthesia, but methoxamine (Vasoxyl) hydrochloride appears more effective than ephedrine or methamphetamine (Desoxyephedrine) hydrochloride in correcting severe pressure falls of over 60 mm. Hg. Chlorpromazine-induced hypotension is no problem in the operating room, where patients with lowered metabolic activity are exposed to a high-oxygen atmosphere and liberal amounts of intravenous therapy.

A CASE OF CORTICOTROPIC HORMONE-INDUCED PSYCHOSIS TREATED WITH PROMAZINE HYDROCHLORIDE

Dean J. Plazak, M.D.

The usual psychological response to the administration of adrenocorticotropic hormone or the various corticosteroids is described as deviation and lability in mood, ordinarily towards euphoria.

Many theories have been advanced as to the mechanism of this and other more intense psychological responses. Among these theories are the concept of disturbance of biochemical equilibrium, a sudden shift in electrolyte balance, interference with the "feed-back" control mechanism of the pituitary gland, and sudden change from one adaptive level to another.

When the emotional reaction is more intense, symptoms of irritability, distractability, a general sense of alarm, intense anxiety and even panic are seen. Occasionally the patient develops an overt psychotic reaction. These varying emotional responses are usually short in duration but have been reported as persisting as long as six months. The reactions of longer duration are thought to represent adjustive devices defending against inadequate psychic adjustment to the sudden changes in metabolic and adaptive level.

Any of these reactions may occur quite independently of the patient's usual level of apparent emotional stability although the content of the mental response to the administration of the drug will be related to the content of their personality structure.

Reactions as severe as overt psychosis have been reported following a single dose of 20 mgs. of corticotropic hormone and abrupt change or cessation of dosage of this hormone or of any of the corticosteroids has frequently been found to precipitate a severe emotional response.

Appropriate alteration of dosage of these medications usually is sufficient therapy but occasionally more intensive psychiatric treatment has become necessary.

The patient described in this report was transferred to the neuropsychiatric service suffering from what appeared to be an acute panic of psychotic proportions with onset three days following the administration of a single dose of corticotropic hormone. She had been receiving regular daily dosages of from 30 to 50 mgs. of various corticosteroids for the preceding seventeen months. At the time of her transfer it was decided to begin a clinical course of a newly introduced phenothiazine derivative (promazine hydrochloride) to determine its effect on her psychotic state.

Report of a Case

A 29 year old white female was admitted to the U. S. Naval Hospital, Bethesda, Maryland, on December 20, 1955. Her chief complaint was one of symptoms of recurrent spontaneous hemorrhages into the skin of her arms, legs, abdomen and face of two years' duration. Onset was after a tooth extraction in July 1954.

Previous laboratory evaluations of her disorder in other Naval hospitals established the fact that her blood plasma was not deficient in any of the normal usual clotting factors but contained an excessive amount of some material found in both her serum and plasma, which was able to inhibit clotting of normal plasma. It was heat-stable and non-dialyzable, and acted in the first stage of coagulation to prohibit conversion of prothrombin, that is, a circulating anti-thromboplastin. Laboratory evaluations of this substance, carried out by Dr. N. R. Shulman at the Naval Medical Research Institute, revealed that trypsin used *in vitro* corrected the clotting defect in the patient's blood. This suggested that the anticoagulant was a proteolytic inhibitor, since trypsin combines strongly with these. Such an anti-coagulant with similar properties and action was recently isolated from normal human plasma.

Prior to clinical trial, trypsin was given in intravenous infusions to dogs *in vivo* with no noticeable anti-coagulant effects, in amounts required to completely correct the patient's clotting defects *in vitro*.

The patient then received eight infusions of a twice crystalline preparation of trypsin, 260 mgs. in all, over a nine week period.

There were no noticeable clinical effects other than complaints of flushing, tachycardia, and headache at the time of infusion. Epinephrine and slowing of the infusion remedied these. The bleeding and clotting time returned to normal and she had no further hemorrhages.

Prior to discharging the patient from the hospital it was decided to gradually discontinue administration of various adrenal corticosteroids that had been intermittently administered since December of 1954 and continuously since December of 1955. On April 6, she was given an intravenous infusion containing 20 mgs. of corticotropic hormone preparatory to reducing her daily dosage of adrenal corticosteroids.

The following day the patient, who ordinarily was rather tense, anxious and had ill forebodings as to her ultimate prognosis, gradually became unusually euphoric, elated, overly optimistic, and energetically assisted with small tasks about the ward. Within three days she began to report disturbing dreams suggestive of severe sexual conflict and attack, and gradually appeared more tremulous, irritable, and anxious to a degree of undifferentiated panic. She became suspicious of the entire medical staff and withdrew to her room. Her personal appearance deteriorated rapidly. Various sedatives and ataractic agents were utilized without apparent success over the next three days. During this period of time, she was receiving about three-fourths of her usual adrenal corticosteroid dosage and receiving no further corticotropic hormone.

She became so intensely disturbed with her severe panic, feelings of impending doom, and fear of others, that by April 13 it was considered advisable to continue her care on the psychiatric service and she was transferred. It was felt that she was suffering from an acute undifferentiated psychotic panic, induced by the introduction of adrenal corticotropin and associated with the sudden change in her dosage of adrenal corticosteroids.

On admission to the psychiatric service she appeared confused, mildly disoriented, unable to concentrate, could not eat or sleep, took little care of her personal hygiene, had strong suicidal ideations, and was excessively concerned over her status to the point of panic. The disturbing dreams continued. It was considered that she could be experiencing visual hallucinations.

On the afternoon of her transfer she was administered 100 mgm. of promazine hydrochloride intravenously, over a period of five minutes. Within that period of time she commented that she felt relaxed for the first time in several days and her loss of excessive concern and reduction of tension was apparent. She fell into a light sleep-like state from which she was easily aroused by soft-spoken voice. She began eating that evening and slept well that night. She was given an additional 150 mgms. oral promazine hydrochloride at bedtime that night and 100 mgms. four times a day orally thereafter. The following day she resumed normal activity, took care of her personal appearance, continued to eat and sleep well, had no further symptoms of anxiety or panic and reported no further disturbing dreams.

She continued to receive 100 mgms. of promazine hydrochloride four times a day and was discharged from the hospital within ten days on that medication. During this time she was able to approach a long standing marital problem never before discussed, and her motivation to return to her home, previously poor, markedly improved. She has remained free of the symptoms and signs displayed while hospitalized, and was last interviewed two months following her discharge.

Discussion

Phenothiazine derivatives are considered to have several sites of action. It has been theorized that they may have an inhibiting action on the diencephalic centers or may exert a dampening affect on the arousal mechanism in the reticular substance. These agents have been found to successfully reduce aggressiveness, severe anxiety and fear in both experimental animals and human subjects.

Corticosteroids and corticotropic hormone are thought to bring about an acceleration of the rate of biochemical interchange and to promote mobilization of energy for cellular work. This effect is considered to constitute a source of instinctual tension and either institutes a drive to discharge energy or creates increased need for instinctual satisfaction. This manifests itself in varying psychic symptoms indicating strong response of the arousal mechanism and excessive sympathetic discharge or adrenergic response. If the individual's increased needs cannot be met, various psychic defense structures may be erected to avoid intense anxiety, possibly ultimately of psychotic magnitude. In this particular patient, the onset of the psychic response of psychotic symptomatology was occasioned by her inability to tolerate the sudden alteration in adjustive level due to the sudden reduction in her daily dosage of corticosteroids and the simultaneous introduction of corticotropic hormone.

It appears that administration of a pharmacologic agent which would counteract strong adrenergic reactions and excessive response of the arousal mechanism should obviate the need for the utilization of a psychotic defense structure as a defense. A phenothiazine derivative, promazine hydrochloride, was utilized successfully for this purpose in this patient.

This clinical experience indicates that those ataractic drugs which are derivatives of phenothiazine might well be given further clinical trial in the treatment of transient emotional disorders occasioned by the use of corticosteroids or corticotropic hormone.

Summary

A single case history is presented, involving the successful utilization of a new phenothiazine derivative (promazine hydrochloride) in the treatment of an ACTH-induced transient psychotic reaction.

The pharmacologic basis for this treatment is discussed.

CHLORPROMAZINE, NEW INHIBITING AGENT FOR PSYCHOMOTOR EXCITEMENT AND MANIC STATES

H. E. Lehmann, M.D., and G. E. Hanrahan, M.D.

Throughout its history psychiatry has been faced with the therapeutic problem of controlling acute and chronic states of psychomotor excitement. Much has been achieved with the advent of systematic pharmacological sedation. More recently the introduction of electroconvulsive treatment has augmented our capacity to handle successfully most of the excited states refractory to sedation by drugs. There remain, however, a number of cases in which one meets particular difficulty in controlling excitement either because of undesirable side-effects of the treatment itself or because of the patient's persistent tendency to relapse. It is the purpose of this article to report on our experiences with a new drug which seems to possess specific properties for the psychiatric management of excited states.

The first clinical investigations with this drug were carried out and published in France, where it is known as Largactil, or 4560 R. P. It is known by the same name in Canada. In the United States it is referred to as chlorpromazine, or Compound 2601-A. Chlorpromazine has been developed in the Rhone-Poulenc Special Research Laboratories during research on potentiating agents in anesthesia.

Pharmacology

Chlorpromazine is a phenothiazine derivative with the following formula:

$$CH_2CH_2CH_2N(CH_3)_2 \cdot HCl$$

Its chemical designation is 3-chloro-10(3-dimethylaminopropyl)phenothiazine hydrochloride. The molecular weight is 335.320; the melting point, 179-180 C. It is highly soluble in water, chloroform, and ethyl and methyl alcohol. A 5% aqueous solution is stable for at least 24 hours and has a pH of 4.9. It is a gray-white crystalline powder, which is photosensitive and will change color when exposed to light.

It is chemically related to promethazine (Phenergan) and diethazine hydrochloride (Diparcol), which are also phenothiazine derivatives and are used as antihistaminic agents and in the treatment of Parkinsonism.

In a group of dogs given 20 mg. per kilogram daily for a month the mortality was nil. Chlorpromazine produced a type of depression in animals which increased progressively with the dose. Hypnosis has never been observed.

The drug has a pronounced antiemetic action and in dogs decreases the vomiting frequency following administration of apomorphine hydrochloride, 40 to 100%.

The vasopressor activity of small doses of epinephrine in cats is reversed by chlorpromazine, which possesses a mild adrenergic blocking activity. It does not modify in any way the hyperglycemia produced by epinephrine. The drug inhibits the secretion of gastric juice and reduces the incidence of gastric ulcers in rats in which a ligature of the pylorus has been performed.

A hypothermic effect is observed in rats, in which the body temperature drops 1-6 C. after the administration of chlorpromazine.

The drug exhibits a moderate antihistaminic activity. A marked potentiating effect is observed when it is administered in combination with sedatives, general anesthetics, analgesics, and ethyl alcohol.

Blood levels and elimination of the drug were studied experimentally with rabbits and reported by the Poulenc laboratories. After oral administration of a dose of 250 mg. per kilogram, the blood concentration rose to its highest level of 8 mg. per liter in three hours. The total quantity excreted by the kidneys in three days represented only 7-8% of the intake, suggesting that the major proportion of the drug is metabolized in the organism before it reaches the kidneys.

Physiological Effects in Humans

The most striking effect of the administration of chlorpromazine in humans is a pronounced drop in blood pressure, which may vary from 20-40 mm. systolic and 10-30 mm. diastolic, according to dosage and individual response. While the blood pressure tends to remain below the normal level of the individual subject, one observes frequent fluctuations upward and downward. A compensatory tachycardia is usually observed as the pulse rate rises from 10-40 beats per minute. A distinct pallor is noted in most subjects, and many exhibit miosis.

The majority of our patients evidenced mild hyperthermia, with ranges from 99 to 101 F. for the first few days of treatment. In each case the fever subsided spontaneously, and in some instances was followed later by hypothermia, with the temperature ranging between 96 and 98 F.

The respiratory rate is not influenced by the drug. Dryness of the mucous membranes and nasal congestion are frequent findings, particularly at the commencement of therapy. Urinary frequency is commonly observed and is possibly due to increased renal blood flow. There is often a tendency to constipation. The appetite remains very good, and most patients gain weight during treatment.

Patients receiving large doses of chlorpromazine exhibit definite motor retardation, with an unsteady gait, while the facial expression becomes rather wooden and the general appearance resembles that of Parkinsonism but there is no muscular rigidity. With smaller doses these phenomena are less pronounced. There is usually marked drowsiness, which may increase to the point of somnolence. Deep and superficial reflexes may be unaltered or slightly depressed.

These symptoms are reflected in the patients' statement that they feel cold, drowsy, faint, and weak. The effects of the drug persist for about 48 hours after termination of treatment.

Administration and Dosage

Delay, Deniker and Harl were the first clinicians to employ chlorpromazine as the sole drug in psychiatric conditions. Similarly, we have used the drug by itself rather than in combination with other antihistaminics or sedatives because of the obscuring effects of "potentiation" which chlorpromazine then produces. Deschamps has administered the drug in conjunction with promethazine and barbiturates.

Patients differ considerably in their reaction to chlorpromazine. Administered parenterally, the drug is much more effective than when given orally. Tolerance develops rapidly and requires an increase in dosage after a few days to maintain a constant level of sedation. In our material we have found it necessary to employ doses which often considerably exceed those used by the French workers.

Depending on the patient's condition, we employ the drug in two ways, as a sedative for severely agitated patients and in states of moderate restlessness. In states of acute psychomotor excitement we have found it effective to begin giving 50 mg. intramuscularly twice a day, with use of 50 mg. orally two or three times a day. If the patient refuses oral medication, the parenteral dose may be increased. The aim is to produce a state of motor retardation, emotional indifference, and somnolence, and the dose must be increased accordingly as tolerance develops. After the first week of treatment the patients remain retarded but are less sleepy. In most cases it has not been necessary to exceed a dose of 800 mg. per day, while some patients may require only 100 mg. or less daily. The course of treatment may last from three days to four weeks. We have not observed withdrawal symptoms even when the drug is abruptly discontinued, although it is advisable to reduce it gradually. It should be noted that parenteral administration is more reliable in its effects than oral administration.

In less pronounced psychomotor restlessness or emotional tension, such as that seen in long-standing anxiety states, senile agitation, and certain behavior disorders, the administration of the drug may have to be continued for two or three months, and in these cases 25 to 50 mg. two to four times a day is given orally. With this amount the patients are not drowsy once tolerance has developed and are able to remain active and composed.

Intravenous administration of the drug requires dilution with isotonic saline because of its relatively low pH and the danger of damaging the venous enothelium. Intramuscular administration is safe but somewhat painful, and for this reason it is recommended to dilute the drug with distilled water, saline, or procaine. In none of our patients did abscesses develop at the site of injection.

Blood pressure, pulse rate, and temperature are charted at least twice daily. Results of urinalysis, including tests for bile, and body weight are recorded every week. A simple and sensitive liver function test should be done at the beginning of treatment. In our material the cephalin-cholesterol flocculation test has been used.

No special diet is required. The patient's appetite remains good as a rule, and laxatives may be necessary if constipation develops. Bed rest is recommended, at least during the first week, if larger doses are employed, because of the orthostatic hypotension which develops in most cases during treatment and which may lead to syncope in ambulatory patients. It is important to note that ordinary analeptics seem to have little effect on the depression of the autonomic and central nervous systems produced by chlorpromazine. Caffeine, aminophylline, and phenylephrine (Neo-Synephrine) may be tried, although in most cases lowering the patient's head and elevating the legs will suffice. Pentylenetetrazol (Metrazol) and nikethamide (Anacardone; Coramine) are contraindicated if chlorpromazine has been given previously. One of our patients who had collapsed owing to orthostatic hypotension and the resulting cerebral anemia was given 2 cc. of nikethamide by error and developed a series of generalized convulsions, from which he recovered within an hour. Precautions should be taken against upper respiratory infections because of the dryness of the mucous membranes which often develops in the course of treatment.

The following is an outline of our ward procedure:
1. Give deep intramuscular injection; do not administer intravenously.
2. Dilute 1 cc. of the drug with 1 cc. of isotonic saline.
3. Rotate sites of injection (right and left deltoid, right and left buttock, and right and left lateral aspect of thigh).
4. Do not inject more than 2 cc. at one place.
5. Start patient on "bedside notes."
6. Encourage patient to remain in bed.
7. Make weekly urinalyses (check for bile) and body weight determinations.
8. Give no other medication while patient is on chlorpromazine, except on special order.
9. Chart blood pressure, pulse rate, respiration rate, and temperature every 12 hours.
10. Give regular diet.
11. Protect patient against cold.
12. Give enema if necessary.
13. In case of syncope or collapse, place patient in horizontal position with legs elevated. Do not give nikethamide or Metrazol.

Psychological Effects

Chlorpromazine has a pronounced inhibitory effect on certain functions of the central nervous system. Patients receiving the drug become lethargic. Manic patients often will not object to bed rest, and patients who present management problems become tractable. Assaultive and interfering behavior ceases almost entirely. The patients under treatment display a lack of spontaneous interest in the environment, yet are easily accessible and respond as a rule immediately and relevantly to questions even if awakened from sleep. As Delay and Deniker described them, they tend to remain silent and immobile when left alone and to reply to questions in a slow monotone. We can confirm the observations of these authors that patients receiving the drug are often aware of their improvement without showing any euphoric reaction.

Some patients dislike the treatment and complain of their drowsiness and weakness. Some state that they feel "washed out," as after an exhausting illness, a complaint which is indeed in keeping with their appearance. Others, however, appreciate the peculiar effect of the drug which allows them to relax from ideational pressure. One manic patient stated after her recovery that with the drug she soon lost the feeling: "I had to live my whole life in one day." Another patient suffering from long-standing anxiety described thus the effect of small doses of chlorpromazine on her feelings: "It was like a chairman taking control of a meeting where everybody previously had been shouting at once."

Although a patient under the influence of chlorpromazine at first glance presents the aspect of a heavily drugged person, one is surprised at the absence of clouding of consciousness. The higher psychic functions are preserved to a remarkable degree, and the patients are capable of sustained attention, reflection, and concentration.

In a series of eight experimental subjects, tests of reaction time, hand steadiness, tapping speed, digit span, and digit symbols (Wechsler-Bellevue subtest) were given one and a half hours before and one and a half hours after the administration of a dose of chlorpromazine sufficiently large to promote definite somnolence. In three subjects the reaction time was significantly shortened; in two, prolonged; in three, unchanged. Hand steadiness was improved in two subjects, impaired in none, unchanged in six. Tapping speed showed the most pronounced impairment, being slowed down significantly in four subjects, accelerated in one, unchanged in three. Digit span was improved in five subjects, impaired in two, and unchanged in one. The digit symbol test was improved in six subjects, impaired in one, and unchanged in one. There was noted, then, definite improvement of functions involving attention and learning as tested in digit span and digit symbols, while coordination and speed of sensory-motor reaction also tended to improve under the test condition, rather than deteriorate. The only test reflecting impairment of function in 50% of our subjects was the tapping speed, which calls for an almost unstructured repetitive motor performance, the speed of which depends almost entirely on the subject's inner motivation, without extraneous stimulation or clue to the success of performance.

With three of these subjects the experiment was repeated a few days later after administration of 3 grains (0.195 gm.) of secobarbital (Seconal) sodium. They showed the typical effects of barbiturate sedation, namely, almost uniform impairment in all tested functions. Yet it was noted that two of these three patients appeared less sleepy after secobarbital than after chlorpromazine.

Thus, it becomes apparent that the sedative effect of chlorpromazine is not associated with clouding of consciousness, impairment of judgment, or disinhibition of affect. One has the impression that this drug promotes an attitude of sober resignation and of critical reflection, even in acutely disturbed patients.

We can state that in our experience chlorpromazine is the only powerful sedative whose action is restricted to a selective inhibition of drive without producing disinhibition of affect at any level of dosage.

RESULTS

This report is based upon our experience in the use of chlorpromazine at the Verdun Protestant Hospital. Seventy-one psychiatric patients, ranging in age from 18 to 82 years, were treated over a period of four months.

The most gratifying results were obtained in the group of manic-depressive patients in the manic or hypomanic state. Psychomotor excitement is usually reduced significantly within 24 hours, and sleep at night is often restored within the same period. Only in the odd case may the addition of minimal doses of other sedatives be required, the effect of which is greatly enhanced by chlorpromazine. Feeding problems disappear rapidly, and the patient soon becomes cooperative to nursing care. The psychiatrist is surprised to find his manic patients amenable to reason. The average duration of treatment for these patients varied from two to five weeks. Although some patients appear to be asymptomatic within a few days, it is advisable to continue the treatment for some time in order to avoid relapses. In keeping with good practice in managing the institutionalized manic patients, we have retained our patients in the hospital for at least two to three weeks after all symptoms have subsided and medication has been discontinued.

The drug is of unique value in the symptomatic control of almost any kind of severe excitement. This includes catatonic schizophrenia, schizoaffective conditions, epileptic clouded states, agitation occurring in lobotomized patients immediately or several months after surgery, and organic-toxic confusional states, as frequently observed in uremic conditions and senile psychoses. A single intramuscular dose of 50 to 100 mg. will usually control most states of excitement. If it is used in conjunction with other sedation, caution must be observed because of its potentiating effect.

In a few cases we had the impression that the immediate administration of the drug for three or four days prevented a psychotic breakdown in patients with a history of one or more psychotic episodes who were exhibiting their typical prodromal symptoms.

Emotional tension is well controlled by comparatively small doses of 50 to 200 mg. daily, amounts which have been administered without untoward effects to some psychoneurotic patients over a period of several months. A 82-year-old woman, whose agitated delirium had proved refractory to all other therapeutic methods, has been successfully controlled by the drug for a period of more than four months, without untoward effects. The possible toxic effect of chlorpromazine on the liver, however, requires caution when used for long periods of time, especially in patients with impaired liver function. The only death reported in the literature occurred during the treatment of a patient with severe delirium tremens and cirrhosis of the liver.

Most of the patients who showed no lasting improvement with the drug were chronic schizophrenics presenting considerable deterioration. We have not observed a direct influence of the drug on delusional systems or hallucinatory phenomena. Delay and associates reported one failure in the treatment of a cortisone-induced manic-confusional state, although they stressed the excellent effects of chlorpromazine in other acute attacks characterized by confusion.

Our therapeutic results are summarized in the accompanying Table.

We are particularly impressed with the favorable results in our manic-depressive patients in a chronic manic state, all of whom had been continuously manic or hypomanic for more than a year and had previously failed to respond to standard therapeutic procedures or had had only brief remissions. In some of these long-standing cases recovery with chlorpromazine may not be immediate, the improvement gradually progressing for a month or two after termination of therapy. In acute manic states chlorpromazine therapy usually leads to recovery in a shorter time than is required with other, established treatment procedures. It is generally known that the rapid remissions that follow electroshock therapy often are short-lived, while relapses following chlorpromazine therapy are not frequent.

In four patients, all manic-depressives in the manic phase and over 45 years of age, we observed an interesting inversion of clinical manifestations, as the patients under treatment with the drug became depressed after a brief remission, which lasted only a few days. The depressed state responded in the typical manner to electroconvulsive therapy, requiring only four to six electroshocks to effect a lasting recovery.

We have observed that psychiatric patients who fail to show the typical physiological changes of drop in blood pressure, rise in pulse rate, and slight fall in body temperature also often fail to give a satisfactory therapeutic response. It should be noted, however, that cardiovascular and thermal responses

*Therapeutic Results with Chlorpromazine**

	Averted	Recovered	Much Improved	Improved	Unchanged	Still Under Treatment	Total
Schizophrenia	2	..	3	9	7	1	22
Schizoaffective	..	..	1	2	..	..	3
Manic, acute	2	8	2	7	..	3	22
Manic, chronic	..	4	1	3	1	3	12
Psychoneurotic	..	1	..	1	2	..	4
Postlobotomy	..	..	..	2	1	1	4
Mental deficiency	..	..	..	..	1	..	1
Senile psychosis	..	..	..	3	..	..	3
Total	4	13	7	27	12	8	71

* Averted means arrest of imminent psychotic attack during prodromal stage; recovered, sustained cessation of symptoms within 40 days; much improved, reduction of symptoms to the point where the patient is able to leave hospital within 40 days; improved, sustained lessening of symptoms within 40 days but patient unable to leave hospital.

during the first few days of treatment can be very unstable, until a new equilibrium is established. Elderly patients, however, frequently fail to demonstrate the relative tachycardia at any time, although their therapeutic response may be satisfactory.

Chlorpromazine has sometimes given results when other treatments, including insulin and electric shock, have proved of no avail or have not produced complete remission. It is of particular value in patients who during a course of electroconvulsive therapy become violently excited. The fact that it does not produce emotional disinhibition gives chlorpromazine a special place in the treatment of acute hysterical agitation, where ordinary sedation might bring about further loss of control. Our material does not include cases of addiction, but one would expect it to be of value in managing withdrawal symptoms because of its dependable sedative action, most of which is free from euphoric effects.

On the other hand, the new drug should not be expected to be a cure-all in psychoneuroses. If moderate oral doses of 100 to 200 mg. per day do not give satisfactory relief from tension, higher doses will usually be of no avail. If traumatic factors cannot be excluded from the environment and major conflicts persist, chlorpromazine can only be considered an adjuvant to psychotherapy.

Toxicity

It is our belief that chlorpromazine must be administered under close medical supervision, since the drug is capable of producing undesirable side-effects in a certain number of persons. As has been indicated, we consider the use of the drug as a therapeutic procedure which preferably should be carried out in a hospital setting. Although safe outpatient treatment with this drug is possible, one must warn against unrestricted use of chlorpromazine as a sedative.

In our clinical material, about half the patients showed slight changes in the cephalin-cholesterol flocculation, a number of these being of questionable significance; 30% showed changes in total serum protein values and albumin-globulin ratios, most of them to a very minor degree. The sedimentation rate increased in about 50%, the changes remaining within normal limits in many cases. We observed no impairment of kidney function as measured by blood urea nitrogen values. Urinary findings remained normal throughout the period of administration. Hemoglobin and red and white cell counts were not altered significantly. Increased susceptibility to upper respiratory infection was noted and was probably related to the dryness of the mucous membranes. Delay and Deniker assume a generally lowered resistance to infection, but we have not encountered any serious complications of this type in our material.

Nausea, anorexia, and epigastric distress have been observed by us in 8% of the patients. Allergic reactions, as manifested by urticaria or asthma, occurred in 13% of cases. These latter complications are interesting, inasmuch as the drug is reported to have powerful antiemetic properties and belongs in the class of antihistaminics. The allergic manifestations subside when the drug is discontinued. Gastrointestinal complications were not considered an indication to termination of the treatment.

In three patients treated for two, three, and four weeks respectively, jaundice developed, which appeared to be of toxic origin, with the attendant blood and urine abnormalities. These patients were symptom-free within 10 days after the drug was discontinued and a supportive dietary regimen instituted. Their cephalin-cholesterol flocculation tests were negative after two to three weeks.

Several patients were treated while ambulatory for four months with doses up to 200 mg. per day, without showing any untoward effects.

Comment

To justify its addition to the voluminous list of therapeutic agents in psychiatry, any new drug might be analyzed from the following aspects:

(a) Does it control symptoms as well as or better than other established treatments?

(b) Does it compare favorably with regard to ease of administration and unpleasant side-effects?

(c) Is there less risk associated with its use?

(d) Does it improve the underlying pathological condition?

(e) Does it permit sustained psychotherapeutic rapport?

It will be noted that the first four questions may be applied to any therapeutic agent in any branch of medicine, while the last one is of singular significance to psychiatry. Many of us have in recent years lost sight of our essential task of understanding our patients, as we subject them to a sequence of comas, shocks, convulsions, confusion, and amnesia, all of which render them incapable of relating to the psychiatrist in a consistent and meaningful manner.

In the light of the questions formulated, we may consider the two principal psychiatric procedures currently employed in the treatment of the manic state of manic-depressive psychosis, namely, E.C.T. and standard pharmacological sedation, including prolonged sleep therapy, as compared with chlorpromazine treatment.

E.C.T. provides excellent and immediate control of symptoms if administered intensively. It may, however, by its disorganizing effect on the higher brain functions, produce a new set of symptoms, characterized by confusion, restlessness, and aggression. While E.C.T. is one of the simplest forms of treatment, it is associated with the unpleasant side-effect of amnesia. The possible injuries to the musculoskeletal system and the complications that may arise from the use of relaxing drugs also constitute important disadvantages. In addition to its symptomatic effect on psychomotor excitement, E.C.T. terminates many manic attacks, but immediate relapses are frequent. Rapport with the therapist is possible only on the most superficial level, in many cases not at all because of the confusion so often associated with the use of E.C.T.

In prescribing barbiturates, scopolamine, insulin, etc., as symptomatic sedation, failures are not uncommonly encountered because of the disinhibiting action of these drugs. However, their administration is extremely simple, and the patient, as a rule, does not experience unpleasant side-effects. While symptomatic control with these sedatives is associated with few risks, the dangers entailed in prolonged sleep therapy are serious and manifold in nature. To protect the patient against pneumonia, hyperpyrexia, and cardiovascular collapse, elaborate nursing procedures are necessary. The clouding of consciousness resulting from the use of standard sedation hampers the therapist in maintaining rapport, even though repressed material may be released from the unconscious. Nevertheless, it has been claimed that prolonged narcosis is followed by fewer relapses than E.C.T. and is the most efficacious form of therapy in manic states, although its wider application is limited by its inherent dangers and difficult administration.

Chlorpromazine, in our experience, has been the most reliable psychiatric agent in the control of symptoms of psychomotor excitement. Its administration is more cumbersome than E.C.T. or ordinary sedation but much simpler than the complicated procedure required for prolonged sleep. Unpleasant side-effects with chlorpromazine are of minor significance. The use of the drug, particularly for extended periods of time in high doses, may be fraught with some risks, but under adequate medical supervision few difficulties should be encountered.

Chlorpromazine, by operating on the underlying pathological process, is capable of shortening the course of a manic attack. Perhaps the greatest advantage of this drug lies in its power to quiet severely excited patients without rendering them confused or otherwise inaccessible.

The mode of action of chlorpromazine has not yet been established. Several theories have been advanced. It has been surmised that the drug operates through an effect on general metabolism by lowering the cellular O_2 requirements. We have not been able to confirm the findings of Delay and Deniker that basal metabolism is lowered after chlorpromazine administration. Nor could we corroborate their findings of a significant drop in the eosinophile count with chlorpromazine. We therefore do not feel justified at this time in assuming that the drug exhibits its specific effects through the adrenals or any other endocrine glands.

In contrast to barbiturates, chlorpromazine does not appear to alter the basic character of the individual E.E.G. as long as the subject is awake. It tends to produce clear tracings comparatively free from muscle artifacts and tension discharges. This finding is not surprising in view of the fact that the drug seems to have little effect on those psychological functions which have their representation in the cortex, but appears to affect selectively those subcortical structures that are concerned with maintaining psychomotor drive and wakefulness.

One may speculate from the above that cortical metabolism is little affected by chlorpromazine and that the possible site of its action is located in the activating reticular substance, the functions of which have recently been reviewed by Magoun. Because of its ganglioplegic effects, one also would think of the hypothalamus as a locus of its action.

In reflecting on the possible chemical mechanism involved, one notes the close relation of the chlorpromazine formula to that of promethazine. The latter drug has been shown by Himwich to possess antiacetylcholine properties in the neuraxis.

Summary

Chlorpromazine is a new phenothiazine derivative related to certain antihistaminic agents. It has pronounced effects on the central nervous system. In animals, it produces a type of depression which increases progressively with the dose, has strong antiemetic properties, inhibits the secretion of gastric juice, and produces hypothermia.

In man it potentiates the effects of cerebral depressants, lowers the blood pressure, and accelerates heart action. It produces motor retardation, somnolence, and weakness. Allergic reactions occur infrequently. Reversible impairment of liver function may be observed if the drug is used in large doses over extended periods of time.

The lethargy resulting from the drug in contrast to other sedatives is characterized by clarity of consciousness and retained responsiveness, which has been demonstrated by experimental psychological methods. Chlorpromazine, at any dosage, does not produce emotional disinhibition but selectively inhibits drive, which makes it unique among the more powerful sedatives.

In this study chlorpromazine was not used in combination with other sedatives. Doses vary considerably with the individual subject and range from 50 to 800 mg. per day. Prolonged administration requires nursing and medical supervision.

Seventy-one psychiatric patients, ranging in age from 18 to 82 years, were treated over a four-month period. The drug has proved to be of unique value in the symptomatic control of most types of severe psychomotor excitement. Impressive therapeutic results were obtained in acute and chronic manic-depressive patients in the manic phase. Attacks are significantly shortened. Relapses are less frequent than with E.C.T.

Selective inhibition therapy with chlorpromazine is compared with two other standard treatments for manic conditions, i. e., E.C.T. and prolonged sleep. Little is known of the exact mode of action of the drug. A possible mechanism involving acetylcholine metabolism has been considered, and, on the basis of clinical evidence available, the reticular activating system in the brain stem is proposed as the site of action.

LARGE DOSES OF CHLORPROMAZINE IN THE TREATMENT OF PSYCHIATRIC PATIENTS

Frank J. Ayd, Jr., M.D.

Since the initial report of the French psychiatrists on the effectiveness of chlorpromazine in the management of anxiety, tension and psychomotor excitement, this drug has been carefully studied by numerous investigators. All are in agreement about the efficacy of this drug in such conditions as manic reactions, catatonic excitements, panic states, and severe anxiety reactions. The consensus of opinion of those reporting on chlorpromazine is that the majority of patients respond favorably to doses ranging from 100 mgm. to 300 mgm. daily. At present, there are no published reports of clinical observations on the response of patients to massive doses of this drug, although several authors have alluded to their observations in individual cases.

This is a brief report on the effect of large doses of Chlorpromazine, 700 mgm. to 2500 mgm. daily, administered to a group of 25 hospitalized psychiatric patients. Large doses were used for the following reasons: (1) to determine if large doses are more effective than the usual dosage range of 100 mgm. to 300 mgm. daily; (2) to determine if toxic effects are more likely to occur with large doses; and (3) to determine what effect, if any, large doses would have on the central nervous system. The drug was administered intramuscularly and orally. The duration of treatment varied from two weeks to six months. The temperature, pulse, and blood pressure was recorded. Psychiatric and neurologic examinations were repeated frequently, in some instance daily.

The response of these patients to large doses of chlorpromazine was quite varied. Initially all of them were somnolent but could be aroused easily for meals and for psychiatric and neurologic examinations. In the absence of external stimuli these patients would return to their somnolent state. Concomitant with this somnolent state produced by large doses of chlorpromazine, all of these patients manifested some degree of catalepsy. Both the somnolence and catalepsy disappeared when the drug was reduced or discontinued.

Those patients receiving the drug intramuscularly had a slight elevation of temperature, up to 101 degrees in one case. This febrile reaction subsided within five days. It was noted only in those patients receiving the drug intramuscularly and was probably due to a local tissue reaction at the site of injection. The pulse rate either remained within the range of normal variation or else a slight tachycardia was recorded. This latter reaction usually occurred within twenty minutes to one hour after medication. There was an initial drop in blood pressure of 20 to 40 mm of Hg. with a tendency for the blood pressure to gradually return to the pretreatment level even though treatment was continued.

Constipation occurred in every patient. Laxatives usually sufficed to relieve this although practically all patients required at least one enema. An apparent polyuria occurred in every case during the first week of treatment, although this was not verified by an intake-output chart. Generally, the urine was darker in color, especially when the patient had not voided for several hours. This apparent polyuria and discoloration of the urine did not persist beyond the first week or two of treatment, although the urine would be darker than usual sporadically.

The appearance of the patients receiving large doses of chlorpromazine changed within the first three days. All of them had a masklike facies. Their face and eyes became immobile as they lay quietly in bed. Pallor was pronounced. All movements were slow and their speech was monotonous as well as slow. On standing they had a drooped appearance and they walked on a wide base. One patient developed the picture of paralysis agitans within 48 hours after being started on 700 mgm. a day. This patient, a 29 year old white male, with a severe obsessional neurosis, in addition to the pale, masklike facies, exhibited muscular rigidity with flexion of the body, dysarthria, dysphagia, salivation with drooling and disturbance in gait. When he went to sit down, he "drooped" into the chair. His speech was monotonous. All his associative movements were slow. The psychiatric examination did not disclose any psychic change other than those for which he was being treated. There was no impairment of the intellect. There was a slight tremor confined to the head and arms. No cogwheel phenomena could be demonstrated. There were no pathological reflexes.

This Parkinsonian-like reaction persisted for five days. It caused considerable alarm among the nurses and the patients' relatives. It did not progress beyond the picture described above even though chlorpromazine 700 mgm. daily was continued. After five days the dosage of the drug was reduced to 500 mgm. a day and by the eighth day of treatment this Parkinsonian-like reaction subsided completely. The patient became ambulatory and experienced no untoward side effects, although he continued to take 350 mgm. to 500 mgm. daily for the next three months. He is now taking 200 mgm. a day and has been on chlorpromazine for five months.

Aside from the masklike facies, the slowness of movement and the monotonous speech, none of the other patients in this series developed any other symptoms suggestive of Parkinsonism, except one. This patient, a 68 year old white woman, with a severe involutional agitated depression, received doses of chlorpromazine ranging from 300 mgm. to 1000 mgm. daily. While receiving 1000 mgm. a day this patient developed a Parkinsonian-like tremor confined to the right arm. This neurologic finding disappeared when the drug was reduced to 800 mgm. daily. For a period of four months this patient received 700 mgm. to 800 mgm. daily without any neurologic changes that were detectable. Chlorpromazine was abruptly discontinued when her relatives finally consented to EST which produced a prompt remission from her psychosis. This abrupt discontinuation of Chlorpromazine did not cause any observable withdrawal reaction, unless this was masked by the shock therapy.

The masklike facies persisted as long as the patients received large doses of Chlorpromazine. Reduction of the daily dosage below 500 mgm. resulted in a disappearance of this facial expression within a few days. Aside from the neurologic findings in those patients who developed a Parkinsonian-like reaction, no gross neurologic changes were detected in patients on large doses of Chlorpromazine.

Likewise no mental changes attributable to this drug, with one exception, were observed. This exception is that if large doses were given for more than two or three weeks, some patients developed a depression. Usually this depressed effect abated with the reduction or the discontinuation of the drug, although in one case the depression persisted. In this case EST terminated the depression. This occurrence of a depressive reaction with Chlorpromazine illustrates the reciprocal relationship between anxiety and depression in some psychiatric patients. Clinically the effect of chlorpromazine on anxiety seems to be similar to that produced by non-convulsive electrostimulation and insulin sub-coma therapy. All three of these treatment modalities can cause a reduction in anxiety, while at the same time enhancing depression. Those patients who developed depressions while taking chlorpromazine and who were treated with EST experienced a return of some anxiety following shock therapy. This resurgence of anxiety in some shock-treated patients is a common experience.

Based on the experience gained from this study, as well as the results obtained in a much larger series of patients treated with chlorpromazine reported elsewhere, it is concluded that large doses of this drug are no more effective, except in the minority of cases, than the usual dosage range of 200 mgm. to 300 mgm. daily for the disturbed patient. To administer large doses of chlorpromazine with the hope of increasing therapeutic effectiveness has been futile.

Because of the appearance of a Parkinsonian-like reaction in some patients receiving chlorpromazine, it was decided to give this drug to patients with Parkinsonism. Two patients with Parkinsonism, one post-encephalitic, the other arteriosclerotic in origin, were treated with chlorpromazine. These patients derived no benefit from chlorpromazine nor was their Parkinsonism made worse. This corresponds to the experience reported by others.

In my experience large doses of chlorpromazine do not cause any serious toxic effects. Jaundice did not occur in any patient receiving more than 500 mgm. daily. Jaundice has occurred in patients on much smaller doses. Likewise, although two patients in this series developed a Parkinsonian-like reaction, this same reaction has been observed in patients on smaller doses. Although none of the patients in this series developed respiratory infections, such illnesses have occurred in other patients on chlorpromazine and the possibility of respiratory infections in patients on large doses of this drug exists. If large doses of chlorpromazine can cause liver damage, such was not observed clinically in this series of patients, although extensive laboratory studies were not done, mainly because there was no clinical indication for such studies.

Whenever a patient is to receive large doses of chlorpromazine, he should be hospitalized. Close medical and nursing supervision is absolutely necessary.

Strict bed rest should be enforced, even though the patient, at least in the beginning of treatment, usually is somnolent and unable to get out of bed. Temperature, pulse and blood pressure should be recorded. Frequent psychiatric and neurologic examinations are necessary for the early detection of depressive reactions and the Parkinsonian-like reactions observed in this series of patients. In the event a depression, a Parkinsonian-like reaction, or any other toxic reaction should develop, these usually subside when the dosage of the drug is reduced. If any severe reactions develop, the drug should be discontinued, at least temporarily.

Summary

Large doses of Chlorpromazine were administered to 25 hospitalized psychiatric patients. The dosage range varied from 700 mgm. to 2500 mgm. daily. The duration of treatment was two weeks to six months. No serious, persistent toxic effects were observed in the patients treated. One patient developed a Parkinsonian-like reaction of moderate severity while receiving 700 mgm. daily. This reaction subsided when the dosage of chlorpromazine was reduced to 500 mgm. daily. This patient has continued to take chlorpromazine for five months without any undesirable side effects appearing. The other patient developed a transient Parkinsonian-like tremor of the right arm while taking 1000 mgm. daily and this subsided when the dosage was reduced to 800 mgm. daily which the patient took for four months without any undesirable side effects.

The clinical picture of patients on large doses of chlorpromazine resembles that observed in monkeys and cats following bilateral hypothalamic lesions. The patients are somnolent, exhibit some catalepsy, have masklike facies, an apparent polyuria, and slowness of associated movements. These symptoms abate when the dosage of the drug is reduced or the drug discontinued.

One undesirable effect of large doses of Chlorpromazine is the possible production of a depression. Fortunately, this depressive reaction is usually not serious. It abates when the drug is discontinued or the dosage reduced. When the depression persists EST promptly relieves it.

Large doses of chlorpromazine are no more effective than the usual dosage range of 200 mgm. to 300 mgm. daily, except in the occasional patient. To administer large doses with the hope of increasing the therapeutic effectiveness has been futile.

In two cases of Parkinsonism, one postencephalitic, the other arteriosclerotic in origin, chlorpromazine was of no benefit and it did not make the Parkinsonian worse.

Large doses of chlorpromazine should be administered only to hospitalized patients under close medical, psychiatric and nursing supervision.

PSYCHIATRIC EXPERIENCE WITH CHLORPROMAZINE

Willis H. Bower, M.D., Mark D. Altschule, M.D., and Leonard Cook, Ph.D.

Chlorpromazine, 10-(3-dimethylaminopropyl)-2-Chlorphenothiazine, is a new central nervous system depressant which has been used in various conditions including manic depressive psychoses, certain schizophrenias especially if acute and with excitement or confusion, symptoms of drug withdrawal, some psychosomatic illnesses and various conditions with vomiting. Its effects include the following; it alters conditioned reflexes in rats, it depresses the emetic mechanism, and it lowers body temperature.

Oddly enough it was not laboratory observation that attracted the psychiatrists' attention to chlorpromazine, but the findings of Laborit, a French surgeon who used chlorpromazine and other drugs in combination with surface cooling of the body to produce artificial hibernation. Laborit suggested that this resting state, mediated by depression of certain diencephalic regions, stabilized the autonomic nervous system and decreased susceptibility to stress occurring in surgery, in certain infectious states, in cranial injuries, and in psychic trauma. His results in hopeless surgical cases seemed to support his concept. Hamon, Paraire and Velluz, colleagues of Laborit, later successfully used this technic to treat manic patients. Their results were confirmed by Delay, Deniker and Harl who subsequently found that chlorpormazine alone proved useful in managing states of excitement, agitation and confusion. These findings heralded the promising aspects of this new drug in psychiatry.

Results of studies with chlorpromazine on a developed conditioned reflex in rats, as well as results in psychiatric conditions in man are presented here. By linking the laboratory data with the clinical data we do not imply that the developed conditioned reflex in animals is analogous to the conflict-laden conditioning in man which so often leads to neuroses and psychoses. Nevertheless, it seems that certain basic elements are similar.

Animal Studies

Method for Developing the Conditioned Reflex:

Rats learned to avoid an electric shock stimulus—given simultaneously with an auditory stimulus (ringing of a bell)—by jumping on to a wooden pole suspended from the top of the test-box. After repeated trials, the rats responded to the sounding of the bell *alone* in the same way that they did to the electric shock. Thus, a new reflex, a conditioned reflex (response to the bell), was established.

Test Procedure

A colony of rats in which a conditioned reflex had been developed was selected for the test. One group of 12 animals was injected with chlorpromazine (10 mg. per Kg., subcutaneously), while another group was injected with saline. The chlorpromazine-treated animals responded to the unconditioned reflex (shock) but *not* to the conditioned reflex (bell), whereas the control animals responded to *both* the bell and the shock. A third group of 12 animals were treated with phenobarbital and similarly tested. When given phenobarbital in doses sufficient to inhibit the conditioned reflex (100 mg. per Kg., orally), the animals could not respond to the unconditioned reflex (shock). Figure 1 compares the results with chlorpormazine and with phenobarbital in blocking the conditioned reflex.

Clinical Experience

Experience with chlorpromazine indicates that it is an agent capable of strongly influencing the course of some psychiatric illnesses. Present evidence suggests that its greatest use in psychiatric illness is in patients with acute symptoms of increased psychomotor activity, regardless of whether the diagnosis is manic psychosis or acute schizophrenia. Good results have been reported by others in its use in anxiety states, phobias, and some other psychoneuroses. It is often useful in the control of agitation and excitement of chronic schizophrenia, but in such cases induces calm without significant change in the mental content. In agitated senile and arteriosclerotic patients it is frequently helpful in calming of overactivity, decrease in destructive behavior, and increase of ability to sleep.

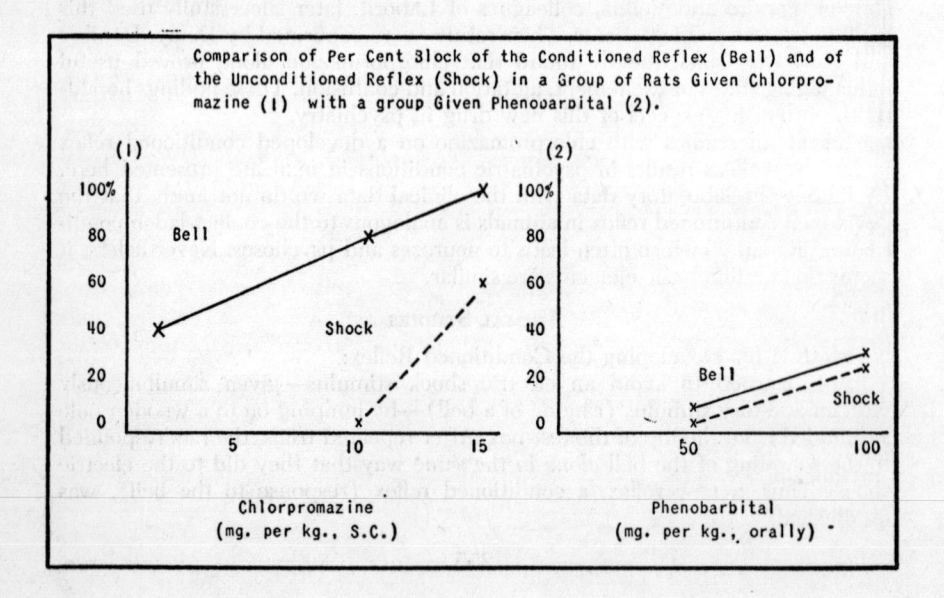

Comparison of Per Cent Block of the Conditioned Reflex (Bell) and of the Unconditioned Reflex (Shock) in a Group of Rats Given Chlorpromazine (1) with a group Given Phenobarbital (2).

Duration of Action

The per cent blockade observed at varying intervals after the administration of chlorpromazine, 10 mg. per kg., subcutaneously, was as follows:

Time	% Blockade	Time	% Blockade
½ hours	25	3 hours	75
1	45	4	50
2	78	24	40
2¼	84	48	0

Fig. 1

In the treatment of acute psychoses with increased psychomotor activity chlorpromazine seems to compare favorably with electric shock as a therapeutic agent and seems to have certain advantages. It is comparatively free from the phenomenon of sudden relapse after improvement. It is also comparatively free from troublesome complications and can be used in patients in whom physical illness precludes the use of electric shock therapy. There is no memory loss nor sudden change in mental content, which is often advantageous when concurrent psychotherapy is being given. Rapid recovery with the use of chlorpromazine following failure of recovery with the use of adequate electric shock in a few cases has suggested that there may be some beneficial interrelationship between the two treatments. A few cases have been treated with concurrent chlorpromazine in low dosage and electric shock with favorable results.

Depression appears not to be helped and often to be made worse by chlorpromazine. When elements of anxiety, agitation, and depression are all prominent, the drug should be used with caution to determine the overall effect. One should be wary that depression may be increased, although anxiety and agitation may be ameliorated.

The treatment schedules outlined here pertain to the use of the drug in hospitalized patients. If chlorpromazine is used in outpatients, oral administration should be used, starting with fairly low dosages, perhaps 25 mg. two times a day. Precautions should be taken lest the patient be taken unaware of the onset of drowsiness while driving, or exposed to hazardous situations. Frequent observation by the physician should take place to guard against any complications going unnoticed.

Typical Patient Response

During the first few days of treatment patients may sleep a good deal or may be drowsy, with slurred speech and drooping of eyelids. If patients sleep, they can easily be awakened. After a few days, the drowsiness usually wears off. Patients then exhibit normal motor activity and show no loss of responsiveness. Destructive and uncooperative patients become manageable, much to the relief of the nursing staff. In addition, sleeping and feeding problems are often largely eliminated, and many intractable patients often become amenable to psychotherapy.

The following case histories indicate some typical results.

Excited Paranoid Schizophrenic

M. N., 27-year-old single woman. Marked neurotic traits in childhood. She showed good imagination but had obsessive rituals and tendencies to be withdrawn. Good student. At age 18 entered college then stopped without completing year. Became depressed and fearful of cancer and death. Thereafter there was a long period of increasing hostility to mother and increasing withdrawal. At age 25 patient thought others were talking about her and had other fantasies. She became insolent and abusive to those about her. She finally became hallucinated, and was hospitalized March 26, 1953. Found to be argumentative, unsociable, disdainful of those she considered inferior to her, and preoccupied with significances of her fantasies and ideas. She became demanding, unreasonable and not amenable to explanation. She was occasionally violent and threatening, biting attendants and having fantasies of killing. She was treated with some electric shock and ambulatory insulin with poor results. None of these treatments were given in three months before treatment with chlorpromazine. Chlorpromazine 50 mg. I.M. t.i.d. started September 24, 1953. No drowsiness but improvement was noted within three days. Dose was reduced to 25 mg. I.M. t.i.d. October 22, then oral dosages 50 mg. q.i.d. starting November 19. Dosage was continued with gradual reductions until finally stopped January 1954. Produced better sociability, relaxation, ability to participate in hospital activities in spite of lack of essential change in quality of thinking. Irritability and unreasonable behavior recurred at time of cessation of chlorpromazine.

Manic-Depressive, Manic

J. T., a 47-year-old single woman, achieved satisfactory education with specialized training as nursery and kindergarten school teacher. Said to be a "born teacher," happy, liked by students, active and restless. Held teaching positions in various places: Japan, England, etc., as well as U. S. During summer of 1952 it was noticed she was very talkative, attracted attention unduly in public, and was extravagant. Thereafter unstable moods of depressive and hypomanic varieties. She was sometimes threatening, sometimes talked of suicide. Acutely disturbed behavior started May 5, 1953. Hospitalized May 10, 1953, and found to be denudative, loud, incoherent, sleepless, constantly pacing and thrashing about. A total of 48 electric shocks given between May 15 and September 28, 1953, with relapse within five days each time if discontinued. There were several relapses with markedly disturbed behavior necessitating return to disturbed ward. Chlorpromazine 50 Gm. I.M. t.i.d. was started October 2, 1953. The patient was quieter by October 7 but still incoherent and slightly drowsy. She started sleeping well, became co-operative and rational in speech by October 9. Discontinued drug temporarily October 13 because of indurations at site of injections. Resumed treatment October 16. Between October 16 and October 19, 1953, she was given chlorpromazine

25 mg. Improvement continued until discharge.

Arteriosclerotic Psychosis

73-year-old woman. Five years prior to admission, she probably suddenly fell and thereafter showed a vagueness and increasing loss of memory. Hospitalized October 23, 1953. Physical findings not remarkable except for generalized arteriosclerosis and enlarged heart. She was talkative, restless, incoherent, and feeble. Chlorpromazine 50 mg. P.O. q.i.d. started March 22, 1954, and stopped March 31, 1954. At that time a geriatric mixture was started with nicotinic acid and metrazol. On April 3, while on this latter mixture, she experienced a convulsion. Geriatric mixture was stopped and chlorpromazine 25 mg. q.i.d. was resumed. During both periods of administration of chlorpromazine, she was somewhat quieter and slept better.

Table I summarizes our results in 30 psychotic patients. It shows that better results can be obtained in the treatment of severely agitated or hyperactive patients than in non-excited, quiet patients.

TABLE I

	MANIC PSYCHOSIS AND SCHIZO-AFFECTIVE PSYCHOSIS WITH MANIC FEATURES	EXCITED SCHIZO-PHRENICS (EXCLUSIVE OF SCHIZO-AFFECTIVE PSYCHOSIS)	MISCELLANEOUS (INCLUDING DEPRESSIONS AND NON-EXCITED SCHIZO-PHRENICS)	SENILES
Good	6	0	1	0
Fair	3	3	1	3
Poor	2	3	8	0
Total	11	6	10	3

TREATMENT SCHEDULES FOR EXCITED PATIENTS

A. *Typical Treatment Schedule*

(1) Start with 50 mg., intramuscularly, every eight hours.
(2) After ten days change to 50 mg., orally, every eight hours.
(3) After five more days reduce to 25 mg., orally, every eight hours.
(4) After three more days, stop.

B. *Variations in Schedule*

(1) Increase to 75 mg., intramuscularly, every eight hours after three days of the initial dosage if excitement persists. When improvement comes, reduce to 50 mg., intramuscularly, every eight hours.
(2) Continue intramuscular dosages, or higher oral dosages, longer than indicated in A if improvement is slow, or if patient begins to relapse with reduction in dosage.

C. *Indications for Withdrawing Drug Other Than Improvement*
- (1) Allergic rash (rare).
- (2) Icterus (rare).
- (3) Development of marked depression.
- (4) Failure to improve after two weeks of therapy.

TREATMENT SCHEDULE FOR AGITATED SENILE PSYCHOTIC PATIENTS
- (1) Start with 25 mg., orally, every 12 hours or 10 mg., orally, every eight hours.
- (2) If necessary, increase gradually to 25 mg., orally, every six hours and then to 50 mg., orally, every six hours.
- (3) Decrease dosage if patient becomes lethargic, drowsy, or depressed. If this happens with small doses, withdraw the drug.
- (4) Withdraw the drug if marked hypotension or hypothermia develop.
- (5) When withdrawing the drug, reduce dosage gradually to prevent possible occurrence of convulsions.

MODE OF INJECTION AND SPECIAL MEASURES
- (1) Dilute chlorpromazine, as withdrawn from the vial, with a diluent consisting of physiologic saline solution containing 1 per cent procaine in the proportion of four drops of the procaine solution to 10 cc. of saline.
- (2) Inject deep in upper outer quadrant of buttock, taking two or three minutes for the injection.
- (3) Massage site of injection for four minutes.
- (4) Keep patient in bed during first few days of I.M. therapy if possible. Orthostatic hypotension may ensue in first three or four days and will increase drowsiness if patient is up and around.
- (5) Moderate drowsiness, with slurred speech and drooping of eyelids often occurs on the second day. It is usually transient. If persistent or severe, dose of chlorpromazine should be decreased.
- (6) Pulse, temperature and blood pressure should be taken at least twice daily as long as the drug is given in any form. Transient hypothermia or hypotension occasionally occur late in the course of treatment.
- (7) Observe patient for rash (particularly if there is a previous history of allergy) and for jaundice, which is rare. If either occurs, they subside quickly when the drug is withdrawn. There has been no evidence of impaired liver function in any of the patients in this series.

EFFECTS OF CHLORPROMAZINE IN PSYCHIATRIC DISORDERS

Irvin M. Cohen, M.D.
University of Texas Medical Branch, Galveston, Texas

SINCE becoming commercially available in the United States in May, 1954, chlorpromazine (Thorazine, S.K.F.) has rapidly achieved widespread usage to a degree seldom accorded a new drug. A rapidly accumulating literature, particularly from Europe where the drug was first introduced, contains reports of its employment in almost every field of clinical medicine. Nevertheless, its ultimate place in therapeutics remains to be determined.

Investigation of the possibilities of chlorpromazine in the treatment of psychiatric illness was begun at the University of Texas Medical Branch in March, 1954. Appraisal of any substance in regard to effects on psychic functions always presents certain difficulties because of the fluidity of diagnostic criteria in psychiatry and the impossibility of accurately quantifying results. In the case of chlorpromazine these factors have been complicated by what appears to be an unusually broad spectrum of application, wide variability of response, and often incomprehensible effects. The range of results has in fact been so wide as to indicate that exceptionally prolonged study will be required before definitive conclusions concerning its efficacy can be reached. This paper is therefore intended as a report of relatively early clinical observations and impressions of the utility of chlorpromazine in the management and treatment of psychiatric disorders, rather than as a detailed statistical analysis of data.

PHARMACOLOGY

Chlorpromazine was first synthesized in France in 1950, during the course of a laboratory investigation of the antihistaminic drugs. It had been found that certain of the phenothiazine derivatives, notably Phenergan, exhibited not only antihistaminic action but hypnotic and anelgesic effects as well and were thus capable of potentiating anesthetics. However, their capacities to do so were too weak to be clinically significant, and a search was made for a compound with greater activity in these directions. Chlorpromazine, a chlorinated phenothiazine derivative like Phenergan but with little antihistaminic action of its own, was found to possess not only the desired properties but also powerful muscular relaxing, hypothermic, and antiemetic activities. Though originally introduced as an adjunct in anesthesia and surgery, its usefulness in psychiatry was quickly recognized. Early clinical trials in the United States began in the latter part of 1952, and on May 15, 1954, it was made available commercially.

The sites of its physiological action are still ill-defined. Clinically the manifestations are referable to all three divisions of the nervous system: central, autonomic, and peripheral, but there is strongly suggestive evidence that the primary effect may be in the diencephalic area. Though the drug produces sleep, it does not seem to do so through depression of the cortex as in barbiturate narcosis. This feature is clinically significant, in that the patient in chlorpromazine sleep can easily be awakened and responds in relevant and coherent fashion, in contrast to the hypnosis of barbiturates where the patient is cloudy, befogged, and even disoriented as a result of cortical depression. In relation to the autonomic nervous system it acts as a ganglioplegic and adrenolytic agent, so that both sympatholytic and parasympatholytic effects, principally the former, are noted. Peripherally it produces a profound muscular relaxation.

Its mode of action is a subject of great speculation. From a strictly psychological perspective one may reason that improvement in the psychological state takes place through some unique method of attack on anxiety as the common denominator of psychiatric illness. It has also been suggested that the drug interrupts conditioned psychological responses in the same manner by which it interrupts conditioned reflex responses. A third explanation may be that psychological illness is in reality based on some yet unknown physiogenic brain dysfunction salutarily affected by the drug.

Material. Experiences reported in this study cover a period of 9 months, and have been drawn from a series of approximately 1000 cases. Case material included patients hospitalized on the Psychiatric Services of the John Sealy Hospital and at St. Mary's Infirmary, and outpatients of the Neurology and Psychiatry Clinic of the John Sealy Hospital. All were being treated for psychiatric illnesses of various types. Although other methods of therapy were often used in conjunction with chlorpromazine, the observations described are those which are regarded as peculiar to the drug.

Clinical Applications

1. NAUSEA AND VOMITING. With rare exceptions, psychogenic nausea and vomiting have responded favorably to the administration of chlorpromazine. It was also effective in cases of nausea and vomiting due to physical disease coexisting with psychiatric symptomatology. Specifically, these have included cases of carcinomatosis, pregnancy, acute alcoholic gastritis, and dumping syndrome. In one case of dumping syndrome following sub-total gastric resection, emptying time on roentgenographic examination was found to have returned to within normal limits during treatment with chlorpromazine. It was also found to be useful in relieving nausea and vomiting occasionally accompanying insulin shock therapy and electro-convulsive therapy.

The doses required were consistently small, usually but 25 to 50 mg., three to four times per day, administered orally or intramuscularly as the case required.

2. FUNCTIONAL PSYCHIATRIC DISORDERS. The results of chlorpromazine in the treatments of the so-called functional psychiatric disorders have been highly variable and very individualized, there being little uniformity in degree or quality of therapeutic response. Patients with identical diagnostic labels and

nearly identical symptom pictures have not necessarily derived identical results. Consequently, we have as yet been unable to establish any specific nosological indications for the use of this drug. Improvement apparently did not depend on diagnosis, but rather on the presence or absence of certain clinical features in the illness. Thus we have found the best results occurring in those cases in which the most prominent manifestations have been (1) agitation, (2) anxiety, or (3) aggression. It is probably safe to say at the present level of our knowledge of the mode of action of this drug that it is principally of use in symptomatic control. However, in some cases in which dramatic results have occurred, one almost suspects that there may be some actual curative effect, the nature of which is still unknown.

Agitation. It is in the reduction and control of agitation that chlorpromazine has proved most useful. The term agitation is used here in the connotation of an increase in motor activity, ranging from moderate motor restlessness to violent excitement. Hyperactivity of this sort is most commonly seen in psychotic patients and consequently usually presents some problem in management. Prevention of exhaustion and maintenance of nutrition under such circumstances are often difficult, so that intravenous sedation and tube feedings may be required, procedures which themselves are not without hazard. In such situations chlorpromazine has proved to be of singular value. Its capacity to convert highly disturbed behavior into docile tractability has remained an impressive phenomenon. Typically, approximately 30 to 40 minutes after intramuscular injection of 50 to 100 mg. of chlorpromazine, the disturbed patient is noted to lie down and fall asleep. The facies is sallow and pale, respiration is slow and deep, blood pressure is reduced, and pulse rate is increased. Despite the depth of sleep, the patient may be awakened easily; if the patient cannot be awakened another factor other than chlorpromazine is present. The patient responds to questions in brief but adequate manner and passively follows commands, quickly falling asleep when left alone. Control of behavior has been maintained with repeated injections. However, in the case of highly disturbed patients, out of caution we have generally not depended on chlorpromazine alone, but have subsequently instituted electroshock therapy because of the proven efficacy of this method. Agitation has been relieved in less disturbed patients without the necessity of combining it with electroshock treatment. This approach has been most frequently indicated in those patients having severe myocardial damage or similar contraindications to electroshock treatment. The diagnostic categories showing disturbed behavior in which chlorpromazine has been applied with success include paranoid and catatonic schizophrenia, agitated depression, and the manic phase of the manic-depressive psychosis.

Anxiety. Patients who complained of "nervousness," tension, vague feelings of unrest, and similar indicators of the presence of freely floating anxiety generally responded well to chlorpromazine. In contrast, patients who displayed little anxiety, or who were withdrawn, derived little benefit. Results were also poor if the anxiety was fixated to an organ or situation, or if there was secondary gain from symptoms in the form of familial sympathy or over-indulgence. Thus it has been of value in the anxiety states, panic reactions, acute obsessional neuroses, and some cases of schizophrenia. Results were ordinarily disappointing in hysteria, the usual depressions, hypochondriasis, obsessive-compulsive and phobic neuroses, and chronic (simple) schizophrenia. In successful cases a type of relaxation and calmness was induced which apparently differs from that produced by narcotics and barbiturates. Whereas in the latter there is temporary replacement or alteration of reality with some degree of clouding of the sensorium, chlorpromazine reduced the level of emotional tension with little loss of efficiency. In addition, by virtue of its complex pharmacodynamic effects, there was diminution of many distressing autonomic symptoms. Purely as a sedative it functioned efficiently in 50% to 60% of cases in which anxiety was marked. Complete remission of symptoms has occurred in about 10% to 15% of neurotic patients treated with the drug alone.

Aggression. In a significant number of cases, chlorpromazine has been noted to exert a curious specificity against thoughts and actions of an aggressive quality. It should be noted that ideation and behavior of this character are nonspecific, and may appear in any category of psychiatric illness. The mode of expression, however, assumes many forms. Thus, hostility may be manifested as excessive irritability in any hysteric, or in persecutory delusions of the paranoid schizophrenic. It may more directly reflect the particular underlying conflict, as in the example of the inhibited man plagued by feelings of inadequacy who becomes an expansive, bellicose manic. This aspect of the drug's action has been most evident in the resolution of hypomanic and manic phases of the manic-depressive psychoses, and particularly in some cases of paranoid schizophrenia. In the latter we have seen remarkable instances of complete remission of symptoms, disappearance of paranoid delusions, and production of insight into the nature of the illness. The following examples may be cited. One patient, who in the past had remitted on a program of combined electroshock and deep insulin therapy but had relapsed, remitted once again on chlorpromazine alone. Another patient, who had not responded to electroshock therapy, deep insulin coma therapy, or lobotomy, completely remitted on the drug alone. Large doses were a consistent requirement in all such cases. The action of chlorpromazine in the management of states of anxiety and agitation can perhaps be easily understood on the basis of its sedative properties, but its ability to attack this class of symptoms is difficult to comprehend.

3. ORGANIC PSYCHIATRIC DISORDERS. Our experience in the use of this drug in organic psychiatric states has been limited to the treatment of post-alcoholic delirium tremens, agitated senile-arteriosclerotic psychoses, postencephalitic psychoses, and post-traumatic personality disorders.

Its use in delirium tremens has been very encouraging, there being strong indication that the duration of delirium is materially reduced when the drug is used. In each case the drug was used in conjunction with the usual routine of fluid-glucose-electrolyte replacement, diet, therapeutic vitamin regimens, and anticonvulsant drugs. The necessity for administering barbiturates and paraldehyde has almost been eliminated, thus obviating the possibility of replacing alcoholism with habituation to these sedatives.

Very satisfactory results were obtained in the management of senile and arteriosclerotic patients manifesting protracted agitation or periodic excitement. Sedation of the aged patient often poses a difficult problem. Barbiturates occasionally aggravate excitement, effects may be unsustained, or such large amounts are required that their use is accompanied by risk of respiratory depression. In the aged patient only small amounts of chlorpromazine have been required to produce a tranquilizing effect. Reduction in hyperactivity was unfortunately the only improvement obtained in these cases, the mental status remaining otherwise unchanged except where malnutrition as a result of refusal to eat was a factor.

One case of postencephalitic psychosis has been treated, the only benefit being in the sphere of control of behavior. In 3 cases where personality disorders followed head injury, irritability was moderately reduced.

Dosage

To date we have been unable to establish any standard dosage requirement for the treatment of any particular psychiatric illness. Therapeutically effective dosage has proved to be an individualized quantity, to be determined entirely on the basis of clinical response. Thus, the principle of increasing the dosage to the level of therapeutic effectiveness or appearance of toxic signs has been found to be the most reliable guide during administration. Dosage level and severity of illness apparently bear no interrelationship. A highly disturbed patient suffering from delirium tremens might require but 50 mg. four times a day, given intramuscularly, whereas an anxious neurotic might require 800 mg. per day for control of symptoms. Furthermore, following the establishment of a therapeutically effective dosage level, either tolerance or diminished requirement may develop, so that elevation or decrease of dosage may be required during the course of therapy.

In our series it was found that larger dosages were required than those described in previous reports. We believe that many failures with chlorpromazine can be attributed to the fact that insufficient dosage had been used. We have found clinically effective levels to lie more frequently in the range of 200 to 800 mg. daily than within the previously recommended range of 50 to 200 mg. daily. In general, the dosage required for improvement of neurotic disorders has been approximately 200 to 600 mg. daily, whereas psychotics have usually required at least 400 to 800 mg. daily. Improvement usually occurred within the first 2 to 3 weeks after treatment had begun; in some cases improvement was obtained later when the dose had been elevated to a higher and hence therapeutically effective level. To date the maximum dosage which we have administered has been 2250 mg. daily. Other investigators have reported giving as high as 3400 mg. daily without appearance of toxic signs.

Rapid effect can be obtained by intramuscular administration; however, repeated injections have been accompanied by the development of marked soreness and tenderness of the site of administration. Our custom in the treatment of highly disturbed patients or in patients in whom rapid effect was desirable has been to administer 50 mg. intramuscularly every 4 to 6 hours. If this dose was found to be inadequate for control of symptoms subsequent doses might be increased to 100 mg. each. If satisfactory response was obtained in 24 to 72 hours by this route, oral medication was partially or totally substituted. Oral dose was increased thereafter each day as indicated. In cases where extremely rapid control of symptoms was not necessary, as was true in most neurotics and psychotics, the oral route was used exclusively. Hospitalized patients were begun on 50 mg. every 6 hours, the dose being increased each day or every other day. In non-hospitalized patients, in an effort to ascertain the intensity of side-effects which might develop, the initial dose has been 25 to 50 mg., one to four times per day, increasing in increments of equal quantity to the desired therapeutic level.

At times it has become necessary to administer barbiturates to patients receiving chlorpromazine. It has been found in such cases that barbiturates in the usually recommended oral doses can be given with safety, notwithstanding the reported potentiating action of chlorpromazine.

The question of how long treatment should be continued has remained unsettled. In general, psychotics and severe neurotics have been placed on maintenance doses, whereas treatment of most neurotics has generally been discontinued simultaneous with symptomatic relief.

Side-Effects

The side-effects of chlorpromazine are numerous and varied, and have appeared in one degree or another in almost every patient to whom the drug has been administered. Although temporarily distressing to the patient, they have not necessitated discontinuation of treatment unless extremely severe. Most appeared early and were independent of the dosage level. However, side-effects of a different character developed 2 or 3 weks after treatment had begun in approximately 10% to 15% of the patients. In contrast to the early side-effects which were of temporary duration, the later side-effects tended to be persistent and could more nearly be correlated with the increasing dosage.

The most common subjective complaints noted during the early phases of treatment included dizziness related to postural changes, profound and often annoying weakness, lethargy, dryness of the mouth, and nasal congestion. Less common but not infrequent were a burning sensation in the esophagus, nausea and vomiting, and constipation. Objectively the most impressive finding was fall in blood pressure. This occurred most dramatically following parenteral administration. Usually within 30 to 40 minutes after injection readings would drop 30 to 50 mm. systolic and 20 to 30 mm. diastolic, associated with compensatory tachycardia. Despite this precipitous fall, there was no case of circulatory collapse in any of our patients. Hypotension also developed during oral administration, but was more commonly of an orthostatic type. Lowered blood pressure was quite temporary with rapid return to former levels as treatment progressed. Syncopal attacks were rare and occurred only in cerebral arteriosclerotic psychotics, who were naturally more sensitive to momentary cerebral vascular hypotension. Hypersomnolence occurred at all levels, but usually began when oral doses of greater than 200 mg. daily were given. Generally there was no interference with nocturnal sleep, even though diurnal sleep might have been as much as 10 hours. Although sedation of this type was useful in disturbed patients, it often distressed otherwise ambulatory patients. In the latter case small doses of sympathomimetic drugs were sufficient to counteract it. Other early findings included facial pallor, hypothermia or hyperthermia, and slowing of movement.

Late effects included excessive appetite, blurring of vision, intense pruritus, photosensitization, rest tremor, and increased sexual urge. Quite often a sudden spike of fever, not associated with evidence of infection or leukocytosis, took place. Swelling of the breasts and secretion of a colostrum-like fluid from the nipples were occasionally noted in female patients.

Complications

Of greater concern were certain side-reactions which we arbitrarily classed as complications, mainly on the basis of their potentially serious quality. However, with the possible exception of a single case, recovery has been spontaneous and rapid. No deaths directly attributable to the drug occurred in this series.

The most frequent complication was dermatitis, which occurred in about 10% of cases. Though occasionally preceded by intense itching, unresponsive to antihistamines, it usually appeared suddenly about 2 to 3 weeks after treatment had been started and was unrelated to dosage level. Most commonly it was in the form of a maculopapular rash confined to the sides of the neck and upper chest. Spread to the trunk and extremities occurred in about one-third of these cases. Somewhat less frequently it occurred as an erythema multiforme, at times associated with either swelling of the face or generalized edema. Generalized urticaria was noted occasionally. With the exception of those cases in which there was an accompanying edema, the dermatitis usually cleared in about 3 to 4 days despite an often florid appearance. In no case was it necessary to resort to steroids. Chlorpromazine was discontinued only when the eruption was generalized or when there was intense subjective distress. In most of these cases it was subsequently reinstituted with no recurrence of the dermatitis in any case. One patient who had become photosensitive developed a maculopapular rash on exposure to sunlight, which subsided within 2 hours after return indoors.

Jaundice occurred in 6 patients (less than 1%) in this series. Results of laboratory studies in these instances consistently indicated an obstructive process within the biliary system, and no evidence of cellular damage. In the majority of cases icterus appeared approximately 3 weeks after chlorpromazine had been instituted and was not related to dose. Usually the patient complained of mild general malaise, persistent or intermittent nausea, occasional vomiting, and vague abdominal pain. The succeeding clinical course in each case was uneventful, disturbing symptoms disappearing within several days, icterus clearing within 2 to 3 weeks. Treatment was of a supportive nature, consisting mainly of withdrawal of the drug, intravenous glucose when indicated, therapeutic vitamin regimen, and high-carbohydrate, high-protein, low-fat diet. In one case the drug was reinstituted without recurrence of the jaundice. Cohen and Archer reported that prolonged administration of chlorpromazine was not accompanied by hepatotoxic effects, and have concluded that the appearance of jaundice is a random effect, in all probability based on an allergic reaction to the drug.

A most interesting and perhaps significant complication has been the occasional development of Parkinsonism with typical masking of the facies, stooped posture, loss of associated movements, rigidity, and tremor. Rigidity has been more prominent than tremor. These cases have appeared in any age group, usually when dosages exceeding 400 mg. daily were given. The syndrome has cleared in 5 to 14 days following withdrawal of the drug. However, in one patient the syndrome persisted until his death from uremia some 4 months later.

Other complications noted have been dependent edema, one instance of nonfatal anaphylactoid reaction, and 2 deaths due to pneumonia. The latter may be regarded as an indirect but preventable complication; both were elderly patients who in all probability suffered pulmonary hypostasis as a consequence of chlorpromazine-induced hypersomnolence.

Fatal agranulocytosis has recently been reported by Boleman. Rare instances of leukopenia and eosinophilia have been encountered in this series, but agranulocytosis has not occurred.

Summary

Variability in clinical response and wide range of effects have made evaluation of chlorpromazine as a therapeutic agent in psychiatry difficult. From a nosological standpoint, the spectrum of this drug has included psychiatric illnesses of all classifications. However, experience in 1000 cases of psychiatric disorders of both functional and organic etiology has indicated that it is most effective if there is evidence of (1) agitation, (2) anxiety, or (3) aggression, irrespective of the specific diagnostic entity in which the manifestation may appear. In approximately 60% of the cases in this series improvement was derived, which varied in degree from mere reduction in intensity of symptoms to apparently complete resolution of illness. Only with extended observation will it be possible to determine if the latter represents temporary remission or absolute recovery. The dosage that may be required is a highly variable quantity which must be individualized and determined strictly on the basis of clinical response. It is believed that many failures with chlorpromazine can be attributed to the fact that inadequate dosages are used. In this series effective dosage for neurotics has been in the range of 200 to 600 mg. daily, whereas psychotic patients have generally required 400 to 800 mg. daily. As much as 2250 mg. daily has been administered without toxic effects. Side-effects of one sort or another have occurred in almost every patient, but only rarely did treatment have to be discontinued because of them. Those which appeared very early were generally transient and unrelated to dosage level, while those appearing during the later phases of treatment when doses were higher tended to be persistent. Complications involving widely dissociated organ systems have been observed, but all have proved to be benign, despite often immediately alarming proportions. Fatal agranulocytosis has recently been reported but has not been observed in this series.

THORAZINE IN THE TREATMENT OF ACUTELY DISTURBED PSYCHOTIC PATIENTS

Gordon R. Forrer, M.D.
Clinical Director, Northville State Hospital, Northville, Michigan

There are presently well over thirty papers in the literature on the use of Thorazine in the treatment of various medical, surgical and psychiatric conditions. Chemically, the drug is related to the antihistamines, but its actions differ from antihistamine type drugs in a number of regards. Primarily, it is a central nervous system depressant and, secondarily, has a mild antispasmodic and adrenalytic activity. It potentiates hypnotics, sedatives, narcotics, anesthetics and alcohol. It appears to act at the cortical and subcortical levels in the cerebrum and on the diencephalon. Its sedative effect is thought to be the result of interruption of impulses passing between the diencephalon and the cerebral cortex. Animal studies indicate that some degree of tolerance to the drug develops, and our clinical impression in the use of Thorazine with patients supports this. It has a wide margin of safety for clinical use, although it has been reported that an obstructive type jaundice develops in 1 to 2 per cent of patients receiving it over a prolonged period of time.

D. Elks, writing in the *British Medical Journal* of September 4, 1954, studied the effects of Thorazine on chronically overactive psychotic patients. He used only 150 milligrams a day, except in a few patients who received 300 milligrams a day transitorily. Of his twenty-seven patients, nine showed an increase in weight from 11 to 34 pounds in twenty-two weeks. Seven of the patients were considered definitely improved, and eleven slightly improved. Improvement did not become apparent until after three or six weeks of continuous medication. The affective group appeared to respond slightly better than the schizophrenics. Patients became quieter, less tense, and less disturbed by their hallucinations and delusions, and more amenable to the suggestions and care of the nursing staff. Three patients of the twenty-seven were thought fit for parole, though none was considered fit for discharge. In none of the cases was the content of the psychosis changed. Schizophrenic patients continued to be subject to delusions and hallucinations, the affective swings of the hypomanic patients continued at intervals normal to each patient, and the chronically agitated melancholics did not themselves admit to any improvement in their mental state. He felt that the relief afforded by the chlorpromazine thus was principally symptomatic.

Garmany, May, and Folkson, writing in the Department of Psychiatry, Westminster Hospital, described the use and action of chlorpromazine in psychoneuroses. They had eighteen cases where tension was predominant and improvement occurred with medication. Results in patients with predominant obsessional symptomatology were poor. They could not confirm the findings of Sigwald and Bouttier concerning the relief given by chlorpromazine to patients with obsessional, depressive, or phobic symptoms. They did concur on the value of the drug in alleviating tension, both in its affective and muscular sense. They suggested that a combination of chlorpromazine, psychotherapy, and what they speak of as "relaxation treatment" appears to give the best results obtainable in the treatment of the tension state. Lancaster combined chlorpromazine and insulin in the treatment of eleven patients. They concluded that the drug caused apparent, but not significant, decrease in the total number of insulin induced anxiety symptoms, and altered the type of these symptoms. Palpitation and tachycardia were increased; perspiration, flushing, anxiety, restlessness, epigastric sensation, and tremor were diminished. Chlorpromazine did not influence the action of insulin on blood sugar levels. A combination of insulin and chlorpromazine was found to be useful in controlling refractory excited patients who were not controlled by either drug alone when administered in dosages of 50 milligrams three times a day. They felt the combination was useful in making more manageable patients who become excited during insulin coma treatment.

We should like to report here our experience with the use of Thorazine in varying dosages in thirty chronically disturbed psychotic patients. When the project was initiated, it was decided to administer the drug to patients who were disturbed, and who, because of this fact, were management problems on the ward. Initially, the dosages were rather low, being approximately 75 milligrams per day, but with the rapid gains in experience with the drug, our staff members began rapidly stepping up the drug dosage so that one patient received 500 milligrams per day, the bulk of them receiving between 100 and 200 milligrams per day. The drug is prepared for both intramuscular injection and as tablets. Many of the patients would take the drug by mouth, but in those instances when they would not, the drug was given by injection intramuscularly and the almost universal experience with these thirty patients was that after a few days, the patients would willingly take tablets and injection was no longer necessary. The drug was not given on the basis of diagnosis, but rather on the basis of clinical evidence of marked intrapsychic disturbance. It soon became apparent that low dosages were essentially ineffective in the management of patients who were markedly disturbed, and it was necessary to administer larger amounts. A rule of thumb was that a dose was sufficient to cause the desired result.

When the dosage was sufficient, there was usually improvement in the patient's personal appearance within a short period of time; in general, one week after effective dosage levels had been achieved. Where many had been untidy and incontinent and unkempt, they began to dress more neatly and show more attention to their personal appearance. Somewhat more striking was the change in their behavior. Patients who had been assaultive, destructive, and combative showed improvement in their behavior, becoming much quieter or only showing agitation. In general, the trend of the drug effect was to quiet the hyperactivity which was common to the majority of this series. So far as the patients' activities were concerned, the Thorazine seemed to have a desirable tranquilizing effect. It was found in those instances where patients could be helped to overcome their initial disturbance, and could be gotten to occupational or recreational therapy or work therapy, that they could continue the new activity even when the Thorazine was discontinued. It was likewise found that patients given Thorazine alone without any additional therapeutic measures frequently relapsed to their previous disturbed condition when the Thorazine was discontinued. It was as though Thorazine acted as a therapeutic lever enabling the physician to shift the patient into a more productive, more healthy activity. We found very little change in the mental trends of patients receiving the drug. They continued as previously, although they did not have the active force behind them that was noted before Thorazine was given. Paranoid delusions continued unabated, but tended to be less spontaneous and elicitable only on questioning. Two patients with obsessive-compulsive symptoms showed no change in this behavior. We found that there was some change in the affective area, with patients becoming less hostile, inappropriate or depressed when under the influence of Thorazine. It should be understood that this is quantitative rather than qualitative and that the essential psychopathological process was not in any way altered by the administration of the drug.

A certain amount of tolerance seemed to develop to the drug. For example, one patient who was gradually built up to a dosage level of 400 milligrams a day had the drug discontinued because the supply ran short. When the drug became available again in a few days, she was placed at the same dosage level and showed marked side effects with drowsiness and sleepiness. This seems to indicate that some tolerance develops as long as the patient is on the drug, but disappears in a short time. The small dosage level in the tablets made administration somewhat difficult, and taking the medication was referred to jokingly as, "It was like eating a handful of popcorn." A 100 milligram tablet is currently available which makes administration simpler.

The over-all impression of the effect of Thorazine on this group of thirty disturbed psychotic patients is as follows: no patients became worse, eight patients showed no improvement, seven patients showed slight improvement, eleven patients moderate improvement, and four patients marked improvement.

Side effects were noted in eight patients (somewhat less than one-third the total) a figure somewhat higher than that recorded in the literature. Five of the patients complained of drowsiness, with three of this group of five complaining of the additional symptoms of dizziness. These reactions did not seem to correspond with the dosage level which ranged in these particular individuals from 50 milligrams a day to 500 milligrams a day.

Of the remaining three who had side effects, these were somewhat more serious. One, at a dosage level of 200 milligrams a day, showed marked facial puffiness and a mild generalized macular rash with pruritus. This disappeared within seventy-two hours after the drug was discontinued. The second of these three patients initially showed nausea, vomiting, and syncope, and at the maximal level of 400 milligrams a day, experienced a pruritic, macular rash on the face and back and a slight generalized facial edema. This toxic effect disappeared within twenty-four hours after withdrawal of the drug. The third patient of these three experienced an intercurrent temperature elevation and complained of pain in the substernal notch. She was on a dosage level of 200 milligrams a day. In summarizing the side effects, then, approximately one-third of all patients had side effects and 10 per cent of all patients had side effects of serious to moderately serious degree. One patient, not included in this series, was given Thorazine in withdrawing her from dilaudid addiction. At a dosage level of 300 milligrams a day, the patient showed no withdrawal symptoms, and the drug apparently modified or prevented nausea and vomiting which is common with withdrawal and allayed her anxiety. There was some dizziness which she experienced and difficulty in focusing her eyes, a symptom not complained of by any other patient.

There seems to be little question but that Thorazine has a place in the armamentarium of the psychiatrist. However, it is not a magical drug which can be dispensed with the idea that the drug itself will cure the patient or insure his improvement. When combined with other measures, however, it seems to have real promise. In a number of patients, particularly the ones who showed marked improvement, the patients were able to engage in work at the hospital, go to occupational therapy, or take part in other activities which previously had been impossible for them because of their disturbed state. When the Thorazine was withdrawn, those patients who had made movement and progress in other areas remained improved, whereas those who had not moved in other therapeutic areas for the most part relapsed. Dosage level was very important in achieving good results. Our highest dosage level was 600 milligrams per day, but for the most part, patients benefited by approximately 300 milligrams per day.

From our rather limited experience with the drug, and from a review of the literature on its use, it would seem that Thorazine has a tranquilizing effect without altering the basic structure of the psychosis. It provides a valuable tool for the psychiatrist in assisting the disturbed psychotic patient to engage in more productive and healthful activity.

EFFECTS OF CHLORPROMAZINE ON CHRONIC LOBOTOMIZED SCHIZOPHRENIC PATIENTS

Harry Freeman, M.D., and Herbert S. Cline, M.D.

There have been numerous articles attesting to the therapeutic efficiency of chlorpromazine in psychoses. There has also been a notable dearth of controlled studies utilizing placebos to evaluate the role of the enthusiasm of the psychiatrist, the ward personnel, and the patients themselves. A search of the literature has noted only two, those of Gardner, Hawkins, Judah, and Murphree, and of Kovitz, Carter, and Addison, both dealing with chronic schizophrenic patients.

The present study is of the double-blind variety, in which the effects of chlorpromazine and placebos on two matched groups of chronic schizophrenic patients were noted. It was not intended, primarily, as a therapeutic investigation but was organized to determine the threshold dose of the drug which would produce an effect distinguishable from that obtained on administering placebos.

The technique used in evaluating the status of the patients was as follows: After an interview, a modification of the Malamud-Sands Rating Scale—15 items—was scored to determine the effects upon various phases of the clinical picture. This scale is shown in Table 1. The deviation from the normal in each item is rated on a six-point scale on either side of the base line and a total score obtained by the addition of the numbers for each item. The first seven items can be observed directly, and the next eight can be determined from the responses during the interview. In a general way, the gradations on the left represent those attitudes which are directed away from the subject, and those on the right indicate internally directed forms of behavior. The higher the score, the more abnormal is the clinical status of the subject. The chief value of the rating is that it represents an attempt to quantify changes in the various elements in the behavior of the patients over the period of the study.

The subjects of the investigation were chronically disturbed schizophrenic patients on whom lobotomies had been performed after failure of all previous therapies. There were 20 male patients, divided into two groups and matched primarily on the basis of means of the rating scores and secondarily on the basis of age, duration of hospitalization, and years since lobotomy. One group was given placebos and the other group chlorpromazine, but the identity of the medication was unknown to the psychiatrist doing the ratings (H. S. C.), the ward personnel, and the patients. The medication was given solely by mouth and twice daily, in individual envelopes, so that the identity and the

TABLE 1.—*Psychiatric Rating Scale*

Function	6	5	4	3	2	1	Base Line	1	2	3	4	5
Appearance	Bizarre		Decorative		Overmeticulous			Slovenly	Untidy			Smearing
Motor activity	Excited		Agitated		Restless			Underactive	Retarded			Stuporous
Mimetic expression	Incongruous		Dramatizing		Exaggerated			Stiff	Waxy flexibility			Mask-like
Responsivity	Anaclitic		Suggestive		Dependent			Stubborn	Resistive			Negativistic
Hostility reactions	Destructive		Combative		Belligerent			Self-depreciating	Self-mutilating			Suicidal
Socialization	Disruptive		Meddlesome		Outreaching			Shut-in	Isolated			Inaccessible
Attention	Uncontrolled		Markedly distractible		Moderately distractible			Preoccupied	Digressive			Completely withdrawn
Speech	Incessantly productive		Push-of-speech		Overtalkative			Undertalkative	Retarded	Blocking		Mute
Mood	Exhilarated		Euphoric		Enthusiastic			Somber	Despondent			Deeply depressed
Affect	Inappropriate		Explosive		Labile			Inadequate	Bland		Flat (rigid)	
Feeling	Panic	Anxious	Tense		Supersensitive			Phlegmatic	Dull		Apathetic	
Perception	Hallucinations		Illusions; pseudo-hallucinations		Exaggerated intensity			Self-observation	Hypochondriasis	Conversions		Somatic hallucinations
Thought processes	Fragmented		Alogical; paralogical		Illogical			Rationalizing		Obsessive hair-splitting	Obsessive doubt	
Subjective reorganization	Cosmic (omnipotence)	Delusions	Delusion of grandeur	Ideas of persistence	Ideas of inference	Ideas of reference		Ideas of inferiority	Self-accusatory	Somatic delusions	Nihilistic	
Insight	Negation of problem	Probably exogenous		Recognition of probability without concern	Shifting of blame			Self-hypercritical	Add. of nonexisting problems	Despairing self-blame	Attitude of complete helplessness	

dosage of the tablets was known only to one of us (H. F.). The placebos, of course, had an appearance identical with that of the drug.

RESULTS

The results of the study are shown in Figure 1. Here are depicted the mean scores for the placebo and chlorpromazine groups in successive weeks. The chlorpromazine was administered in a dosage noted at the bottom of the Figure, 200 mg. daily for the first four weeks, 400 mg. daily for the next two weeks, 600 mg. daily for the next two weeks, 800 mg. daily for the next three weeks, and then placebos for the next four weeks.

The mean scores show a sudden drop in the first week of treatment, then a variable degree of fluctuation over the next seven weeks, but no consistent change. It was for this reason that the dosage was varied. It was not until the

TABLE 2.—*Means and Ranges of Variables Used in Matching Patients in Placebo* and Chlorpromazine* Groups*

	Placebo Mean	Placebo Range	Chlorpromazine Mean	Chlorpromazine Range
Chronological age	36.3	23-49	38.4	30-57
Years in hospital	11.2	4-27	9.4	4-17
Years postlobotomy	7.5	1-16	8.2	1-13
Pretreatment rating score	31.4	19-38	34.0	27-48

* Ten patients each.

dosage had been increased to 800 mg. daily that the chlorpromazine group showed a decrease in its mean score. This was noted within a week and continued to drop irregularly in the next two weeks. It is evident, then, that for this group of patients the threshold dosage lay between 600-800 mg. daily. At the end of three weeks of medication at this level of dosage, the patients who were taking chlorpromazine were given placebos. For three weeks there was no essential change in the mean score, but during the fourth week the score rose again above the level noted preceding the 800 mg. dosage period. It is apparent that the "tranquilizing" effect of the drug lasts between three and four weeks after the medication is omitted.

There are several points of interest in this trend which may be described in more detail. Initially, the chlorpromazine group had a slightly, but not significantly, higher score than the placebo group. This was due primarily to the fact that the ratings for "motor activity," "appearance," "affect," and "subjective reorganization" (delusions) were higher. During the first week of the study the scores dropped in both groups, but in the chlorpromazine-treated patients there was a greater fall in these same items, so that the mean scores for the first week of medication were the same. The decrease in scoring may be pri-

Fig. 1

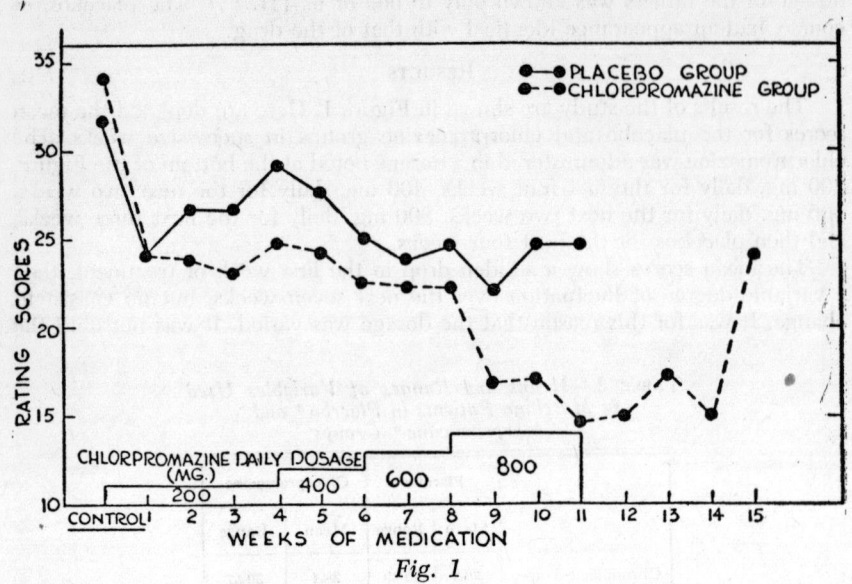

marily due to the enthusiastic hopefulness of both the psychiatric personnel and the patients at the onset of a new therapeutic study, so that the patient-doctor rapport was increased and the abnormal phenomena either seemed not so abnormal or were less obviously displayed. Certainly, the gross scores per subject showed a lessening in 9 of the 10 patients in each group, indicating a universality of operating factors.

Following the initial drop in scores there is a secondary rise which reaches its maximum in the fourth week of the study and which is more marked in the placebo-treated group. This increase was present in six of the nine patients in each group. The other patients in each group showed a decrease. The distribution of trends for each group was the same, but one of the chlorpromazine-treated patients (on a dosage of 200 mg. daily) showed such a marked decrease in scores as almost to offset the increases in the six.

The reason for the increase in scoring is obscure. The patients were living on three different wards, an equal number from each group on each ward. It would, therefore, be unlikely that some factor common to the hospital environment would affect patients on different wards. It is also difficult to presume that an endogenous variability would affect 12 out of the total group of patients simultaneously. It would seem more likely that the variable factor may be the judgment of the psychiatrist.

At any rate, the general level of scores for each group was essentially the same from the first to the eighth week of medication, so that we may conclude that the dosage of chlorpromazine up to this point was not sufficient to affect the group as a whole. At a dosage of 800 mg. of chlorpromazine, the values for the two groups differentiate.

TABLE 3.—*Sums of Scores in Placebo-Treated and Chlorpromazine-Treated Groups for the Three Weeks Before the 800 Mg. Daily Dosage Was Begun and Differences Between These Sums and Those Obtained During the Three Weeks at a Daily Dosage of 800 mg.*

	Placebo Group			Chlorpromazine Group	
Subject No.	Sum of Scores Before 800 Mg. Dosage	Difference in Sums of Scores Under 800 Mg. Dosage*	Subject No.	Sum of Scores Before 800 Mg. Dosage	Difference in Sums of Scores Under 800 Mg. Dosage*
1	83	−13	1	54	0
2	37	−13	2	87	0
3	58	−6	3	28	+8
4	107	−1	4	87	+18
5	43	0	5	59	+20
6	78	+2	6	18	+20
7	75	+8	7	88	+23
8	89	+8	8	73	+25
9	97	+19	9	70	+34
10	68	+21	10	76	+40
Median	76.5	1.0†		71.5	20.0†

* Plus signs indicate improvement in score.
† Difference between corresponding values for chlorpromazine and placebo groups is statistically significant. p = 0.02. Mann-Whitney U-test.

The data have been analyzed to determine the significance of the difference between the two trends. In order to include the variation observed previously and achieve a more reliable base line, for each subject the sum of the scores obtained during the three weeks before the 800 mg. daily dosage was introduced (weeks 6 to 8) was compared with the sum of the scores obtained during the three weeks on the 800 mg. daily dosage. The difference between the two sums was computed for each subject. The values are seen in Table 3. For the placebo-treated group the median value for the three pre-800-mg. weeks was 76.5; for the chlorpromazine-treated group, 71.0. There is no statistically significant difference between the two figures. The median difference[1] between these values and the sum of the scores obtained in the 800 mg. daily dose period was +1 for the placebo group and +20.0 for the chlorpromazine group. The differences between these values is statistically significant, the probability being 0.02. This difference between the two groups of patients is not affected by the initially higher values for the placebo-treated group because (*a*) there was no significant difference between the pre-800-mg. dose values in the two groups; (*b*) there was no relationship between the initial levels and the shift in values during the 800 mg. daily dose period. It should be noted at this point that this statistical technique is conservative, since it takes into account the trend before the medication has achieved its maximum effect at the end of the three-week period of medication at the 800 mg. dose.

As the medication, at what we consider an adequate dosage, was given for only a short period of time, a therapeutic judgment would not be very valid but

---
[1] Positive changes indicate improvement in the score.

is given for what it is worth. On the basis of the rating scale, in the placebo group, seven showed no improvement and three showed a mild degree of improvement. Of the chlorpromazine group, five showed a mild improvement and five showed a moderate degree of improvement, the latter referring purely to better hospital adjustment. One patient in each group was in seclusion throughout the whole study, and each showed a similar degree of mild improvement. In view of the similarity of numbers in each group showing a slight change, it should probably be considered that this level of improvement in drug-treated patients should be attributed to the altered environmental situation.

Four of the chlorpromazine-treated group showed an improvement in their scores before the 800 mg. daily dosage level was reached. Two had shown a mild improvement, one at the 400 mg. dosage level and one at the 600 mg. dosage level, with no further improvement at the larger dosage levels. Two had shown a moderate degree of improvement, one at 200 mg., with no further improvement, and one at 400 mg., with further improvement at the 800 mg. dose.

In order to determine what elements of the rating scale changed during

TABLE 4.—*Changes in Ratings for Individual Items in the Three Weeks Before the 800 Mg. Dosage of Chlorpromazine Was Begun as Compared with Changes for the Three Weeks During the 800 Mg. Daily Dosage, with Comparison of these Changes in the Two Groups*

Item	Chlorpromazine Change	P Value	Placebo Change	P Value	Chlorpromazine vs. Placebo, P Value
Appearance	10	....	8	....	....
Motor activity	−2	....	0	....	....
Mimetic expression	19*	0.05	2	....	0.10
Responsivity	22*	0.02	0	....	0.05†
Hostility reactions	17*	0.05	0	....	....
Socialization	18*	0.01	3	....	0.05†
Attention	13	....	2	....	....
Speech	10*	0.05-0.02	7	....	....
Mood	0	....	−3	....	....
Affect	4	....	−1	....	....
Feeling	10*	0.05-0.02	−2	....	0.07
Perception	13*	0.02	0	....	0.05†
Thought processes	28*	0.001	−2	....	0.05†
Subjective reorganization	10	....	−5	....	....
Insight	15	....	4	....	....

* Difference between sums of rating scores for individual items for three weeks before 800 mg. dose of chlorpromazine is instituted and those obtained during the three weeks at the 800 mg. dose is statistically significant by Wilcoxon's test for paired replicates.
† Difference between corresponding values in individual items for chlorpromazine- and placebo-treated groups is statistically significant by the Mann-Whitney U-test.

this period of maximum dosage, we have used the same technique as that for the individual total scores, namely, to add the scores for each item before the 800 mg. dosage was instituted and compare it with the ratings during the three weeks this dosage level was maintained. The results are shown in Table 4.

In the placebo-treated group, none of the changes were significantly different from one another, indicating a completely random variation. For the chlorpromazine-treated group, there were eight items that showed significant trends from their base line in the direction of improvement (positive changes)—mimetic expression, responsivity, hostility reactions, socialization, speech, feeling, perception, and thought processes. However, if the variation in the placebo group is taken into consideration, significant differences are found in only four—responsivity, socialization, perception, and thought processes. Again, it should be noted that this technique is conservative in that it takes into account the improvement before the maximum has been reached, thus diminishing the magnitude of the trends. At any rate, it is encouraging that in these chronic, lobotomized schizophrenic patients there is improvement not only in interpersonal relationships (as shown by the first two items) but also in the intrinsic psychotic processes in so far as this can be detected in the psychiatric interview.

As has been noted in Figure 1, once the medication has been omitted, there is a reversion to a previous score, or even above it, between the third and fourth weeks. The individual scores showed this "rebound" in all the subjects, although three of the five patients who had previously shown a moderate degree of improvement clinically maintained this level during the period in which the chlorpromazine was omitted. A study of the individual items shows this same trend. In Figure 2 is shown a comparison of the changes in the items while the patient was taking chlorpromazine (800 mg. daily dose) (week 8-week 11); with those after omission of the drug for four weeks (week 11-week 15). On the left is shown the decrease in values under this dosage; on the right, the increases after omission. It may be seen that, with the exception of "speech" and "attention," all the items on the right changed about as much as or more (in the opposite direction) than the ones on the left. The most striking reversals are seen for "subjective reorganization" (delusions), "affect," "perception" (hallucinations), "motor activity," and "hostility reactions." Thus, in both thinking processes and ward behavior the patient reverted to his previous behavioral characteristics, evidence of a merely suppressive effect of the drug.

So far as untoward effects were concerned, no serious ones were noted in this small group. Complete blood counts, taken every two weeks throughout the study, showed no consistent change. Three patients showed some degree of unsteadiness, one of whom exhibited a mask-like facies. These patients had shown only a slight improvement, while the five who were moderately improved showed no abnormal symptoms. Thus, there seemed to be no relationship between clinical improvement and drug toxicity. Withdrawal of the drug resulted in a prompt disappearance of such symptoms.

It was previously mentioned that in four patients improvement in the rating scale was evident at lower doses than 800 mg. The reason for this is unknown. There was no relationship between the threshold dosage and age, duration of

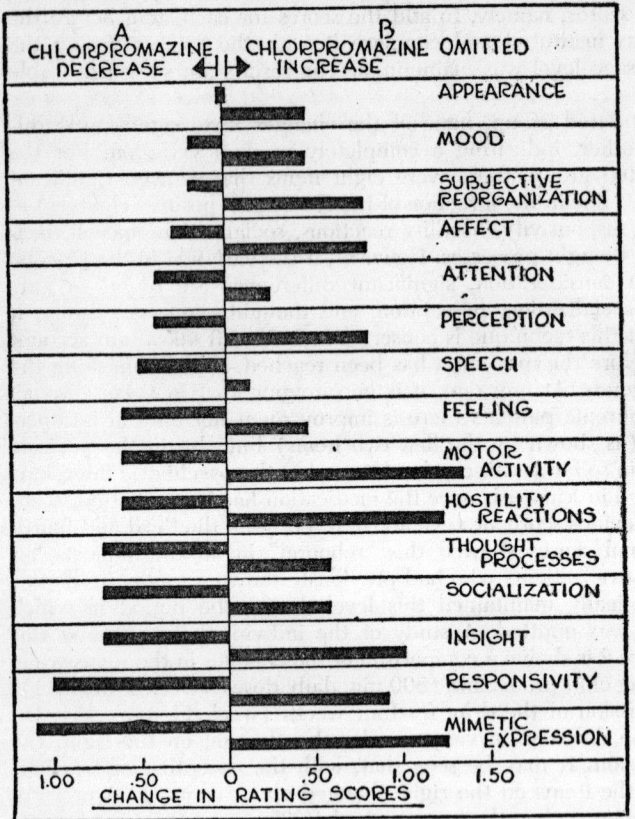

Fig. 2.—Changes in mean rating scores for each item: (A) during chlorpromazine therapy (800 mg. daily for three weeks), and (B) during omission of chlorpromazine for four weeks.

hospitalization, years since lobotomy, or the clinical status as evidenced by the rating score.

Comment

It is evident from the trend over the 11-week period that the administration of any substance, no matter how innocuous, coupled with the inevitable increased attention, results in some degree of improvement in behavior even in long-institutionalized schizophrenic patients. Such improvement is evident early and soon reaches a limit. A drug demonstrates its potency only when its therapeutic results exceed the point attained by the placebo situation. For this reason, "slight" or "mild" degrees of improvement should be questioned as being solely due to pharmacological effects of the medication.

In this study the effective oral dose of chlorpromazine has been found to be between 600 and 800 mg. daily. This amount is somewhat higher than those used in the other controlled studies with a chronic schizophrenic population, one at 100-400 mg. and the other at 500 mg., but is far lower than that employed in some therapeutic studies, e. g., Kinross-Wright, in which the average dose was 2400 mg. It may well be that had the lower dosage levels been maintained for a longer time than two weeks a change in the rating scale would have been noted. On the other hand, 9 of the 10 patients showed changes in the rating scale within one to two weeks after the institution of a given level of dosage, so that on the basis of consistency it would seem that the results obtained were valid. The reasons for the wide variation in therapeutic dosages are obscure.

The rapid onset of changes in behavior at this level of dosage (within a week) and the duration of effects once the medication was discontinued (four weeks) suggest that the maintenance dosage may be intermittent rather than constant, with a consequent economic saving and a minimizing of complications.

The most encouraging result of this study was the significant improvement in thought processes and the reduction in hallucinations. For this to occur in chronic psychotic patients argues for a better prognostic outlook than has hitherto been considered possible with any other form of therapy.

Summary

Twenty male lobotomized schizophrenics, who had been hospitalized an average of 10 years, were divided into two groups matched for age, duration of hospitalization, years since lobotomy, and psychiatric status (Malamud-Sands Rating Scale). One group was given placebos and the other chlorpromazine by mouth, on a double-blind basis. When the chlorpromazine dose was increased to 800 mg. daily, the scores on the rating scales for the two groups were differentiated, the placebo group showing little or no change, whereas the chlorpromazine group showed a significant trend to betterment in their scores. An analysis of 15 items which were used in the rating scale showed that on 4—responsivity, socialization, perception (hallucinations), and thought processes—the improvement in the chlorpromazine group was statistically significant.

THE INFLUENCE OF CHLORPROMAZINE ON PSYCHOTIC THOUGHT CONTENT AND MECHANISM

Douglas Goldman, M.D.
Longview State Hospital, Cincinnati, Ohio

It was soon evident to most of us engaged in work with chlorpromazine that we were not dealing with just another sedative or "tranquilizing" agent, but that we were observing effects of considerable specificity on the psychopathologic manifestations in mental illness. Such effects were not restricted to illness of recent origin, but could be achieved even after 15 or 20 years of continuous chronic illness.

The most rewarding theoretical formulations from these observations can be achieved only by adoption of a fresh point of view and setting aside the strained sophistries and verbal calisthenics which have served to obscure and stand in the way of understanding the mental illnesses with which we as physicians must deal as effectively as possible. Patients upon whom these observations have been made were patients in a state hospital, with the addition of a few from private practice. All were severely ill, and necessarily classified as psychotic or severely psychoneurotic. Many had been ill for years, and many represented the "back-ward" population of the state hospital. Most of the common classifications of psychotic illness are included. The word "diagnosis" in its proper medical sense hardly seems to apply in the present state of our knowledge.

To date, we have treated about 750 patients with chlorpromazine. Illustrative examples from our material are being discussed without any attempt to elaborate any numerical conclusions.

Treatment in practically all patients is by oral administration of chlorpromazine. The minimal dosage level is 50 mg. every 8 hours, the maximum usually 500 mg. every 8 hours, and the mean dosage is 150 to 200 mg. every 8 hours. The changes to be described have occurred within the first few days of administration of the drug in the earliest instances, and after 5 to 8 months of administration of the drug in those patients whose changes took place at a slower pace, usually associated with long duration of the psychotic process. In describing the effect of chlorpromazine on the elements of psychopathology, verbally expressed thought content, or, in lieu of such expression, performance, behavior, or adaptive activity, the outline shown in Table I will be pursued.

The remarkable effect of chlorpromazine on acute delirious states has been noted by all workers. One interesting example is that of patient Mark B., who

TABLE I: Psychopathologic manifestations influenced by chlorpromazine
> Acute Delirium
> Acute Psychotic Excitement
> Acute Psychotic Depression
> Chronic Psychotic Reactions
>> Hallucinations and Delusions (sensory manifestations)
>> Motor Manifestations
>> Social Manifestations
> Psychoneuroses

served as his own control. He was first treated for early delirium tremens in the prechlorpromazine days. He recovered with vigorous treatment with large doses of Vitamin B fractions, and moderate sedation, with transient appearance to him of hallucinatory giraffes on the third and fourth days. He remained dry for almost a year, and then entered another alcoholic debauch of even greater intensity of several months' duration. His appearance on the second admission to the hospital was worse, tremor more pronounced, etc. With the help of chlorpromazine, 50 mg. q.i.d., he was able to leave the hospital on the fourth day, without having experienced any faunal invasion. The marked amelioration of sensory distortion, motor incoordination, and excitement by chlorpromazine is clearly demonstrated. Even more remarkable was the consequence of this relief. He was able to discuss the family disturbance which had prolonged the last bout of alcoholism. His wife had become pregnant by another man. With his improvement he adopted an attitude that was reasonable and civilized beyond anything that might have been expected. He and his wife worked out the plan whereby she would have the child and arrange for its adoption and they would continue their marriage and rearing of the child they had had together.

Acute psychotic excitement likewise was among the first recognized indications for the use of chlorpromazine. Robert W. was admitted to the state hospital in a highly excited homicidal state. His eyes were red and bulging, face suffused, restraint required. This patient was loud, screamed that he would kill someone, and communicated his sincerity in this purpose to attendants and other personnel. Chlorpromazine administration was begun very soon after his admission. When the patient was presented to the staff 4 days later, receiving 100 mg. chlorpromazine every 8 hours, the clinical picture had been transformed completely. He exhibited a whimpering, guilt-ridden state of anxiety and apprehension, with no aggressive features, no need for restraint. In the course of 2 more weeks of hospitalization, this patient had quieted down, had lost his anxiety almost altogether, was able to discuss his illness and his future plans in an objective and rational manner. This patient is illustrative of the mechanism of projection and displacement of hostile drives, without actual delusional or hallucinatory content. Again, however, there is sensory and perceptive distortion behind this mechanism.

Acute psychotic depression has been found to be the most likely reaction to fail to respond to chlorpromazine, particularly when the depression is "pure" and not accompanied by agitation and anxiety. However, such patients under the influence of chlorpromazine require fewer and milder electric shock treatments. Vivian T. illustrates this point. After only slight improvement under chlorpromazine from a depressed state in which, among other symptoms, she thought herself unworthy of her husband and children, she failed to improve further. After only 3 electric shock treatments, she had achieved her previous warmth and spirit. In this patient, as in most depressed individuals, there seemed to be much less of the perceptive and motor defect which seems to presage benefit from chlorpromazine.

The chronic psychotic reactions, particularly schizophrenias and related conditions, present a formidable challenge to all drugs and to all theoretical formulations. It is unnecessary to consider a great number of illustrative cases individually in detail. Besides, any worker who has assiduously followed an adequate number of such patients under chlorpromazine treatment for a number of months can supply details from his own experience, of hallucinations, voices, visions, and odors which have disappeared or appreciably diminished; of delusions of being "royalty" which have merged with the common herd; of delusions of being a "great healer" which have themselves been healed; of delusions of marital infidelity which melted into conjugal trust; of "poisoned" food which became wholesome and palatable; of ideas that "people seemed to be pigs" that presently turned into the insight that such ideas were "stepping stones to insanity."

TABLE II: Delusions and Hallucinations

Stopped	74
Denied	25
Changed	88
Persisting	38

Table II shows numerically an experience with delusions and hallucinations under chlorpromazine treatment. Even the hallucinations and delusions which are mitigated rather than relieved are of interest. Voices are no longer obscene, are more pleasant, become merely "mental suggestions," or can now be "ignored." "Motor" manifestations in chronic psychoses are equally benefitted by chlorpromazine. Muteness, even of many years' duration, gives way to communicative ability which is often warm and astonishingly indicative of insight. Mannerisms and rituals present for many years give way to cooperative helpfulness and even employment, and assaultiveness changes to "peaceful coexistence" at the very least. The effect of chlorpromazine on certain "social" qualities in so-called deteriorated patients is often the earliest evidence of benefit. Soiling and wetting cease, and there is neatness of clothing and eating habits not previously evident. A pair of identical twins of whom only one received the medication dramatically demonstrated the contrast between the acceptable treated member of the pair and the revolting untreated one. The unifying observation which relates to all of these patients is that there is, in every case, improved appreciation of reality associated with resolution or improvement in the perceptive defect.

The psychoneuroses, which have been considered the prime examples of purely "psychogenic" mental disorder, have responded to chlorpromazine treatment strikingly in many instances. I shall only mention two examples.

Charles W. had for over two years experienced persistent and totally disabling pain in his lower back, following an industrial injury. After a brief period, three weeks, of what now would be considered mild dosage, 25 mg. t.i.d. of chlorpromazine, the pain disappeared. Arlene P. for years had been obsessed with fear of contamination and dirt; she was a characteristic and typical "hand-washer." She went through all of the exhausting ritual of decontamination in every conceivable situation. Electric shock was, of course, ineffective. After approximately 4 months of chlorpromazine, she had gained weight, and had a friendly smile with no fear evident in her countenance. She indicated that she thought her idea about contamination, and the need to protect herself by frequent hand-washing, was a "foolish notion." In these patients the perceptive defect involved the "body image," but in other respects the defect was of the same order and intensity, and had the same destructive effect on personality, as the defect in psychotic individuals.

One other observation must be briefly detailed. This concerns two patients who had failed to respond to electric shock treatment, or to insulin, or both, who subsequently improved almost to recovery with chlorpromazine treatment. But they could not free themselves of remaining mild symptoms. The remaining symptoms were not of psychotic proportions. In one patient, instead of hearing "voices" she had "evil thoughts" which related to unpleasant early life experience. In the second patient, severe paranoid delusions had disappeared entirely, and had given way to insight, but a partly disabling "free floating" anxiety could not be overcome. In both these patients the development of perceptive acuity under chlorpromazine apparently precluded return to the psychotic reaction. Fortunately, both responded to a few electric shock treatments, and have maintained adequate adaptations with occasional (1 per month) electric shock treatments.

The unifying concept which is offered as a working hypothesis, and not as a demonstrated fact, is that in all of the psychopathologic manifestations described there is a defect in ability to perceive, elaborate, and interpret the sensory stream and to organize and control the motor outflow. These are the functions of normally adaptive consciousness in a healthy organism. Recently reported work of Himwich and Rinaldi and others indicates that the midbrain reticular formation with its adjacent analogues is the structure primarily affected by chlorpromazine as well as other drugs which we are considering. The studies of Penfield, Magoun, Lindsley, Jasper and others in the last few years indicate that it is in this area of the brain that the functions of consciousness are chiefly executed.

It seems reasonable to relate observed reactions in psychotic individuals, physiologic studies on the site of action of the drug, and studies indicating this site to be related to important manifestations of consciousness. Clinical psychotic illness may, therefore, be considered as a manifestation of varying degrees of qualitative and quantitative disturbance of consciousness, amenable to many approaches to some degree. None has thus far been more rewarding than treatment with the new drugs, both from the clinical therapeutic and the theoretical view.

CLINICAL TRIAL OF A NEW PHENOTHIAZINE COMPOUND: NP-207

Vernon Kinross-Wright, M.D.,
Department of Psychiatry, Baylor University College of Medicine,
Texas Medical Center, Houston, Texas

The successful introduction of chlorpromazine into psychiatric treatment has prompted an intensive study of phenothiazine derivatives. NP-207 was synthesized by the Sandoz Laboratories in Switzerland, and was selected from a number of other related compounds for clinical trial. The structural formula is compared with that of chlorpromazine in Figure 1. The chemical formula is 3-chloro-10/2'-(N-methyl-piperidyl-2")-ethyl/phenothiazine hydrochloride (Figure 1).

The animal pharmacology of NP-207 generally resembles that of chlorpromazine. It shows well-marked anti-cholinergic action upon the isolated

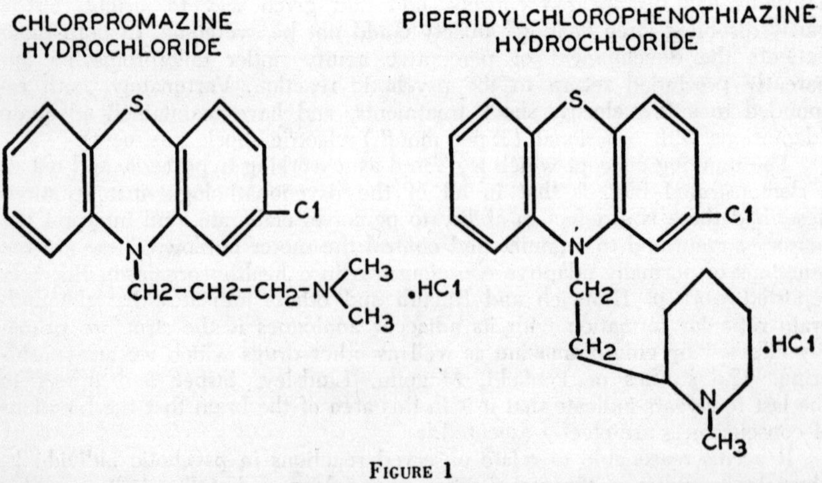

FIGURE 1

intestine of the guinea pig. It causes a prolonged fall in blood pressure in the cat; adrenolytic activity is also demonstrable in the guinea pig. It shares with chlorpromazine the properties of histamine antagonism and potentiation of barbiturate anesthesia in mice; it also potentiates analgesics. A hypothermic and anticonvulsant action have likewise been demonstrated in animals. The oral toxicity to both rats and mice is about half that of chlorpromazine.

Materials and Methods

Thirty-two patients admitted to the psychiatric in-patient service were selected for trial. Fifteen of the patients were chosen because they had either failed to respond to chlorpromazine, Frenquel, or reserpine, alone or in combination, or had relapsed. The remainder were selected at random. Ages ranged from 17 to 65 years. Twenty-seven of the patients were female and five male. Eleven were Negroes. Twenty-three of the patients were schizophrenics. The other patients comprised a scattered sample of the psychiatric spectrum.

It should be stated here that the author has used chlorpromazine as a standard in judging the efficacy of other phenothiazine derivatives. The dosage schedule was, therefore, on an empirical basis; modeled after that used for chlorpormazine. A parenteral preparation of NP-207 was not available. Most patients were started on 50 mg. NP-207 orally four times daily with increase of 200 mg. a day at one or two day intervals up to a maximum of 1000 mg. daily. The first patients in the series were given as high as 2800 mg. a day, but it soon became apparent that such high doses were unnecessary. The average daily dosage for all patients was in the region of 400 mg. daily, a much lower figure than is used with comparable patients on chlorpromazine.

Duration of treatment varied from three to 74 days, with an average of 34 days. Total quantity of the drug received by each patient ranged from 56,000 mg. to 900 mg., with an average of 20,000 mg.

The first 24 patients were observed carefully for changes in alertness, amount of sleep, blood pressure, and body temperature. They were also given a complete white count, urinalyses, and three liver function tests at four day intervals. Serum bilirubin, alkaline phosphatase, and thymol turbidity estimations were selected as being most likely to reveal early hepatic dysfunction.

Results

NP-207 bears a general family resemblance to chlorpromazine in its clinical effects. Table I indicates that its therapeutic efficiency is of the same order as that of chlorpromazine. However, it must be remembered that almost half of the patients in this series had failed to respond satisfactorily to the latter drug. For comparable results with NP-207, daily doses of only one-third to one-half those of chlorpromazine were required. The duration of treatment was somewhat more extended, but this was probably due to lack of initial parenteral administration.

Unlike chlorpormazine, NP-207 was described by the patients as a pleasant medicine to take. It rarely induced feelings of being "washed-out" and lacking in energy. The patients were noticeably more alert and active. There was no evidence of a disturbance in consciousness or motor performance in any dosage (except one patient who became confused), either by clinical or psychological examination.

Except on doses above 1600 mg. daily, patients did not complain of drowsiness. However, they slept better and there was a definite increase in the

TABLE I: Clinical Results with NP-207

	Number of Cases	Remission	Social Recovery	Improved	Unchanged or Worse
Schizophrenia					
Catatonic	4	1	1	1	1
Hebephrenic	5	—	3	1	1
Simple	1	—	—	1	—
Paranoid	6	1	4	1	—
Chronic	5	—	2	3	—
Acute Undifferentiated	2	1	1	—	—
Depression (Psychotic)	3	1	2	—	—
Mania	1	—	—	—	1
Mental Deficiency	1	—	—	—	1
Chronic Brain Syndrome	1	—	—	—	1
Hysteria	1	—	1	—	—
Drug Intoxication	2	2	—	—	—
Total	32	6	14	7	5

amount of nocturnal sleep even on smaller doses.

None of the subjects experienced gastro-intestinal symptoms. Observations were not made which might indicate that NP-207 has anti-emetic properties.

A few of the subjects mentioned dizziness with higher doses. However, serial blood pressure recordings failed to show a hypotensive effect. Both blood pressure and pulse rate remained strikingly constant throughout.

There was no clinical evidence of a hypothermic action of NP-207.

All liver function tests fell within normal limits except in one patient who showed a consistently elevated serum alkaline phosphatase. There were no other signs of hepatic dysfunction, but this patient was a moderately severe diabetic. The cause of the abnormal serum phosphatase was not established, but was not considered attributable to NP-207.

White cell counts were normal throughout. No one in the series showed changes in renal function.

Neither dermatitis or antineurotic edema was observed. No patient complained of photosensitivity or photophobia.

Fine tremor was noticeable in some of the patients. Even on doses over 2000 mg. daily there were no signs of Parkinsonism. The patient with a chronic brain syndrome became confused while on 600 mg. daily. However, he had been confused before, and has been similarly affected since the drug was withdrawn.

It has been mentioned above that the anti-psychotic effect of NP-207 is similar to that of chlorpromazine. Successful patients show an increased responsiveness, become more sociable, and develop a more normal affect, often within a few days. Delusional patterns recede, and in some disappeared completely. These effects were more noticeable in the acutely disturbed schizophrenics, but striking improvements were noticed in the chronic group, too. Best results were achieved with the paranoid group.

The group of depressed patients is too small to permit conclusions; however, all improved, and without the apparent initial deepening of depression usually seen with chlorpromazine treatment.

NP-207 does not act as rapidly on delirious patients, but again this might well have been due to the lack of parenteral dosage.

Thus far, NP-207 appeared to be a very satisfactory therapeutic agent with almost no side effects. However, on the 41st day of treatment, one patient (diagnosis—hysteria), who had been discharged from the hospital, complained of blurring of vision which in a few days progressed to total inability to see. Repeated ophthalmological examination was thought to be negative and a diagnosis of hysterical blindness made. An unsuccessful attempt was made to hypnotize the patient, but during a pentothal interview she was able to see quite well. A second patient (diagnosis—paranoid schizophrenia) developed similar symptoms, and also within a few days said she was totally unable to see. Negative ophthalmological findings and other factors led to the same diagnosis of hysterical blindness. In the first case, NP-207 was stopped within four days of the first complaint; and in the second, continued in a diminished dosage for two weeks. Six weeks after the initial complaint of the first patient, repeated fundoscopic examination revealed a deposition of brownish-black pigment on both retinae. It was most marked peripherally, but extended up to the optic disc, sparing the macula. The pigment was in the form of discrete clumps without evidence of vascular or choroidal involvement. Visual fields showed a marked constriction, but with sparing of central vision. Dark adaption was greatly impaired. The disc was reddened but not swollen. The retinal vessels were normal or perhaps slightly constricted. These changes first appeared some twelve weeks after the commencement of NP-207, and six weeks after its discontinuance. The retinal changes did not resemble any known pathological condition of the retina, but seemed to be a new form of toxic retinitis.

About the same date, the other patient mentioned above and three more were found to have developed varying degrees of the same condition. NP-207 treatment was discontinued on all patients.

Twenty-eight of thirty-two patients developed retinopathy, though symptoms were only recognized by two patients in retrospect (Table II).

Sixteen cases were considered mild with some night blindness, moderate reduction in visual fields, and retinal pigmentation with reddening of the disc.

Four cases showed extensive pigment deposits and impairment of visual activity.

Eight patients became nearly blind, had almost complete obliteration of the visual fields, and showed severe retinal changes.

The degree of retinal involvement appears to be related more to the daily dose of drug than it does to the duration of treatment. Table III illustrates the relationship between retinal changes and total amount of NP-207. Retinitis occurred in patients who had taken as little as 9000 mg. of the drug. The first appearance of retinitis varied from 31 days to 83 days after the beginning of treatment. These patients have received intensive treatment with

TABLE II: INCIDENCE OF TOXIC RETINITIS WITH NP-207
(As of 9/10/55)

Severe	8 patients
Moderate	4 patients
Mild	16 patients
Normal	2 patients
Not examined (presumed normal)	2 patients

TABLE III: RELATIONSHIP BETWEEN TOXIC RETINITIS AND TOTAL AMOUNT OF NP-207 TAKEN

Total Amount NP-207	Total No. of Cases	Retinitis (%) Severe	Moderate
40-55,000 mg.	5	80	20
25-40,000 mg.	7	29	29
10-25,000 mg.	12	15	8
Under 10,000 mg.	8	—	40

corticothrophins, corticosteroid, and vitamins A, B-1, and B-12. Supportive group therapy was instituted for a majority of the patients.

The retinal pathology has not been associated with other delayed side effects.

DISCUSSION

A critical evaluation of NP-207 is scarcely possible until the outcome of the retinal toxic effects has been established. It will not find a place among the psychiatric therapies. However, from a research point of view, the clinical trial of the drug provides valuable data.

Firstly, its therapeutic effects, judged by so brief an experience, appear to be at least comparable to those of chlorpromazine, the chemotherapeutic agent of choice for schizophrenia. Although the chemistry and the animal pharmacology of both drugs are similar, the dissimilarity of clinical side effects is noteworthy. Prior to the onset of eye symptoms, NP-207 appeared to be a more satisfactory drug than chlorpromazine and far superior to other derivatives of the phenothiazines. The lack of discomfort associated with taking the drug, absence of allergic reactions, and Parkinsonism were especially important.

Secondly, it has produced a unique form of toxic retinopathy which was first encountered by two investigators in Switzerland. A detailed account of the toxic retinopathy is to be given by Drs. E. L. Goar and M. Fletcher. This condition is unusual, also, in that it is not associated with other toxic effects, appears even after the drug is stopped, and occurs in a very high percentage of subjects. The pigmentation of the retina is a primary change. It does not follow obvious damage to the optic nerve and is not a chorio-retinitis, even though the nerve head has been reddened in every case. The premonitory symptoms are those of retinitis pigmentosa. But while the early distribution of pigment corresponds with that of retinitis pigmentosa, the characteristic "bone-corpuscle" appearance of the latter is lacking. One Swiss investigator reports a considerable regression of pigment and a lessening of visual symptoms. We are currently endeavoring to reproduce the retinal lesions in animals, and also are investigating our patients for disturbance of melanin and porphyrin metabolism.

Conclusions

Trial of a new phenothiazine derivative, NP-207, has produced very favorable initial clinical results in a group of 32 psychiatric patients.

The study was discontinued because of the late incidence of toxic retinitis in a high percentage of subjects. The outcome of this is yet unknown.

Addendum

All cases have shown improvement. This has been rapid in some and extremely slow in others, depending on the degree of involvement of the eyes. Improvement is still continuing after five months.

The mild cases have normal vision with a few persistent field defects, and are showing recession of the pigment. Of the moderately severe cases, one is normal and three are asymptomatic.

Three of the severe cases are asymptomatic, two have moderate visual difficulty, and four still have marked loss of vision.

The good psychiatric results have been maintained. However, group therapy may have contributed to this.

CHLORPROMAZINE TREATMENT OF MENTAL DISORDERS

Vernon Kinross-Wright, M.D.
Department of Psychiatry, Baylor University College of Medicine,
Houston, Texas

Chlorpromazine, a derivative of phenothiazine, was developed in France by the Rhone-Poulenc Research Laboratories. Under its trade names of Largactil and Megaphon it has been the object of much interest and experimentation in Europe, during the past 2 years. In this country where it is known as Thorazine it has been accepted for its superior antiemetic properties. More recently it has been used in the treatment of psychiatric disorders.

PHARMACOLOGY

Courvoisier, *et al*. have conducted extensive animal and chemical investigations and find that chlorpromazine exhibits the following properties: (1) Anticholinergic action; (2) antiadrenergic action; though there is no inhibition of the hyperglycemic response of adrenalin; (3) central effect which is sedative, anticonvulsive, hypothermic, and antiemetic. The drug is also said to lower the metabolic rate. (4) There is a mild antihistaminic and local anesthetic activity. (5) The compound potentiates certain drugs, especially morphine and barbiturate derivatives.

The fate of chlorpromazine in the organism is unknown but probably it is degraded in the liver. Little is excreted through the kidneys.

The work of Moyer, *et al*, in this country indicates that chlorpromazine in dogs is a hypotensive agent which decreases peripheral resistance with a variable effect upon cardiac output. These authors found no evidence of acute renal toxicity, though parenteral administration increased sodium and water excretion.

CLINICAL STUDIES

There appears to be considerable variability in the human response to chlorpromazine. The central depressant effects have been universally noted. There is usually a striking drop in blood pressure, particularly during the first few days of administration of the drug, with a compensatory tachycardia. Changes in body temperature, basal metabolism, urinary excretion have been variable. Other effects of sympathetic and parasympathetic inhibition have been noted. Increase of appetite may occur. No significant changes in the body biochemistry have been reported.

Clinical Uses

Chlorpromazine has been used in Europe for a wide range of conditions in the fields of surgery, anesthesia, gynecology and medicine. It was introduced into psychiatry in combination with barbiturates in prolonged sleep treatment. Hamon, *et al.* first used chlorpromazine alone in the treatment of manic illness. Their good results were reproduced by Delay and his associates, who have treated a variety of psychotic patients with success. Of the increasing number of publications, mention should be made of that of Staehelin and Kielholz in Switzerland and more recently of Lehmann and Hanrahan in Canada. Improvement, and often cure, has been described in practically every type of mental illness. As might be expected with a new therapy dosages and uses have differed considerably, but most authors have agreed that initial parenteral administration speeds up improvement. Treatment has been continued for months in some cases.

The present study concerns an unselected group of admissions to the psychiatric service of a general hospital together with a lesser number of outpatients, 95 in all. A majority of the patients received initially a minimum of 50 mgms. of chlorpromazine intramuscularly 4 times daily. The effects of the drug are cumulative and it is usually possible to switch to oral dosage after a few days. Intramuscular administration is often painful and produces marked induration at the site of injection, particularly if the solution escapes into fatty tissue.

The total daily amount of chlorpromazine may be increased by as much as 100 mgms. *per diem* until optimum effect is achieved. Increasing familiarity with the effects of the drug has led to the use of higher dosages. In one case improvement was delayed until 1,600 mgms. a day had been given for 10 days. However the average therapeutic dose for psychotic patients is about 800 mgms. each 24 hours. In neurotic patients and in children treatment is started by the oral route and in doses as low as 30 mgms. daily. Once improvement was manifested medication was given solely by mouth and progressively reduced over a period of weeks. In a few patients who showed a tendency to relapse higher dosage was again instituted.

Although most of the expected clinical phenomena were observed during treatment there was a surprising inconstancy in degree in different patients. All the patients who responded to chlorpromazine showed an initial somnolence from which, however, they could be easily aroused. After the first few days of treatment the lethargy decreased. Some patients presented a rather striking similarity to patients a few days after prefrontal lobotomy—a fact remarked on by some of the European writers.

In spite of the lack of spontaneous activity, patients are fully oriented and even severely withdrawn patients showed a rapid increase in their contact with reality. Some said that they had never felt so relaxed and very few of the psychotic patients made any complaints about the treatment. Neurotic patients on the other hand were aware of the hypotension and described themselves as "lightheaded, dizzy, and faint." None of the patients experienced frank syncopal attacks but these have been reported elsewhere. Some patients complained of a dry nose and mouth. Nausea and epigastric distress occurred occasionally in patients on oral therapy though this was somewhat unexpected in view of the well-established antiemetic properties. Three patients mentioned aching eyes and experienced some difficulty in focusing on close objects. Occasionally injection is painful and in these cases procaine is added. While on intramuscular dosage many of the patients exhibited a marked grayish pallor which is quite characteristic.

The hypotensive response was always apparent, the systolic pressure often dropped by 40 to 60 points and diastolic reading by as much as 40 points. In no case was it found necessary to withdraw chlorpromazine on this account even in ambulatory patients. Two of the patients were hypertensive before treatment and in both of these blood pressure dropped to normal levels without bad effects. After the withdrawal of chlorpromazine the blood pressure returned to pretreatment levels within 48 hours.

The compensatory tachycardia is often conspicuous but does not worry the patients. One woman suffering from an anxiety state commented on it but said that it was not nearly as unpleasant as the palpitations she had experienced for years.

No consistent temperature changes were noted. A consistent reduction of body temperature did not occur. In 5 cases there was a marked elevation of temperature for a few days during chlorpromazine administration, without leucytosis or other clinical findings. These patients had few complaints and the pyrexia promptly subsided when chlorpromazine was discontinued. In 2 cases replacement of the drug was accompanied by return of the fever for a short time. Measurement of metabolic rate was not attempted but there was no clinical evidence of significant decrease. Increase of appetite was the rule and some patients became ravenously hungry and gained weight. This was true even where other signs of clinical improvements were meager.

Sleep was greatly improved in almost all the patients in spite of the fact that those on large intramuscular dosage were lethargic throughout the day. Improved sleep is often associated with heightened dream activity. It is worth noting that the total sedative requirements for the service have been greatly reduced since this new treatment was instituted. Also worth mentioning is the strange, striking quiet which has come over the ward with its population of acutely disturbed patients. On one occasion when supplies of the drug were exhausted this was brought home to us with particular emphasis.

When patients are on chlorpromazine the vital signs and blood pressure are recorded at 6 hourly intervals. All barbiturate sedation is avoided. When necessary, paraldehyde, whose action does not seem to be potentiated by chlorpromazine, is used for sedation. As part of an investigation into possible hepatic toxicity many patients are given a battery of liver function tests before and every 4 days during treatment. Electrocardiogram and a thorough physical examination are prerequisites of treatment.

RESULTS

Table 1 briefly summarizes the results obtained to date with 95 patients. Many of these patients are still receiving chlorpromazine on an outpatient basis and are continuing to make progress. Some have been under treatment for over 3 months. Others have required but a few doses to relieve their major symp-

TABLE 1
Results of Chlorpromazine Treatment

	Total	In remission	Much improved	Slightly improved	Unchanged
Schizophrenia	29				
Paranoid		4	5	2	3
Hebephrenic		1	2	1	
Catatonic		1	3	1	
Simple					1
Unclassified		2	3		
Depression	18				
Manic depressive		4	2	1	
Reactive		1	4	2	1
With cerebral vascular disease		1			
Involutional melancholia		1	1		
Mania	2	2			
Anxiety State	9	2	4	3	
Hysteria	8				
Conversion		1	2	1	2
Dissociation		2			
Delirium	10				
Bromide		1			
ACTH		1			
Alcohol		5			
With organic brain disease		2	1		
Psychosis	2				
Unclassified			1	1	
Posttraumatic Neurosis	5		2	3	
Alcoholism	2		1	1	
Psychopathic Personality	2				
Aggressive			1		
Inadequate				1	
Emotional Immaturity	1				1
Neurodermatitis	1		1		
Childhood Behavior Disturbance	3	1	1	1	
Narcolepsy (Idiopathic)	1		1		
Convulsive Disorder	2		1		1
Total	95	32	36	18	9

toms. In agreement with general experience states of psychomotor excitement and agitation have been quickly controlled with 200-400 mgms. daily. This seems to be true regardless of the type of psychomotor excitement. In one case of schizophrenic excitement, and one case of acute mania, however, chlorpromazine did not ameliorate the symptoms. The addition of 3 electric shock treatments on successive days produced a prompt remission in both these patients. This experience was duplicated with another case of involutional melancholia. It seems as though the combination of EST and chlorpromazine does well in certain instances since all 3 of these patients had had previous attacks of lesser severity, which has required a greater number of EST's for improvement. Delirious states are notably responsive, often clearing up in a matter of hours. The series includes cases of toxic deliria due to alcohol, bromides, ACTH, and brain lesions.

The results in the schizophrenic patients have been gratifying, particularly in those with paranoid symptomatology. Of 14 paranoid schizophrenics, only 3 were not improved. Six of these have already returned home and are making good adjustments. In 3 patients with delusional ideas the hallucinations seem to have entirely disappeared. The following case history is illustrative:

A 32-year-old colored, married female was admitted because of combativeness, refusal to wear clothes, ideas of being poisoned, hearing persecutory voices, and generally disorganized behavior of 4 months' duration.

Patient had an unhappy childhood and had always been introverted with compulsive habits, episodes of nervousness and severe dysmenorrhea. She was highly ambitious and never made friends, always hypersensitive and suspicious. Four months prior to admission the patient accused her husband and sister of trying to poison her, made violent assaults on her husband. She believed her mind was being controlled by others, heard voices plotting to kill her, was unable to sleep and refused to care for herself.

On admission she was acutely disturbed and presented a picture of paranoid schizophrenia. Physical examination was unremarkable and laboratory findings within normal limits. Her condition grew worse during first 4 days; totally disorganized in behavior with many paranoid ideas, she was extremely belligerent. She was given chlorpromazine 50 mgm., I.M., q.i.d. After 6 days there was slight lessening of activity and paranoid delusions but she was still very disorganized, slept little, but ate better. Chlorpromazine was increased to 100 mgm., q.i.d. Within 24 hours there was marked improvement, she seemed euphoric, slept well, and ate with enormous appetite. There was moderate hypotension. Within 48 hours the patient was rational and cooperative, sleep rhythm was restored. Oral chlorpromazine was substituted after 4 days with continued improvement, and tapered off over the next 10 days. Patient continued to improve. She was discharged 23 days after admission in good health. She was friendly toward her husband, had no ideas of persecution or reference, showed good affect and had some insight into her illness. She has continued to do well at home.

All the cases of depression have shown some improvement and several have returned home and are doing well. Depressed patients, particularly those who showed much psychomotor retardation, did not demonstrate the striking results seen in the schizophrenic and manic group. However, improvement in depressed patients is often masked by the effects of chlorpromazine itself, and only when it is withdrawn or reduced in amount is the improvement apparent. The following case history is illustrative:

A 42-year-old married, colored man was well until 3 years ago, when he broke his ankle at work. Following this he was confused for 3 weeks and was thought by his doctor to have had a cerebral vascular accident. Since then he has been seclusive, nervous, and progressively more depressed, profoundly depressed in the past few months. He would not eat, slept little, cried, and read the Bible. He talked frequently of suicide, complained of backache. He had not been able to work.

On admission the patient presented a picture of retarded depression. Physical examination showed B. P. of 240/118 with hypertensive heart disease and grade ii retinal arteriosclerosis. Routine investigation and liver function tests were within normal limits. EKG showed left axis deviation; x-ray of spine was negative. Diagnosis was depression secondary to hypertension and possible cerebral vascular accident.

The patient remained depressed and almost mute for the first 10 days. During this period his B.P. dropped to an average of 210/110. Chlorpromazine was instituted, increased gradually by 50 mgm. steps each day up to 200 mgm. daily, by mouth (to avoid sudden hypotension). The patient improved at once; appetite increased and he slept well. He had no diurnal lethargy and was more sociable. Blood pressure dropped in 24 hours to 130/90 and in one week to 120/70. He was discharged 17 days later on 75 mgm. daily with B.P. 110/80. He was cheerful and considering a return to work. He had no complaints referable to reduction in B.P. He continued to have backaches but did not spontaneously mention this.

Among the neurotic group response has been more variable. Most of the patients report some improvement but as mentioned above the side effects of chlorpromazine sometimes cause patients to refuse larger doses. The improved sleep habits and increased appetite in this group suggest that chlorpromazine would be of value as an adjuvant to psychotherapy. This case of conversion hysteria, though, appears specially noteworthy.

A 31-year-old married, white mechanic was referred because of painful paralysis of the left leg, nervousness and headaches of 3 months' duration. His symptoms developed 30 minutes after a heavy truck transmission had fallen on his abdomen and left leg. His previous adjustment had been good though there were marital difficulties and he had been living for some months previously in a setting of tension on this account.

Following his accident he had been conservatively treated. Aside from the paralysis and extensive bruising there were no injuries. Neurological examination was negative except for stocking anesthesia of the lower extremity. He received osteopathic treatments and when these did not help was given a bad prognosis. After seeing several other medical men he was finally referred for psychiatric help by his lawyer. A diagnosis of conversion hysteria with tension state was made and psychotherapy instituted some 3 months after injury. Probably because of the compensation and legal issues the patient did not progress. Sodium amytal interviews were unrewarding. For over 5 months after his accident his leg was still paralyzed and very painful. He developed numbness in his right leg, was repressed, and losing weight. He entertained paranoid ideas against his physicians.

He was hospitalized and treated with chlorpromazine, 200 mgm. daily by injection. He became extremely drowsy for 24 hours. The next day he said that his leg no longer was numb and that he felt good. By the third day he was ambulatory with a slight limp. He was happy and elated over his improvement. He continued to improve while chlorpromazine was tapered off over a 2-week period. Three weeks after the termination of treatment he was back at work, eating and sleeping well. He stated that he had never felt so well in his life. He had fair insight into his illness and was unconcerned about the possible loss of a large financial settlement.

Two patients with convulsive disorders associated with behavioral disturbance are included in the series. One of these has fewer seizures with chlorpromazine than on any other anticonvulsant regime. This finding has been noted by others.

Few undesirable reactions other than those attributable to the physiological effects of chlorpromazine have been encountered so far. Moyer, et al. in a study of renal and hepatic functions have found no evidence of toxicity in their patients who were, however, on smaller dosage. They also did not find abnormalities of the electrocardiogram or blood elements attributable to the drug. Lehmann and Hanrahan noted slight changes in liver function tests in some of their patients with clinical evidence of hepatic dysfunction in 3. In this series no conclusive evidence of hepatic toxicity has been found, even in patients with pre-existent liver damage of moderate degree. This aspect of chlorpromazine is being more extensively investigated.

Three patients developed more or less generalized skin eruption of an urticarial nature associated with malaise. More powerful antihistamines did not bring relief, but in each case cessation of chlorpromazine for a few days only allowed the skin to clear. One schizophrenic patient became very euphoric with outspoken erotic tendencies which subsided with discontinuance of treatment for 10 days. Two patients on high doses developed coarse tremor, muscular rigidity, and immobile expression. This Parkinson-like syndrome disappeared quickly after reduction of dosage.

There do not appear to be any absolute contraindications to chlorpromazine treatment. It should be used with caution in patients with hepatic, cardiac or renal disease and in those who have recently taken barbiturates or opiates.

Comment

Chlorpromazine has a diverse pharmacological action on the human organism. A considerable body of evidence has been accumulated pointing to its therapeutic efficacy in many kinds of mental disorders. It is a drug of low toxicity even in large doses and one which may be administered over long periods of time without an undesirable increase of tolerance.

It appears to be a highly effective agent for controlling psychomotor excitement of all kinds without the undesirable effects of the standard methods and maintaining the patient in a fairly accessible state at all times. Its action on other types of mental illness is not so remarkable but is certainly worthy of further investigation, particularly in the chronic schizophrenic patients in whom most treatments are unrewarding. Facilitation of communication together with a remarkable objectivity towards significant ideas and feelings has occurred in many of this group.

Speculation about the mode and site of action of the drug seems premature but such evidence as there is suggests that it is a subcortical one. While in the initial states of treatment there is a definite resemblance in the behavior of these patients to those who have been lobotomized there are none of the deficit found in the latter. Neither the dosage nor the mode of administration of the drug is in any way standardized. The initial results obtained in Europe and this country have been satisfactory enough to justify a thorough clinical investigation of chlorpromazine and a search for even more powerful related compounds.

OFFICE TREATMENT OF PAIN AND PSYCHIC STRESS: THE USE OF A NEW TRANQUILIZING AGENT

Jack R. Wennersten, M.D.

The effective relief of stress and pain—whether somatic or psychic in origin—calls for flexibility and ingenuity. Individual responses to stress make it imperative that the regimen of treatment be adaptable when pain is complicated, or increased, by anxiety. Time-honored sedative and hypnotic preparations, while often useful in controlling somatic and psychic complaints, may lead to addiction and may be unsuitable when nervous depression must be avoided. In addition to the excessive demands that such agents may place on impaired cardiovascular, biliary and renal function, the patient is often forced into an unnecessary dependence on others for his care. There has long been a need for agents that would decrease the importance—to the patient—of his pain and anxiety, and yet would not be depressant in their action or place an extra load on systems already damaged by disease.

TRANQUILIZERS

The introduction of "tranquilizers" has helped to solve this problem, but indications for their application have not been clarified. Chlorpromazine is especially suitable for the treatment of serious mental illnesses. Meprobamate is helpful in relieving neuromuscular tension and less effective in dealing with mental or emotional stress. We recently undertook a study of Compazine, a non-analgesic, non-hypnotic drug reputed to relieve psychic stress and awareness of pain, without depressing central nervous system function or over-extending the work of organ systems impaired by disease.

This white, granulated powder: 2-Chloro-10-[3-(1-methyl-4-piperazinyl)-propyl]-phenothiazine Dimaleate is available in 5 mg. coated tablets, and appears to be more effective, at low doses, than chlorpromazine in its tranquilizing and antiemetic actions.

EVALUATION OF FORMER INVESTIGATIONS

Several hundred physicians have reported on 4105 patients treated for nausea and vomiting of various etiologies; for mental and emotional stress; for behavior disorders; for pain of organic disease; and for menopausal distress, mild postpartum depression and unspecified symptoms.

The usual daily dosage was less than 20 mg., given over periods varying from one day to three months. Side effects, seen in 12% of the patients, were for the most part mild, and all disappeared when the drug was discontinued.

No patients developed blood dyscrasias or jaundice. Slight drowsiness, which often disappeared as therapy was continued, was the most prominent side effect.

According to the preliminary tabulations, 1,429 of the patients suffered, without concurrent physical symptoms, from such mental and emotional problems as anxiety and hysteria, phobias, obsessive-compulsive reactions, premenstrual tension, emotional stress and neurotic depression. Results in 73% of these were excellent or good, 14% fair, and 13% poor. Of the 934 patients whose symptoms were obviously psychosomatic in origin—headaches, gastrointestinal upsets, minor aches and pains—71% experienced excellent or good results, 16% fair, and 13% poor. Nausea and vomiting associated with pregnancy, uremia, operative procedures, drug administration and psychogenic stress were the complaints of 1,034 patients. The drug yielded good or excellent results in 76% of these cases, fair results in 11%, poor results in 13%.

Of the 156 patients suffering from cancer, arthritis, neuralgia, dysmenorrhea, migraine, rheumatism and other diseases, 70% found marked relief from the associated pain. In another group (151 patients) which included chronic behavior and personality problems such as alcoholism and drug addiction, good or excellent results were obtained in 68%. Of the 401 patients experiencing unspecified depression, menopausal disorders, postpartum depression, and other symptoms not easily categorized, 74% obtained good or excellent results.

METHOD

It was on the basis of such preliminary reports that 50 patients were selected for this study. Ten had arthralgia, chest pain, abdominal pain or headaches associated with organic disease, such as chronic fibrositis, coronary artery disease, tertiary syphilis, osteoarthritis and essential hypertension; two of these suffered from postoperative pain. Twenty-six had headaches, rectal pain, burning sensations, indigestion, chest pain and abdominal pain and cramps that were primarily psychic in origin. This group included such diagnoses as menopause and male climacteric, senile depression, nervous indigestion, psychoneurosis with anxiety reaction, chronic gastroenteritis, chronic cholecystitis and neurocirculatory asthenia. In none of these cases was there any demonstrable pathologic change. The complaints of three other patients—while not involving somatic pain—indicated psychic stress expressed as nervousness, fear, syncope, dizziness, melancholia, physical exhaustion, peculiar cutaneous sensations, insomnia, insecurity and hysteria. Eleven patients were treated for nausea and vomiting associated with pregnancy.

The ages of these patients ranged from 12 to 78 years, averaging 41.4 years. There were 38 females and 12 males in the group. Their complaints had lasted from three weeks to 20 years. Compazine was administered in oral dosages ranging from 5 to 40 mg. daily, over periods of 4 to 11 weeks, averaging 7.6 weeks.

RESULTS

Evaluating the effect of any drug on emotional or mental stimuli is difficult, for the findings usually must be based on subjective statements. The patient's feeling of well-being may vary from week to week according to the stress he encounters. In this study, fortunately, I was able to evaluate the drug more objectively, for all cases had been treated, with varying degrees of response, with other medications.

I categorized the response as excellent when all symptoms were abolished permanently; as good when the patient was pleased with the effective, but temporary, abatement of symptoms; and as poor when there was little or no improvement.

Of the 50 patients in this study, 31 (62%) obtained excellent results—prompt, complete relief from their pain or psychosomatic complaints; 17 (34%) obtained partial symptomatic relief, and two (4%) showed little or no improvement. In most cases 5 mg., given three or four times daily, was an adequate dose.

The drug was used to treat the nausea and vomiting associated with pregnancy in 11 cases: 10 obtained excellent relief shortly after the first dose. In the other case, transient morning nausea persisted but the vomiting was controlled. As the drug was continued, the nausea disappeared.

The only side effects, noted by 10 patients, were drowsiness, dizziness, headaches and insomnia. In general, side effects were mild and transient. In only one case did headaches and dizziness make it necessary to discontinue the drug. In another patient, dizziness disappeared as the medication was continued. In the 33 cases followed by laboratory studies, there was no decrease noted in the hemoglobin concentration, nor was there any evidence of bile in the urine.

Discussion

The fact that 48 (96%) of the 50 patients in this study obtained relief of their symptoms is significant, especially in the light of favorable findings of other investigators. It is encouraging that several of these patients obtained relief from chronic pain that had been unresponsive to other sedative or tranquilizing therapy. The drug was effective in reducing the pain—or the awareness of it—and in increasing mobility of the joints in cases of chronic arthralgia and osteoarthritis.

One of these patients, a woman, 61 years of age, announced—after a 20-year history of pain, stiffness and nervousness that she now felt well, had more energy and could move around more freely to do her work. An arthritic patient, 76 years of age, who had complained of pain and stiffness in her hands and knees for ten years, obtained more relief than with any previous medication, including steroid hormones and analgesics. Fear, anxiety, apprehension and melancholia disappeared as these patients became less tense, and their lives took on more meaning as they felt like being active again. In some cases the drug proved itself a valuable adjunct to therapy for illness of organic origin, for patients whose anxiety had been relieved showed more response to curative therapy. Furthermore, headaches, abdominal discomfort of psychosomatic origin and nausea and vomiting cleared rapidly.

Adjunct in Angina Therapy

The drug was given to six patients with hypertension and myocardial infarctions, when apprehension was a serious problem. In all these cases, its addition to the therapeutic regimen produced excellent or good results. In one case, a man, 57 years of age, had had coronary artery disease since January 1951, when a cerebrovascular hemorrhage occurred with coronary occlusion and myocardial infarction. For five years he had complained of chest pain after exercise, heavy meals or excitement. After 16 days of treatment—in addition to routine cardiac therapy—he was having fewer attacks of chest pain, and these were less severe. After 11 weeks of treatment, all symptoms had disappeared. It is evident that Compazine succeeded in reducing the pain and frequency of anginal attacks by relaxing the patient and eliminating his emotional stress.

Reduces Frequency and Intensity of Headaches

Just as the drug was found to be helpful in cases of angina, it was effective in reducing the frequency and intensity of headaches of essential hypertension—by enabling the patient to relax and to avoid building up tension. A woman, 67 years of age, had a two-year history of labile essential hypertension that dated from the death of her husband. Although no organic cause had ever been demonstrated, she was highly nervous, and her headaches, fatigue and apprehension often became almost completely disabling. Hydralazine hydrochloride, barbiturates and tranquilizing agents had failed to give consistent relief. However, she showed marked improvement when Compazine was administered as an adjunctive measure, and continued to improve to the point at which her symptoms were almost completely abated and she was feeling "fairly well."

It was encouraging that only two of the group failed to derive any benefit from the drug. One of these, a woman, 34 years of age with a 16-year history of psychoneurosis, had severe bouts of symptoms that had failed to respond to treatment with sedatives and other tranquilizers. She had complained most recently of severe head pain and dizziness which she supposed were increased by the drug. She refused to continue the medication. Subsequently, it became necessary to provide psychiatric care. The other patient, a woman 44 years of age, had menopausal distress for one year—hot flushes, headaches, dizziness, "nerves" and rectal pain (for which a proctologist could find no cause). Estrogens and amphetamines, given concomitantly, increased her nervousness, dizziness and rectal pain, and the medication was discontinued.

In two instances, the drug reduced the pain and anxiety following operative procedures. Both patients obtained excellent results within a short time and their symptoms did not recur.

Conclusion and Summary

Compazine seems to be a valuable agent for use in a general office practice and is usually effective in dosage of 15 to 20 mg. daily. It is my conclusion that this new agent can control psychosomatic symptoms—make them seem less important to the patient who depends on them—reduce anxiety and tension—and decrease the awareness of pain associated with organic disease. As such, it becomes a valuable adjunct to treatment of the underlying organic disease and, in psychosomatic disorders, may make counselling and psychotherapy more effective.

When Compazine was used to treat pain and psychosomatic disorders of 50 patients, 31 patients noted rapid, complete relief; 17 showed partial improvement; and two failed to benefit. The most effective dosage was 5 mg., given three or four times daily. Transient drowsiness, dizziness and insomnia were the only side effects noted by ten patients.

PROMAZINE HYDROCHLORIDE IN THE TREATMENT OF CHRONIC CATATONIC SCHIZOPHRENICS

Clarke W. Mangun, M.D., and Warren W. Webb, Ph.D.

Veterans Administration Hospital, Roanoke, Virginia

Promazine hydrochloride (hereinafter referred to as promazine) is a phenothiazine compound which differs from chlorpromazine hydrochloride in that promazine does not have a chlorine atom substituted on the phenothiazine ring. Fazekas *et al.* have found promazine to be effective in the management of acute drug and alcohol induced syndromes and in calming acutely disturbed psychotics (manic depressives and agitated schizophrenics). Mitchell confirmed the findings of Fazekas *et al.* in the management of acute alcohol induced syndromes.

Purpose of the present study was to make an initial assessment of the effectiveness of promazine in the treatment of chronic, regressed, catatonic schizophrenic patients.

METHOD

Previous treatment methods had been unsuccessful with the 30 patients in this study. Twenty-seven of the 30 had been treated with electric convulsive therapy and/or with insulin coma therapy, and three of these 27 had also undergone a prefrontal lobotomy. Age range was from 25 to 63; median age was 35. Years continuous hospitalization ranged from 1 to 20; median was 10.

Method of drug administration was primarily oral with only occasional intramuscular injections. Dosage was started at 50 mg., q.i.d., was stepped up by 50 mg. every three days until the fourth week when a dosage of 450 mg., q.i.d., was reached. At this time, there was a four-day break in the drug supply so that the dosage was reduced to 450 mg., b.i.d., for one day; to 50 mg., b.i.d., for one day; to nothing for two days; then back to 100 mg., t.i.d., for one day; to 100 mg., q.i.d., for one day; then to a maintenance dosage of 200 mg., t.i.d.

Behavioral evaluation was accomplished by three procedures: (1) Each patient was seen for a clinical psychiatric interview immediately prior to treatment, again 3 months after treatment began, and again 6 months after treatment began. At the 3-month and 6-month interviews, a clinical judgment was made as to degree of change from the patient's pre-treatment level of adjustment. This judgment of change was stated in terms of the usual clinical judgment scale, i.e., marked improvement (thinking, affect, and behavior approaching normality), moderate improvement (more comfortable, less of a management problem, no longer mute, etc.), slight improvement (noticeable improvement in any particular), and no change. (2) A standardized interview was developed wherein 30 specified behaviors were observed for and then checked as to presence or absence. Each behavior was assigned a weight of one. Total score for this standardized interview could, then, range from zero to 30. Those behaviors were selected on the basis of their relative simplicity so that even minimal changes in behavior could be discriminated. This interview was conducted at the same intervals as the clinical psychiatric interview. Inter-rater reliability was high, rho = .96. (3) The Ward Observations section (items 41-62, excepting items 46, 49, 51, 54, 59, 61) of the Multidimensional Scale for Rating Psychiatric patients was completed by the psychiatric aide at the same time intervals as the above procedures. A total scale points deviation from the normal pattern (possible scores zero to 40) was obtained from this scale. These procedures provided us with three independent evaluations of behavioral change which are referred to as the clinical psychiatric, standardized interview, and ward behavior, respectively.

RESULTS AND DISCUSSION

Table 1 shows the changes from pre-treatment to 3 months and from pre-treatment to 6 months as determined by the three procedures. Plus values represent gains, and minus values represent losses in total score. The changes in patient behavior are in the direction of improvement and are statistically

TABLE 1.—CHANGES IN BEHAVIOR WHILE ON PROMAZINE MEDICATION

Clinical Psychiatric			Standardized Interview			Ward Behavior		
Change	3 mos.	6 mos.	Change	3 mos.	6 mos.	Change	3 mos.	6 mos.
Improvement								
Marked	0	0	+13 up	0	0	+18 up	0	0
Moderate	6	6	+8 to +12	3	3	+11 to +17	1	1
Slight	6	9	+3 to +7	10	16	+4 to +10	8	7
No change	18	14	−2 to +2	16	9	−3 to +3	19	20
			−3 to −7	1	1	−4 to −10	2	0
			−8 to −12	0	0	−11 to −17	0	1
N	30	29*		30	29*		30	29*
Mean change	—	—		2.13	3.52		1.53	2.24
t	—	—		3.13	5.42		2.11	2.82
P	—	—		<.01	<.001		<.05	<.01

* One patient lost by transfer for treatment of pulmonary tuberculosis.

significant. Practical significance (as contrasted with statistical significance) was also deemed an important yardstick for assessing the value of a treatment method, however, and by this yardstick there was little about which to become enthusiastic. The average gain was minimal. There were no dramatic recoveries or even striking improvements. Correlations among the three evaluation procedures were quite low (median r = .23), suggesting that they tapped minimal variations in different aspects of patient behavior. From these considerations of the data, it is doubtful if any practical therapeutic significance can be ascribed to promazine medication (alone and in the dosages here prescribed) with long-term catatonic schizophrenic patients. It was the clinical impression of the senior author and ward personnel that the patients may have become somewhat more relaxed during the treatment period, but increased relaxation alone in chronic catatonic patients is a difficult variable to assess.

A comment in regard to methodology may be appropriate in the discussion at this point. In this study, each subject served as his own control. Had we been able to conclude from our data that therapeutic gains of practical significance had accrued during the course of treatment, then a follow-up study with matched control subjects would have been indicated in order to parcel out the effects of such variables as patients' knowledge that they were receiving a new medication, increased attention from personnel, and experimenter bias. A recent study by Hall and Dunlap presents a clear discussion of the hazards in making positive conclusions from drug studies without adequate safeguards of a controlled design. In our design, the limited number (local) of specifically designated chronic, regressed, catatonic schizophrenic patients were conserved in one experimental group of sufficient size so that what may have occurred with treatment was given ample opportunity to occur. Since we have concluded from the data that any practical therapeutic advantage of the medication (as prescribed and with chronically ill subjects) under study is doubtful, a controlled follow-up study is not indicated.

Side Effects

Though it was not our primary purpose to study the physiological side effects of promazine, the usual precautions in administering a new drug preparation were adhered to, and the consequent observations are, accordingly, presented as a matter of record.

There was an average increase in weight of eleven pounds ($P < .01$) during the first three months of treatment and an additional average increase of five pounds ($P < .01$) during the second three months. The weight gain was more often regarded as a desirable rather than an undesirable side effect. With few exceptions, resting blood pressure, alkaline phosphatase, white blood count, and differential counts all showed minimal changes during the study. Diastolic pressure showed a slight average drop from 75 mm. Hg to 71 mm. Hg during the first three months. Neutrophils showed a slight average increase from 59 per cent to 63 per cent during this interval. Alkaline phosophatase showed a slight average increase from 3.30 to 4.17 Bodansky units during this interval. From pre-treatment to six months there were no average trends of any importance in any of these variables (alkaline phosphatase was dropped from the routine laboratory test schedule after the first three months).

First toxic symptoms occurred with one patient fainting at the 200 mg. daily level and again at the 600 mg. daily level. At 800 mg. daily, another patient fainted. Upon reaching the 1,400 mg. daily level, two patients developed marked generalized tremor and fell to the floor. One of these patients was placed on a reduced maintenance dosage of 800 mg. daily and experienced no further difficulty.

The second of these two patients suffered a linear skull fracture from his fall. Promazine medication was discontinued, and he was given penicillin, vitamin C, and intravenous dextrose. On the sixth day after his fall his white blood count was 2,750, neutrophils 0, lymphocytes 99, monocytes 1. He had a 48-hour rise of temperature reaching a maximum of 105° (R). He received further treatment with penicillin and was given three blood transfusions. Neutrophils reappeared on the eighth day, and on the eleventh day the white blood count was 8,450 with a normal differential. The cause of this agranulocytosis was presumed to have been the administration of promazine, but the possibility of other factors in the etiology such as skull fracture or an intercurrent virus infection was considered. On the 31st day after skull fracture, the administration of promazine was cautiously resumed and built up to a dose of 600 mg. daily, which he has subsequently received for a period of five months without difficulty of any kind.

Upon reaching a dosage level of 1,800 mg. daily, four more patients developed marked tremor. Two of these fainted; one became hyperactive.

It was at the 1,800 mg. level that there was a 4-day break in the drug supply. Upon withdrawal, five patients showed transient vomiting. One patient showed repeated vomiting and was given 100 mg. promazine intramuscularly with relief. Two other patients showed marked agitation upon withdrawal. After the drug supply was renewed and medication was resumed, symptoms of vomiting and agitation were relieved.

During the last three months of the study and with a median maintenance dosage of 600 mg. daily, there has been no recurrence of any toxic symptoms. At no time have there been any such complications as jaundice, dermatitis (of either patients or personnel), edema, or Parkinsonism. Treatment interval was from October to April so that the patients were not exposed to severe insolation. With the few intramuscular injections there was no local tissue reaction even in doses up to 250 mg. in 5 cc. of water.

Summary and Conclusions

A new phenothiazine derivative, promazine, was administered to a group of 3 chronic, regressed, catatonic schizophrenic patients (median years continuous hospitalization: ten) in an initial assessment of its therapeutic effectiveness with such patients. Dosages were stepped up to 1,800 mg. daily, then reduced to a maintenance dosage of 600 mg. daily. The treatment period extended over six months. Behavioral evaluation was accomplished by three independent procedures: Clinical psychiatric judgments, a standardized interview, and ward observations. The changes in patient behavior were in the direction of improvement and were statistically significant. The average gain was minimal, however, and there was no individual instance of marked improvement. It is our conclusion that little or no therapeutic efficacy of practical significance can be attributed to promazine medication (as administered in this study) with the chronic, regressed patients under study.

Side effects were of no consequence at dosage levels up to 1,400 mg. daily. At a level of 1,400 to 1,800 mg. marked tremor developed in six patients. Tremor was followed by fainting in four of these six. Reduction to a maintenance dosage relieved these symptoms. One instance of agranulocytosis developed which responded to withdrawal of promazine and appropriate treatment. With adequate safeguards this patient was again placed on promazine with no ill effects.

Through a break in the drug supply, the patients were two days on reduced dosage and two days with no medication. Six patients showed vomiting upon withdrawal which cleared upon resumption of treatment. Such complications as jaundice, dermatitis, edema, and Parkinsonism have not been noted.

In view of the extreme chronicity and general lack of agitation of the patients under study and the low order of toxicity observed (relative to that reported in the use of chlorpromazine), it is suggested that promazine be tried with a less chronic and more disturbed group of schizophrenic patients.

THE USE OF CHLORPROMAZINE IN PSYCHOTHERAPY

H. L. Newbold, M.D., and W. David Steed, M.D.
Veterans Administration Hospital, Hines, Illinois

Since the discovery of chlorpromazine (also known as Thorazine, Largactil, Megaphen, Compound 2601-A, and R. P. 4560) in France in 1950, it has been quickly accepted by physicians as a valuable drug in certain psychiatric disorders, especially those disorders in which anxiety, aggression or agitation is a prominent symptom. It is now a well-known fact that the drug was discovered while seeking a more efficient antihistamine preparation. In 1952, its action on psychiatric patients was reported in the French literature, and it quickly came into general use on the continent. The first reports came out of this country in 1954, and in May, 1954, it became commerically available in the United States.

Following the initial reports there appeared a number of papers on the use of the drug. Although the authors have cited only a few of the reports, all of the published material had one thing in common: Each evaluated the drug on a group of patients, and the results were tabulated in terms of the whole group rather than in terms of the individual. In fact, these studies were made in terms of a large group of patients, and the findings presented the statistical changes which took place in the group. These studies failed to describe what happened psychodynamically with individual patients.

Purpose and Method

The purpose of this study was to make detailed observations of individual patients undergoing Thorazine treatment. The authors chose patients who were in regular psychotherapy. Careful observations were made on appearance, behavior, emotional reactions, content of thought and sensorium, before, during, and after chlorpromazine therapy. The conflicts and the mechanisms of defense were also studied. Behind this purpose lay the idea that it might be possible to reach some conclusions about the use of chlorpromazine in psychotherapy. Since detailed studies are time consuming, it was not felt possible to include more than four patients in this initial effort.

The four patients were all men, hospitalized in the Veterans Administration Hospital at Hines, Illinois. They were started in psychotherapy (three times weekly) several weeks before a placebo or chlorpromazine was administered and followed by the same therapist three times weekly in regularly scheduled 30-minute psychotherapeutic sessions throughout the study.

Each of the patients was given a 10-week period of treatments with Thorazine and an equal period of time with placebo. The placebos looked exactly like the chlorpromazine and were given in the same amounts at comparable stages in the treatment.

Chlorpromazine—50 mg. daily for 1 week, followed by:
Chlorpromazine—100 mg. daily for 2 weeks, followed by:
Chlorpromazine—200 mg. daily for 3 weeks, followed by:
Chlorpromazine—400 mg. daily for 4 weeks.

The second group was given a chlorpromazine placebo on the same routine as above. Neither the patient nor the psychotherapist knew which group was on the drug and which was on the placebo.

At the end of a 10-week period, the groups were reversed, i.e., the first group was placed on the placebo, and the second group was given the chlorpromazine as scheduled above. This reversal was made immediately. At the end of the last day of the 10-week period, the one type of pill was discontinued and the next morning the build-up of the other was begun.

It will be noted that the chlorpromazine was gradually built up from 50 mg. daily to 400 mg. daily, and held there for four weeks. When the drug was discontinued, it was cut off suddenly in order that the effects of the medication could be observed more clearly.

This study was arbitrarily terminated two weeks after the last medication (chlorpromazine or placebo) was discontinued regardless of the fact that the patients were continued after this in psychotherapy.

Patients in Study

Perhaps it will give a clearer picture of the study if a brief summary of the history of each patient is given.

1.S was a 26-year-old white, single, male, who lived at home and ran the farm for his elderly father and mother in addition to working as a part-time carpenter. He had been rather sterile in his interpersonal relationships all of his life. However, he remained psychologically compensated until a few months before his younger brother was released from the Army. It has never been clear what the patient's deep feelings were about his brother, although it was obvious that the brother was more favored, more aggressive, and more vocal than the patient. It is quite possible that the patient looked upon the return of his brother to the farm as a threat. The younger brother would take the patient's place as a leader, and, in effect, the patient would be working for his younger brother.

In any case 1.S began developing a depression before his brother's return. This was characterized by a feeling of hopelessness. His main complaints were about pains in his body and the fatigue associated with it. Because of the discomfort and the fatigue, he had been unable to work for over six months. He had consulted several physicians about these symptoms but had not been able to receive any significant relief. He was in the hospital approximately six months before he was started on psychotherapy with one of the authors (H. L. N.). During this period he was seen briefly several times a week on ward rounds. He was quiet and emotionally rather dull and never exhibited any strong affect. He was in group psychotherapy and was active in the regular program (including manual arts therapy).

At the time psychotherapy was initiated, the patient had lost the more dramatic elements of the depression and was complaining less of pains. He felt he was too tired to get a job again and take his place in society, even though he was at this time going to his sister's home in nearby Chicago each week-end on a pass. The psychotherapist observed that he was rather withdrawn. Interviews soon brought out frightening memories of bestiality.

His diagnosis was: Depressive reaction, super-imposed upon an underlying schizoid personality.

2.B was a 32-year-old, white, single, male crane operator who was brought to the hospital shortly before psychotherapy was begun because he had threatened to kill some men at work.

For seven years prior to admission, he had been seen in psychotherapy, one to three times weekly by private psychiatrists. No precipitating factors were found which brought about the deterioration in his condition which necessitated hospitalization.

At the time psychotherapy was started, the patient was having a few auditory hallucinations. He was moderately agitated with ideas of reference, and there was a great deal of somatization accompanied by death fantasies. His ego strength was at such low ebb that he immediately produced a great deal of hostility and homosexual material in therapy. The picture was essentially the same when he was started on this research program.

The diagnosis was: Schizophrenic reaction, paranoid type.

3.K was a 38-year-old, white, married, male draftsman who had always led a very restricted emotional life. He was very religious and claimed he never had any hostile feelings of any kind. "That's not the American way," he would say. He said that he did not enjoy sexual relations with his wife, but did have intercourse "to get a family."

His hospitalization was precipitated by his father-in-law's death. The old man had moved in with the patient about a year previously and had rented out his own house, thus earning money at the patient's expense. The situation was made more tense because the father-in-law suffered from chronic pulmonary edema and coughed a great deal. While in the Army, the patient had been hospitalized for a protracted period of time for observation because of pulmonary scars. The father-in-law's lung trouble stirred up all of 3.K's anxieties in this area.

When the father-in-law died, the patient became very disturbed and left the house in his bed clothes one wintry night. The next morning when the psychotherapist saw him, 3.K had lost his agitation. He was depressed, somewhat withdrawn and admitted having heard threatening voices. His condition was essentially the same when he was started on this research program.

Diagnosis was: Schizophrenic reaction, schizo-affective type with depression.

4.P was a 33-year-old white, single, unemployed male who was discharged from the Navy in 1944 with a diagnosis of anxiety reaction. Upon reviewing the history, it would seem that this diagnosis was justified at that time; however, over the course of years, alcoholism became an increasing problem with this man. For example, he was admitted to the Veterans Administration Hospital, Hines, Illinois, 10 times for severe disturbances associated with alcoholism in the five years preceding this admission. During this period he had worked very little, had been in minor difficulties culminating in his being jailed several times, and had had only one interpersonal tie, which had been severed four months prior to his admission. During the months preceding this hospitalization, the patient had led the life of an alcoholic derelict while living on West Madison Street in the most degenerate environment imaginable.

At the time of this hospitalization, he was intoxicated, had generalized tremors and was suffering from visual hallucinations.

Before starting on the research program, he was free of his hallucinations, was in good contact and was able to follow the therapeutic activities program on the ward.

Diagnosis was: Passive aggressive personality with alcoholism.

Results

Although careful detailed observations were made throughout all phases of the project, it was not possible to point out specific effects of the chlorpromazine during the gradual buildup and the maintenance dosage. All patients got along reasonably well during this time with fluctuations compatible with their total situation.

The abrupt discontinuance of the chlorpromazine, however, brought sudden dramatic changes which could be correlated precisely chronologically with the discontinuance of the chlorpromazine. Sudden dramatic changes were present at this time in each of the four patients, regardless of whether the chlorpromazine was followed immediately by placebos. Furthermore there was no dramatic change when the placebos were discontinued in any case. The changes which occurred on termination of the chlorpromazine are delineated below for each individual patient.

1.S (the farm boy, part time carpenter, who was diagnosed as depressive reaction in a schizoid personality) had more energy immediately after the chlorpromazine was discontinued. He was less depressed, his dreams seemed more real to him, guilt feelings showed up in the dreams for the first time, he stated he was full of feelings (affect) which was very different from his usual self, he talked more freely in therapy, he had more anxiety, and for the first time he discussed his future and the possibility of obtaining employment.

It is interesting to note that this man looked upon the medication as a threat to him. It made him more lethargic and psychologically impotent so that it seemed to him that his depression was returning. Later when the placebo dosage was started, he protested against taking it. At that time he stated he did not want the medication, that he would rather put up with his tension (which had come upon having the chlorpromazine withdrawn) than to feel constantly tired.

He actually did feel tired again when placed on the placebo; however, this cleared up in a few days and there was no sudden change noted when the placebo was later discontinued.

2.B (the crane operator diagnosed as a schizophrenic reaction, paranoid type) cried for the first time in therapy on the day after chlorpromazine was discontinued. He was generally more active both physically and psychologically, and there was an increase in the warmth of his interpersonal relationship with the therapists. He dreamed for the first time. When he had homosexual preoccupations, he was able to say "to heck with them" (evidence of more ego strength), he talked of future plans for the first time, he had some insomnia and a few somatic complaints, he helped out on the ward work for the first time, and he would listen to the psychotherapist's comments with much more interest.

This man had no change in his psychological status after the placebo was discontinued.

3.K (the inhibited draftsman with a diagnosis of schizophrenic reaction, schizo-affective type) exhibited a marked change the next day after the chlorpromazine was discontinued. To sum it up, he disintegrated. During the course of therapy, he had lost the depressive aspects of his illness, he had been in good contact on an open ward and had been taking week-end passes home even though his personality had remained about as rigid as before.

However, after the chlorpromazine was discontinued, he became very depressed and was retarded in his speech, movement and thought. He was certain that he was about to die. He developed the delusion that his wife was dead and another woman, similar to her, had been substituted in her place. His wife, a woman very devoted to him, asked that he not be given any more week-end passes because of this strange behavior. He became confused, was unable to follow the program on the open ward, and had to be returned to a more regulated environment.

There had been no change in his condition when the placebo was discontinued.

4.P (the man who had been wandering up and down West Madison Street, chronically intoxicated, with the diagnosis of passive-aggressive personality, with alcoholism) had adjusted well to the open ward routine, was generally friendly and had established a close emotional relationship with the therapist and was attempting to deal with problems of hostility.

As soon as the medication was discontinued, he became very hostile. This was such a problem with him that he could hardly concentrate on his work in manual arts therapy. He slept poorly and his tremor returned. He was argumentative with the hospital personnel and with other patients. At this time he became angry because some of the other patients would get the newspaper which came to the ward every morning and he would have to wait his turn to read it. He began buying his own paper and, after reading it, would tear it into little pieces and throw it away. While in therapy session he would became so angry that he could not follow a train of thought or help work through his dream material.

Discussion and Conclusions

It is noted that the close psychotherapeutic relationship demonstrated no impairment of intellectual functioning during the course of chlorpromazine treatment, nor any change in the intellectual abilities when chlorpromazine was discontinued. However, all patients showed evidence of a marked accentuation in feelings when chlorpromazine was discontinued. 4.P had exhibited prominent feelings of hostility well controlled during chlorpromazine therapy. When the drug was stopped, the hostility became incapacitating. In another, depression had been the predominant affect, but it was not incapacitating during chlorpromazine therapy. When this therapy was discontinued, he developed a psychotic reaction, schizo-affective type with depression. Another cried and dreamed for the first time after being removed from chlorpromazine. These observations indicate stronger affect. This latter patient also became mildly insomniac and showed a new anxiety about somatic symptoms, associated with an increase in psychic and physical activity. The authors feel that these symptoms can be attributed to an increase in affect.

The other patient described himself as full of feelings, including anxiety. Dreams were more real and guilt showed in them for the first time. This patient, though inhibited in his expression of feelings, certainly expressed them more than at any time in his hospitalization. We believe that the affect which had been mobilized by the psychotherapy was expressed only after the chlorpromazine was discontinued.

It would appear to the authors that chlorpromazine in some way masks the affect and thus reduces the amount of anxiety experienced by the ego. This would seem to fit very well with the studies which have pointed out that disturbed wards are quieter when chlorpromazine is used. With less affect and therefore less anxiety, there is less acting out of the affects and less need for defense mechanisms.

The role of chlorpromazine in psychotherapy can be discussed from the standpoint of these four patients and also this theoretical standpoint.

In the four patients discussed here the affect was much increased when the chlorpromazine was discontinued. The question arises whether this was helpful in the psychotherapy. It is noted that 3.K and 4.P were unable to deal with problems psychotherapeutically after discontinuance of the chlorpromazine. Attempts at psychotherapy had to be dropped with 3.K. On the other hand, 1.S and 2.B made more rapid progress after being removed from chlorpromazine treatment.

Psychotherapy requires that mutually meaningful communications be established between the patient and the therapist. Many factors, of course, influence this. A common variable is the degree of disturbance of the patient. If the disturbance is too great, then the psychotherapy is impeded or is ineffective. On the other hand, unless there is some disturbance, experienced as discomfort by the patient, there is no motivation for psychotherapy by the patient.

It appears to us that we experienced several types of situations in this project. 3.K and 4.P seemed to deal more effectively with psychotherapy while receiving relatively large amounts of chlorpromazine. When the medication was discontinued, they were too disturbed for psychotherapy. 1.S and 2.B, on the other hand, did better after being removed from chlorpromazine. Their anxiety was notably increased at this time, but they did not become disorganized and the psychotherapy seemed more effective.

The results of this investigation suggest that chlorpromazine is useful in psychotherapy when it reduces internal disturbance enough to allow good contact with the therapist. On the other hand, psychotherapy may be impeded by a dosage which is high enough to dull the effects and/or the motivation for treatment.

PRELIMINARY REPORT ON FIVE HUNDRED PATIENTS TREATED WITH THORAZINE AT ROCHESTER STATE HOSPITAL

Benjamin Pollack, M.D.

The use of thorazine was first begun in Rochester (N. Y.) State Hospital in June 1954, but the vast majority of treated patients there have been on this therapy for a period of one to nine months at the time of writing. The group treated has comprised 170 male and 330 female patients, a total of 500. Most of them have been in the hospital a considerable time. Each patient has been carefully followed, with periodic summary charts. The observations in this paper are the result of personal evaluations by the author, as well as by the physicians in charge, by the supervisor of nurses of each service, and by nurses and attendants who have been in frequent contact with the treated patients.

Patients were selected from every service in the hospital and free choice in the selection was given to the physicians in charge of the services. Various forms of treatment procedure were used in each service, both as regards dosage and type of administration. In general, an attempt was made to choose patients with "mobile emotion" directed toward themselves or others. Thorazine was administered, likewise, to a number who were usually or constantly in restraint or seclusion. Various studies were instituted, and the results will be outlined later in this paper.

Comparison with Lobotomized Patients

An attempt was made to evaluate the use of thorazine as a prognostic test for patients upon whom prefrontal lobotomy operations were contemplated. It would appear that thorazine is a valuable aid in determining the choice of patients for such operations; but, as a matter of fact, lobotomies have been indefinitely deferred for some patients because of the marked improvement in them following treatment with thorazine. It is important to realize that these patients had previously been treated with insulin, electric shock, or other types of therapy—with temporary, slight, or no results. Some patients were treated who had demonstrated only transient improvement following prefrontal lobotomies and who had then continued with their disturbed behavior or their delusional ideas. A number of such patients have been maintained in a stable state by thorazine. No tendency to increased convulsions was noted with its use.

Comparison with Electric Shock

There is apparent emphatic unanimity of the medical staff of this hospital about the efficiency of thorazine as contrasted with electric shock. A group of patients who required maintenance electric shock to retain improvement was placed on thorazine. With pratically no exceptions, they could be maintained in as good or better condition than when on electric shock. Some who had remained in the hospital because they needed maintenance doses of electric shock have left on home visits or have been transferred to better wards since they have been receiving thorazine; and they have continued to maintain improvement without additional shock. A small number have been treated with both thorazine and electric shock. Experience at Rochester is limited in this field, but it would appear that thorazine does not potentiate, or change in any way, the dosage of electric shock required. There is a growing list of patients who previously failed to respond to electric shock but who have shown rather astonishing improvement with continued therazine treatment. This group consists, for the most part, of patients who were formerly described as regressed. Many of them were irritable and resistive and were cared for in restraint or seclusion on the disturbed wards.

Since thorazine has been given on the continued treatment services, the number of electric shock treatments has decreased tremendously. Before thorazine was used, there was a daily average of 300 patients treated with electric shock; at the present time, the average is only nine so treated; and these are suffering from retarded depressions or involutional melancholia.

Indications

Thorazine acts by facilitating communication and permitting an objective viewpoint of the stresses and difficulties which are upsetting the individual. Thus, it is useful in situations associated with anxiety, fear, apprehension, suspicion, certain depressions, and hypochondriacal states. Observers at Rochester are in general agreement that agitated, openly hostile, aggressive, excited, overactive, anxious, fearful, and resistive patients show a high response to this medication. It would appear that with certain exceptions much the same favorable prognostic signs that have been used to select prefrontal lobotomy patients can be used to select patients for thorazine. Favorable cases are patients with purposeful, aggressive or sadistic tendencies. Others are those with anxiety, mood swings, obsessive-compulsive tendencies, hysterical, and hypochondriacal manifestations. Patients with paranoid states, with much emotional instability in chronic functional or organic psychoses, may show very good responses, but there are many unexplained failures. It may be that some of these are due to inadequate dosage. Catatonic states with fluctuations, particularly those in which there is stupor or excitement, mutism, or refusal to take food, appear to indicate a good response. Chronic psychotic states which show periodic remissions spontaneously, or under electric shock, or which are maintained in remission by electric shock or ambulatory insulin, likewise show generally excellent results with Thorazine. Patients who have chronic psychotic states, with periodic fluctuations in mood or in intensity of their reactions to their psychoses or in their delusions or hallucinations, do well under treatment. Occasionally, chronic psychotics with purposeless periods of excitement that are not apparently related to exogenous or endogenous stimuli may show improvement.

Some patients, ill for a long time, showed initial improvement with thorazine and then relapsed within a week. However, continued treatment resulted in improvement again, and apparent reintegration occurred. This was particularly notable in behavior changes, rather than in content of psychosis, although, in many patients, delusional contents gradually became less marked as the patients felt more comfortable. This period of reintegration was associated with a gradual reduction in the intensity of delusional content. In a number of patients this was rather marked, so that finally hallucinations and delusions either entirely disappeared or their presence was difficult to elicit.

Effect on the Use of Restraint

A group of 85 patients who had histories of restraint or seclusion for many years was selected for treatment. At the time of writing, 42 of these patients have been out of restraint or seclusion for a month or more, 32 still require one or the other most of the time, and the remaining 11 patients now require either treatment infrequently.

Continued experience has definitely shown that thorazine is a very effective agent in reducing the amount of restraint and seclusion needed. With the use of thorazine extended throughout the entire hospital, a great deal of the restraint previously used has been eliminated, particularly during the daytime. Most of the restraint that is still being used, is for nonpsychiatric reasons, and at night for restless, feeble, bedridden, elderly patients. On many services restraint has been almost entirely abandoned. Again, it must be emphasized at this point that, coincident with the use of thorazine, other measures must be instituted, so that the patients' activities, and particularly their aggressive impulses, are utilized in more productive and beneficial fields.

Involutional Psychoses

The writer has been impressed with the effect of thorazine on patients with involutional psychosis, both melancholia and paranoid types, where there is fairly marked emotion or signs of motor restlessness, particularly if associated with much anxiety or apprehension. Fear in such patients, which is expressed in the form of delusional material and kinetic outflow, seems also to lead to favorable results. In the present series, the number of patients with this diagnosis is too small to make any but general observations, but it would appear that results with thorazine may not be proportionately so effective or so rapid as those with electric shock. It must be remembered that many thorazine-treated patients were those who had not shown sustained results with electric shock. However, about 50 per cent of such patients responded favorably to thorazine. Including the more acutely ill patients in the figures, 88 per cent displayed significant improvement in behavior and 71 per cent in their psychoses. Improvement in this group was maintained either when thorazine was used alone or when it was given following series of electric shock treatments. Such patients may be maintained at home with thorazine.

Outpatient Treatment

Thorazine has been used on patients who have applied for voluntary admission to the hospital. Patients who were not too depressed, agitated, or suspicious for a trial to be made were given thorazine and advised to remain out of the hospital. It seems evident that hospitalization can be avoided in the majority of carefully selected patients, where the co-operation of the patient and his family can be obtained. A number of such patients have been treated without complications. At least half of these patients were well known to the staff, as they had previously been admitted to the hospital. Some of these latter patients would not co-operate because they knew what electric shock had done for them in the past and insisted upon admission to the hospital for this treatment. They thus took thorazine in a perfunctory manner and in a few days returned, stating that the drug was ineffective and demanding hospital readmission. Many such patients were continued on thorazine after readmission with effective results. Thorazine has also been continued on patients leaving the hospital on convalescent care. Maintenance doses of 50 to 100 mgs. are given once or twice daily. It is felt that the medication should not be discontinued when the patient leaves the hospital, since there are many additional stresses which he will encounter in adjustment at home and which make medication at least temporarily essential to maintain stability. At present, 103 patients who have been treated with thorazine are at home, either on convalescent care or discharged after voluntary admission. Thorazine medication when given to patients out of the hospital is always accompanied by a warning concerning the dangers of driving a car or working with machinery. A number of patients who have shown a tendency to relapse while on convalescent care have been

Table 1. Distribution by Diagnosis of 103 Patients Now Out of the Hospital

Diagnosis		Per cent
Schizophrenia		53
Catatonic	22	
Paranoid	26	
Hebephrenic	5	
Manic-depressive psychosis		7
Manic	4	
Depressive	3	
Involutional psychosis		17
Melancholia	11	
Paranoid	6	
Arteriosclerotic and senile psychoses		7
Psychoneurosis		11
Psychosis with psychopathic personality		3
Psychosis with mental deficiency		2

treated with thorazine; and, in the majority of such patients, a return to the hospital has been avoided. The distribution by diagnosis of thorazine-treated patients on convalescent care or discharged can be seen from Table 1.

TREATMENT OF ELDERLY PATIENTS

A number of patients diagnosed as having a senile psychosis or psychosis with cerebral arteriosclerosis have been treated with thorazine, and in 78 per cent of them, favorable responses have been noted. These were seen particularly in patients who were extremely agitated, restless, hostile, or resistive. A word of caution should be introduced that this drug is not as innocuous as perhaps has been assumed in the treatment of elderly patients, particularly of those who show unstable vascular systems or who have histories of myocardial disorder. At Rochester, six elderly patients receiving thorazine died of cardiac disease. It is not clear whether the drug played a role in these deaths, but the number is proportionally large, and would indicate that perhaps thorazine, by depressing the blood pressure and slowing the circulation, breaks down the cardiovascular balance of the body. In five of the six, there were sudden cardiovascular collapses after the drug had been taken for periods ranging from two days to three weeks. In at least two, it is felt that Thorazine may have been implicated. All six had some type of cardiovascular disease—compensated in some cases. All had been adjusting to the drug generally satisfactorily and had become quiet and fairly co-operative. Each of the six, without warning, showed a sudden change, characterized by labored respirations and rapid pulse rate; and death followed shortly. One patient, who had had a previous myocardial infarct and who had been in a marked state of excitement for some time, showed a good response to thorazine for some weeks and then died suddenly. Unfortunately, this is the only one of the six upon whom there was an autopsy.

One patient, aged 61, diagnosed as having a psychosis with cerebral arteriosclerosis, had been showing a good response to thorazine for two weeks. She had become quiet, co-operative and alert, and had lost much of her confusion. Then she suddenly had a series of convulsive seizures, during which she seemed to be critically ill. She was unconscious and in a state of collapse. Before thorazine administration, her blood pressure was 220/106; afterward, 146/90. It is pure conjecture, but it is possible that even a minor drop in blood pressure in elderly hypertensive patients may lead to premature thromboses in either the cerebral or coronary arteries. There have been no convulsive seizures in young patients.

In some of the confused, elderly patients there has been—coincident with improvement in their excited, restless states—a loss of confusion and delusions. It would appear that reducing physical overactivities tends, in certain patients, to cause an improvement in the mental state. This may, of course, result from decreasing the amount of blood required by the muscles, and, at the same time, permitting the patient to eat a better diet.

BLOOD PRESSURE CHANGES

An attempt was made to follow blood pressure changes; but they did not reveal any definite or consistent findings. In most patients, particularly where there was much restlessness or emotional drive, the systolic blood pressure fell—with a less marked fall of the diastolic blood pressure. In many regressed schizophrenics, very little change was noted. In the majority of patients, the diastolic blood pressure returned to almost its pre-treatment level, while the systolic pressure varied from very marked changes to minimal changes a week to two months after treatment. In some patients, however, rather marked falls occurred, such as one to 80/60 in a patient whose pressure had previously been 124/80. It was impossible to predict from blood pressure alone which patients would complain of such hypotensive symptoms as weakness, fainting, dizziness, or headaches. Some appeared entirely comfortable with their lower blood pressures, while others complained of dizziness and headaches, particularly on rapid movement.

As previously mentioned, extra care should be used in administering this drug to elderly patients. It should be pointed out that there were variable responses in the blood pressures in this group, with little correlation between blood pressure changes and clinical symptoms. Many elderly persons treated were either extremely restless, ambulant patients, or were overactive, bedridden ones.

There was one case of tachycardia, in a 35-year-old woman who had essential hypertension and whose blood pressure at the beginning of treatment was 190/110. After three days with thorazine, she developed a tachycardia with a pulse rate of 144, coincident with a continued fall in blood pressure, which dropped to 140/80 on the sixth day. When treatment was discontinued, the blood pressure rose for three days, and the pulse rate fell. On the fourth day after treatment ended, the blood pressure was 190/110, and the pulse rate varied between 80 and 90.

Dosage

The drug can be given either orally or intramuscularly. As far as can be determined there is no advantage in the latter procedure, except where it is impossible to give medication by mouth. For the vast majority of patients the daily initial dosage was 200 mgs.; this was increased every three days by 25 to 50 mgs. until the maximum response was obtained. Most patients were maintained at daily dosages between 200 and 400 mgs.; occasionally 600 mgs. were given. Larger dosages appear unnecessary and do not produce additional improvement. It seems better to begin with doses in the higher range, since complications seem less marked and less prolonged, and hypotensive symptoms with headaches, dizziness, and feelings of weakness seem to vanish much more quickly than with smaller dosages.

In elderly patients much caution was used, and, where possible, they were kept in bed for the first few days of treatment. For the most part, they were treated with the smaller doses, since it was quickly learned that more than 200 mgs. made such patients very drowsy. A very few patients who were almost continuously excited seemed to show no response to this drug. Most of the failures probably resulted from inadequate dosage. In the present series, the physicians in charge noted behavior improvement in 88 per cent of all treated patients according to the observations of the physicians in charge of these patients. In an independent survey, the supervising nurses judged that 83 per cent of such patients have shown behavior improvement. This is a surprising consistency of findings. Thorazine was given both orally and intramuscularly. Oral dosages were between 100 and 600 mgs. daily, and the intramuscular dosages between 100 and 400 mgs. daily.

Initially, thorazine was administered—whether orally or intramuscularly—four times a day because of the impression that its action was short-lived and probably would not persist for longer than six hours. This impression had been obtained from experience elsewhere—it had been demonstrated that thorazine had an anti-emetic effect lasting for six hours on antabuse-alcohol reactions. It would appear, after various trials, that the action of thorazine persists for a much longer period. The dosage schedule is now altered so that patients start on this medication with doses only twice, or at the most three times, a day. As far as can be judged, the results are as effective as with more frequent dosage. Maintenance doses are now of various types. One group of patients who have shown sustained improvement now get 50 mgs. each, twice a day; another group, 50 mgs. once a day; and a third group, 50 mgs. every other day.

At first, patients receiving intramuscular injections remained in bed for an hour after treatment. Most of these were chronic, regressed schizophrenics. They developed few complaints following injections, however, and at present are not put to bed but are allowed up and about. There have been no hypotensive reactions in this group.

COMPLICATIONS AND SIDE EFFECTS

Many patients on the larger doses complained at first of some dizziness, weakness and lethargy. They could readily be aroused, however, and would quickly become alert on stimulation or conversation or when their attention was sustained by external and environmental events. In a few—particularly in the older group—drowsiness was such that it was necessary to administer small doses of dexedrine, 5 mg., once or twice a day. In the vast majority, drowsiness, weakness, lethargy, and complaints of headache and dizziness disappeared in three to four days. In a small number, these symptoms were present at all times within 15 minutes to one-half hour after intramuscular injection or one hour after oral ingestion, but the symptoms quickly disappeared and generally did not persist for more than an hour. While there was no apparent tolerance built up, symptoms gradually decreased in intensity, and in the majority of patients disappeared after the first or second week of treatment. Patients with symptoms did not appear confused, and there was no obvious intellectual impairment.

In the entire series of 500 patients, only four markedly severe hypotensive reactions with fainting attacks occurred. These quickly responded to bed care and required no further treatment. Thorazine treatment was continued, and the hypotensive effects disappeared.

One case of agranulocytosis appeared suddenly in a patient who complained of sore throat and malaise. The white blood count was only 550 cells, all lymphocytes. The patient died the following day.

Dermatitis. Seven nurses who had given intramuscular injections of thorazine developed dermatitis of the hands, and in two cases, of the face also. There was a maculopapular rash on the hands, or on the hands and face, with some slight edematous reaction, which might be on the face or the back of the neck. Besides these seven nurses, two others developed a scaly, marked erythematous reaction on the hands. This was treated with hydrocortisone because of its severity. Nurses giving intramuscular injections of thorazine have now been instructed to wear gloves. A generalized dermatitis developed in 3 per cent of the patients treated, mostly within two weeks of treatment. This consisted of a maculopapular rash which began at first on the hands, face, and neck, and later spread to the chest, occasionally to the back, and frequently to the legs. In most of these patients this was intensely itchy. They were treated with antihistaminics and by cessation of thorazine treatment.

Jaundice. Clinical and obvious jaundice occurred in 4 per cent of the total series. The ages of the patients affected varied from 46 to 82. This jaundice was not accompanied by marked symptoms, except for complaints of itching of the skin, and of course, obvious discoloration of the skin and sclera. If elevation of temperature occurred, it was minimal, and no active treatment was required. The icteric index and van den Bergh tests indicated an obstructive type of jaundice. Patients were re-treated with thorazine after the dermatitis or jaundice disappeared; and, except for two, there was no return of the complication. In addition to the patients just described, a number had yellowish discolorations of the sclera without corresponding skin changes. They were continued on treatment with no aggravation of jaundice. Several liver biopsies were done on patients with jaundice, disclosing swollen bile canaliculi which had become invaded by lymphocytes. There was no evidence of necrosis, cirrhosis, or parenchymal damage.

Other Side Effects. A number of patients complained of rather marked dryness of the mouth. No cases of Parkinsonism developed, perhaps because the dosage level never exceeded 600 mgs. pr day. A few patients complained of gastritis after treatment, and a few likewise reported constipation. Some of the younger women stated that their menstrual periods—while they were on thorazine—were free from painful cramps experienced previously. A few patients developed a rather grayish facial pallor, and this seemed to be associated with a wooden expression. There were few complaints of "grippe-like" states. Some patients complained of blurred vision, of tremors of the extremities, of feeling faint, weak, slowed-up or unsteady. Others reported that their reactions and their skill in fine work were impaired. Although the drug produced tremors in some patients, choreiform movements were almost entirely controlled in three out of six patients who had Huntington's chorea.

Need for Total Push Program

It is important to remember that the medication is only one step in the treatment of the patient. The drug makes the patient more accessible to psychotherapy and to a total push program. In this, occupational therapy, recreational therapy, habit training, and social acclimatization and competition play vital roles in a process of continuing and final rehabilitation, especially in patients who have been ill for long periods.

The patients themselves appreciated their improvement, and questioning would bring out such statements as: "I feel relaxed"; "I am comfortable"; "I feel good"; "I don't seem to worry any more"; "my troubles don't seem so great." Many patients became more communicative in a normal fashion and lost their previous reactions to trends or their oversensitivity to environmental or endogenous stimuli.

Effect on Employees' Morale

A byproduct in research programs like this—and one which should be stressed and which plays an important role—is the stimulus given to the ward personnel in the treatment of patients. The ward personnel are extremely enthusiastic about this medication. Various comments are: "The ward seems quiet"; "there appear to be no annoyances on the ward"; "the work seems more interesting because the patients can talk and react as individuals." This stimulation of the personnel plays an important role in the individual treatment afforded by them to the patients and has awakened the interest of attendants and nurses in therapy. The attempt has been made to increase and maintain such interest by assigning small tasks so that ward workers can feel that they play some part in the research and therapeutic program. They have been assigned to write individual reports and observations on the patients on their services, to take blood pressures and pulse rates, and to discuss frequently the aims and objectives of the treatment, some of the signs of improvement, and possible complications which might occur. Although both intramuscular and oral administration have been used, there has been little complaint by the personnel of the additional work.

Case Summaries

The following brief summaries illustrate the changes that have occurred in some of the treated patients:

M. D.

This woman was admitted to Rochester State Hospital in 1941 at the age of 38 with a history of four previous admissions, on all of which she had been diagnosed as a manic-depressive, manic type. During her most recent hospitalization, she had shown very frequent attacks of excitement, with overactivity, flight of ideas, distractibility, and elation. At times she was destructive, assaultive, impulsive, noisy, and frequently required restaint.

Thorazine treatment was begun on October 27, 1954, at which time 50 mgs. was given four times a day. Initially, this was given intramuscularly, and, then, as the patient became more co-operative, orally. On November 1, she was quiet, agreeable, co-operative, and out of restraint. On November 15, she was still receiving 200 mgs. per day. She had continued to be ambulatory, cheerful, co-operative and quiet, and was able to care for herself. Restraint had not been required since the beginning of treatment. Her blood pressure before treatment was 128/88, and a half-hour after treatment it was reported as 124/92. On December 6, her conduct was exemplary; she was now pleasant, friendly, quiet, co-operative and slept well. She is being maintained on 50 mgs. of thorazine, given once daily.

R. A.

This 43-year-old woman was admitted to the hospital on January 30, 1950 with a history of an illness of possibly seven years duration. She was diagnosed as suffering from dementia praecox, paranoid type. She had a grandiose delusional system, with many ideas of persecution, which became much more extensive with the passage of years. Several courses of electric shock treatment brought only temporary improvement in her behavior. At all times, however, her paranoid delusions persisted. She was seclusive, irritable, constantly preoccupied, and at times assaultive without provocation. She generally took no part in ward activities.

At times, there was a temporary improvement in the intensity of her reaction, and she would leave the hospital for a short period, but would always have to be returned. She had not been out of the hospital for three and one-half years when thorazine treatment was begun on October 30, 1954 with 100 mgs. daily. This was quickly increased to 200 and then 300 mgs.; and, finally, by November 15, she was receiving 400 mgs. per day by mouth. On November 13, she was reported as having improved markedly in behavior, in that she was less resistive and irritable and had begun to mingle with some of the others on the ward. It was also noted that she began to take part in recreational activities. Her delusional content was still present, unchanged, but she showed an increasingly better adjustment to her surroundings and gradually became much more friendly.

On December 14, she was seen to have lost all her restlessness; she seemed calm and relaxed. She recalled her delusions and seemed surprised that she had entertained them. She is now cheerful, friendly, and causes no difficulty. She was released on convalescent care on December 23, and placed on a maintenance dosage of 200 mgs. per day. She has continued to maintain her improved state for the three months she has been home at the time of this writing.

R. D.

R. D. is a 57-year-old woman who was admitted to Rochester State Hospital on October 1, 1953 with a history of five electric shock treatments at a general hospital for a disorder which had been present for over a month. At the time of admission, she was sullen, resistive, thought her food was poisoned, and frequently refused to eat. She appeared agitated and restless and thought imaginary machines were going to cut off her fingers. She was actively hallucinated and expressed many delusions of persecution. Her diagnosis was involutional psychosis, paranoid type.

For a year before thorazine was instituted, she had required frequent seclusion. She had received 70 electric shock treatments without any obvious improvement. On October 27, 1954 she was placed on thorazine and the dosage was gradually increased from 300 mgs. intramuscularly to 500 mgs. intramuscularly on November 1. On November 10, she was seen to be markedly improved; she had become pleasant, co-operative, agreeable, and caused no difficulties. On November 24, she continued her improved state on oral medication of 200 mgs. per day.

On December 16, it was noted that she was still markedly improved; she was pleasant, friendly, neat and tidy, and no paranoid trend could be elicited. She had good insight and was appreciative of the improvement which had occurred. She was placed in convalescent care on this date and was given 100 mgs. of thorazine daily while at home. She was recently placed on 50 mgs. per day and has continued to be well in four months at home.

M. F.

M. F., an 82-year-old woman, was admitted to the hospital on September 10, 1954, diagnosed as senile psychosis, with an agitated depression of three months' duration which had not responded to electric shock given in a previous hospitalization. She had had a previous admission to another state hospital in 1946 for an attempted suicide. On the present admission, she showed memory defects for recent and remote events; she was disoriented for time and place, but her personality seemed to be fairly well preserved. She was restless, overtalkative, paranoid, suspicious, resistive, and at times assaultive. On September 15, she was started on 75 mgs. of thorazine daily by mouth. On September 30, she had improved markedly; her restlessness and insomnia had disappeared, and she seemed co-operative and normally productive. There were no complaints, she felt well and her previous trend had disappeared. She was released from the hospital on January 29, 1955 and is still out of the hospital.

Results

The largest group treated consisted of schizophrenics, who comprised 285 of the total series of 500. No patients were included in Table 2 who had not had at least a month of treatment. Some of the group had been maintained on regular doses of electric shock, but many patients who formerly were resistive to all treatments are included. Some of these demonstrated rather dramatic and unexpected improvements on thorazine. Some displayed prompt improvement in behavior, but the effect upon the psychosis was not so evident until after one or two months. In some, the psychosis seemed to disappear gradually, and in others to collapse suddenly. Many were able to discuss their previous trends and actions with surprisingly good objective recall. The following table indicates the results of treatment in schizophrenic patients without consideration of the duration of psychosis:

The decided changes in behavior indicated by the groupings from "much improved" to apparently normal behavior were thus shown by 67 per cent of

Table 2. Schizophrenia—285 Patients

Result	Behavior Per cent	Psychosis Per cent
Recovered (social)	10	4
Markedly improved	21	7
Much improved	36	22
Improved	19	18
Unimproved	14	49

the treated schizophrenics. The psychosis in this group was noted as varying from "much improved" to socially "recovered" in 33 per cent of the patients.

When the series is broken down according to the duration of psychosis, the results become much more significant, indicating, as was expected, that the patients ill for less than one year had much better prognoses than those ill from one to five years. This contrast in prognosis was very marked when the group that was ill five years or more was contrasted with the group ill for a shorter period. This is particularly evident in the degree of recovery from psychosis and is somewhat less marked in improvement of behavior.

It is recognized that diagnosis alone is no indication for treatment with thorazine. As it has already been pointed out, the behavior, particularly the emotional

Table 3. Results According to Duration of Psychosis in 285 Treated Schizophrenics*

Result	Under 1 year B**	Under 1 year P**	1 to 5 years B**	1 to 5 years P**	Over 5 years B**	Over 5 years P**
Recovered (social)	43	21	20	9	4	2
Markedly improved	29	29	28	23	21	4
Much improved	14	21	23	17	42	23
Improved	7	0	20	17	19	20
Unimproved	7	29	9	34	14	51
	100	100	100	100	100	100

*Of the total of 285, the under-1-year group was 7 per cent; the 1-to-5-year group, 20 per cent; the over-5-year group, 73 per cent.
B**,—Behavior. P**—Psychosis.

reaction, of the patient appears to be the crucial indication for such therapy. It might however be of interest to indicate the results obtained by the use of thorazine in the other diagnostic categories shown in Table 4. These should be interpreted as indicating significant trends. Table 5 summarizes the results for the whole 500 patients.

SUMMARY

1. In a group of 500 patients treated with thorazine from one to nine months, an over-all behavior improvement was noted in 89 per cent. The behavior improvement was obvious (much improved to social recovery) in 74 per cent. The total improvement in psychosis was 60 per cent, with obvious improvement (much improved or better) in 44 per cent.

2. Much improved to apparently normal behavior was noted in 85 per cent of the treated manic-depressive and a much improved to socially recovered state occurred in the psychoses of 80 per cent of these same patients. Of 285 treated schizophrenics, obvious improvement in behavior was seen in 67 per cent, and a similar change in psychosis in 33 per cent. When the schizophrenics were broken down according to duration of psychosis, it was seen that there was an obvious improvement in psychosis in 71 per cent of those who had been ill for one to five years. and in 29 per cent of those ill for five years or

Table 4. Results by Diagnostic Categories Other Than Schizophrenia

Manic-depressive psychosis	B* Per cent	P* Per cent	Involutional psychosis (Melancholia and paranoid)	B* Per cent	P* Per cent
Recovered (social)	50	30	Recovered (social)	17	13
Markedly improved	15	35	Markedly improved	46	21
Much improved	20	15	Much improved	25	37
Improved	5	5	Improved	8	21
Unimproved	10	15	Unimproved	4	8

Psychoneurosis	B* Per cent	P* Per cent	Arteriosclerotic and senile psychoses	B* Per cent	P* Per cent
Recovered (social)	18	5	Recovered (social)	6	0
Markedly improved	44	48	Markedly improved	14	8
Much improved	21	22	Much improved	58	14
Improved	4	4	Improved	14	20
Unimproved	13	21	Unimproved	8	58

Psychosis with epilepsy	B* Per cent	P* Per cent	Psychosis with mental deficiency	B* Per cent	P* Per cent
Recovered (social)	25	0	Recovered (social)	27	18
Markedly improved	50	25	Markedly improved	37	28
Much improved	13	38	Much improved	9	27
Improved	12	25	Improved	27	0
Unimproved	0	12	Unimproved	0	27

Psychosis with alcohol, drugs, psychopaths	B* Per cent	P* Per cent	Psychosis with mixed organic brain disease	B* Per cent	P* Per cent
Recovered (social)	69	46	Recovered (social)	0	0
Markedly improved	15	31	Markedly improved	29	14
Much improved	8	8	Much improved	29	14
Improved	0	8	Improved	14	29
Unimproved	8	7	Unimproved	28	43

B—Behavior; P—Psychosis.

Table 5. 500 Patients—All Psychiatric Diagnoses Treated

	Behavior Per cent	Psychosis Per cent
Recovered (social)	15	7
Markedly improved	25	15
Much improved	34	22
Improved	15	16
Unimproved	11	40

more. The over-all quality of the improvement was very much greater in those sick one year or less. Of these, 21 per cent were considered socially recovered; of those sick one to five years, 9 per cent, socially recovered; and of those sick five years or more, only 2 per cent. In the involutional group, both melancholic and paranoid type, 88 per cent displayed much improvement or better in behavior and 71 per cent much improvement or better in psychosis. In the senile and arteriosclerotic group, 78 per cent showed obvious improvement in behavior, and 22 per cent in psychosis.

3. The dosage ordinarily varied between 200 and 400 mgs. No advantage was noted for intramuscular over oral administration. The effective duration of thorazine's action appears to be much longer than was previously believed. It would appear that the drug is just as effective when given twice daily as when given oftener. Comparatively large initial doses produce fewer complications than smaller doses. There appears to be no advantage in giving doses in excess of 400 to 600 mgs.

4. The use of thorazine and the substitution of this drug for electric shock treatment has reduced the number of patients receiving electric shock to nine, from a daily pre-thorazine level of 300. In most psychoses, thorazine appears to be as effective as electric shock. Possible exceptions are certain retarded depressions and involutional psychoses. A number of chronic patients improved with thorazine after electric shock failed.

5. The best results appear to be obtained in patients with labile emotionality that is directed actively toward the environment or toward the patient: agitated depressions, active paranoid schizophrenia, and manic types of behavior associated particularly with overactivity, hostility, and aggression. Patients who show anxiety, apprehension, or fears of some type seem to respond well. A number of patients in whom there appeared to be no outward anxiety or aggressive tendency improved unexpectedly.

6. Thorazine should be used with certain precautions in the treatment of elderly patients with myocardial diseases.

7. Jaundice occurred in 4 per cent of the treated patients, and dermatitis in 3 per cent. Recurrences were noted in only two patients when they were retreated after the complications had disappeared. Seven nurses giving intramuscular injections of thorazine developed contact dermatitis of a rather severe degree.

8. An attempt to evaluate the blood pressure changes was inconclusive. There appears to be, in the majority of patients, an initial fall, at least in the systolic blood pressure, and to a lesser degree in the diastolic.

9. Patients released from restraint or seclusion totaled 50 per cent of those treated.

10. Thorazine, used as a prognostic test for the selection of patients for prefrontal lobotomy operations, resulted in improvement in a certain number of patients, so that this operation was no longer required for them.

11. Thorazine may be used on an outpatient basis to reduce the number of hospital admissions. Patients on convalescent care, likewise may be maintained on this drug.

12. Thorazine must be administered under the supervision of a physician

to carefully selected patients. Thorazine is no cure-all and must be accompanied by psychotherapy and other techniques used in treatment, since the drug facilitates communication and allows objective viewing by the patient of his difficulties.

13. Thorazine is only one additional tool which has been added to the treatment of mental disorders.

CHLORPROMAZINE IN THE TREATMENT OF NEUROPSYCHIATRIC DISORDERS

N. William Winkelman, Jr., M.D.

The management of anxiety, agitation, and manic states in psychoneurotic and in psychotic patients is a problem inadequately solved by current therapeutic measures. Moreover, conditions such as severe obsessive-compulsive neuroses, chronic hypochondriasis, chronic schizophrenia, and agitated senile states are not consistently amenable either to convulsive or coma therapy or to psychoanalysis and other means of psychotherapy. To control the ever-increasing incidence of psychiatric disturbances, additional therapeutic aids are needed.

Recent studies conducted in Europe suggest the usefulness of a new drug, chlorpromazine, for managing and treating psychoneuroses and psychoses. Chemically it is 10-(y-diethylaminopropyl)-2-chlorophenothiazine hydrochloride. Laboratory investigations revealed that this compound possessed diverse pharmacological activity. Provocative from a psychiatric standpoint was its ability to abolish conditioned reflex responses in animals.

Chlorpromazine was developed in France and was first studied by French and other European investigators in surgery and then in obstetrics and psychiatry. Observations by Delay, Deniker, and Harl that this compound controls psychomotor excitement in psychotic patients have been confirmed by Cossa and co-workers. In this country, Friend and Cummins recently reported its use as an antiemetic agent.

This study was undertaken to assess the usefulness of chlorpromazine in relieving increased psychomotor activity seen in tension and anxiety states, mild to severe agitation, and hypomanic and manic behavior, as well as its usefulness in treating patients with delusions, hallucinations, and various obsessive-compulsive-phobic conditions. It was also given to patients with epilepsy and paralysis agitans.

MATERIAL

One hundred forty-two patients received chlorpromazine for two to eight months. Sixty-five were psychoneurotics. 5 had psychophysiological disorders, and 15 were ambulatory schizophrenics seen either in private practice or on an outpatient basis at Sidney Hillman Medical Center, Philadelphia. Twenty-seven agitated, senile patients were treated in a hospital for the aged, and 10 agitated and manic psychotic patients were treated in a psychiatric hospital. In addition, 12 patients with neurological disorders and 8 patients, who served in a dosage range study, were given the drug. Half of the hospitalized and the ambulatory groups had previously received psychiatric treatment that included symptomatic sedation with barbiturates, group and individual psychotherapy, carbon dioxide therapy, electroconvulsive therapy, and insulin coma therapy; the other half had not previously received psychiatric treatment. Clinical characteristics of the group, expressed as major symptoms according to standard nomenclature, are listed in the table. In general, the symptom complex of the psychoneurotic patients was one of anxiety, palpitations of the heart, insomnia, profuse sweating, urinary frequency, decrease or loss of libido, gastrointestinal disturbances,

Results of Therapy with Chlorpromazine

	\multicolumn{5}{c}{Degree of Improvement}	Total No. of Patients
	4	3	2	1	0	
Psychoneuroses *						
Anxiety reactions	4	29	23	6	5	67
Obsessive reactions	1	3	2	..	2	8
Phobic reactions	1	2	2	..	2	7
Depressive reactions	1	1	5	3	2	12
Conversion reactions	5	9	14	5	12	45
Impotence	2	2	..	..	..	4
Stammering	..	1	1	2	1	5
Psychophysiological reactions (psychosomatic) *	1	1	2	..	1	5
Schizophrenia *						
Hallucinations	1	1	..	1	1	4
Delusions	2	2	..	2	1	7
Agitations	2	2	..	1	..	5
Senility with agitation *	8	7	3	2	1	21
Neurological disorders *						
Psychomotor epilepsy	1	..	..	..	1	2
Grand mal epilepsy	1	..	..	..	1	2
Petit mal epilepsy	..	..	..	..	2	2
Paralysis agitans	..	..	..	2	4	6
Manic-depressive-manic †	..	1	1	.	.	2
Senility with agitation †	3	3	..	..	..	6
Schizophrenia †						
Hallucinations	..	..	1	1	2	4
Delusions	..	2	2	..	..	4
Agitation	2	1	1	..	..	4

* Chlorpromazine given orally
† Chlorpromazine given parenterally.

dizziness, headaches, generalized aches and pains, and, in many cases, an obsessive-compulsive-phobic syndrome. The senile group showed all degrees of agitation with behavior problems, restlessness, and insomnia and was difficult to manage.

Dosage

In the nonhospitalized and the agitated senile patients, therapy was begun with an oral dose of 75 mg., 25 mg. with each meal. They were told that they might become drowsy during the first four to seven days of treatment, but that they should continue to take the drug since this effect would gradually diminish. The patients were re-examined weekly. At the end of the first week of treatment, the dosage was gradually increased, depending on the patient's response, until clinical improvement was obtained or excessive drowsiness occurred. If drowsiness interfered with the patient's normal activity, the dosage was decreased to 10 mg., three or four times daily. Patients received the drug for from 8 to 32 weeks and could be satisfactorily maintained on dosages of 30 to 150 mg. a day. Patient response to the drug varied considerably. Some patients responded well to 30 to 50 mg. a day; others required 150 mg. Some patients given 50 mg. a day became drowsy to the extent that it interfered with their normal activity, while others did not become drowsy when given 150 mg. a day. Hospitalized psychotic patients were given 25 mg. intramuscularly four times daily for the first two or three days and 50 mg. intramuscularly four times daily thereafter. The dosage was adjusted, increased or decreased, to maintain the patient in a resting or even a somnolent state.

Results

The patient's clinical response was judged in three ways—self-appraisal, comments from friends and family, and psychiatric evaluation. So that the effect of chlorpromazine on the components of the illness, as well as on the illness as a whole, could be judged, each patient's total illness was divided into its signs and symptoms. The response was rated as 4, absence of symptoms; 3, marked improvement; 2, moderate improvement; 1, slight improvement; and 0, no improvement. Results of treatment, in relation to major signs and symptoms, are summarized in the table.

Severe anxiety and tension states responded well with chlorpromazine. Of 67 patients manifesting typical severe anxiety reactions, 56 showed improvement ranging from moderate to complete relief of symptoms. Those patients who did not improve after taking the drug for three weeks usually did not improve with further treatment. Most patients reported that after one week they began to sleep better and to feel more refreshed on awakening. Anxiety was markedly reduced and often was replaced by a sense of well-being. Physical complaints decreased too; musculoskeletal symptoms that had persisted for years gradually diminished as did gastrointestinal symptoms. Improvement in mood was observed in patients who had been irascible, short tempered, and irritable. Patients who formerly waited for appointments by impatiently pacing up and down now sat quietly and waited their turn.

Five of six patients with phobic reactions reported at least moderate relief, and in one case the relief was complete. Six of eight psychoneurotic patients with obsessive thinking experienced moderate to complete relief. One patient who had had a 10 year history of severe obsessional and phobic symptoms, with great tension and marked urinary frequency, was unable to hold a job. Attempts at psychotherapy were futile, and frontal lobotomy was seriously considered; however, after taking the drug for four weeks, her phobias and urinary frequency disappeared and she started psychotherapy. Another candidate for lobotomy, a 28-year-old woman with a long history of disabling fears, phobias, and plaguing obsessional thoughts, who visibly gasped for air constantly, showed total relief of all symptoms after three weeks' treatment. This relief has been maintained for 16 weeks by a dosage of 100 to 125 mg. a day. These results suggest that no obsessive patient should have a frontal lobotomy until he has first been given chlorpromazine medication.

Twenty-seven senile patients who exhibited agitation, severe anxiety reactions, belligerence, difficulty in handling, or delusional reactions and who had been unsuccessfully controlled with the usual sedatives were treated with chlorpromazine. For three to seven days after they were given oral doses of the drug, half of the patients became aggravated. Shortly thereafter, a dramatic beneficial effect followed. Twenty-one of the 27 patients became markedly improved and remained improved during the two months they took the drug. Before treatment, the condition of two patients in this series had become so extreme that they had been considered for placement in a state mental institution. While receiving the drug, they improved greatly and were then described as "ideal patients" by the nursing staff. These results, though preliminary, indicate that chlorpromazine is superior to phenobarbital or other barbiturates for relieving agitated and belligerent destructive states in elderly persons. Six other senile patients who were extremely agitated and unable to sleep were successfully controlled when given a dose of 25 mg. intramuscularly.

Chlorpromazine appears to calm the patients without depressing their mental processes as the barbiturates do. And the risk of suicide appears considerably less with chlorpromazine than with barbiturates. Deniker told of a patient who attempted suicide by taking 30 tablets (750 mg.), lapsed into a coma-like state, but recovered uneventfully within a few days without the aid of analeptics.

Eight moderately to markedly agitated psychotic patients were adequately controlled with doses of 50 to 75 mg. of chlorpromazine intramuscularly, three or four times daily. Oral doses of 100 mg., four times a day, failed to quiet them. In one schizophrenic patient, a complete reversal of paranoid delusional features and of hallucinations occurred. Another elderly paranoid schizophrenic patient, who was so belligerent and nasty that she cursed vilely when anyone entered her room, was given 50 mg. of the drug intramuscularly three times a day. Attendant nurses reported afterward that the patient was less belligerent and more friendly to the staff than she had ever been in her several years' stay at the sanatorium. Two other psychotic patients, who were not hospitalized, were given oral doses. One of them, who had a rather sudden onset of paranoid delusions, ideas of reference, and auditory hallucinations with marked anxiety had a complete reversal of symptoms when given an oral dose of 25 mg. four times a day. Another paranoid patient with marked anxiety reactions said the medication "made him more like himself," and, though his delusions were still present, he did not seem to be bothered by them.

Six patients with epilepsy were treated with chlorpromazine, and, although four did not benefit from the drug, results were singularly good in the two other patients. A patient with intractable psychomotor epilepsy had been experiencing about three seizures a week while receiving diphenylhydantoin (Dilantin) sodium, phenobarbital, and Mesantoin (3-methyl-5,5-phenylethyl hydantoin).

The neurosurgical staff had recommended a temporal lobotomy for this patient. During the period that this operation was being considered chlorpromazine was added to the regimen and, until the supply of chlorpromazine ran out, the man had no seizures (for two months). This seemed to demonstrate the potentiating effect of chlorpromazine on other drugs, especially its effect on the barbiturates as reported by Courvoisier and Fournel. Another epileptic patient who has had grand mal seizures for 33 years has been maintained fairly comfortably with a regimen of diphenylhydantoin and phenobarbital; however, she continued to have biweekly seizures and could not tolerate an increased dosage. Chlorpromazine was, therefore, added to the regimen, and, since then, she has been free of seizures for three months. From these two cases, one can hardly generalize; however, the results are interesting and warrant further study. Six patients with paralysis agitans were given chlorpromazine, but no significant change was observed. No improvement or potentiating effects were observed when the drug was given with Rabellon (a compound of belladonna alkaloids) and trihexyphenidyl (Artane).

It was observed that with short-term therapy the beneficial effect of chlorpromazine lasted for two to four days after its administration was stopped. With long-term therapy (three to six months), the beneficial effects of the drug usually persisted after therapy had been discontinued for two to five months.

Side-Effects

Some degree of drowsiness was reported by almost all patients when they started taking the drug. In most cases, this effect diminished or disappeared by the end of the first week of treatment. Drowsiness could usually be counteracted by giving 5 mg. of d-amphetamine (Dexedrine) sulfate or 180 mg. of caffeine citrate with the morning and noon doses of chlorpromazine. Twenty per cent of the patients reported dryness of mouth; 10% complained of a bad or bitter taste in their mouths. Fifteen per cent of the patients remarked that they had experienced an increased frequency and intensity of dreaming. These dreams were vivid and filled with emotional content. Constipation was reported infrequently. In two patients in whom urticarial dermatitis developed, this side-effect cleared during the second week of treatment in one and had almost cleared by the 14th day of treatment in the other, but this patient discontinued medication at that time.

In three patients who had taken chlorpromazine for approximately two to five weeks jaundice developed, but subsided when administration of the drug was discontinued. It is unknown, at this time, whether this was a true toxic effect. Liver biopsy of one of these patients revealed the presence of chronic liver damage and suggests that the drug may precipitate jaundice in patients with impaired hepatic function. In England, in a few patients in whom administration of chlorpromazine was discontinued because of jaundice, the drug was given again when the condition subsided, and it was tolerated without a recurrence of the disorder. Intense investigation is under way in this series of patients to determine whether chlorpromazine is implicated in liver dysfunction.

A fall in blood pressure was observed in seven of eight patients after they were given an intramuscular injection of 50 mg. of chlorpromazine. The resultant hypotensive effect varied from 5 to 60 millimeters of mercury systolic, and 5 to 25 millimeters of mercury diastolic. Although in some cases the drop in blood pressure was marked—the greatest drop occurred in hypertensive patients—there appeared no danger of shock. It is well, however, to follow the example of Deniker and other European investigators who instruct their patients to remain lying down after receiving the drug parenterally. Local reactions at the site of injection appeared minimal. No significant change was observed in blood cell counts routinely made on patients in this study.

Possible Mode of Action

Chlorpromazine affects the central and autonomic nervous system and exhibits diverse pharmacological actions. It possesses depressant properties, alters conditioned reflex responses in animals, reduces blood pressure and body temperature, blocks apomorphine-induced vomiting and intensifies and prolongs the action of barbiturates, narcotics, ether anesthesia, muscle relaxants, and ethyl alcohol. Although its mode of action has not been clearly defined, Laborit and co-workers believe that chlorpromazine modifies or interferes with synaptic transfer of excessive psychomotor excitement between cortical areas and the diencephalon so that conscious perception of, and pattern of reaction to, personality-disturbing stimuli are altered. In the present study, it was observed that, when given parenterally and in sufficient doses to psychotic or severely obsessive patients, the drug produced an effect similar to frontal lobotomy. Patients who had been severely agitated, anxious, and belligerent became immobile, wax-like, quiet, relaxed, and emotionally indifferent; unlike persons who have received barbiturates for sedation, they remained responsive when spoken to and could easily be awakened if they fell asleep. From the side-effects produced, it seems likely that the drug modifies sympathetic ganglionic and post-ganglionic functions as well.

Tolerance

Two-thirds of the patients experiencing drowsiness became tolerant to this side-effect of the drug, whereas only two of the patients in the series had partial tolerance to the beneficial action of chlorpromazine. These effects are being studied further; however, at this point it is probable that there exists no relation between tolerance to its beneficial action and tolerance to its side-effects.

Because chlorpromazine has transient soporific properties, it is possible and often desirable to give the medication before bedtime, for in this way a troublesome side-effect can be used advantageously while tolerance to it is developing. Since patient response varies considerably, the optimum dose for each patient is best determined on an individual basis. In general, however, the following regimen can be used to reduce the drowsiness that occurs during the first days of treatment. The patient should be instructed to take a 25 mg. dose one-half hour before bedtime for the first three days. While tolerance to drowsiness is being developed, this side-effect can be used constructively, for patients will often fall asleep easily and quickly and will feel refreshed on awakening. On the fourth day patients should begin taking 25 mg. with breakfast as well as

25 mg. at bedtime until they can tolerate this dosage without undue drowsiness. After this, the dosage should be increased; the patient should take the drug with the evening meal, as well as before bedtime and with breakfast. Depending on response, the dosage can be increased further by instructing the patient to take the drug with each meal and at bedtime.

Conclusions

From the results of this study, it can be said that chlorpromazine (10-[y-diethylaminopropyl]-2-chlorophenothiazine hydrochloride) has a definite place in the treatment of neuropsychiatric patients, both by the general practitioner and by the psychiatrist. Chlorpromazine should not be considered merely a chemical restraint that has no real effect on the patient's illness; on the other hand, it cannot be used as a panacea for all psychiatric ills. Although it should never be given as a substitute for analytically oriented psychotherapy, it must be considered a true therapeutic agent with definite indications. The drug is especially remarkable in that it can reduce severe anxiety, diminish phobias and obsessions, reverse or modify a paranoid psychosis, quiet manic or extremely agitated patients, and change the hostile, agitated, senile patient into a quiet, easily managed patient.

* * *

An Appraisal of Chlorpromazine

A preliminary report on the present investigation was published in the *J.A.M.A.* on May 1, 1954, at which time certain clinical findings were observed and conclusions reached concerning the use of chlorpromazine in the treatment of psychiatric disorders; 142 cases were reported. The present paper continues that study, and reports 1,090 psychiatric patients treated with chlorpromazine and followed up to three years.

Although only recently introduced, chlorpromazine has become one of the most widely used and discussed compounds in the world. Remarkable claims have been made for it in both the lay and the medical literature. On the other hand, some observers have reported less effectiveness than that generally claimed. Furthermore, there have been reports of serious side-effects that could contraindicate use of the drug almost entirely. All this is confusing enough to warrant a drastic reevaluation and clarification of the precise risk and a general, realistic appraisal of what can and what cannot be expected from the drug, based on this series of 1,090 psychiatric patients which, we believe, has been followed longer than any other in the United States...

1. Chlorpromazine is a highly effective drug in many psychiatric entities, more effective in some than in others, and in groups of patients suffering the various syndromes, although its exact effectiveness cannot be predicted in the individual patient.

2. It is more effective in severe symptomatology than in mild, and is most effective when there is overactivity in any subdivision of psychomotor

activity, such as anxiety, agitation, panic, hostility, manic behavior, phobic activity, obsessional activity, and delusional and hallucinatory activity. Acute emotional illnesses have a better prognosis than chronic illnesses; chronic hypochondriasis and personality problems offer very poor prognosis.

3. Since its exact effectiveness cannot be accurately predicted, chlorpromazine must be initiated on a 6-8 week trial basis. Each case must be evaluated for treatment separately. To predict, the clinician should evaluate the patient's disease entity as a whole and also the individual symptom reactions. In this way, the clinician should be able to predict approximate results in perhaps 2/3 of the patients, provided the diagnostic and symptom evaluations are correct.

4. When the decision to use the drug has been made, it must be used in an optimum manner. As is true with insulin in diabetes, liver in pernicious anemia, and the antibiotics in infection, a small amount is essentially worthless.

5. However, chlorpromazine is a potent drug and its use should be considered "chlorpromazination," rather than just a routine administration. Chlorpromazine therapy is as sensitive and skilled a procedure as insulin is for the diabetic, anticonvulsives for the epileptic, or digitalis for the cardiac. This is illustrated by experience with the 85 patients who stopped taking chlorpromazine because of the negative psychological response. These patients were chronically ill, fearful, and highly suggestible. Their reactions occurred during the early months of the investigation, and we soon learned that it is necessary to start treatment with small dosages and build up gradually in this type of patient in order to avoid such reactions. Resistance to psychotherapy makes effective use of chlorpromazine all the more important for these patients.

6. Before the therapeutic test is made, the clinician must decide what additional treatment is necessary for the most complete and effective management of the individual problem. In thinking of treatment, the clinician should consider 4 factors: (1) The probable benefit to an individual patient from the drug; (2) the achievement of adequate dosage to initiate treatment, to build up, to reach optimum dosage, and to maintain; (3) the length of treatment probably to be required; (4) the additional treatment necessary for the most effective management in view of the: diagnosis, prognosis, age, resistance, duration of symptoms, intelligence, psycho-dynamics, ability to communicate, ability to achieve insight.

7. Chlorpromazine therapy should be thought of as either primary or secondary treatment. Primary treatment employs the drug as the most basic therapy available. Secondary treatment employs it as an ancillary and more symptomatic treatment. Its use in the agitated delusional paretic is secondary to the high-dosage penicillin therapy. In the psychoneuroses this concept is particularly important. Certain types of patients are known to respond well to psychoanalysis or other well-oriented psychotherapies. Use of the drug in these is, of course, secondary, and much can be said concerning this use. In elderly patients or those with low intelligence, with too great resistance, or with inability to communicate verbally, the drug becomes of

necessity the primary therapy. In the acute, agitated, unapproachable schizophrenic the use of the drug is primary, unless electroconvulsive therapy is administered.

8. The drug has considerable use as a secondary treatment with psychoanalysis or psychotherapy. However, the more classical psychoanalysts give three objections. They contend, first, that partial relief of anxiety will remarkably decrease the motivation for psychotherapy. I do not believe that this is so; however, each case must be individually judged. Good treatment should be motivated by more than anxiety. However, the skilled therapist can adjust the chlorpromazine dosage so that anxiety can be rather accurately regulated. It is ideal to reduce anxiety so that the patient will be able to work in treatment and be able to use ego functions unencumbered, and yet not be so symptom-free that he will not be motivated to continue therapy. If the drug is at least partially successful in this aspect, the patient will certainly proceed in treatment with intensity. In schizophrenia the drug helps foster the therapist as a kind, helpful, giving, parental figure. The second objection, that the patient will regard the medication as the primary treatment and psychotherapy as secondary, is not particularly valid. If the drug is given, the therapist should explain to the patient that it is to be considered something to help temporarily relieve certain symptoms while the main treatment is going on. In fact, most patients in therapy already know this. The third objection, that the drug implies that psychotherapy is not necessary, does not come up, if the explanation is given. Incidentally, the vivid dreams full of emotion are often helpful in the psychotherapeutic approach.

9. In my original paper I suggested that the drug could be well used by the general practitioner. I now believe that he should treat patients with chlorpromazine only after being certain of the exact diagnosis and being thoroughly familiar with the therapeutic procedure. Better still, the situation should be discussed with a psychiatrist as to diagnosis, prognosis, and treatment of choice. If indicated, a consultation concerning a therapeutic trial should be carried out; this can be done by the practitioner and save referral. If referral is made after this, then the therapeutic trial does not have to be repeated. The greatest tragedy of management by the general practitioner is that many patients will never benefit from a basic psychotherapy attitude toward treatment.

10. To achieve optimum chlorpromazine therapy in the psychoneuroses, combined chlorpromazine-well-oriented-psychotherapy should be instituted. Chlorpromazine should not be eliminated but continued indefinitely, according to the patient's clinical status. If withdrawal is necessary, it should be slow, taking a week or more, depending on the level of dosage.

11. Chlorpromazine may be used instead of convulsive therapy in the acute agitated states of schizophrenia, manic-depressive psychosis, or the psychoses of organic origin. It markedly reduces risk, the need for seclusion, and various restraints; and it can frequently be used to care for acute episodes or acute exacerbations at home and save the expense of hospitalization.

12. Chlorpromazine can be used at home for treatment in all except the

most extreme situations, and many patients can even remain at their jobs; 40% of patients who would formerly have been hospitalized were treated as outpatients.

13. Pure depressions do not respond to the compound.

14. The relapse rate after withdrawal was considerable: 80% in 6 months. This rate was markedly reduced (in half) if the patients were also being treated by psychotherapy.

15. Maintenance therapy must be continued indefinitely, unless the basic pathology is altered. A certain percentage who live successfully and have a real ego-reorganization on this basis can in time be taken off the drug. Slowly diminishing the drug over a few days is suggested after maintaining the patient on it for at least 6 months. If any symptom recurs during dosage reduction, dosage should be returned to its former level. Some patients can be maintained on dosages smaller than the optimum dosage. Trial and careful observation will determine this.

16. Two control studies with phenobarbital prove the marked superiority of chlorpromazine.

17. Control studies showed that a placebo has 35% effectiveness, but this is far short of the 84% effectiveness of chlorpromazine.

18. Undersirable side-reactions do not contraindicate the drug when it is clinically indicated, especially as primary treatment.

19. Suicidal outpatients should certainly be given chlorpromazine instead of the barbiturates, because of the great margin of safety. Suicidal attempts were made by 3 patients who took up to 1,250 mg., with only a 3-day sleep resulting.

20. Since there are available today many dozens of drugs that have a depressing action on the central nervous system, classification of them becomes increasingly difficult. *Ataractic* and *tranquilizer* could essentially be used to describe them all. At the present time our knowledge is probably insufficient to label each group with precise boundaries. Considering its site of action, its chemical structure and character of action, we can describe chlorpromazine as a reticular formation or diencephalic depressant, a phenothiazine derivative, an "ascending depressant," or an indifference-producer.

21. Freud and many others showed that the difference between the "normal" and the neurotic is a quantitative one. Anxiety is certainly an important component of healthy mental functioning and plays an important role in the adjustment of the organism to reality, just as muscle tones readies the body for physical action. A tranquilizer should not be used unless the anxiety is actually pathologically increased, and the degree of anxiety reduction should be regulated carefully so that the organism will be able to respond in a healthy manner to environmental stimuli, and yet not over-respond abnormally to either exogenous or endogenous stimuli. Let us, as physicians, not take away the already impaired ability of the neurotic to respond to his environment with awareness and effective action.

22. The conversion hysteric and the tranquilized patient have something in common. Whereas the patient with conversion hysteria has "la belle indifference" concerning his paralyzed right arm, the tranquilized patient

has a rather generalized indifference. This suggests that the two conditions stand in a relationship which might give us a lead to further understanding of the anatomical-physiological-psychological relationships. The energy of anxiety is certainly combatted by the drug; whereas, it is bound or "converted" by the hysterical system.

23. The author feels that a study of a large series of patients is an important and necessary approach to the investigation of drugs. This has been the approach of the investigations up to this time. A really intensive study of a small number of patients also seems important, but no such studies have been reported in the literature. I have studied 6 patients during the course of 200-300 hours of psychotherapy. An investigation of the intrapsychic changes that could possibly be attributed to a drug appears to me to be of real importance. This study is in its preliminary stages and will be published at a later time. The investigation is exceedingly difficult. Tentatively, a reduction in the drive of id impulses and in superego rigidity and strictures occurs; with a reduction in the energy of these traditional enemies, the ego has less of a conflict to handle. Therefore, the ego can function more smoothly, coping with reality more effectively.

24. We are dealing with an exceedingly complex arousal mechanism involving anatomically not only the reticular formation, but also a whole interconnecting system of cortical and subcortical structures. This system has to do with the response of the organism to stimuli, both external and internal. It appears that the signs and symptoms of anxiety arise in response to any evidence of threat to continued intactness and feelings of stability and constancy of the organism.

This "anxiety reflex," which probably becomes a conditioned reflex and acts upon the general principles of such a reflex, is probably mediated through part of the reticular activating system. It appears to be one of the deepest, most automatic, and most primitive responses of the organism. A tranquilizer such as chlorpromazine produces a chemical inhibition of the arousal system and of the "anxiety reflex." This theory in no way contradicts psychoanalytic thinking. Threatening internal stress from emotional conflicts between two or more institutions or structural components of the psyche—ego, id, and superego—probably resides in areas of the brain connected to the activating system. If the energy created by such a conflict extends over to the activating system, anxiety results, unless it is combatted either by solving and eliminating the emotional conflict psychoanalytically or by chemical action on the structure of the arousal mechanism.

CHLORPROMAZINE AND RESERPINE, AND THEIR RELATION TO OTHER TREATMENTS IN PSYCHIATRY

Lothar B. Kalinowsky, M.D.

There is no other field of medicine so much in the public eye as psychiatry. This easily leads to exaggerated reports in newspapers and magazines, and some psychiatrists and hospitals are using this interest on the part of the lay press somewhat too liberally. At a time when only few of us were acquainted with European reports on chlorpromazine and reserpine, these drugs were presented to the general public as "miracle drugs" and as a revolution in psychiatry. Under these circumstances it is difficult for non-psychiatrists to form an opinion on the actual value of such treatments, and it happens too easily that the failure to see miracles leads to the suspicion that this is "just another racket in psychiatry." Let me say from the start that drugs like chlorpromazine and reserpine do not perform miracle cures in any of the psychiatric conditions for which they are used but that they are revolutionizing because they represent the first successful attempt at removing mental symptoms pharmacologically.

Chlorpromazine is a derivative of phenothiazine, an antihistaminic containing carbon, hydrogen, nitrogen and sulphur in its molecule. It was introduced in France in 1950 for use in anesthesia, and as early as 1951 its sedative effect in psychiatric patients was noted. In the psychiatric clinic in Paris, Delay and Deniker introduced chlorpromazine, known in France and in many countries including Canada under the name of Largactil, under the term of "artificial hibernation treatment." The same term "Winterschlafbehandlung" had been used in German psychiatry for chlorpromazine under the trade name of Megaphen but lost popularity when, in 1953, it became known in this country under the name of Thorazine. It had been noticed in anesthesia as well as in psychiatry that the drug reduced metabolism, lowered the temperature and decreased the blood pressure, and thus the terms "neuroplegic agent" and "neurovegetative stabilizer" were introduced for this drug which obviously had a central effect quite different from other drugs used in psychiatry, including the barbiturates. These neurovegetative side reactions do not interefere to any extent with the administration of chlorpromazine. In particular the hypotensive effect disappears so fast that, contrary to Rauwolfia derivates, chlorpromazine has no value in the long-term treatment of hypertension. The only unpleasant side effect of neurovegetative origin is the occurrence of orthostatic collapse which is seen more often in patients after intramuscular and still more intravenous injections and which is probably due to vasodilation. It is important to keep the patient in a prone position, at least after the first injections which makes adequate medication with this drug more a hospital precedure than is usually recognized. Another feature of this drug which recommended it for use in anesthesia is the potentiation of other drugs such as barbiturates. In psychiatry this potentiating effect, in my experience, make it necessary to avoid the intravenous injection of sodium amytal or pentothal in patients under chlorpromazine medication.

One of the most frequent complications is a classical picture of Parkinsonism with masque facies, loss of associated movements and all the other symptoms seen in Parkinson's disease. In some observations of my own, symptoms appeared which are not seen in Parkinson's disease. These patients suffer under a terrible restlessness in their legs which forces them to walk day and night or step from one foot to the other continuously. It may take several weeks after discontinuation of Thorazine for this Parkinson syndrome to clear up. The theory has been expressed that the effect on deeper centers of the brain which causes the Parkinsonism is also responsible for the therapeutic effect of the drug. It has been claimed that the best therapeutic results are obtained where a Parkinson syndrome occurred, and in France, where most psychotic syndromes are localized in the diencephalon, this concept found many followers. A parallelism is seen between the slowing down of motor function and of emotional responsiveness of the patient, both being localized in the same area of the brain. A more generally accepted theory is that chlorpromazine depresses the hypothalamic mechanisms including those concerned with emotional responsiveness. This toning down of emotional expression is said to explain the improvement of emotionally disturbed patients.

Less frequent than Parkinsonian symptoms is the much discussed complication of jaundice which experimentally could not be explained by hepatic toxicity. Choluria and clay-colored stools make the clinical picture undistinguishable from obstructive jaundice, and surgical intervention as reported by Brandt and Dallos from this group, is much more frequent than it appears from the literature. Some biopsies showed edema without changes of the parenchyma; others saw inflammatory and degenerative changes in liver cells and thrombi in the bile ducts. The occurrence of jaundice does not seem to depend on the amount given as daily dose nor on the duration of chlorpromazine medication.

Also to be mentioned are toxic skin manifestations in the sense of a dermatitis. Exposure to sunshine predisposes to such skin conditions. They are also seen in nurses who come in contact with these drugs. Both jaundice and dermatitis often disappear in spite of continuation of treatment, and they usually do not recur if treatment is reinstated. Changes in the blood picture have been described but observations are contradictory. Most frequent harmless side effects are feeling of a stuffed nose and an unpleasant grogginess which will be discussed later.

In 1953, when the first clinical reports on chlorpromazine began to appear in France, Swiss psychiatrists in Zurich-Burghoelli started experiments with reserpine, an alkaloid derived from the Indian plant Rauwolfia Serpentina which had been used in India against insanity for a long time, and described by Indian physicians in medical journals in 1931. It was produced chemically by Ciba, and first applied for hypertension. When some Indian patients reported about it to Swiss psychiatrists, they tried it successfully in psychiatric patients. It soon occurred to them that results were almost identical with those obtained with chlorpromazine including most of the complications and side effects, although the chemical structure is quite different. It was a strange coincidence similar to the one that had occurred once before in psychiatry, when insulin and convulsive therapy had been discovered independently within a year.

The following discussion of the psychiatric indications and results will deal with them jointly. If any difference can be identified, it is that reserpine makes patients slightly more depressed than chlorpromazine, and this may be the reason why it seems that reserpine is losing out somewhat to chlorpromazine. An advantage may be that chlorpromazine, injected intramuscularly, sometimes gives painful infiltrations, although never leading to abscess, while reserpine gives no infiltrations. In the gastrointestinal tract chlorpromazine constipates, while reserpine causes diarrhea and more unpleasant nausea and vomiting. These are the reasons why chlorpromazine is easier to take by mouth, and reserpine by injection. Undoubtedly it is an advantage that we have two drugs with almost the same efficacy, and that we are able to use them interchangeably whenever we run into difficulties with one of them as, for instance, in cases developing jaundice under Thorazine this can be replaced by Serpasil which undoubtedly is less damaging to the liver.

The best technique in applying chlorpromazine and reserpine is not yet quite established. The usual dosage in psychiatry lies considerably beyond the amounts given by general practitioners for various complaints of their patients. In this country oral medication with Thorazine is more customary than by injection. A minimum of 25 mg. q.i.d. is usually given and quickly stepped up to 300-600 mg. in hospital patients, but, of course, less in ambulatory patients. In some cases 1000 mg. are necessary to achieve the desired effect, and Kinross-Wright in Texas gives daily doses of 4000 mg. without untoward side effects. It is the general impression that side effects do not necessarily depend on the amount given. In Europe intramuscular injections are preferred in the beginning of a treatment course for at least a few days. In Switzerland, where the sleep treatment introduced by Klaesi is still being used and is only replaced by the new drugs, patients are kept in a dark room in a sleeplike condition from which, however, contrary to prolonged barbiturate narcosis, they can be easily awakened. After a few days the injections are replaced by oral medication, and this is kept up for several weeks even in patients who show an immediate improvement. The superiority of parenteral application seems obvious, and I prefer to start with a few intramuscular injections even in ambulatory patients whenever feasible. Reserpine in the form of Serpasil is frequently given in tablets of 25 mg., while Thorazine is prescribed in 25 mg. tablets. This is inadequate, and 1 mg. tablets of Serpasil correspond better to the 25 mg. Thorazine tablets. There are few comparative studies available, but one was undertaken in Zurich-Burghoelzli, and it was found that a daily dose of 200 mg. chlorpromazine compares with a daily dose of 10 mg. of reserpine. If this is given as an initial dose in hospital patients an increase to 300 mg. chlorpromazine and 15 mg. reserpine was usually sufficient. In this country, where reports are mostly based on disturbed chronic patients, doses are usually higher.

Results

A discussion of results with chlorpromazine and reserpine must take into account and explain why extremely enthusiastic reports come from our rather conversative mental institutions, while practicing psychiatrists are increasingly dissatisfied in their work with these drugs. It must be explained, too, why the much-publicized reports from some of our hospitals go far beyond results obtained in otherwise far more therapeutically minded European institutions. These contradictions are best understood when results in various types of psychiatric patients are discussed separately. Such separate discussion of psychiatric entities will be equally necessary in order to determine the relation of the new drugs to our previous methods of shock treatments and psychosurgery as well as psychotherapy. We find it practical to deal separately with acute schizophrenia, chronic schizophrenia, depression and other affective disorders, organic psychoses and finally neuroses and borderline cases between psychoses and neuroses.

There is no convincing evidence that the drugs are specific for any particular psychiatric illness. Symptomatically they reduce restlessness, excitement, disturbed and aggressive behavior, anxiety and tension. The patient becomes more indifferent, which means that those who feel threatened by delusions and hallucinations become less disturbed by such psychotic experiences. These effects of the drugs explain why they have been applied in all types of mental conditions because their indication does not depend on the diagnoses as much as on the symptomatology of a given patient. After this general statement a discussion of the various psychiatric disorders mentioned before will be undertaken, in order to delineate the results obtainable with these drugs, and furthermore to discuss where other treatments are more indicated than the new drugs.

Schizophrenia, as the most frequent mental illness, has been the main object of studies with chlorpromazine and reserpine in our mental hospitals. Acute schizophrenic episodes with disturbed behavior for the last twenty years, could be brought under control relatively well by insulin and convulsive therapies with Metrazol or electric shock. The acute symptoms can be equally well controlled by the new drugs, but the decisive question is whether or not a lasting remission of the schizophrenic illness can be obtained. There is no agreement yet on this question. If the medication is discontinued after the patient has quieted down, he usually relapses into his previous psychotic state. Attempts have been made to continue treatment for weeks and months. There are no comparative studies available for patients treated only with the drugs and patients treated with insulin or electric shock. However, it is the impression of those experienced in the treatment of schizophrenia for the last few decades that insulin and electric shock treatment lead to better and longer-lasting remissions in schizophrenics. The danger, which has not been sufficiently stressed, is that a patient is being kept fairly well adjusted under constant medication with the drugs, but in the meantime the period during which shock treatments are effective passes by unutilized. It is a known fact that both insulin and electric shock treatment are most effective during the first six months after the outbreak of a schizophrenic psychosis, and this time should not be lost on experimentation with medication which affects the most disturbing symptoms rather than the underlying disease.

Our therapeutic considerations are quite different in chronic cases of schizophrenia. It has often been stated that the drugs lead to fairly good remissions in patients who have failed under insulin and electric shock. This is perfectly true, though somewhat misleading. Patients who have failed to show lasting improvement under shock treatments were either given up, or they were treated with an occasional shock treatment, so-called maintenance electric shock treatment, after which they relapsed within a week and the shock treatment had to be repeated every week. These patients can now be controlled much better with medication. They are able to adjust to the hospital. It is this group of chronic schizophrenics in which the most spectacular results have been reported. Noisy hospital wards with disturbed patients have become quiet since the introduction of the drugs. We also hear that the number of restraint sheets and jackets could be reduced to half, but we should realize that this can be accomplished also with more and better personnel because in Europe hospital restraint had not been in use long before we entered psychiatry. In any event, the progress made in the management of patients in the hospitals is obvious. It is equally obvious that occupational and work therapy, so important in the treatment of chronic psychiatric patients, can be applied much more successfully with the help of these new drugs which, contrary to the barbiturates, do not cloud the patient's sensorium. It is furthermore obvious that thanks to the combination of drug treatment with work therapy as well as psychotherapy, a greater number of patients can be prepared for a better adjustment outside the hospital and eventually returned to the community, where continuation of drug therapy helps them to maintain their improvement.

It should be mentioned that the so-called primary symptoms of schizophrenia, namely, thinking disorders and emotional flatness, cannot be influenced by the drugs, but they are equally untouched by the shock treatments. The place of the two new drugs in schizophrenia might not be entirely settled, but there is no doubt that they add considerably to our therapeutic armamentarium in this serious disease, the otiology of which is still unknown and for which we cannot yet hope for an otiological treatment.

A few words should be added to the place of psychosurgery, namely, lobotomy and similar operations, in the treatment of schizophrenia after the introduction of the new drugs. There is a great similarity between the effect of the drugs and of the operations in that both give patients a more detached attitude toward their psychotic manifestations such as delusions and hallucinations. Therefore, the term "chemical lobotomy" has been used for these drugs in France. Of course, the difference is that the dosage of the drugs, if they slow down the patient too much, as they often do, can be reduced, while the effect of a lobotomy, if it has changed the patient's personality too much, is irreversible. It has been more and more recognized that lobotomy performed on chronic schizophrenics with some degree of deterioration does not yield as good results as in some other groups of psychiatric patients. Therefore, we are glad that the application of lobotomies in chronic schizophrenic material could be reduced since the introduction of the new pharmacological treatments. However, there are still many patients who cannot be kept on sufficient medication, especially after they have been discharged from the hospital. Thus, lobotomy still has its indication in individual cases, and we remain grateful that this surgical procedure is one more means in the treatment of schizophrenia.

Manic-depressive psychosis is the second group of the so-called functional psychoses. In these patients, who show either manic excitement states or depressive episodes, the manic excitement can be well controlled by the medication. All workers in the field agree that this is the most convincing indication for Thorazine and Serpasil. This is all the more gratifying as electric shock used so far in these conditions is not quite as reliable in the manic as it is in the depressed state of such patients.

The depressed phase of the manic-depressive psychosis as well as other depressions including involutional depressions are disappointing as far as their response to chlorpromazine and reserpine is concerned. Chlorpromazine might relieve the agitation of an agitated depression but not the depressive affect and thoughts. Reserpine may even increase the depression. There is mounting evidence that reserpine produces depressions in patients who received this drug for hypertension or other conditions. These depressed states do not always clear up when reserpine is withdrawn, and some workers, including myself, had to give electric shock treatment to patients who had become depressed under long medication with Serpasil. Contrary to some much-publicized reports the evidence is convincing that in depressions electric shock continues to be the treatment of choice. In practically all depressions undergoing electric shock today, attempts with drug therapy have preceded such treatment, and, thus, the evidence of lack of efficacy of the drugs in the depressed patient is overwhelming. It is an interesting sideline that depressive affect also remained uninfluenced by psychosurgery. In patients under chlorpromazine or reserpine it is important to discontinue the medication for several days before electric shock can be instituted. Fatalities due to sudden fall in blood pressure during the electric shock convulsion have been reported to me in several unpublished instances when electric shock had been given during Thorazine or Serpasil medication. Lately, one such fatality has been published, and the combination of electric shock with Thorazine or Serpasil must be warned against, all the more as no evidence has ever been brought forward that this combination is more effective than pharmacotherapy and shock therapy given subsequently. In depressions without agitation attempts with chlorpromazine and reserpine can be omitted because the waiting period between withdrawal of the drug and administration of electric shock increases the suicidal risk which is ever present in these patients.

A vast field for the new drugs with their symptomatic effect on psychotic excitement is represented by the various organic psychotic syndromes. Here the results are remarkable, and thanks to them it is possible more often than before to keep a temporarily disturbed patient in a general hospital. This is of great importance in postoperative confusional states as well as in infectious diseases with brief psychotic episodes which can all be well controlled with the new drugs. The same is true for toxic conditions such as beginning delirium tremens, where it is so important ot keep the patient under good medical supervision on a medical service rather than sending him to a psychiatric institution.

In alcoholism as well as drug addiction the usefulness of the new drugs is even greater because withdrawal symptoms can be prevented entirely by Thorazine or Serpasil, while they themselves do not lead to addiction and, thus, can be withdrawn easily as soon as the patient has no more urge for the originally used drug or alcohol.

Another important therapeutic field for the new drugs is represented by arteriosclerosis and senile psychoses. The temporary excitement states of these patients, which are often the reason for their hospitalization and which also make their management in the hospital more difficult, can often be controlled with chlorpromazine and reserpine. Senile patients overcrowd our mental hospitals, and 30 per cent of all admissions are already coming from this group. The importance of pharmacological treatment of the most disturbing symptoms in these patients will not only help the individual and his family but will be of the utmost social importance for the most serious problem of our state hospitals. Mention should be made of many other organic mental conditions whose most disturbing symptoms can be influenced by the drugs, such as disturbed and aggressive behavior in epileptics and certain groups of mental defectives.

The last group to be discussed are the psychoneuroses. The neurotic patient falls even more into the domain of the general practitioner and non-psychiatrist-specialist. For this group you will prescribe the new drugs in the same way as you prescribed phenobarbital or other barbiturates in former times. Unfortunately, the neurotic represents the type of patient with the least predictable therapeutic results. I cannot discuss this group without stressing the importance of a proper diagnosis. It is a great difference whether you are dealing with a neurotic patient whose neurotic complaints happen to be fixed in his throat or his heart or his stomach, or whether you are dealing with a depressed patient who happens to have a variety of similar physical symptoms but whose underlying psychiatric condition is a depression. It is only in the first mentioned patient that you can expect improvement with the drugs, while the second patient will lose his various somatic complaints only if his depression is cleared up by means of a few electric shock treatments. The same is true for patients with anxiety who will respond well to the drugs if they are suffering from a pure anxiety neurosis but not from an agitated depression with anxiety. Tension and anxiety as symptoms, however, are well influenced by the drugs. The more serious cases of neurosis, especially the obsessive-compulsive neuroses, do not respond well. Reports on the effect of the drugs in neuroses and in all types of ambulatory patients are still too few to draw final conclusions. In our own experience and in that of some reliable colleagues results are not very satisfactory. The unavoidable side effects of the drugs frequently tend to aggravate the condition of the neurotic, who especially regards the feeling of detachment and depersonalization caused by the drugs as evidence of approaching insanity; or he may add other side effects to his list of neurotic or psychotic complaints. On the other hand, some remarkable results can be achieved in neurotics at least for some period of time. The unsolved problems in this new field were well demonstrated to me by a recent case, where severe obsessive-compulsive symptoms, present for twenty years, disappeared under Thorazine for several months until an occasionally observed, so-called paradoxical reaction with restlessness and depression occurred, symptoms which this patient had never experienced before. In neurotic patients of mild and severe degree alike, it is certainly indicated to make an attempt with the drugs, but it is much more difficult to obtain maximal results in these usually ambulatory patients. Results are better in hospialized psychoneurotics where higher doses of the drugs can be applied. In the very severe neurotics with chronic-neurotic symptomatology results are disappointing. This is particularly true for those borderline cases which Hoch and Polatin described as pseudoneurotic schizophrenia and for which psychosurgery continues to be the last therapeutic step with extremely gratifying results.

In milder neuroses the drugs are of great symptomatic help if the patient is willing and able to accept some of the unpleasant side effects. The drugs have also been found to be useful as a means to make patients more accessible to psychotherapy, although some psychoanalysts object to any somatic treatment in psychiatric patients. It is obvious that drugs which relieve or reduce tension and anxiety facilitate psychotherapy. It is also more and more recognized that any medication which makes it easier for the patient to tolerate his neurotic symptoms, can be of great help in the adaption of such patients to their personal and social problems.

As general practitioners you will have better results with chlorpromazine than, for instance, with drugs like Miltown if you are willing to give sufficient amounts of at least 100 or 200 mg. If you encourage the patient to continue the medication in spite of some discomforts, he will overcome the side effects, and you will achieve improvement in a variety of patients without having to send them to a psychiatrist.

My purpose was to show that psychiatry has reached a state where many different treatments are available. The therapeutic nihilism of former years is gone. Not only did we become active therapists; it is no longer justified to use one single type of treatment for all psychiatric patients. It is also no longer a proper procedure to try one somatic treatment in all schizophrenics regardless of symptomatology and stage of disease. Psychiatrists must learn to do what is common procedure in all other fields of medicine: to select the right type of treatment for the right type of patient. The new drugs undoubtedly enable us to be still more selective in the choice of the proper treatment for many psychiatric patients.

A CRITIQUE OF THE TRANQUILIZING DRUGS, CHLORPROMAZINE AND RESERPINE, IN NEUROPSYCHIATRY

Harry Freeman, M.D.
Director of Research, Worcester State Hospital, Worcester, Massachusetts

The advent of the tranquilizing drugs has aroused a ferment in psychiatric quarters that to the laity has implied the coming of the millennium in this phase of medicine. In view of the history of previous somatic therapies with similarly enthusiastic claims, it behooves the medical profession to evaluate the present results with a judicial and skeptical eye. It is the purpose of this paper to review the highlights in the literature on these drugs. The paper will be confined to the results obtained through the administration of chlorpromazine and reserpine, since other drugs have been reported in too few cases to be capable of adequate assessment.

Double-Blind Studies

Despite the intense optimism expressed by many clinicians concerning the therapeutic efficacy of the drugs, there has been some opinion that the results obtained were due, to some extent, to the enthusiasm that attends the advent of any new therapy on the part of the medical and ward personnel and even of the patients.

A survey of the literature shows the publication of about a dozen articles in which the drugs have been tested by the double-blind technic in which, unknown to the personnel dealing with the patients, one group of subjects received the presumably potent agent and the other a placebo. In several cases this initial procedure was followed by an alternation of the drug and the placebo between the two groups, and in a few cases by an alternation of chlorpromazine, placebo and reserpine in the same patients.

The daily doses of reserpine usually ranged from 2 to 5 mg., but up to 10 mg. was given in one study. The period of medication was usually four to six weeks. The daily doses of chlorpromazine ranged from 100 to 600 mg. but in one study was 800 mg., and the usual period of medication was about eight weeks.

In all these studies, using the double-blind method, except one, either chlorpromazine or reserpine was noted to have effects in behavioral improvement superior to those found in the placebo-treated groups. In the single study in which no difference was found the dose of reserpine (2 mg. by mouth) may have been too small to alter the behavior of the patients. The subjects in these studies numbered about 300 in the reserpine-treated groups, 400 in the chlorpromazine-treated groups and about an equal number in the placebo-treated groups. With the exception of one study, which included 150 patients exhibiting anxiety states, the majority of the other cases were of the chronic schizophrenic type in which the possibility of spontaneous improvement during the short period of study was extremely slight.

There is no question that this review of the literature indicates that the behavioral improvement after the administration of these drugs is definitely beyond that produced by suggestion. Approximately two thirds of the patients showed some degree of improvement on the drug, whereas usually less than a third of the placebo-treated patients showed any improvement and, on the whole, this was to a less marked degree than that in the previous group. Very few striking improvements were noted in the drug-treated group, but this may be attributed in part to the relatively modest dosage and in part to the relatively brief time in which they were employed.

Among these studies were six in which both drugs had been employed in contrast with placebos. Each drug was tested on the same patients in two and on different patients in the other four. In five of these studies, one with the same patients and four with different groups of patients, the percentage of improved cases seems to have been about the same for both drugs. In the sixth trial reserpine seemed to give a somewhat higher percentage of improved patients than chlorpromazine—56 per cent vs. 42 per cent. On the whole, however, in this limited series, the two drugs seemed to be equivalent in therapeutic effect.

SCHIZOPHRENIA

Dosage

The application of the drugs to schizophrenic patients, who number half the mental-hospital population, is discussed first.

There is not too much uniformity of dosage in chlorpromazine. There have been, in general, three dosage schedules, which may be labeled as low (150-400 mg.), moderate (500-900 mg.) and high (1000 mg. and up). In each group there appears to be roughly the same degree of improvement, though the advocates of the higher dosages claim better results because of this. Sainz, for example, notes that in patients with chronic catatonia receiving 300-500 mg. daily, little if any improvement was seen, whereas 31 of 39 others receiving increasing amounts improved remarkably, 6 showing social recovery. Kinross-Wright advocates an intensive treatment with rapidly increasing dosages up to 4800 mg. daily for eight to ten days.

In general the dosage is usually increased from an initially lower level until the patient has shown improvement, maintained at that level for a varying period and then gradually decreased to a maintenance level. The average dose is about 500-600 mg. daily, divided into three or four doses. The average maintenance dose is about 100-200 mg. daily.

For reserpine the usual dose is initially 5-10 mg. intramuscularly, with about 3 mg. by mouth for a week to ten days, after which, if the patient has improved, the parenteral dose is discontinued. Much higher doses have been given. Sainz has administered 240 mg. of reserpine within twenty-four hours without inducing deep catatonic conditions or significant hypnosis. A diminishing dose is also used as the patient improves. The drug can be given once or twice daily.

Duration of Treatment

In the acute cases the treatment is maintained until the patient has definitely improved, or up to at least two months. In the chronic cases the treatment should be continued for six to eight months before it is concluded that no benefit is derived. Goldman, for example, notes that in patients hospitalized for less than five years and treated for less than two months, the rate of recoveries and social remissions is 19 per cent whereas in those treated for over two months this value increases to 56 per cent. Similarly, Hollister states that increasing the dose of reserpine from 1-4 mg. daily in one group to 2-8 mg. in another group raised the rate of improvement (moderate to marked) from 30 to 54 per cent. Although improvement may be noted in less than a week a maximum degree may not be achieved for many months when the patient has been hospitalized for a long time.

Duration of Hospital Stay

The duration of the psychosis, as measured by the length of hospital stay, is an important factor in influencing the degree of clinical improvement. In the opinion of most investigators the longer the duration, the less likely the possibilities of all grades of improvement, and this is seen most strikingly in the number of patients who are sent out of the hospital in a state of remission (no residual symptoms) or social recovery (slight residual symptoms). In the acute cases these two grades of improvement range between 43 per cent and 79 per cent whereas in the chronic stage of the psychosis, the values are decidedly lower, decreasing to 5 per cent to 32 per cent. Obviously, it would be necessary to maintain the treatment for a longer time in the chronic patients.

Clinical Results

For the vast majority of investigators the administration of chlorpromazine and reserpine has produced definite behavioral improvement in the majority of schizophrenic patients. Violent, agitated, anxious, assaultive, denudative patients have, on the whole, shown a decrease in aggressive behavior, a lessened responsiveness to disturbing hallucinations and delusions and an increased degree of socialization with other patients, as well as with ward and medical personnel. This lessened emotional tension has allowed for more contact with the physician, the nurse and the occuptional and industrial therapist. Granted this degree of improvement, which, from the point of view of the hospital administrator and of the patient, is quite important, the question arises how the number of patients being sent out to resume their normal degree of activity in the community compares with that obtained in patients under other methods of treatment. Even if the discharge rate is no more than with custodial care, electroshock, insulin coma or lobotomy treatments, the simplicity, economy and lesser emotional turmoil would make the drug treatment preferable so long as there were no high percentage of untoward effects.

Unfortunately, most of the figures for improvement obtained after drug treatment are cited as if the patients existed in a therapeutic vacuum. Disregarding for the moment the bias that therapists tend to assume toward a new method of therapy, the fact remains that in most well run mental hospitals a definite percentage of patients are discharged to the community in a condition approximately that observed before they became ill. For this I shall have to draw on figures obtained in Alexander's review of the literature in 1953

TABLE 1. *Effects of Various Types of Therapies in Schizophrenic Patients.*

Type of Therapy	No. of Patients	Complete Remission Combined with Social Remission %
Custodial & supportive treatment*	11,080	19
Convulsive shock*	7,357	29
Insulin coma*	9,483	48
Lobotomy†	1,211	18
Chlorpromazine	1,517	34
Reserpine	897	22

*Figures derived from Alexander.
†Figures derived from Greenblatt et al. Freeman & Watts, Walker and Great Britain Board of Control.

(Table 1). In 11,080 schizophrenic patients with varying periods in the hospital complete and social recovery was obtained in 19 per cent. This figure is the base line against which all other methods of therapy must be compared since it is invariably present. In 7357 schizophrenic patients treated with convulsive-shock therapy, the rate of complete and social recovery is 29 per cent. In 9483 cases of schizophrenia treated by the insulin-coma technic, the figure is 48 per cent. In 1211 patients treated with lobotomy, the value is 18 per cent. In 1517 cases that I have obtained from the literature, the figure is 34 per cent for chlorpromazine. For reserpine (897 cases) there is a corresponding figure of 22 per cent. The figures for lobotomy must be evaluated on the basis that this technic was a last resort in patients who had not improved by any other method of treatment.

It seems evident, then, that of all the forms of somatic therapy, insulin-coma treatment has the highest remission rate, and indeed Bleuler and Stoll believe that this method brings a more lasting and basic psychotherapeutic accessibility than the drugs do. At any rate, two facts are evident: despite the widespread change in behavioral manifestations—that is, the "tranquilization"—the percentage of recovered cases with drugs is roughly comparable to that obtained by the shock treatments; and reserpine is not as effective as chlorpromazine in producing recoveries. The superiority of chlorpromazine over reserpine is further attested by a survey Margolis recently made, in which 19 of 22 psychiatrists with extensive experience with the two drugs preferred chlorpromazine. He mentions that Azima, in a report of a recent international colloquium on

chlorpromazine, notes the same over-all preference for this drug.
Ideation Content
As has been mentioned, there is general agreement on the behavioral improvement in patients on these medications. There is less agreement about whether the intrinsic psychotic mechanisms have been affected. It could be safely assumed that in the patients sent home with complete or with social remissions there has been a reinstitution, to at least a marked degree, of the prepsychotic personality. In the other patients, who have lost their aggressive or hostile behavior, the disappearance of hallucinations and delusions, and the reconstitution of fragmented thinking is still in doubt. Some authors speak of a disappearance of these phenomena, others of a lessening of their intensity, and still others of no change in the ideational content. This point, as yet, is unsettled, and it is probably safer to assume that in nonrecovered patients there is greater indifference to these phenomena. This feature, in itself, is of value since the lesser interaction of the patient to his disturbing ideational content may weaken the intensity of the emotional drive that tends to perpetuate the existence of the abnormal thought content.
Subtypes
Of the various subtypes of schizophrenia, many authors have noted the superiority of results in the paranoid and catatonic over those of the hebephrenic patients. In many cases this is stated as a flat impression, but in some publications a statistical breakdown is shown. I have been curious enough to

TABLE 2. *Effects of Chlorpromazine and Reserpine Therapy in Subtypes of Schizophrenia.*

Subtype	No. of Patients	Marked or Moderate Improvement
		%
Paranoid	317	54
Catatonic	322	37
Hebephrenic	153	33

compile some of these figures and offer these as a sample of moderate to marked degrees of improvement in the three subtypes with either drug (Table 2).

It is evident that the paranoid cases show the best results, with the catatonic next. However, the difference between the catatonic and hebephrenic types is probably of no significance. The result is interesting, though not definitive, since of the three categories one would have expected that the catatonic variety, with its impulsive outbursts, should show the greatest degree of change. On the other hand, it may be that the reason for the superiority in results of the paranoid group may lie in their relatively better integration and easier restoration to a normal level. One would have anticipated much poorer results in the hebephrenic group, but there may have been some selection here in that the most disturbed patients were chosen for treatment out of a larger sample of burnt-

out and vegetating persons.
Tolerance to Drugs
In the usual course of treatment the dose is increased to a maximal therapeutic level, depending on the clinical course, and then gradually reduced. No tolerance to the medication, such as a need for increased dosage, is noted by the majority of authors during the course of treatment. This point is further strengthened by the fact that, as the patient improves, the dosage can be reduced while the clinical improvement is maintained. On the other hand, Sainz has stated that a tolerance to chlorpromazine appears in all cases as shown by the fact that an increase in dosage of 20-50 per cent is needed between the second and third months of treatment to maintain the patient. Rees and Lambert have found that even after the initial improvement has been achieved, relapses occurred under constant dosages of chlorpromazine in 78 of 117 cases of anxiety states. Neither investigator used high dosages, and this phenomenon might appear only when the dosage level was at a critical or threshold stage.

A problem that is undergoing a good deal of discussion is that of the duration of treatment needed to prevent relapses. Approximately 33 per cent of all patients sent out of state hospitals under previous forms of therapy have had to return. What happens to the drug-treated patients? It is the general consensus that those with acute cases, after a prolonged tapering-off process, should be sent home without medication but that many of those with chronic cases, particularly those without striking improvement, should be kept on maintenance doses of 100 mg. of chlorpromazine or 2-3 mg. of reserpine. Barsa and Kline state that in some patients on reserpine the therapeutic effect lasts only as long as the drug is administered. Pennington notes that 20 per cent of the discharged patients treated with reserpine returned to the hospital, most of them because they stopped taking the drug. Freyhan states that 32 per cent of the improved schizophrenic patients relapsed after termination of treatments, a third of them in less than a month. I have already mentioned the results of Rees and Lambert, in whose improved patients 66 per cent relapsed despite continued treatment. On the other hand Goldman and Stephens and Pollack found that only 5-6 per cent of the chlorpromazine-treated discharged with medication had to return as compared with 30 per cent of those treated by other methods.

This problem can only be solved in the future. It is probably wisest to omit the medication in the cases of recent origin and continue it in the chronic or recurrent cases. So far as the individual episode is concerned retreatment after relapse usually results in the previously noted level of improvement, so that not too much is lost if the relapse occurs because of the discontinuance of the drug. Periodic observations of the patient must be made, however, to prevent or treat any of the complications.

MANIC-DEPRESSIVE PSYCHOSIS

In manic attacks, general experience agrees that the drugs are very effective in diminishing the psychomotor agitation. Approximately a half to two thirds of the cases show excellent results. According to Goldman the manic episode subsides as quickly as after electroshock treatment and even more rapidly according to Delay and Deniker. There is an occasional dissenting note. Bennett found no effect comparable with that obtained with electroshock. Sainz states that in 17 patients there was a reduction in activity in all, but 4 went into a depressed phase and all relapsed after discontinuing medication. In general, however, manic excitement seems to be one of the most favorable states for the employment of the drugs.

The case is somewhat different for depressions. The vast majority of investigators agree that the drugs are of little value and that electroshock treatment is the technic that should be used. When there is marked agitation with the depression this phase subsides, but the underlying psychomtor retardation remains. As a matter of fact, the depression may be intensified, especially by reserpine, since Hollister *et al.* have noted in 7 normal subjects that 1 mg. daily caused a mild depression; Freis described 5 cases of depression in patients with hypertension taking reserpine (2 with suicidal trends), and Gosline and Kline, in 100 acute cases treated with reserpine, noted a 9 per cent incidence of depressions, half of which were suicidal. Margolis, in a recent survey of the literature and of psychiatric practice, collected a total of 177 cases of depression that had been treated with reserpine. Undoubtedly, in many cases other factors besides the drug influenced the onset of the depressive state, but the number of cases is certainly large enough to warrant care in its use in depression-prone persons.

Aged Patients

The aged now form approximately a third of the state-hospital admissions and present many problems from the point of view of confusion, restlessness, combativeness and irritability. In these cases dosages should be started at a low level, 10-25 mg. of chlorpromazine three times a day, rising to a possible maximum of 200 mg. or 1-3 mg. of reserpine daily. The published results have been in general good, half to three quarters showing a definite improvement in behavior, with the result that some can be sent home to their families on small maintenance dosages. The results seem to be better when there is definite agitation, since Settel reports improvement in 40 out of 48 with irritability and apprehension compared with a similar change in 22 out of 41 with depressive features. It is not to be expected that the cerebral changes will be affected by the medication, but the improvement in behavior will make life easier for such fragile patients, their relatives and hospital personnel.

Psychoneuroses

The results of treatment in the psychoneuroses is quite variable. In the anxiety states in which there is marked tension there is general agreement that about a half to two thirds of the patients do well, although Bennett found only a sedative effect in 5 out of 9 patients. Sabshin and Ramot note only a moderate quieting affect in 20 per cent, and Kinross-Wright says that although sleep, appetite and muscle tension improve, there is rarely a cure. The results seem to be more specific for the emotional tension than for reorientation of the patient's ideational content.

In hysteria, compulsive-obsessive neuroses, hypochondria and psychosomatic complaints the therapeutic effects have been in general poor, with occasional exceptions. In cases characterized by depression the results are mixed.

The dosages usually employed are 40 to 400 mg. of chlorpromazine or 1 or 2 mg. of reserpine. These dosages are small in comparison with those employed in the psychoses, but are limited because of the apparent lesser tolerance to the somnolent effects of the drugs in nonpsychotic patients.

Mental Retardation

The drugs have also been of definite value in hyperactive, destructive, aggressive, mentally retarded patients of all ages. In children the dosages have been 75 mg. of chlorpromazine or 1-2 mg. of reserpine. In adults the doses have been somewhat lower than the level used in schizophrenic psychoses. Approximately 50 per cent of them improve in behavior while the drug is maintained. In children the reduction in hyperkinetic behavior can result in an improvement in the intelligence quotient (owing to the diminution in distractibility). Again, the treatment is symptomatic but at least has beneficial behavioral effects.

Delirium

Acute delirious states associated with alcoholic intoxication respond favorably to either drug. Initially, the drugs must be given parenterally in doses of 2.5-5.0 mg. of reserpine or 50 mg. of chlorpromazine, but when the patient quiets down, as he usually does within an hour, the other doses may be given orally. The patients are quiet, without the somnolence and confusion characterized by treatment with paraldehyde or the barbiturates. Although the acute stage is easily managed, Sainz has found in 17 cases of chronic alcoholism that the administration of chlorpromazine relieved the anxiety but did not prevent the patients from drinking.

Complications

Each drug has a long list of possible complications or side effects, but only a few are of any importance. Practically all are reversible with discontinuance of the medication, and some do not reappear on retreatment with the specific drug. So far as the complications are concerned, there is a factor of individual idiosyncrasy in most of them, although the influence of varying dosage cannot be discounted in some.

For chlorpromazine the side effects described are local tissue irritation (when injections are used), potentiation of effect of narcotics, sedatives or alcohol, sensitivity of aged or debilitated patients, constipation, galactorrhea, transient hyperthermia or hypothermia, dermatitis, confusion, convulsions, hypotension, jaundice, Parkinsonism and agranulocytosis. Only the last seven are of any importance, and only the last is dangerous. A toxic-confused state has occasionally been noted by Kinross-Wright that calls for discontinuance of the drug. Dermatitis, which may be troublesome not only to patients but also to nurses—in as many as 10 per cent of those handling the material. It is treated by ACTH or steroids but according to Margolis does not necessitate interruption of therapy. The hypotension is orthostatic and can be minimized if the patient rests for an hour in bed after a dose. Jaundice occurs in a variable number of cases and has been reported in as many as 8.3 per cent. The rate of jaundice with higher doses (500 mg. and up) is on an average 1.4 per cent, with lower doses less than 1 per cent. The jaundice is a benign condition, but some investigators continue the therapy and find that it diminishes. Others interrupt the treatment and reinstitute the drug and find that the jaundice does not recur. Convulsions have occurred in intensive chlorpromazine therapy but can be readily avoided by reduction of dosage. Parkinsonism usually follows higher dosages. Some investigators, such as Goldman and Kinross-Wright, consider it desirable to arrive at this stage and merely utilize anti-Parkinsonian drugs. It is easily controlled by reduction in the dosage. In my opinion, there is no more rationale in considering this complication a necessary accompaniment of the therapy than considering the production of Cushing's disease a desirable component of steroid therapy. In addition the somnolence and inco-ordination that accompany this syndrome go beyond the unique tranquilizing effects of the drug and approach the effect of heavy barbiturate therapy. The most serious complication is agranulocytosis. This is rare, occurring in 1 out of 50,000 to 100,000 patients, but it cannot be lightly disregarded.

Reserpine has less serious untoward effects. These include drowsiness, fatigue, nasal congestion, diarrhea, bradycardia, hypotension, increased salivation, edema, convulsions, confusion and the Parkinsonian syndrome. The last three indicate overdosage and require diminution of the drug. Barsa and Kline, like Goldman, do not consider the development of the Parkinsonian symptoms as necessitating a diminution of dosage, but continue with accessory drugs to combat this. The tendency to depression with reserpine has already been discussed.

Combination of Drugs and Electroshock Therapy

A final point to be mentioned is the combination of the two drugs in cases not responding to either, or the combination of one of the drugs with shock therapy. One is in sympathy with the clinician who is hard pressed to produce improvements in patients, but at present there is no scientific evidence that a combination of the two drugs will do better than either one. Regarding the utilization of either one of the drugs with shock therapy or insulin therapy, the literature has already shown a certain number of cases with serious complications and deaths in drug-shock combinations, and this method must be approached with great caution.

Discussion

There is little question that the utilization of the tranquilizing drugs has resulted in a definite behavioral improvement in many patients exhibiting aggressive, hostile, antisocial trends. From this point of view there has been a mild revolution in mental institutions in the decreased use of shock therapies, in the activities of the patients and in the appearance of the wards. Unfortunately, there are no statistics as yet about the effect on the economy of the hospitals to validate this point.

There is no definite evidence that the drugs affect the ideational content of the psychoses or even of the psychoneuroses. They diminish the emotional expression of the abnormal thought content, but it is questionable whether the underlying psychic turmoil is affected. This lessening of emotional tension is of value in many cases, particularly in those of recent onset, in that it conserves physical and psychic energy and allows the patient to reorient himself to reality. On the other hand, a recent paper describes 14 cases in which further psychotic deterioration or enhanced anxiety was produced by treatment with these drugs because the submissiveness that followed psychologically threatened the patients in whom activity was the sole means of expressing their emotional conflicts. In other words, in some patients, restraint by any method, chemical, electric or surgical, may be of more benefit to the hospital than to the person concerned.

It is at this point that one may mention the desirability of psychotherapy in association with the treatment. The drugs afford a unique opportunity for intensive psychotherapy of patients in whom such an approach was previously impossible. The practical question arises regarding how this additional therapeutic aid will be obtained in mental hospitals at present inadequately staffed.

Finally, I wish to make one further comment. The effectiveness in altering behavior beyond the factor of suggestion has been attested in chronic patients in the double-blind studies I have previously mentioned. There have been no similarly controlled studies in acute admissions. This would require a very large number of patients, in the thousands, because of the higher improvement rate than in that of chronic cases. Nevertheless, it is the only method by which the effects of these agents on number of remissions, number of relapses and duration of hospitalization and ideational content can be properly evaluated. It would have to be an elaborate program but one that would make possible an estimation of the true value of these drugs at least a decade before the usual trial-and-error methods determine their true place in treatment.

THE USE OF CHLORPROMAZINE AND RESERPINE IN PSYCHOLOGICAL DISORDERS IN GENERAL PRACTICE

H. Azima, M.D.

Within the last three years, we have been witnessing the appearance of new pharmacological substances which, according to the editorials of leading magazines and newspapers, have revolutionized the field of psychiatric treatment. According to these sources, the new drugs have provided us with psychiatric aspirins to alleviate the mental aches of patients and eliminate their psychopathology.

Unfortunately, psychiatry, as yet, cannot fulfil all these expectations. The question may arise in the minds of the general practitioners, who are professionally closest to the psychosomatic field of human complaints, as to what is the real value and true therapeutic position of these drugs, which we may designate as "psycholeptic"[1] and of which reserpine and chlorpromazine are the two important ones. The general practitioner may ask about the value of these drugs in his daily practice in treatment of psychologically deviant behaviour, and what he can expect from them. The purpose of this paper is to clarify, if possible, some aspects of these questions. However, before doing this, it may be worth while to discuss very briefly what these drugs are, how they are used in strict psychiatric practice, and their expected complications.

PHARMACOLOGY

Chlorpromazine and reserpine are chemically quite different. Chlorpromazine is a phenothiazine derivative chemically quite close to antihistaminic substances, such as Phenergan and Diparcol (used in treatment of Parkinsonism). It has a marked adrenergic activity, a moderate cholinergic activity, and a weak antihistaminic action. Its main effect is an inhibition of sympathetic mediated autonomic functions. It has an inhibitory effect on diencephalic autonomic structures, which regulate temperature, metabolism and other vegetative activities. It is a potent hypotensive agent and is also a valuable antiemetic.

Reserpine is an alkaloid fraction of the roots of any one of several species of plants of the genus *Rauwolfia* (named for Leonard Rauwolf, a German physician and botanist, who described this plant in 1582). Reserpine's action is also inhibitory and consists of a reduction of the activity of the central sympathetic

---
[1] Meaning "reducing psychological tension."

mechanism. However, it appears that the reserpine inhibition is mediated in part through the cortex, while chlorpromazine more particularly inhibits midbrain structures. Regardless of these neurophysiological differences, both drugs have an inhibitory effect on some psychomotor and affective states of the organism, chlorpromazine being more rapid in its activity.

Dosage and Indications

In psychiatric practice, chlorpromazine is used in doses from 50 to 2,000 mg. or more a day, reserpine from 0.5 mg. to 20 mg. daily. It is legitimate to say that in psychiatric cases seen in general practice the average daily dose does not need to exceed 200 mg. for chlorpromazine and 3 mg. for reserpine.

The strict psychiatric indications for these drugs are all states of excitation and tensional rise, particularly manic states and acute psychotic states associated with agitation and excitation.

We will now consider the situations in general practice where these two drugs may be used beneficially.

1. *Prevention of some psychotic relapses.*—This problem arises in two different situations: (a) The situation where patients live far from a psychiatric centre, or their financial means do not allow them frequent trips to these centres. In these cases, prolonged administration of reserpine or chlorpromazine over periods of years (two or more) after the patient has been discharged from a psychiatric centre may maintain an improved level of functioning, and, in some instances, may prevent the outbreak of acute episodes. The general practitioner may undertake or supervise this prolonged treatment in association with his important psychological supporting role. It should be noted that this prolonged treatment necessitates two or three visits a month, not only to give support to the patient and establish a warm relationship, but also to detect any complications that may arise. (b) The situation where the patient has not received this prolonged form of drug treatment. In some of these cases, occasionally an acute psychotic episode can be aborted if the patient is seen at the very onset of the attack and moderate doses of chlorpromazine or reserpine are given. Many patients, particularly maniacal ones who have experienced recurrences of their symptoms before, can detect the emergence of a new outbreak long before it clinically becomes evident. Drug therapy at these stages may abort the full-blown clinical picture. In some schizophrenic states the relatively sudden emergence of irrational anxieties may be the harbinger of an acute psychotic episode. Here too, drug therapy may occasionally arrest the progression of the syndrome.

2. *Pre-admission management of psychiatric cases.*—In many cases of acute agitation and excitation (manic state, acute agitated schizophrenias, agitated depression with suicidal tendencies), immediate admission to a psychiatric hospital is impossible, because of lack of beds or distance, and the patient has to wait several days. In many such cases, the ordinary sedatives and hypnotics do not and cannot control the patient, and a situation of great stress for the patient and his family may arise. In many of these cases, chlorpromazine or reserpine, alone or administered in conjunction with other sedatives, may foster a rapid decrease of agitation and excitation and a smoother period of

waiting, and prevent disruption of family organization and routine.

3. *Pre-admission management of non-psychiatric cases.*—In this category we may include all those patients who are worried, and very anxious about hospitalization for causes other than psychiatric illnesses. Among these we may think of patients waiting for major surgical operations which entail some mortality and some morbidity. Psycholeptic drugs may be of some benefit in these cases. By decreasing anxiety and tension in such patients, one may be able to prepare them better for surgery, and organize a better postoperative recovery in an atmosphere of lowered anxiety and apprehension. Since chlorpromazine is used extensively in many centres as pre-anaesthetic and anaesthetic medication, in needed cases the medication may be administered a few days earlier. Anxiety arises, in some cases, in relation to anticipated mutilation or loss of an organ. Regardless of the deeper psychological significance of this loss, anxiety in itself, if intense, may hamper organized preoperative and postoperative planning of the patient's social undertakings and roles. It is conceivable that the anxiety-reducing capacity of psycholeptic substances may be used to prevent this disorganization.

4. *Management of severe somatic illnesses.*—In this category we consider especially those patients suffering from advanced and incurable cancers. Psycholeptic substances may be beneficial through their pain-reducing capacity, and as well as lessening tension and anxiety, they may permit a cooler appraisal of the situation and the development of a "let us enjoy what is left of it" attitude. What was said about the anxiety over loss of organs in surgery holds true for the total loss of the organism. If the anxiety of annihilation and death can be decreased, it is evident that life in these cases may be tolerated better and with less suffering. We know that in some instances these drugs (particularly chlorpromazine) produce a kind of blunting of experience, where the perceptions lose their sense of self-belongingness, and the harrowing nature of experience is neutralized and becomes less alarming. This kind of psychological state is, from a humanitarian point of view, beneficial for patients who harbour incurable diseases, and allows a more comfortable existence.

5. *Social anxiety.*—There has been recent evidence indicating that in states of social disorderliness, panic and agitation, administration of psycholeptic substances either to the leader or to the member of a group, or to individuals confronting a social group, will increase the managing and controlling power of the leader or member. Cases have been cited of officers in combat and judges in trial settings who, because of intense anxiety and tension, have felt unable to manage a stressful position, but under psycholeptic substances were better able to control themselves and the situation. It is conceivable that, particularly in small communities, outbursts of what can be called mass agitation and hysteria could be controlled by administration of these drugs. Pierson, a French North African psychiatrist, reported that on one occasion he was able to control the disorderliness and hysterical reaction of a small group of people who were caught in a riot by giving them small doses of chlorpromazine. He thought that the drug decreased the tension, apprehension, and hysterical reactions of each member to a sufficient degree to allow the suppression of the riot.

Evidently the speculative nature of these observations is stronger than their scientific value. However, they indicate the possibility of a sociological use of our psychopharmacological knowledge. It would appear that the general practitioner, who is most likely to be involved in social situations, is the one who can test these speculations and investigate their validity.

6. *Miscellaneous.*—In this category we include only two conditions, headaches and addictions. The problem of headaches is too complex to allow a unified conception, and it would be erroneous to think that these psycholeptic substances can play a major role in their treatment. But there are cases of intractable headache, in which pent-up and undischarged hostility plays a large role, where benefit may be gained from these drugs. The temporary alleviation of the headache may allow the possibility of instituting other forms of treatment, particularly psychotherapy.

As regards the problem of addiction to alcohol or otherwise, many reports have indicated the valuable contribution that psycholeptic drugs can make. They allow in many instances a rapid withdrawal, and cut down considerably postwithdrawal complications and symptoms. They are valuable also in the treatment of delirium tremens, which may become an acute emergency. In this case, these drugs are of great value to the general practitioner, who probably will see the patient first.

The therapeutic value of psycholeptic drugs in premenstrual tension states and in the management of labour may be mentioned here.

COMPLICATIONS

We will consider briefly those complications which are of some importance and may become troublesome.

Chlorpromazine complications.—Of these, we should mention sudden collapse because of drop in blood pressure, the treatment being simply to make the patient lie down; allergic cutaneous manifestations, which will respond to a decrease in dose or cessation of the drug; liver damage; and Parkinsonism. Alteration of liver function occurs in 5 to 10% of cases with or without jaundice. It occurs usually within the first four weeks of treatment. The histological changes are in the bile ducts, and are cholangiolitic in nature, while liver cells are not altered. The liver returns to normal shortly after cessation of the drug. We have found that one liver function test, alkaline phosphatase determination, is a fairly reliable index of liver changes in chlorpromazine therapy. If this test is repeated once a week, and if there is a gradual rise in three successive readings, there is a fair possibility that jaundice will develop, and the drug should be stopped.

Parkinsonism occurs in 3 to 5% of cases, usually in the third week of the therapy. It will disappear within a month of cessation of treatment. It is always transitory, with no sequelae.

Reserpine complications.—In addition to its general systematic effects (hypotension, stuffiness of the nose, etc.), some extra-pyramidal signs are occasionally seen which some investigators have called Parkinsonism. Actually, this does not appear to be a "true" Parkinsonism and disappears with decrease in dosage. Because of the reports of two cases of rupture of stomach by Bleuler in patients receiving reserpine, caution is recommended when the drug is used in patients suffering from gastric disturbances.

Summary

To summarize, the so-called psycholeptic drugs, chlorpromazine and reserpine, have a wide variety of application, but they are by no means curative agents. They do not treat the cause, but are symptomatic medications which may arrest the evolution of some psychopathological sequence of events within a particular psychiatric syndrome, or in relation to other disorders. They are indications of a new era in psychiatric and psychosomatic therapy, but they are far from constituting the penicillin period of psychiatry. We should not let our enthusiasm accelerate unduly the vehicle of our scientific accuracy.

USE OF CHLORPROMAZINE AND RESERPINE IN MENTAL DISORDERS

Mark D. Altschule, M.D.
Assistant Clinical Professor of Medicine, Harvard Medical School

The last three or four decades have seen great progress in the treatment of mental disease by physical means. Syphilis of the brain and pellagra, both of which were formerly responsible for many admissions to mental hospitals, are no longer serious problems in America, owing to the development of specific cures for them. Insulin and electroshock have been useful in the treatment of manic-depressive and, to a lesser extent, schizophrenic psychoses. Hormones also have been helpful in patients with depressions or with post-partum psychoses.

A few years ago two chemical agents, chlorpromazine and reserpine, were introduced; they have already changed the practice of psychiatry. These drugs are currently called "tranquilizing agents" and will probably continue to be so designated, even though their action is not the induction of the state of serene security that the word "tranquility" connotes. It would more accurately describe their action to call them "deturmoilizers" or perhaps "apatheticatory agents." Irrespective of what they are called, however, there is no doubt of their beneficial action.

The effects of these drugs in man cannot be accurately evaluated, for several reasons. In the first place, there are no specific laboratory findings in schizophrenic or manic-depressive psychoses. All abnormalities thus far observed in these conditions—and there are many—are found in other diseases as well. However, these nonspecific physiologic evidences of illness are helpful in assessing the effects of the treatment of mental disease.

Another fundamental difficulty in evaluating these effects is that the origin—and even the symptoms—of mental disease cannot yet be satisfactorily explained on a physiologic basis (or on any other basis). Fragmentary evidence pertaining to the mechanism of anxiety is available; these data have been reviewed elsewhere and need not be detailed here. All that can be said with any confidence about the mechanism of anxiety is that it can be produced by intravenous infusions of epinephrine in doses too small to cause circulatory changes and that it can be produced by electric stimulation of the temporal lobe. Stimulation of this general area may also be followed by mood changes. The abnormal general awareness of internal and external stimuli exhibited by patients with mental disorders is probably related to changes in the function of the ascending reticular activating system, whose functions were defined by Magoun. The mechanisms of the hallucinations described by such patients are not well understood; schizophrenic hallucinations are different in character and content from those that occur in normal subjects who have received hallucinogenic drugs. The mechanisms of delusions and of the loss of the ability to think abstractly—symptoms of the more serious mental disorders—are complete mysteries (as are the mechanisms of normal thought). It is evident, therefore, that no evaluation of the "tranquilizing" drugs can be based on their effects on the physiologic mechanisms of mental disease.

It is known that these drugs counteract in animals the electrophysiologic effects of various hallucinogenic agents, such as adrenochrome, lysergic acid and bufotenin. However, this fact is irrelevant to the present discussion; these substances do produce hallucinations in man, but it is not valid to regard schizophrenia as due to the presence in the body of some such substance. Not only are these hallucinations different from those of schizophrenia but also they are accompanied by electroencephalographic changes, which are uncommon in schizophrenia. Moreover, the normal subjects who have these induced hallucinations are able to discuss them calmly and objectively while experiencing them, unlike patients with mental disease, to whom their spontaneous hallucinations are real experiences. In addition, giving these agents to patients with schizophrenia does not aggravate the symptoms that they have at the time: the symptoms are changed or disappear, or new ones appear, but the specific clinical pictures exhibited are not made worse. The study of these hallucinogenic agents will undoubtedly increase knowledge of normal and abnormal neurophysiology, but it will probably not reveal much about the origin of schizophrenia.

Unfortunately, the favorable effects of the tranquilizing drugs can be described only in terms of behavior, and this circumstance makes objectivity difficult, since it involves value judgments. A semblance of objectivity is imparted to clinical evaluations of mental disease by the use of rating scales that employ numbers; nevertheless, these ratings are still based on personal judgments and cannot ever be objective. Value judgments depend largely on cultural bias—for example, some rating scales designate increased sociability and conformity as indicative of improvement, whereas these changes might be taken as evidence of mental disease in some parts of New England.

Moreover, the clinical evaluations must be made by the attendant psychiatrists. Under these circumstances other sources of error inevitably arise: the psychiatrists did not know the patients before the illness began, and consequently they can never define the degree of return toward normal; psychiatrists who have spent many years working with the discouraging problems of chronic psychosis are likely to overrate small improvements; many state hospitals are in isolated communities, and since the staff members spend most of their time with the patients, they may gradually develop a somewhat distorted view of what is normal; and some psychiatrists are so much under the influence of some specific dogma as to become poor judges of behavior—statements and actions by patients that some physicians might regard as evidence of serious mental disease might be considered evidence of insight (and, therefore, of improvement in the patient) by some psychiatrists.

In particular, cultural phenomena influence the discharge rate of patients from mental hospitals: the tolerance of the community to which they return is a controlling factor. Some of the most favorable published reports on the effects of chlorpromazine and reserpine originated in parts of the country where community tolerance is high, or perhaps where the difference between people inside and outside mental hospitals is smaller than elsewhere.

A final difficulty in clinical evaluation of therapeutic measures in psychiatry deserves some comment: it is probably impossible for one mind to characterize another mind satisfactorily, since it is impossible for any operation to describe an operation similar to itself. Accordingly, psychiatric evaluations based on judgments of thinking and behavior must always be inadequate.

Pharmacologic Considerations

The chemical formula of chlorpromazine shows the relation of the drug to some others (Fig. 1). Diparcol and Parsidol are not much used in this country;

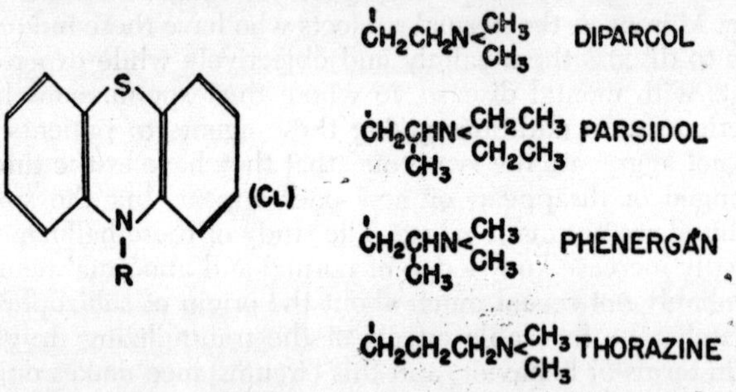

FIGURE 1. *Chemical Relations of Chlorpromazine.*

the one is of some benefit in Parkinson's disease, and the other paralyzes the automatic nervous system. Phenergan is a well known antihistaminic; the fact that it causes drowsiness has led some workers to conclude that much of its effectiveness in allergic states was due to its sedative action.

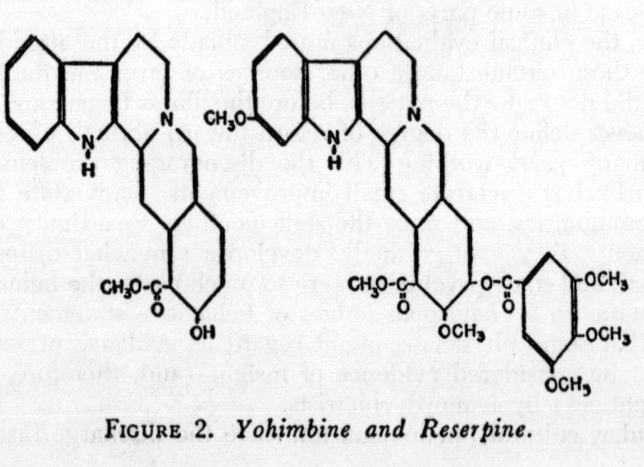

FIGURE 2. *Yohimbine and Reserpine.*

The New Chemotherapy in Mental Illness

Reserpine (Fig. 2) is closely related to yohimbine, which in the past was reputed to be an aphrodisiac but is not much used at present. Reserpine contains an indole nucleus and is therefore related to the hallucinogenic drugs, adrenochrome, lysergic acid, bufotenin and harmine—and also, of course, to serotonin (Fig. 3).

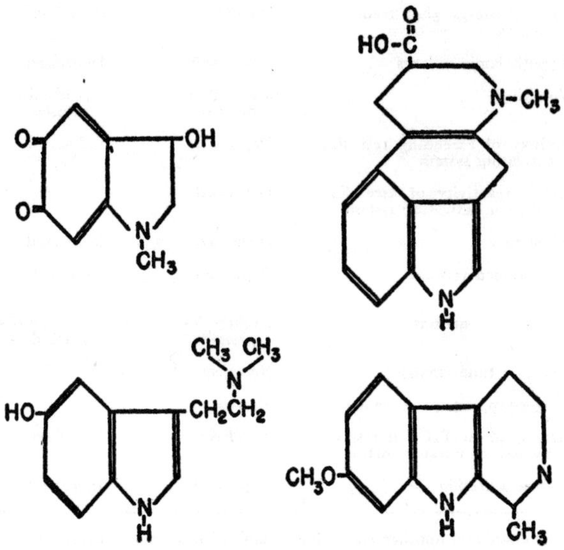

FIGURE 3. *Adrenochrome, Lysergic Acid, Bufotenin and Harmine.*

The effects of chlorpromazine and reserpine on transmission or their action in counteracting the effects of hallucinogens on transmission through synapses in various parts of the animal brain will not be discussed here; such data are available but cannot yet be related to clinical phenomena.

Reported observations on neurophysiologic changes induced by the drugs are summarized in Table 1.

Some of these findings are not yet securely established, since they have not been corroborated. In addition, it is not clear what bearing the phenomena listed above have on the clinical changes induced by the drugs. Of particular interest regarding behavior, however, are the observations that chlorpromazine inhibits conditioned reflexes without greatly affecting avoidance responses whereas reserpine does not affect conditioned reflexes but does inhibit avoidance responses evoked by frightening stimuli.

The action of chlorpromazine in depressing the reactivity of the ascending reticular activating system is also of interest in that it may explain the drug's effectiveness in allaying the hypersensibility that often occurs in neurosis.

TABLE 1. *Pharmacologic Data.*

Type of Action	Chlorpromazine	Reserpine
Hypotensive effect	Rapid'	Slow*
Adrenolytic action	Moderate	None
Sympathetic-ganglion transmission	No effect	No effect
Hypothalamic reflexes	Depressed*	Depressed
Vomiting	Markedly depressed	Slightly depressed
Activity of ascending reticular activating system	Depressed	Enhanced
Reflex reactivity of ascending reticular activating system	Depressed	?
Sham rage	Depressed	Depressed
Conditioned reflexes	Depressed	No effect (short of narcosis)
Avoidance reactions	Slightly depressed	Markedly depressed
Reaction time (man)	No effect	?
Finger-tapping speed (man)	Slowed[1]	?
Release of ACTH and responsiveness of adrenal cortex	No effect	No effect
Gastric secretion	Depressed	Increased

*Yohimbine, another Rauwolfia alkaloid, has some adrenolytic potency.

Clinical Effectiveness

The drugs are highly effective in self-limited psychotic syndromes associated with hyperactivity and restlessness; these syndromes include manic disorders, schizoaffective states and some cases of early schizophrenia. The drugs are sometimes used in depressions accompanied by extreme agitation (for the control of the latter symptom), although it is recognized that they may exacerbate, or sometimes produce, depression. Chlorpromazine is probably the drug of choice in all such syndromes, since it usually works more quickly than reserpine; in fact, the latter often produces excitement before it quiets the patient. Chlorpromazine is usually given by intramuscular injection for a few days, after which oral medication is instituted. If chlorpromazine fails to quiet the patient, reserpine may be given in addition. The use of the drugs has greatly changed the treatment of these disorders. The patients eat and sleep well almost from the start, and their spontaneous recovery is thereby hastened; moreover, nurses and attendants are freed from the necessity of standing constant watch over excited patients (each of such patients formerly kept as many as three or four attendants fully occupied). In the absence of accurate data on the life histories of these syndromes, it cannot be stated how many of the patients greatly helped by the drugs would not have shown similar improvement with the older methods of treatment.

Another acute syndrome that is greatly benefited by these drugs is delirium tremens, as are the closely similar syndromes that accompany withdrawal in drug addicts. Delirium tremens is a serious disease (15 to 55 per cent of patients who had it in a large municipal hospital died of it); the introduction of "tranquilizing" drugs has simplified the treatment and apparently improved the outcome in patients with this disorder. Similarly, the acute anxiety exhibited by addicts deprived of narcotic or barbiturate drugs can be greatly ameliorated through the use of chlorpromazine or reserpine. These drugs should be given parenterally in such cases.

Occasional patients with catatonia are greatly benefited—at least so far as the catatonic syndrome is concerned—when treated with reserpine; however, they remain schizophrenic.

Results of the use of chlorpromazine for the control of the symptoms of anxiety are difficult to evaluate; many neurotic patients are so suggestible that they report improvement, temporarily at least, after being given almost any medication. However, in most patients with severe recurrent anxiety or with some of its manifestations—including some types of headache and muscle spasms of the neck or back—the drug ameliorates these symptoms. Even more striking is the diminution of the hypersensibility—awareness of and hyper-reactivity to external and internal stimuli—that commonly accompanies neurosis. Most patients with these disorders report lasting benefit when given moderate doses by mouth.

The situation is different in the chronic psychoses. Patients with senile psychoses, with chronic schizophrenic or manic psychoses or with severe behavior disorders, in whom destructiveness, assaultiveness, aggressiveness and noisiness constitute therapeutic problems, often show improvement of these symptoms when given chlorpromazine or reserpine. One may be effective where the other is not, and it cannot be predicted which will work in any given case. These drugs have greatly improved the general status of patients with these syndromes: the use of electroshock treatments may be decreased by 75 per cent and that of lobotomies by 100 per cent, and the decline in destructiveness makes it possible to provide the patients with a more nearly normal environment. On the other hand, probably no more than 15 or 20 per cent of these patients can be discharged; the delusions persist in all, as do hallucinations in most. The biochemical disorders that occur in chronically psychotic patients are not ameliorated, even when there is striking clinical improvement—in their behavior, that is,—not in their thinking (Fig. 4).

It is evident that chlorpromazine and reserpine change psychotic patients but do not cure them. In acute disorders the drugs create circumstances that favor spontaneous remission; in chronic psychoses they greatly improve behavior, permitting discharge in a few cases and improvement of hospital environment in most of the others. These comments apply only to the findings reported in the literature so far. There is no way of knowing whether the use of the drugs over a period of years will benefit a majority of chronically psychotic patients enough to warrant their discharge.

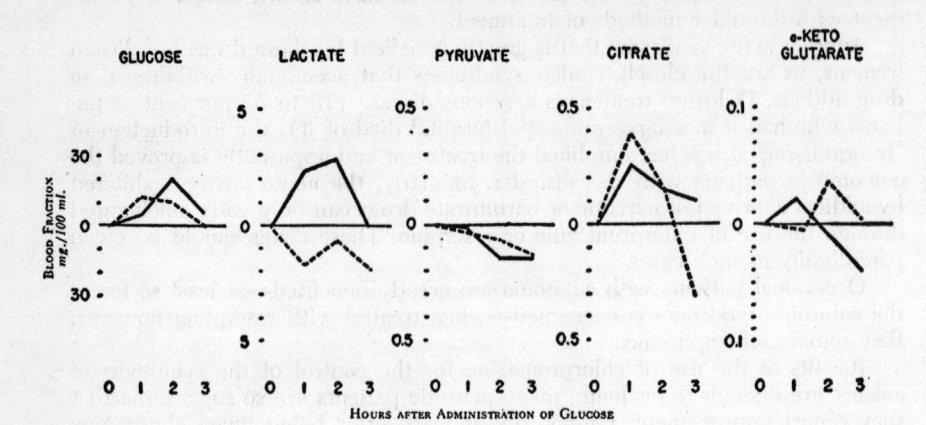

FIGURE 4. *Changes in Blood Carbohydrate Fractions in a Chronic Schizophrenic Patient after Oral Administration of 100 Gm. of Glucose.*
The solid lines indicate curves obtained before treatment; the broken lines indicate curves obtained while the patient was improved on reserpine. Only the curves for citric and alpha-ketoglutaric acid were abnormal before treatment, and they remained so.

At any rate, the changes in status of the patients will make it possible to answer a number of questions. Among these are the extent to which residence in the abnormal environment of the wards for chronically violent patients impairs the patients' chances of recovery and the validity of the claim (often made but never substantiated) that chronically psychotic patients would recover if their intractability did not prevent intensive psychotherapy.

SIDE REACTIONS AND THEIR ABSENCE

Chlorpromazine causes jaundice in about 1.5 per cent of patients who receive large doses by mouth; parenteral injection apparently does not have this effect. This suggests that during oral administration the drug either becomes excessively concentrated in the liver or is changed in some way by the alkaline pH of the intestinal juices. The jaundice usually disappears quickly when the drug is stopped; its course is apparently more prolonged in patients who are malnourished. Rashes also occur in some patients (often those with previous histories of allergies). In a series of over 200 patients no blood dyscrasias occurred—perhaps because no patient received more than 300 mg. a day (Fig. 5 and 6). Agranulocytosis has been reported in rare cases in patients who received large doses. Parkinsonism may also appear in patients given large doses; it wears off quickly when the drug is stopped. Weakness, dizziness and fatigue are often precipitated by the intramuscular use of chlorpromazine; these symptoms are probably of hypotensive origin. Drowsiness may occur when large doses are given by any route. Nasal congestion, dryness of the mouth and constipation are often experienced, but these are usually minor in degree.

Reserpine has no effect on the skin, the liver or the blood. It too produces weakness, dizziness and fatigue. Nausea, vomiting and diarrhea are common;

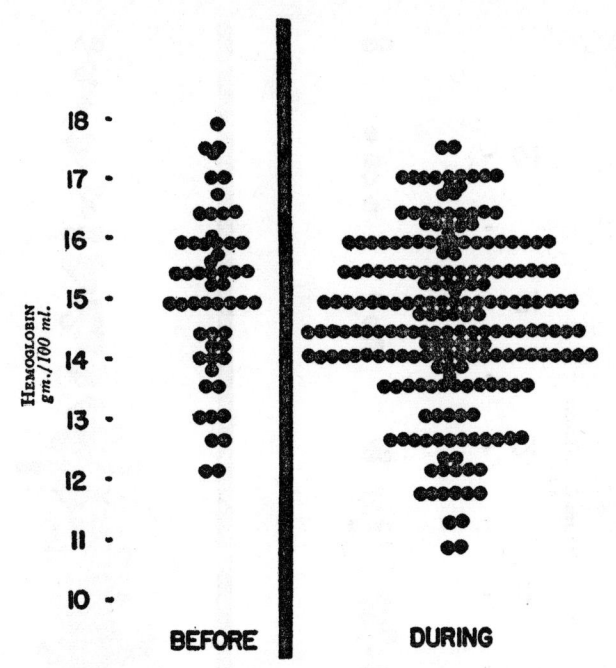

FIGURE 5. *Blood Hemoglobin Concentrations in 55 Patients before and during Treatment with Chlorpromazine. The apparent slight fall during treatment is specious, being due to relaxation of the venospasm commonly encountered in emotional disorders.*

Parkinsonism, nasal congestion and dryness of the mouth also occur. In addition, the drug often causes nightmares and erotic behavior; when given in large doses it usually causes transitory excitement in the second week of treatment. Increased gastric secretion and, occasionally, perforation of gastric ulcers have been reported to occur when large doses are given. (Chlorpromazine decreases gastric secretion.)

Except for the jaundice caused by chlorpromazine and the gastric perforations caused by reserpine, none of the complications of their use are very important. In fact, the absence of serious complications is noteworthy. Of particular interest is the ability of patients to take enormous doses of reserpine and large doses of chlorpromazine with little or no lasting hypotensive effect. This is probably due to the abnormal vasoconstrictor activity of their autonomic nervous systems.

Chlorpromazine and reserpine have changed psychiatric treatment greatly in the last two or three years; as far as can be judged at present, their chief value in therapy is that they produce conditions favorable to recovery in acute,

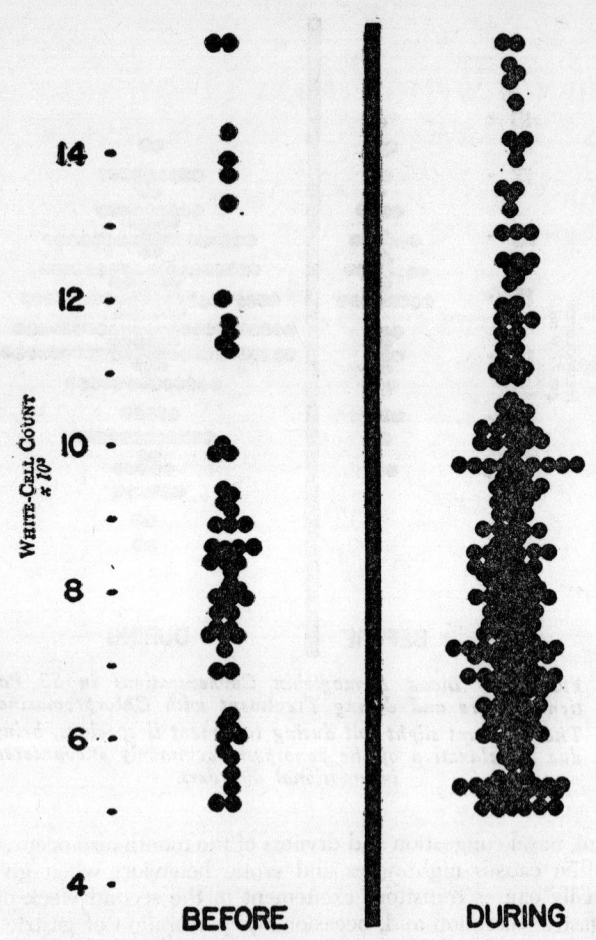

FIGURE 6. *White-Cell Counts in 55 Patients before and during Treatment with Chlorpromazine.*

self-limited psychoses, ameliorate anxiety in many syndromes and make behavior, if not thinking, more nearly normal in chronic psychoses.

I am indebted to Roscoe B. Doughty, Ph.D., of the Science Information Department, Smith Kline and French Laboratories, Philadelphia, for assistance in the preparation of this review.

EXPERIENCE WITH THE USE OF CHLORPROMAZINE AND RESERPINE IN PSYCHIATRY

With Especial Reference to the Significance and Management of Extrapyramidal Dysfunction

George W. Brooks, M.D.
Senior Psychiatrist, Vermont State Hospital, Waterbury, Vermont

The introduction of the tranquilizing or ataraxic drugs in the treatment of mental illness during 1954 resulted in widespread research in the use of these agents and numerous publications of the findings. Varying results have been obtained, and diverse programs for administration have been suggested. Despite differences in dosage ranges and duration of therapies, most practitioners who have used the ataraxics recognize their role in providing symptomatic relief in many types of psychiatric disorders and in facilitating the introduction of adjunctive therapies and the management of patients. Some practitioners believe that the drugs have brought about or helped bring about interruption or alteration of basic psychotic processes, particularly in schizophrenia. The ataraxics, depressants of the central and autonomic nervous systems, appear to act chiefly on subcortical areas of the brain. To these agents, many clinicians have added milder stimulants to overcome concomitant therapeutic effects or side reactions.

Although ataraxics had been in use at the Vermont State Hospital since May, 1954, they were not used extensively until early September of the same year. All told, 386 female patients began treatment with ataraxics before September 1, 1955. This report concerns the experience with this group through January 11, 1956, and represents over 40 per cent of the total number of female patients treated during the period of study. During the early months of this study most patients were selected because they presented some problem of disturbed behavior. However, as experience increased, the group was expanded to include a number of nondisturbed patients of various types.

MATERIALS AND METHODS

Of these 386 patients, 187 received chiefly chlorpromazine, 67 chiefly reserpine, and 132 a combination of the two. Since these drugs were administered at an early stage of their research, it was necessary to use imagination and courage in the regimens and vigilance in following the patients. The use of such medications as trihexyphenidyl (Artane), methyl-phenidylacetate, mephenesin, benzotropine methanesulfonate (Cogentin), diphenhydramine (Benadryl) and thonzylamine (Neohetramine) to control side effects of the ataraxics required that the drug combinations or dosages be changed as often as 20 to 25 times in many patients. As a result, the figures on dosage regimens do not easily lend themselves to statistical evaluation.

The usual daily dosages for the ataraxics were 300 mg. of chlorpromazine or 3 mg. of reserpine, or in combination, 150 mg. of chlorpromazine and 1 mg. of reserpine. Not more than 800 mg. of chlorpromazine or 30 mg. of reserpine or 450 mg. of chlorpromazine and 3 mg. of reserpine were given in one day.

The duration of treatment has ranged from one to sixteen months. It is planned to continue treatment indefinitely for a number of patients with more chronic disorders. In 204 of 386 patients at least minimum signs of extrapyramidal disorder were detected; this reaction is discussed below. To counteract it, trihexyphenidyl, 5 to 15 mg. daily, in 151 cases, or methyl-phenidylacetate, a new drug not yet on the market, 30 to 120 mg. daily, in 27 cases, or a combination of the two, in 26 cases, was added to the dosage of ataraxics.

TABLE 1. *Status of Patients on January 11, 1956, by Diagnostic Group.*

Diagnosis	Totals	Patients Released Off Drugs	Patients Released On Drugs	Patients Very Much Improved in Hospital	Patients Much Improved in Hospital	Patients Moderately Improved in Hospital	Patients Not Improved	Patients for Whom Drugs Stopped	Patients Who Died
Schizophrenia:									
>5 yr. in duration	176	13	29	12	61	46	3	8	4
<5 yr. in duration	50	29	11	2	5	0	0	1	2
Manic reaction:									
>5 yr. in duration	8	0	1	0	2	3	0	2	0
<5 yr. in duration	22	19	1	1	0	0	0	0	1
Psychoneurosis	17	9	6	0	1	0	1	0	0
Personality disorders	11	11	0	0	0	0	0	0	0
Acute brain syndrome	5	5	0	0	0	0	0	0	0
Chronic brain syndrome	55	0	0	0	8	16	1	13	17
Epilepsy	8	0	2	0	2	3	1	0	0
Mental deficiencies	13	0	0	0	5	4	0	4	0
Depressions:									
With electroconvulsive treatment	14	14	0	0	0	0	0	0	0
Without electroconvulsive treatment	7	0	1	0	1	3	0	2	0
Totals	386	100	51	15	85	75	6	30	24

RESULTS

The over-all results are summarized in Table 1. It is evident that varieties of acute reactions respond most readily to these drugs. They do not seem to be of dramatic value in chronic reactions except in schizophrenic and paranoid reactions, or psychoneurotic and personality disorders with anxiety. Of patients with schizophrenic or paranoid psychoses who were ill for five years or longer, 164 were able to continue a course of treatment. Forty-two have been discharged. Of these, 10 had had deep insulin-coma treatments, and most others had had one or more courses of electroconvulsive therapy. Twelve, still in the hospital, are very much improved and expected to go home soon. Sixty-one are much improved to the point of enjoying social activities and engaging in useful occupations. Forty-six are improved in the sense that they are quiet, tractable and co-operative with ward routine. Only 3 are unimproved. As in other treatment programs, paranoid and catatonic schizophrenias responded somewhat more readily than other types.

There were 50 patients with schizophrenic or paranoid reactions who had been ill for less than five years. Of these, 40 are now out of the hospital, another 2 are very much improved and about ready to leave, and 5 are much improved.

Fifty-five patients suffering from chronic brain syndrome[1] have responded less favorably. None have been discharged, only 8 are much improved, 13 have had to be taken off the drugs, and 17 have died.

These drugs seem to be specific for acute manic reactions. The results with chronic manic reactions have been disappointing.

The ataraxics were of considerable value in controlling anxiety, agitation and acute delirious reactions accompanying electroconvulsive treatment of depressions.

The administration of chlorpromazine or reserpine or both is the treatment of choice in schizophrenic or paranoid reactions, in psychoneurotic or personality disorders with anxiety and in acute brain syndromes. In these cases 50 per cent of patients able to continue treatment have been discharged. Another 31 per cent are much or very much improved. Of patients with these disorders who have been mentally ill for less than five years, 80 per cent have been discharged, and an additional 9 per cent are much improved.

Of the 151 patients now in the community, 90 have been out of the hospital for more than six months, and 122 for more than four months. The remaining 29 have been released during the past four months.

Of the 151 patients who have been released from the hospital, 109 received chiefly chlorpromazine, 15 were treated with reserpine alone, and 27 with a combination of the two.

In this series, 24 patients died during the course of the study, but this represents no significant change in either the death rate or the pattern of causes in the female service. There is no indication, in 23 of these cases, that death was connected in any way with the use of the medications. Only 15 of these patients had received ataraxics during the two weeks before their terminal illness. Of the 24, 17 were over seventy years of age, 13 being over eighty. Seventeen of the group suffered from chronic brain syndromes. The chief causes of death were respiratory and circulatory: 10 died of bronchopneumonia, 5 of circulatory disturbances, and 2 of cerebrovascular accidents. One patient died of perforated duodenal ulcer a day after beginning to receive 3 mg. of reserpine daily.

The usually reported side effects of the ataraxics were encountered in this study. In the group taking chlorpromazine, a variety of rashes developed in 48; 2 of these were severe exfoliative dermatitis, which occurred before those administering treatment were alert to this possibility. Thereafter, the adminis-

---

[1] The terms "acute" and "chronic" brain syndrome follow the official classification adopted by the American Psychiatric Association in 1950.

tration of antihistaminics for two or three weeks controlled all these skin disorders, usually without reduction in the dose of chlorpromazine. In 3 patients mild leukopenic reactions developed on chlorpromazine therapy; 2 were continued on the drug with satisfactory increase in blood counts, and 1 was shifted to reserpine. There were 3 cases of jaundice with chlorpromazine, but 1 patient has been receiving the drug again for six months without signs of recurrence. Among the patients on reserpine, 15 had gastritis with anorexia and some nausea and vomiting. In 4 patients taking trihexyphenidyl a toxic delirium occurred, subsiding within a day or two of withdrawal of the drug or reduction of dosage. Five patients had a return of excited behavior with methyl-phenidyl-acetate.

Discussion

The results of the study are more impressive in terms of qualitative improvements in the patients and in hospital routine than in those of quantitative or statistical analysis of this experience. Particularly impressive has been the striking facilitation of communication with patients with chronic schizophrenia. Even before the patients began to lose their hallucinations and bizarre ideation, it became possible to talk directly with the person behind the disease. As the malignant mental trends began to fade, a peculiar type of objectivity and insight, such as had not been seen before, developed. The patients were able to talk about their strange experiences in the way normal poeple recount bad dreams. After the hallucinations had disappeared, several patients referred to them in words similar to these: "It's hard to describe what it's like to be insane—it's something like being in a bad nightmare all the time."

One of the most encouraging results has been the release from the hospital of the 42 patients with severe schizophrenic or paranoid reactions that had lasted for more than five years. Twenty-four have been out for more than six months. Seventeen had been suffering from mental illness for over ten years, 1 for twenty years, and 1 for thirty years. Twenty-nine of these patients have been continued on medication outside the hospital. Thirty-five are productive members of the community. Five are making a marginal adjustment. Only 2 have relapsed at home and may be returned to the hospital soon. These patients were treated for two to ten months before they were able to leave the hospital. Most required four to six months of treatment. Of these patients, 23 received chlorpromazine, 6 reserpine, and 13 a combination of the two.

The detection of extrapyramidal dysfunction in 204 patients has led to two interesting observations. In the first place the initial sign of improvement often coincides with the onset of obvious extrapyramidal disorder. This onset varied from four weeks to four months in patients receiving only one of the ataraxics, but tended to occur in two to four weeks in those receiving a combination of the two drugs. Before a more extensive and detailed survey of patients for this reaction was made, obvious signs had been noted in 18 per cent of those on reserpine, 30 per cent of those on chlorpromazine, and 56 per cent of those on the combination. The other observation was that the patient's immediate progress was enhanced when extrapyramidal dysfunction was relieved. Slowness of motion, loss of some associated movements, loss of facial mobility and some cogwheel rigidity were regarded as minimum signs. These were relieved by the addition of trihexyphenidyl or methyl-phenidylacetate or both to the regimen. The patients' muscles loosened up, they complained less of lameness and fatigue, their mood improved, and they more readily participated in re-education efforts. After a number of other medications had been tried, trihexyphenidyl was added for 151, methyl-phenidylacetate for 27, and both for 26 patients. Of 232 patients still on ataraxics, 80 per cent are receiving these drugs as well.

Before the occurrence of extrapyramidal signs became a consideration, many patients had left the hospital; however, of the 181 still under medication in the hospital, 89 per cent showed some dysfunction. A variety of disorders developed, including 3 cataleptic states with a suggestion of oculogyric crises, 2 cases of spasmodic torticollis, a number of cases of extreme restlessness, with constant aimless motions suggestive of chorea, and many cases of sialorrhea. All responded favorably to the addition of trihexyphenidyl or methyl-phenidylacetate, or a combination of the two, to the medication schedule. In a few cases it was also necessary to reduce the dose of ataraxics. It was believed that careful attention to the management of extrapyramidal dysfunction contributed greatly to the progress of many patients.

As far as I know, only one other investigator, Haase, has reported a comparable occurrence of extrapyramidal dysfunction among patients treated with large doses of ataraxics. He reported signs and symptoms of Parkinsonism in 88 per cent of his patients. In his series this effect was carefully studied by extensive analysis of changes in handwriting. He postulated that the changes in extrapyramidal function are the essential effect ("Eigenwirkung") of the drugs on the central nervous system. My opinion has been that signs of Parkinsonism heralded the particular effect being sought. However, it was found that the therapeutic effects were not dependent on extrapyramidal dysfunction. On the contrary, alleviation of such dysfunction, as soon as it occurred, sped the progress of recovery.

Although, as noted above, most of the 386 patients in this study had presented considerable problems in behavior, a few were very withdrawn, quiet, seemingly "comfortable" patients with schizophrenia. Some of these chronically ill patients did not show any great improvement until as much as six months after the beginning of the treatment. It has been believed that a trial of treatment lasting less than six months would be inadequate for any chronic, severe psychotic condition.

The qualitative changes wrought in mental-hospital practice have been impressive. The disturbed wards no longer deserve the name. Restraints and seclusion have been practically abolished. Departments of recreational, occupational and industrial therapy have been strained to the utmost to provide for the vastly increasing number of patients who are able to participate in these activities. Destruction of clothing and bedding has been greatly reduced. Many patients who had not been properly dressed in years are now neat and clean. The wards smell better. The atmosphere in those for "deteriorated" and "disturbed" patients at mealtime is strikingly changed; meals are now a comparatively quiet, pleasant interlude.

A total of 51 patients in this series have continued receiving medications outside the hospital. The majority of these return to the hospital at least once a week at first, for an interview and a prescription or a supply of medicine for a state-supported patient. A few have been followed primarily by their own physicians or private psychiatrists.

The most pressing problem for the future is the rehabilitation of the 73 much improved patients with chronic schizophrenic or paranoid disorders that had lasted for more than five years. Many in this group have lost all contact with the community. A few have been divorced as "incurably" insane. The families of some have died, or drifted away. A small beginning in a co-operative program with the Division of Vocational Rehabilitation has been made. Jobs have been found for 3; The Division of Vocational Rehabilitation is working with 6 others who are out of the hospital and 16 others who are still inside. It is recognized that there is a need for a far more ambitious, extensive and imaginative program of research in comprehensive public-health medicine, in co-operation with the Division of Vocational Rehabilitation, mental-health clinics and other agencies under the direction of the University of Vermont College of Medicine, to study community resources and attitudes and search for the most effective methods to fit these people back into productive life in the community.

SUMMARY

Chlorpromazine, reserpine and a combination of these two agents (in a ratio of 150 mg. of chlorpromazine to 1 mg. of reserpine) have been employed as standard medications in 386 psychotic female patients for a period of sixteen months at Vermont State Hospital. Most of these patients were agitated or showed antagonistic attitudes. A number of anti-depressant drugs, particularly trihexyphenidyl and methyl-phenidylacetate, have been added to the dosage regimens of many patients to control side effects of the ataraxics.

One hundred and fifty-one patients have been discharged; 15 others are awaiting discharge; 85 are much improved, though still in the hospital; and 75 are improved, being quiet and co-operative with ward routine.

Qualitative improvement in many psychoses was likewise impressive. The drugs appeared to facilitate communication with patients with chronic schizophrenia. A peculiar type of objectivity and constructive insight was noted in many cases. In this series 36 patients failed to respond to treatment or had to be taken off the drugs, and 24 died during this period. The death rate was normal in comparison with that in previous years.

The occurrence of extrapyramidal dysfunction was usually followed by initial signs of improvement in the patient's psychosis. The chlorpromazine-reserpine combination tended to produce this dysfunction more frequently and sooner than either drug alone. The patient's progress was enhanced when this dysfunction was relieved by trihexyphenidyl or methyl-phenidylacetate, which are now in use for this purpose in 80 per cent of the drug-treated patients.

Conditions within the hospital have been significantly improved: disturbed wards have been virtually eliminated; the atmosphere of dining halls and living areas has been transformed; and psychotherapeutic and sociotherapeutic facilities are being widely utilized. These results emphasize the need for social agencies to help the hospital restore to society patients like the 73 who are being retained largely because their families can no longer absorb them after five years or more of mental illness.

AMBULATORY AND COMPARATIVE TREATMENT OF THE ANXIETY NEUROSIS SYNDROME WITH CHLORPROMAZINE, PHENOBARBITAL AND DIMETHYLANE

Wallace Marshall, M.D.

Anxiety neurosis is defined as "a psychoneurosis characterized by emotional instability, apprehension, and a sense of utter fatigue; caused by incomplete suppression of emotional problems. It is associated with visceral phenomena such as tachycardia, palpitation, nausea, a sense of suffocation, diarrhea, tremors, and perspiration. Also called 'anxiety state'."

Some authorities regard anxiety neurosis as a form of "psychasthenia" in which fear is the predominant symptom as are other obsessions such as fear of saying or doing wrong acts. Musser states that "a general nervous irritability (or excitability) is regularly associated with the anxious expectation or dread. . . . Fluctuations occur in the intensity of the symptoms, acute exacerbations constituting the anxiety attack." Musser goes on to state that "neurasthenia and some of the anxiety states, too, are faulty responses—attempts to escape from the difficulties and conflicts of life."

Schneider and Rodis state that the anxiety states are among the most common psychoneurotic manifestations which are characterized by abnormal fear, apprehension, and anxiety. Vasomotor changes are commonly present. They feel that such symptoms are related to past emotional conflicts. These anxiety symptoms serve as a justifiable cause for worry rather than the true and fundamental causes of which the patient is ashamed or to which he will not admit. A good prognosis in such cases can be expected if the patient possesses a reasonable amount of intelligence and also insight and if he desires to rid himself of his unfortunate mental condition.

Malamud feels the etiology of anxiety neurosis is produced by "a primary frustration of or danger to free flow of the vital instincts." He mentions interference with the sexual instinct as a frequent factor in the production of the anxiety neuroses. These conditions, according to Malamud, are produced by "a definite blocking or damming up of instinctive energy and not with a transformation of sexual gratification into new channels."

Overstimulation of neural impulses from various perceptors, which I have termed psychoallergens, can produce an overstimulation of related cortical centers. The physiological process appears to be very similar to the production of allergic states elsewhere in the body economy. For the overexcitation from allergens produces hyperallergic states to the specific allergens which were employed to institute the original reactions. Once a hyperallergic state is produced, even a modicum of the offending allergen is ample to produce a severe allergic reaction. I am sure many physicians can recall cases of such unfortunate responses in many of their patients.

Similarly, once a psychoallergic state is produced in the various recipient cortical centers from excessive psychoallergens, a similar surmenage may well take place. Here is a physiologic basis for abnormal human behavior. For the so-called psychic insults spoken of by many of our psychiatrists can be boiled down to excessive perceptual stimuli which have been allowed to bombard the perceptive cortical centers of learning.

Hence the use of general narcosis at least temporarily shuts off all these cortical centers from further punishment. This effect forms the time-honored Wier-Mitchell treatment as does any medication which depresses the central nervous system.

The process of psychoanalysis can be explained readily by our theory of psychoallergy. Certain painful experiences are reintroduced (mostly through the analyst by recall), and mild psychoallergic reactions are allowed to recur. This process is repeated as is the use of infinitesimal amounts of allergens in an allergic patient. Finally, desensitization takes place since the patient does not react to former painful psychic stimuli.

Psychic stimuli can be most complex in nature, for patients can *learn* to identify those individuals who have committed the psychic insults along with the acts themselves. Hence, it is not unusual for a patient to react unfavorably to certain human characteristics and acts which have become identified with those responsible for the original psychic insults.

It appears that many diverse and sundry agents can produce overstimulation to an individual's cortical centers. Sexual insults do not necessarily exclude the many other causes for such psychoallergic upsets.

Treatment of Anxiety Neuroses

The psychiatric approach to the treatment of anxiety neurosis is to find the offending cause and remove it. This is a time-consuming procedure, especially for those physicians who do not use psychiatric procedures for one reason or another.

The medical or pharmacologic approach to the treatment of such disorders is to use some type of medication which will prevent or block these emotional surmenages by blocking impulses from the hypersensitized cortical centers.

One of the oldest and most commonly used medications is phenobarbital through its general depression of the cortical centers. Of recent date are two new additions to the physicians' therapeutic armamentarium. One of these recent drugs is chlorpromazine (largactyl, Thorazine, SKF-2601A) and the other is Dimethylane (2, 2-diisopropyl-4-hydroxy-methyl-1, 2-dioxolane).

Since phenobarbital has been used for many years for anxiety states, this drug was chosen as our standard or control in order to compare it to the therapeutic actions of the two newer drugs.

The barbiturates have been employed for many years to control the emotional surmenages found in neurotic and so-called "nervous" patients. The recommended dose of phenobarbital is one-half grain. I am sure that many clinicians employ the larger and more used dosage of 1½ grains by mouth.

According to Sollmann "the sedative action of the barbiturates is used to secure sleep, to dull worry and apprehension, to calm nervousness, and to obtain tranquillity and rest in conditions ranging from 'overwrought nerves' through drug addictions, hyperthyroidism, mania, chorea and epilepsy; the narcotic action is used to produce partial or complete unconsciousness in anesthesia, amnesia in parturition; and a hypnotic state suitable for psychiatric analysis. The effects can be readily graded in intensity by dosage, and in duration by the selection of the appropriate barbiturate."

Sollmann cites clearly the disadvantages of barbiturates by stating that "the response is rather variable, markedly so in some individuals." I presume many physicians have noted the same observation with the use of certain opiates. Some patients become stimulated mentally instead of becoming depressed. Other disadvantages from the use of barbiturates, as cited by Sollmann, are that "the hynotic effect is rather preceded by considerable excitement, inebriation and even delirium; and the sleep and hepetude may be undesirably prolonged. Collapse occurs exceptionally."

Mayer *et al*. found that chlorpromazine in doses of 50 mg. three times daily gave "an excellent therapeutic result without exception and the patient felt better on chlorpromazine than on any other regime." Their observations were in varied neuro-psychiatric disorders: 217 patients were neurotic and had other minor mental and emotional disorders, 31 cases exhibited anxiety neuroses. According to Mayer *et al*. two thirds of these cases had excellent results, although drops in blood pressure were not unusual even in some hypertensive cases. Foster *et al*. found that chlorpromazine caused a fall in blood pressure with a rise in pulse rate. They found that the extent of these changes was variable and unpredictable. According to these investigators, the drug possesses a central inhibitory action on vasomotor tone. The exact nature of chlorpromazine's action is unknown, although it is thought that it interferes with the synaptic transfer of excessive psychomotor excitement between cortical cells and the diencephalon. Winkelman found the drug especially remarkable in that it could "reduce severe anxiety, diminish phobias and obsessions, reverse or modify a paranoid psychosis, quiet manic or extremely agitated patients, and change the hostile, agitated, senile patient into a quiet easily managed patient."

Kinross-Wright reported that "among the neurotic group, response has been more variable. Most of the patients report some improvement but as mentioned above the side effects of chlorpromazine sometimes cause patients to refuse larger doses . . ." Trethowan and Scott reported the presence of jaundice as a most serious complication in 3 of their series of cases. Skin rashes occurred in 7 of their cases, while 6 patients developed pyrexia. Other minor side effects were dizziness, thirst, abdominal discomfort, and constipation. Eight patients complained of nightmares. Some drowsiness developed in at least one-half of his patients. Tasker reported a case of agranulocytosis which was caused by the use of chlorpromazine. He suggested that "evidence of sensitivity to chlorpromazine should be treated with respect. Fever, jaundice, and skin eruptions during the early weeks of treatment should be taken as danger signals and should compel repeated examination of the blood, if not withdrawal of the drug.

Ulcerative stomatitis, particularly if it occurs at about the sixth week of treatment, should be an absolute indication for the immediate cessation of chlorpromazine therapy."

Burnstein and Sampson reported a case who suffered a prolonged and gravely severe hypotensive reaction from four 25 mg. doses of chlorpromazine (Thorazine) by mouth. The drug produced a critical shock-like state in a 71 year old white male who also exhibited psychic irritability of three days' duration.

Psychiatric conditions have, of late, been treated with various new pharmacologic products such as mephenesin and its allied group of compounds. Schlesinger *et al.* stated that mephenesin acts on the spinal cord and brain stem. "At certain concentrations it has definite hypnotic effects; at others it is an effective local anesthetic. Its curare-like action seems of minor import, but its ability to depress cortical potentials relates it more closely to the barbiturates ... It may be suggested that its site of action is the internuncial neurones."

Dimethylane, a 2, 2 diisopropyl derivative of dioxolane, was found to have a wider margin of safety and greater activity than mephenesin according to Boines and Horoschak. Dimethylane was found by Kissen *et al.* to control psychomotor agitation in alcoholics. Boines reported the control of anxiety tension symptoms related to the menopausal syndrome. Dimethylane was observed by Boines and Horoschak. Dimethylane was found by Kissen *et al.* to control psynorrhea. These same investigators found that Dimethylane was very effective in improving the symptoms of anxiety in cases of occupational stress.

The success which these investigators experienced with the practically non-toxic preparation, Dimethylane, suggested to this writer that it would be worthwhile to employ it in those cases of the anxiety states which are common in general practice.

It must be quite apparent that these anxiety states are the result of previous hypersensitizations of those cortical areas which received perceptual sensations from the five avenues of perception (sight, hearing, smelling, tasting, and feeling.) A leukotomy interrupts through a surgical procedure the surmenage of cortical potentials from the oversensitized cortical cells. By means of drugs a temporary interruption (medical leukotomy) may occur when phenobarbital, chlorpromazine, or Dimethylane are employed.

Clinical Trial of These Drugs

"A continuous narcosis is of use in the case of the acute anxiety state, as is possible only in the hospital," according to Rorie. He feels that psychotherapy is preferable in such cases. Our series of cases were ambulatory patients, hence hospitalization was avoided to conserve our patients' financial resources.

Six patients with moderately severe anxiety symptoms were placed on chlorpromazine. The initial dose per patient was 50 mg. three times daily by mouth. It soon developed that all the patients in this group complained of (1) drowsiness, (2) inability to cerebrate properly, and (3) lack of proper coordination so that driving their cars was highly dangerous if not impossible. All patients in this group stated that they didn't seem to care much about their personal problems. They reacted sluggishly to their environment, although all patients stated that they did not have any further feelings of anxiety. This change of mental and emotional status was noticed soon after the first day of therapy.

The dose of chlorpromazine was reduced to 25 mg. three times daily by mouth in these six patients. They reported that drowsiness and their reflexes had improved, but three patients noted the return of their anxiety symptoms while three did not experience this difficulty. However, even with the decrease in the chlorpromazine dosage to three 25 mg. tablets per day, all experienced some difficulty in coordination and the partial loss of adequate reflex control. It became apparent that this drug did not appear safe for ambulatory patients because of the partial loss of adequate reflex control. Therefore no further cases were placed on this medication.

Twenty patients with anxiety symptoms were placed on phenobarbital, 1½ grains twice daily. Although this is a much larger dose of phenobarbital than is recorded for the usual amount per dose in many pharmaceutical textbooks, past experience has proved that our daily dose was permissible.

Of the 20 patients on phenobarbital twelve felt somewhat better so far as their anxiety symptoms were concerned. Of these 12 patients, four complained of general grogginess and inability to cerebrate. Eight patients reported no improvement.

The six previous chlorpromazine cases along with 14 new cases were treated with Dimethylane in enteric coated capsules, each capsule representing 250 mg. of the drug. All cases with the exception of two reported marked relief of their anxiety symptoms. All the improved cases experienced no drowsiness, no inability to cerebrate, and no loss of coordination. All cases had rapid relief (except the 2 cases which were recorded as failures) within a matter of 24 hours after taking their first capsule.

However, it was found necessary for these improved patients to continue on Dimethylane since their symptoms of anxiety returned if they went without medication. It seemed necessary to employ two capsules (500 mg.) four times daily. The capsules were administered by having each patient take 2 capsules (500 mg.) after each meal and at bedtime by mouth. Several patients tried to cut the dosage to one capsule (250 mg.) four times daily without proper or adequate results. Their relief from the symptoms of anxiety became manifest only upon the previous recommended dosage of 2 capsules (500 mg.) four times daily.

Report of a Typical Case

This case is cited because this patient first was given chlorpromazine, then phenobarbital, and finally Dimethylane. A 28 year old married white woman, found it impossible to be away from home at any time. She refused to shop at a store or to mingle with people. She continually felt ill at ease with anyone but her immediate family. Her anxiety symptoms occurred following the birth of a daughter six years ago.

Chlorpromazine produced a complete obliteration of old symptoms of anxiety. However, she complained of feeling "drugged and dopy." She found it difficult to hold any trend of thought, and she felt like sleeping continually.

Upon using phenobarbital her symptoms of anxiety returned, although she could carry a good trend of thought. She experienced no difficulty in coordination. She felt tired continually.

When all medication had been discontinued for a week, she was placed upon Dimethylane. She took two capsules of this drug twice daily. The first day her husband suggested that they go for a walk. She agreed, and they stopped at the corner drugstore and had some ice cream. Her husband related that was the first time they both enjoyed going out together since her illness began. She has continued to improve and now shops downtown without the usual feeling of intense fright which had plagued her previously. She is unable to discontinue her medication as yet. This patient has been free of all anxiety symptoms for a period of three months. She lives in a large city and can travel downtown by herself without any difficulty.

Summary

The use of certain pharmacologic preparations depresses the entire hypersensitized cortical areas, thus bringing temporary relief in cases of anxiety neurotic patients. Chlorpromazine apparently produces a deeper disruption than does Dimethylane. Patients in the present series of cases treated with Dimethylane do not report the production of drowsiness, the inability to cerebrate properly, and the lack of proper coordination which appears to be the case with the use of chlorpromazine. Since patients prefer to remain ambulatory for many reasons, the use of Dimethylane is preferred to chlorpromazine. Therefore Dimethylane appears to be the drug of choice in ambulatory patients because of its practically non-toxic properties and its ability to block those cortical surmenages which produce the symptoms of anxiety states. In other words, Dimethylane appears to produce pharmacalogically temporary clinical improvements similar to those which are expected when a leukotomy is performed.

THORAZINE AND SERPASIL TREATMENT OF PRIVATE NEUROPSYCHIATRIC PATIENTS

Frank J. Ayd, Jr., M.D.

Thorazine and Serpasil have proven effective in the treatment of hospitalized psychiatric patients manifesting symptoms of anxiety, tension, agitation, confusion, panic, and psychomotor excitement. The value of these drugs to the private practicing psychiatrist who treats the majority with similar symptoms has yet to be assessed.

This is a report of the findings in the treatment of 300 nonhospitalized private psychiatric patients, 150 of whom were treated with Thorazine and 150 with Serpasil. The patients were selected at random in order to determine the effect of these drugs in the treatment of a variety of psychiatric disturbances.

CASE MATERIAL

Sixty-six men and eighty-four women, ranging in age from 16 to 82, were treated with Thorazine. Sixty-one men and 89 women, ranging in age from 14 to 78, were treated with Serpasil. The dosage and route of administration varied with the severity and acuteness of the patient's condition. The neurotic and moderately disturbed psychotic patients received Thorazine in divided daily doses of 100 to 500 mg. orally or 0.5 to 10 mg. of Serpasil orally. Disturbed schizophrenic and manic patients, who were hospitalized initially, received daily 500 to 2,500 mg. of Thorazine or 5 to 15 mg. of Serpasil, orally and intramuscularly. Parenteral medication was discontinued usually within one week. Unlike intramuscular Thorazine, parenteral Serpasil was not painful.

The appearance of the patient receiving Thorazine or Serpasil is contingent upon the dosage and duration of treatment. Patients started on 300 mg. or more of Thorazine, whether orally or parenterally, sleep for long periods. They can be aroused easily, are mentally alert and in the absence of external stimuli return to their somnolent state. Their skin is pale and warm. Their facial expression resembles the mask-like facies of Parkinsonism. There is an enopthalmus and ptosis of the eyelids suggestive of a Horner's syndrome. The pulse rate is accelerated and the blood pressure may fall 20 to 40 mm. Hg. There is some hypotonia and the patients complain of feeling weak.

The appearance of patients receiving more than 5 mg. of Serpasil initially is similar to that described for those taking Thorazine, with the exception that Serpasil patients have a bradycardia.

These signs of the effects of Thorazine and Serpasil subside when the dosage is reduced. If treatment is continued, the signs abate gradually, even when the dosage is increased.

TECHNIQUE OF THERAPY

Before Thorazine or Serpasil therapy is instituted, the patient and the relatives should be informed of possible side-effects and instructed to report immediately any pronounced change such as grippe-like symptoms, chills and fevers, marked itching, anorexia, nausea, diarrhea, heavy darkening of the urine, or light-colored stools. These instructions prevented anxiety about such symptoms if they occurred and obviated unnecessary phone calls to the psychiatrist, and, as well, insured the early detection of adverse reactions to the drugs, especially jaundice in the patients on Thorazine.

Thorazine is prescribed as follows: Neurotic and mildly disturbed psychotic patients are started on 25 or 50 mg. tablets t.i.d. or q.i.d. The dosage is increased gradually until a therapeutic level for the individual patient is achieved. The patient is maintained at this dose schedule from 2 weeks to several months. When he appears to have obtained maximum therapeutic benefit, Thorazine is discontinued by reducing the dose gradually over 1 to 2 months. In the event of a relapse, he is placed immediately on his previous therapeutic dose. This is not always effective and then larger doses are prescribed. If no favorable change occurs within one month, the drug is discontinued. In a few instances a patient's symptoms recur as the dose is reduced. Such patients are placed on maintenance doses. Six patients, not included in this study, have been taking Thorazine for 16 months without any observable adverse effects from this prolonged medication and with a preservation of improvement.

Acutely disturbed patients are started on Thorazine orally or intramuscularly. For most patients 500 mg. daily for a week or 2 is sufficient to produce a quiescent state permitting their discharge from the hospital. Since the dose of any drug must be individualized some of the patients received as much as 2,500 mg. of Thorazine daily before their therapeutic level was reached. They were then treated in the same manner as less disturbed ones.

Serpasil has one distinct advantage over Thorazine in that it is longer acting and may be prescribed in divided daily doses or the entire daily dose can be taken at one time. It is prescribed as follows: Neurotic and mildly disturbed psychotic patients are started on 0.5 mg. or 1 mg. daily. Some patients take 0.25 mg. after supper and h.s., and others take 1 mg. h.s. Since Serpasil is slower in taking effect than Thorazine, to prevent overdosage, the dose is increased gradually, usually weekly, until the patient's therapeutic level is reached. He continues on this dose until he appears to have achieved maximum benefit. This period lasts from 2 weeks to several months and then the drug is discontinued by gradual reduction of the dose for 1 to 2 months. If a relapse occurs, the patient is restarted on his previous therapeutic dose. If improvement does not result within 1 month, even with increased doses, Serpasil is discontinued. As with Thorazine a small number of patients have required a maintenance dose of Serpasil to prevent a relapse.

Acutely disturbed patients are begun on 5 mg. Serpasil orally and parenterally. Most patients respond to doses of 5 to 12 mg., although a few require 15 mg. daily for a week or 2 before they are subdued enough to leave the hospital. Once the therapeutic level for the individual patient is obtained he is treated in the same manner as mildly disturbed patients.

RESULTS

The therapeutic results obtained with Thorazine and Serpasil are indicated in Table 1. Improved means recovery or symptomatic improvement to a degree that the patient is able to make a satisfactory home, work, and social adjust-

TABLE 1
DIAGNOSTIC GROUPINGS AND THERAPEUTIC RESULTS

Diagnosis	Thorazine Improved	Thorazine Unimproved	Serpasil Improved	Serpasil Unimproved
Schizophrenic reactions				
Paranoid	8	1	7	3
Catatonic	5	—	5	1
Simple	—	1	—	1
Unclassified	2	3	1	2
Schizo-affective	3	1	3	1
Pseudoneurotic	—	1	—	2
Manic-depressive reactions				
Depressed	4	10	2	8
Hypomanic	2	—	3	—
Manic	3	—	1	—
Involutional depression	2	5	1	8
Psychoneurotic reactions				
Anxiety	39	5	35	8
Depressive	1	5	4	6
Mixed	16	7	15	6
Hysterical	2	1	1	3
Hypochondriacal	1	1	—	1
Obsessive-compulsive	3	8	2	9
Senile psychoses	6	—	4	2
Character disorder	2	2	—	4
Total	99	51	84	66

ment. Unimproved means no change or a relapse after initial improvement.

These drugs are most effective in the acutely ill patient, with symptoms due to enhanced central sympathetic excitability, regardless of the diagnosis or the duration of the illness. Chronically ill patients who have no anxiety and who accept their illness with a certain degree of complacency do not benefit from them. Likewise, depressed patients who have no associated anxiety do not respond. Obsessive-compulsive patients often improve initially but with continued treatment relapse. These patients, in particular, vociferously object to the side-effects of these drugs and frequently refuse to take them. They build up intolerable anxiety because the side-effects interfere with the maintenance of their self-imposed standards.

Thorazine and Serpasil make it possible to treat on an ambulatory basis many patients who would have otherwise had to be hospitalized. In the few instances that hospitalization was necessary, patients could be adequately treated in a general hospital or a regular nursing home. After a week or 2 of hospitalization, these patients were treated in the office. Only in severe manic or schizophrenic reactions was commitment to a psychiatric hospital necessary for a few weeks.

Geriatric patients made satisfactory home adjustments while taking Thorazine or Serpasil. Without these drugs they would have been placed in nursing homes, or state or private psychiatric hospitals. With the drugs geriatric patients in nursing homes were able to remain there or return home instead of entering a psychiatric hospital.

It should be emphasized that Thorazine and Serpasil are not specific for any psychiatric illness. They cause symptomatic improvement. They calm the excited, agitated, and anxious patient. As tension is reduced, the patient becomes less concerned with his symptoms and is not preoccupied with any particular train of thought or action. Obsessions, phobias, and delusions may die out for lack of emotional reinforcement or are not verbalized because they do not concern the patient. Hallucinations very often persist but worry him less.

Thorazine and Serpasil are not substitutes for psychotherapy. Patients treated with these drugs are better candidates for psychotherapy and seem to derive

TABLE 2
Thorazine Failures Re-Treated with Serpasil

Diagnosis	Improved	Unimproved
Schizophrenic reactions		
Paranoid	—	1
Simple	—	1
Unclassified	—	3
Schizo-affective	1	—
Pseudoneurotic	—	1
Manic-depressive reactions		
Depressed	—	3
Involutional depression	—	3
Psychoneurotic reactions		
Anxiety	1	2
Mixed	1	1
Obsessive-compulsive	—	4
Character disorder	—	2
Total	3	21

more benefit from it. Neither are they a substitute for insulin coma therapy or electroconvulsive therapy. They have not been of value in the treatment of the endogenous depressions. They are as effective as, and preferable to, ECT for quieting the disturbed patient. In a few instances these drugs replaced ECT entirely. Some patients who failed to benefit from ECT responded favorably to Thorazine or Serpasil. Combined Thorazine-ECT has minimized postshock anxiety and excitement, and has reduced the number of electroconvulsive treatments required by patients.

Therapeutic failures with Thorazine were treated with Serpasil and vice versa. Twenty-four patients who did not benefit from Thorazine were treated with Serpasil and 3 of them improved (Table 2). Twenty-four who did not benefit from Serpasil were treated with Thorazine and 5 of them improved (Table 3).

TABLE 3
SERPASIL FAILURES RE-TREATED WITH THORAZINE

Diagnosis	Improved	Unimproved
Schizophrenic reactions		
Paranoid	2	1
Unclassified	—	2
Schizo-affective	1	—
Manic-depressive reactions		
Depressed	—	4
Involutional depression	—	4
Psychoneurotic reactions		
Anxiety	1	2
Mixed	—	1
Obsessive-compulsive	1	3
Character disorder	—	2
Total	5	19

Combined Thorazine-Serpasil therapy was tried in 10 patients. This combination did not appear to be more effective than treatment with the individual drugs. Combined therapy did cause more frequent and more marked side-effects.

Therapeutic failure with either of these drugs may be due to inadequate dosage or an insufficient period of treatment. It is certain that psychotics, especially schizophrenics, require larger doses for a longer period than do neurotics. This is most probably due to a difference in metabolism between the psychotic and the neurotic.

SIDE-EFFECTS

Thorazine and Serpasil have undesirable side-effects which are seldom troublesome or serious (Table 4). They occur more frequently with Serpasil than with Thorazine and patients complain more about the effects of Serpasil. However, they disappear when the drug is discontinued or the dosage reduced.

TABLE 4
Side-Effects

	Thorazine	Serpasil
Jaundice	Yes	No
Parkinsonism	Yes	Yes
Dermatitis	Yes	No
Photosensitivity	Yes	No
Depression	Yes	Yes
Agranulocytosis	Yes	No
Lactation	Yes	Yes
Weakness & fatigue	Yes	Yes
Aching arms & legs	Yes	Yes
Tremulousness	Yes	Yes
Enuresis	No	Yes
Dizziness	Yes	Yes
Headaches & sinusitis	Infrequent	Frequent
Nasal congestion	Yes	Yes
Dryness of mouth	Yes	Yes
Miosis	Yes	Yes
Constipation	Frequent	Infrequent
Diarrhea	No	Yes
Nausea & vomiting	Infrequent	Frequent
Altered erotic drives	Yes	Yes

The most frequent complaint of patients taking Thorazine or Serpasil is a feeling of weakness, fatigue, or lethargy. This may be counteracted by prescribing Dexedrine, Ritalin, Meratran, or Desoxyn.

The more important idiosyncratic reactions to Thorazine are: (1) Obstructive jaundice—this occurred in 4 female patients in this series, an incidence of 3%. There was no correlation between the dosage of Thorazine and the onset of jaundice which appeared in every case within the first month of treatment. In all but one case, which persisted for a month, the jaundice cleared in 10 days after discontinuation of treatment. Subsequent liver studies have not revealed any residual damage. Two of these patients were retreated with Thorazine and one became jaundiced again. (2) Dermatitis—8 patients (5.3%) developed an allergic dermatitis while on Thorazine. In 3 a generalized maculopapular eruption appeared and, in 5, localized rashes occurred. Two Clistin-RA tablets daily for 3 or 4 days relieved the dermatitis, which did not recur in spite of continued treatment with Thorazine. (3) Photosensitivity—2 men developed erythema of the face and neck whenever they were exposed to the sun. Clistin-RA tablets gave complete relief but had to be taken whenever these patients were so exposed. (4) Lactation—one non-pregnant, 28-year-old woman began lactating 1 month after taking 100 mg. Thorazine daily. This ceased when the drug was discontinued but recurred when she was re-treated with Thorazine. (5) Parkinsonism, depression, agranulocytosis—none of the patients in this series developed any of these reactions. The author has had one 48-year-old woman patient who developed agranulocytosis which responded to ACTH and antibiotic therapy.

The more important idiosyncratic reactions to Serpasil are: (1) Parkinsonism—one patient developed this reaction. It ceased when the Serpasil was reduced. (2) Nasal congestion and sinusitis—more than a third of the patients complained of nasal congestion which was most noticeable in the morning. (3) Visual disturbances—more than a third of the patients mentioned blurring of vision. This was frequently associated with dizziness. (4) Tremulousness was mentioned by almost one half of the patients. Many found this especially annoying and some refused Serpasil because of it. (5) Nausea and vomiting—12 patients complained of nausea especially in the morning. Four had vomiting in addition to nausea. The addition of Thorazine to the medication relieved this in all but 2 cases. (6) Diarrhea occurred in 4 patients. It subsided with reduction of the dose of Serpasil. (7) Aching arms and legs—16 patients mentioned this side-effect. Edema of the ankles occurred in 3. (8) Depression—2 patients developed depressions with obsessive features, which remitted when the dose of Serpasil was reduced. (9) Lactation did not occur in this series, although one woman developed painful swelling of the breasts.

Thorazine and Serpasil may cause a polyphagia, polydipsia, and polyuria. The polyphagia is accompanied by a gain in weight, which may be excessive. In this series weight gains ranged from 2 to 40 pounds, the men gaining an average of 10 pounds and the women an average of 13. Improved appetite, weight gain, and improved sleep were associated with an improvement in the patient's clinical condition. Epigastric distress, anorexia, weight loss, and insomnia occurred only in those patients who did not respond to these drugs.

Discussion

In spite of the experience gained by this study, it is extremely difficult to establish positive indications for choosing Thorazine or Serpasil. The effects of these drugs are similar in many respects. Nevertheless, some patients will respond to the one and not to the other, irrespective of their symptoms. For the present it may be said that Thorazine should be prescribed for those neurotic patients whose anxiety is associated with altered gastro-intestinal function, while Serpasil should be prescribed for those whose anxiety is centered on the cardiovascular system.

The Funkenstein test is an accurate indicator of patients who will respond to Thorazine or Serpasil therapy (Fig. 1). Among our patients, those whose Funkenstein test results indicated enhanced central sympathetic excitability derived the most benefit from these drugs. Thus, patients who reacted with anxiety to adrenergic or cholinergic stimulation, responded to Thorazine or Serpasil. This reaction was seen most frequently in anxiety neurotics; 88% of those treated with Thorazine improved and 81% of those treated with Serpasil.

Thorazine and Serpasil have not been beneficial in depressions and they can cause depressions, which may remit after discontinuation of the drug. Some of the depressive reactions induced by these drugs did not remit spontaneously but did respond to ECT. Since both of these drugs are sympathetic depressants, theoretically they can cause an enhanced hypotensive response to cholinergic stimulation, such as is found in depressed patients. In a previous study, 3 patients developed depressions while taking Thorazine. Prior to the institution of

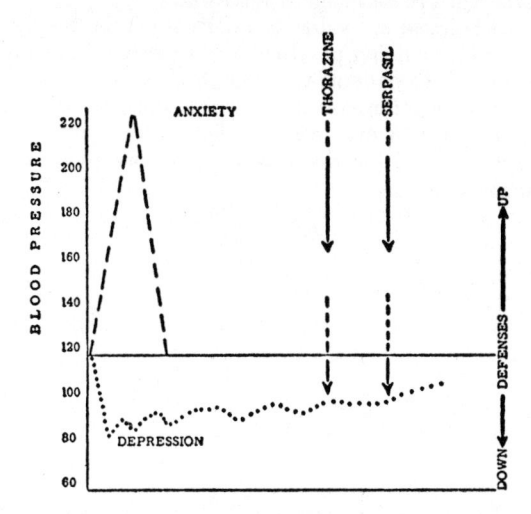

Fig. I.—Epinephrine injection causes varying degrees of elevation of the blood pressure, and may precipitate anxiety. Mecholyl injection causes varying degrees of lowering of the blood pressure; marked and prolonged lowering of the blood pressure by mecholyl is characteristic of depression. The defenses go up with anxiety and down with depression.

A general shift upward on the graph indicates lessening on mecholyl injection, increased reaction to epinephrine, alerting of the defenses, and possible precipitation of anxiety. A shift downward indicates relief of anxiety, lessening of reaction to epinephrine, increase and prolongation of blood pressure fall on mecholyl injection, lowering of defenses, and, finally, possible precipitation of depression.

The way in which Thorazine and Serpasil alter these psychophysiologic constellations is indicated by the solid arrows. (Modified from—L. Alexander: "Treatment of Mental Disorder," Philadelphia; W. B. Saunders, 1953.)

Thorazine therapy the Funkenstein test of these patients showed a normal response to Mecholyl. When the depression appeared the Funkenstein test showed a prolonged hypotensive response to Mecholyl. A third Funkenstein test after Thorazine was discontinued, and the depression over, revealed a normal response to Mecholyl. In the present study 2 patients became depressed while taking Serpasil. Their Funkenstein tests showed the same changes as did those of the patients who became depressed while taking Thorazine.

Summary and Conclusions

This paper reports the findings in the treatment of 300 nonhospitalized private psychiatric patients, 150 of whom were treated with Thorazine and 150 with Serpasil. Their illnesses were diagnosed acute and chronic psychoneuroses, schizophrenic reactions, manic-depressive reactions, senile psychoses, and character disorders. The technique of therapy, the therapeutic results, and the side-effects of these drugs are described. The psychophysiologic action of Thorazine and Serpasil as indicated by changes in the Funkenstein test pattern of patients treated with these drugs is discussed.

Thorazine and Serpasil are valuable additions to the therapeutic armamenterium of the private practicing psychiatrist. Properly utilized, these drugs can: (1) increase the number of patients who may be treated in the office; (2) shorten the period of hospitalization, or make hospitalization unnecessary, thereby reducing the admissions to our overcrowded state psychiatric hospitals; (3) replace or reduce the need for electroconvulsive therapy; and (4) reduce the cost of psychiatric care.

CHLORPROMAZINE (THORAZINE) — RAUWOLFIA COMBINATION IN NEUROPSYCHIATRY

Harold B. Eiber, M.D.
New York Medical College, Flower and Fifth Avenue Hospitals,
New York, N. Y.

The use of chlorpromazine (Thorazine) alone or Rauwolfia serpentina alone in neuropsychiatric conditions has been reported by many authors. At the time of writing, there have been no published reports on the use of the combination of chlorpromazine and Rauwolfia in this type of patient. For the past 18 months this combination has been used with a degree of success in the treatment of moderate and severe essential hypertension. The ease of administration, lack of toxicity and side-effects, and the synergistic therapeutic potentiation suggested the possibility of their simultaneous administration in neuropsychiatric conditions.

This preliminary report is based upon observations on 24 patients with varied neuropsychiatric conditions, none of whom were confined to an institution while receiving this therapy.

METHOD

Preliminary testing with the combination of chlorpromazine and Rauwolfia was begun on patients with schizophrenia, manic-depressive psychosis, senile agitated states, anxiety neuroses, menopausal agitation, epilepsy, primary behavior disorders, and mental deficiency. The subjects were all ambulatory and varied in age from 3 to 92 years.

The diagnosis of each patient had been previously determined by a psychiatrist. All the patients were chronically disturbed, and their behavior patterns had been observed, treated, and documented. Prior therapy included the use of chlorpromazine alone or Rauwolfia sepentina alone, as well as shock therapy, psychoanalysis, barbiturates, and amphetamine.

The patients were placed on the following oral combination:
    Chlorpromazine   25 mg.
    Rauwolfia serpentina 50 mg. (whole root)

The medication was given three to four times daily. In some instances the dose was doubled or tripled. In the cases of smaller, younger patients, the dose was halved. None of the subjects received parenteral treatment. No differences were observed when the whole root of Rauwolfia serpentina was replaced by one of its alkaloids, reserpine.

Results of Combined Chlorpromazine-Rauwolfia Therapy in Neuropsychiatric Patients

No.	Case	Age	Sex	Diagnosis	Previous Treatment	Duration of Chlorpromazine-Rauwolfia Treatment, Mo.	Results
1	K. N.	36	F	Anxiety neurosis	Psychoanalysis Barbiturates Chlorpromazine alone	10	Marked improvement in 3 wk.
2	R. F.	24	F	Schizoid	Shock, lobotomy Barbiturates Institutions	8	Marked improvement in 2 mo.
3	W. B.	6	M	Schizoid	Barbiturates Rauwolfia alone Chlorpromazine alone	6	Dramatic improvement in 1 wk.; able to start school
4	E. S.	33	F	Anxiety neurosis	Barbiturates Psychoanalysis Shock, amphetamine	2	Normal behavior in 3 wk.
5	H. P.	3	F	Schizoid	Institution Rauwolfia alone Chlorpromazine alone	6	Slight improvement after 3 mo.
6	S. R.	46	F	Suicidal	Psychoanalysis Barbiturates Chlorpromazine alone Rauwolfia alone	12	Improved while on combined chlorpromazine-Rauwolfia; no carry-over
7	J. M.	66	F	Anxiety Senile	Shock Barbiturates	2	Marked improvement in 2 wk.
8	R. M.	42	F	Suicidal	Barbiturates Psychoanalysis Institutions	7	Marked improvement in 5 wk.
9	C. B.	36	F	Depression	Barbiturates Shock Rauwolfia alone Chlorpromazine alone	1	Marked improvement in 8 days
10	L. S.	54	F	Anxiety Senile	Barbiturates Amphetamines	10	Marked improvement in 1 mo.
11	D. J.	42	F	Menopausal	Shock Barbiturates Institution	2	Requested and received shock therapy; very little improvement
12	G. B.	44	F	Anxiety Neurosis Suicidal	Shock Institution Barbiturates	6	Normal behavior after 2 wk.
13	S. J.	38	F	Anxiety neurosis	Psychoanalysis Barbiturates Chlorpromazine alone Rauwolfia alone	4	Dramatic improvement in 4 wk.
14	W. A.	43	F	Anxiety neurosis	Barbiturates Amphetamine	13	Marked improvement in 3 wk.
15	R. I.	69	M	Anxiety	Barbiturates	4	Moderate improvement in 2 mo.
16	S. I.	50	F	Menopausal	Barbiturates Chlorpromazine alone	12	Marked improvement in 3 wk.
17	R. H.	33	M	Colitis	Institution Barbiturates	2	Diarrhea worse
18	M. F.	39	M	Anxiety neurosis	Institution Barbiturates Chlorpromazine alone	6	Moderate improvement
19	P. J.	32	M	Functional G. I. disease	Antispasmodics Barbiturates	1	No improvement
20	R. R.	92	F	Anxiety Senile	Choral hydrate Amphetamine Chlorpromazine alone	1	Improvement no greater than with chlorpromazine alone
21	F. B.	60	F	Menopausal	Barbiturates Rauwolfia alone	2 wk.	No improvement; shock therapy required
22	C. P.	44	F	Anxiety neurosis	Barbiturates	10	Dramatic improvement in 10 days
23	C. F.	48	F	Anxiety neurosis	Psychoanalysis Barbiturates Amphetamine Rauwolfia alone	3	Moderate improvement; no greater than with Rauwolfia alone
24	B. M.	52	F	Epilepsy	Barbiturates Diphenylhydantoin Rauwolfia alone	2	Fewer seizures and less anxiety than with Rauwolfia alone

Results

The patients were observed, first, at weekly intervals and, later, at monthly intervals. Of this preliminary series of 24 patients, there were only 3 who did not improve significantly from the effects of the medication. All the remaining 21 patients demonstrated moderate to marked improvement. Unfortunately, there exists no precise method of grading, but an honest attempt was made to evaluate the response from the patient and the family and other general observations. One possible objective yardstick is the amount of time the patient is asymptomatic without recourse to shock therapy or hospitalization.

During the course of therapy, the patients were given, at one time or another, a placebo of similar size, shape, and color. In most of the cases, after a period of 3 to 12 days of placebo therapy, there was an aggravation of symptoms. No attempt at any statistical evaluation is made in this preliminary report. There will be further statistical evidence upon the completion of large-scale studies now being conducted in outpatient departments and psychiatric institutions.

Several cases are briefly presented.

Case 1.—K. N.; anxiety neurosis. A 36-year-old sister of a physician. She had received large doses of barbiturates and amphetamines from her psychoanalyst over a period of nine years. She had a severe anxiety neurosis, was unable to cope with the family, and remained almost constantly confined to her home. She was unable to stay alone, and insomnia was a besetting problem. There was moderate improvement with 300 mg. of chlorpromazine daily alone. Three weeks after the onset of therapy with chlorpromazine and Rauwolfia, her family relationship improved; she could sleep with no sedation, go to the movies, and visit friends. There has been steady improvement over a period of 10 months.

Case 2.—R. F.; schizophrenia. A 24-year-old unmarried woman with a psychiatric history dating back to childhood. She had spent four years in mental institutions, had received several courses of electroshock, and had a lobectomy seven years before. She had been unable to remain away from a mental hospital for more than six months. Results with Rauwolfia alone, and with chlorpromazine alone, were encouraging. Treatment with a combination of the two for a period of two months was rewarded by the ability of the patient to assume a position in her father's store, where she is happy and working satisfactorily.

Case 3.—W. B.; schizophrenia. This 6-year-old boy has been disturbed since infancy. He was destructive, agitated, and uncooperative and could not attend school. There was almost no response to either 100 mg. of chlorpromazine daily or 2.0 mg. of reserpine daily when given singly. One week after start of combined chlorpromazine-Rauwolfia therapy he became more docile and manageable. Two months later he made a fair adjustment in school. Five days after placebo therapy he reverted to an agitated state but was under control within 48 hours after the medication was restored.

Case 6.—R. S.; anxiety neurosis. A 46-year-old woman, separated from her husband, made four suicidal attempts within seven years; she was constantly melancholic and frigid. She showed greater improvement while on combined chlorpromazine-Rauwolfia therapy than when taking either agent singly. She went out of town for a period of one month, during which she neglected to take the medication. Upon her return she took an overdose of barbiturates. Therapy was reinstituted, and she apparently now realizes the importance of continuing with the medication.

CASE 11.—D. J.; severe menopausal symptoms. A 42-year-old woman with marked depression after an artificial menopause. After two months of therapy with both preparations she felt that her improvement was too slow and requested shock therapy. It was thought that there was some degree of amelioration, inasmuch as this patient had requested shock on her own volition.

COMMENT

It is recognized that the psychological treatment of mental illness is dependent on value judgment that the patient is able to exercise as he becomes increasingly aware of the nature of his problems. This raises many questions regarding the use of pharmacological agents, which in many ways diminish value judgments. We do not know, for example, the exact effect of the combination of chlorpromazine and Rauwolfia on the brain. It is possible that this combination may act as a temporary depressant of the frontal lobes of the brain or of the corticothalamic tracts.

There are tremendous difficulties in achieving satisfactory results through the use of psychological treatment alone.

There is also no attempt to minimize the fact that we are dealing with a combination of agents which may hamper judgment, nor is there any attempt on the grounds of expediency to apologize for the use of such agents. There are limitations of psychotherapeutic procedures, as well as limitations of chemical procedures, but it is felt, however, that in this small series of cases a combination of therapeutic agents has been employed that is exceedingly effective in the treatment of many mental conditions.

Of the 21 patients improved, there were 11 who had received chlorpromazine or Rauwolfia singly with moderate improvement. Nine of these 11 showed greater tranquillity, less anxiety, increased cooperation, and fewer symptoms when taking the two agents concurrently.

There were no significant side-effects to warrant cessation of therapy in any of the cases. No jaundice or other toxic manifestation was encountered or reported.

CONCLUSIONS

For the first time, a combination of two therapeutic agents, chlorpromazine and Rauwolfia, is reported for the use of varied neuropsychiatric conditions. It is felt that the two agents, either of which is moderately beneficial when used singly, are mutually synergistic. The marked improvement noted in 21 of the 24 cases suggests the effectiveness of this combination and the advantages over the use of either agent when employed alone. The possibility that this combination may act as a chemical agent on the corticothalamic centers, enabling patients to function at a more satisfactory level, is suggested. The simultaneous use of the two medications appears to be of greater value than when either agent is used singly.

USE OF CHLORPROMAZINE AND RESERPINE IN THE TREATMENT OF EMOTIONAL DISORDERS

William W. Zeller, M.D., Paul N. Graffagnino, M.D., Chester F. Cullen, M.D., and H. Jerome Rietman, M.D.
Institute of Living, Hartford, Connecticut

In the past two years there have been encouraging reports concerning the uses of chlorpromazine [10-(y-dimethylaminopropyl)-2-chlorpromazine hydrochloride] and reserpine (the chief active alkaloid of Rauwolfia serpentina) in the treatment of emotional disorders. Clinical observations thus far have been made mostly on patients in state hospitals.

In general, it has been reported that chlorpromazine and reserpine have a unique calming effect. They have been found to produce a form of sedation without narcosis that causes improvement in the behavior of disturbed, agitated, hyperactive, assaultive, and excited patients, making them more easily manageable. Patients have become quieter, less tense, and more amenable to suggestions from nursing and medical personnel. The need for physical and chemical restraints has been reduced to a minimum. The incidence of accidents and loss or destruction of personal and hospital property has been significantly reduced. The drugs have reduced the need for electroconvulsive treatment, insulin coma treatment, and prefrontal lobotomy in certain patients. Some schizophrenic patients have shown dramatic improvement in their thinking, feeling, and behavior. They have become quieter, less emotionally labile, less concerned about the content of their delusions and hallucinations, and less impulse-ridden in their behavior. Communication of thoughts and feelings to others has improved to such an extent that some of the patients have been more accessible to conventional "interview" type of psychotherapy. Some patients have improved so dramatically that they have been able to leave the hospital after years of confinement. With such consistently favorable reports from various investigators in different parts of the country appearing in the literature, there naturally has followed a wave of hopeful optimism among all individuals vitally interested in the treatment and management of acutely disturbed psychiatric patients.

The purpose of this paper is to present a preliminary report of our clinical experience in treating a group of patients in a 350-bed private psychiatric hospital with chlorpromazine and reserpine. Furthermore, it is the purpose of the present study to determine the ability of each drug to control disturbed ideation, affect (mood), and behavior, to ascertain by the administration of placebo medication whether or not the drugs are responsible for the clinical improvements observed in patients, and to report the incidence of side-reactions and toxic effects of each drug.

METHOD OF STUDY

Fifty-one patients treated with chlorpromazine and 44 patients treated with reserpine comprised an experimental group in which a one-month's trial of placebo medication was evaluated. Forty-four patients receiving chlorpromazine and 37 patients receiving reserpine served as a control group. The patients in the control group were selected at random to match the patients in the placebo group according to diagnosis. Comparison of patients in the experimental (placebo) and control groups according to diagnosis is shown in Table 1. The

TABLE 1.—*Comparison of Patients in Experimental (Placebo) and Control Groups According to Diagnosis*

	Chlorpromazine		Reserpine	
	Placebo	Control	Placebo	Control
Schizophrenic reactions				
Paranoid	15	6	10	11
Catatonic	1	3	0	1
Simple	2	1	0	0
Hebephrenic	1	0	4	0
Acute undifferentiated	2	1	3	5
Chronic undifferentiated	11	7	8	4
Schizoaffective	1	5	0	0
Depressive reactions				
Involutional	2	1	4	4
Psychotic depressed	1	5	2	2
Organic reactions				
Metabolic	0	1	1	1
Senile	8	5	3	3
Other	0	0	1	0
Neurotic reactions	6	6	3	3
Manic-depressive reaction, manic	1	3	5	3
Totals	51	44	44	37

patients in the placebo and control groups were generally comparable with respect to diagnosis, severity and duration of illness, dose of the drugs administered, and duration of treatment. The main distinction between the two groups of patients was that patients in the control group received their medication without interruption throughout the study, whereas patients in the placebo group had placebo medication introduced at some point during the course of therapy. Only one investigator knew which patients were in each group and when placebo treatment was instituted.

Multiple, independent clinical observations were made by members of a research team who were throroughly familiar with the pattern of each patient's illness before drug or placebo treatment was instituted. This research team was comprised of each patient's psychotherapist, members of the nursing staff, and members of the departments of educational and occupational therapy. Each patient was seen by his physician on the average of two to three times per week for interviews lasting 30 to 60 minutes. Each week the physician filled out a special report in which he rated the patient's clinical progress according to selected items of the Malamud and Sands Worcester rating scale. Such items as the patient's appearance, motor activity, aggressiveness, socialization, mood, thought content, and thought processes were evaluated. In addition, the physician was asked to write his own progress note with respect to any changes observed in the patient's ideation, affect, and behavior. Also, from the physician's report such information as dosage, rate of administration, and occurrence of toxic effects or side-reactions was obtained. Members of the nursing staff and departments of educational and occupational therapy made daily progress notes on each patient and submitted their reports separately at the end of each week. Furthermore, the patient's behavior was reported daily to the physician by the nurses at morning and evening conferences.

At the end of each week we reviewed all reports and recorded on a summary sheet such information as patient's name, age, and diagnosis; observable changes in ideation, affect, and behavior; blood pressure; pulse rate; hours of sleep; type and amount of sedation; the use of electroconvulsive treatment, insulin coma treatment, cold wet packs, hydrotherapy, or restraints; and any moves that the patients made to different wards or units of the hospital. From the cumulative data on the summary sheet, improvement or lack of improvement was evaluated by us in each of the three spheres of personality functioning; namely, the spheres of ideation, affect, and behavior. Improvement was rated as: none, slight, moderate or marked. No patients were included in the study who received medicaments for less than a month. Most patients were administered the drugs regularly during the period from September, 1954, to April, 1955. Adequate doses of the drugs were given according to recommended dosage schedules. The majority of patients treated with reserpine received 2 mg. or more daily; those who received chlorpromazine were administered 200 mg. or more daily. Most of the medication was oral, although extremely disturbed and agitated patients received the medicaments parenterally.

TABLE 2.—Comparison of Clinical Results in Experimental (Placebo) and Control Groups

	Chlorpromazine			Reserpine		
	Placebo	Control	"t"	Placebo	Control	"t"
Total patients	51	44	....	44	37	....
Patients who improved with drug but later relapsed while on either treatment	30	5	....	25	6	....
Placebo patients who improved upon resumption of drug	17	..	....	19	..	....
Placebo patients who did not improve upon resumption of drug	0	..	....	1	..	....
Placebo patients whose drug was discontinued in favor of other treatment	13	..	....	5	..	....
Patients who improved with drug but relapsed before placebo treatment	0	..	....	1	..	....
Patients who maintained improvement throughout therapy	14 (27.5%)	31 (70.5%)	4.89*	13 (29.5%)	23 (62.2%)	3.76*
Patients who did not improve	7	8	....	5	8	....
Patients who showed initial improvement, % of total patients in group	86.3	81.8	....	88.6	78.4	....
Patients who relapsed after initial improvement, % of total improved patients in group	68.2	13.9	4.17†	66.6	20.7	2.05†

* Significant at the 0.001 level of confidence.
† Significant at the 0.05 level of confidence.

RESULTS

A comparison of clinical results in the experimental (placebo) and control groups is shown in Table 2. Among the 44 patients in the chlorpromazine placebo group who showed initial improvement with chlorpromazine, a significant number (68.2%) relapsed when administration of the drug was stopped, as compared to the number relapsing among 36 improved patients in the control group (13.9%). Similarly, the relapse rate for 39 improved patients in the reserpine placebo group was 66.6%, as compared with 20.7% for the 29 improved in the control group. Furthermore, at the conclusion of the placebo experiment, the patients who received the medicament continuously showed a significantly greater percentage of improvement than did those patients whose medication was discontinued because of placebo treatment. For example, 70.5% of the patients in the chlorpromazine control group showed improvement at the end of the study as contrasted to 27.5% in the chlorpromazine placebo group. Similarly, 62.2% of the patients in the reserpine control group showed improvement at the end of the study as compared with 29.5% of the reserpine placebo group.

Of 30 patients who improved initially with chlorpromazine but then relapsed after placebo treatment, 13 were changed by their physicians to another form of treatment, so that drug therapy was not resumed. Of the other 17 patients, all improved when drug therapy was resumed. Similar results were observed in the 25 patients receiving reserpine as shown in Table 2, one not improving upon resumption of drug therapy, while medication was not resumed with 5.

Recurrence of symptoms that followed placebo medication occurred sooner in patients receiving chlorpromazine than in those receiving reserpine. In the chlorpromazine placebo patients, relapses usually occurred within 24 to 48 hours; whereas in patients receiving reserpine, the relapse occurred from three to seven days later. Conversely, control of disturbed behavior was obtained more rapidly with chlorpromazine than with reserpine when the drugs were administered orally. With chlorpromazine the time was usually from 24 to 48 hours, whereas with reserpine the optimal clinical effect was usually not obtained for at least a week. However, rapid clinical effect was obtained with both drugs when they were administered parenterally in adequate doses (200 mg. to 400 mg. daily for chlorpromazine and 5 mg. to 10 mg. daily for reserpine). Whenever rapid drug effect was desired, however, chlorpromazine was usually the drug of choice.

Over-all evaluation of the effect that these medicaments had upon ideation, affect, and behavior was made in a larger group of 106 patients who received chlorpromazine and 103 patients who were treated with reserpine. As seen in Table 3 and the figure, the effects of chlorpromazine and reserpine on ideation, affect, and behavior were similar in quality and degree. It was observed, however, that the improvement in affect and behavior was significantly greater than improvement in ideation in the patients studied. For example, Table 4 shows that, in the chlorpromazine group, 78% improved behaviorally and 76% improved affectively, as compared with 53% who improved ideationally. Similarly, in the group treated with reserpine, 74% improved behaviorally and 61% improved affectively, whereas only 38% improved

TABLE 3—*Comparative Effect of Chlorpromazine and Reserpine on Ideation, Affect, and Behavior*

Type of Personality Disorder	No. of Patients	Drug Used*	Ideation NO†	SL	MD	MK	Affect NO	SL	MD	MK	Behavior NO	SL	MD	MK
Schizophrenic reactions	51	C	28	18	4	1	15	28	7	1	12	24	12	3
	47	R	31	13	1	2	20	21	4	2	14	18	12	3
Depressive reactions	17	C	10	6	1	0	8	7	2	0	7	6	4	0
	22	R	15	6	1	0	10	11	1	0	5	12	2	0
Organic reactions	16	C	10	5	3	0	2	9	5	0	2	5	7	2
	15	R	10	4	1	0	5	7	3	0	1	9	3	2
Manic-depressive reaction, manic	6	C	0	0	2	4	0	0	2	4	0	0	2	4
	8	R	1	4	2	1	1	2	4	1	1	1	4	2
Neurotic reactions	8	C	2	6	0	0	1	7	0	0	2	6	0	0
	8	R	5	3	0	0	3	5	0	0	3	3	2	0
Alcohol and drug withdrawals	8	C	0	1	5	2	0	1	5	2	0	1	5	2
	3	R	2	0	0	1	1	0	1	1	0	1	1	1
Totals	106	C	50	36	13	7	26	52	21	7	23	42	30	11
	103	R	64	30	5	4	40	46	13	4	27	44	24	8

* C = chlorpromazine, R = reserpine.
† NO = no improvement, SL = slight improvement, MD = moderate improvement, and MK = marked improvement.

TABLE 4.—*Comparison of Improvement in Ideation, Affect, and Behavior in 106 Patients Treated with Chlorpromazine and 103 Patients Treated with Reserpine*

	Chlorpromazine Improved, %	Difference, %	"t"	Reserpine Improved, %	Difference, %	"t"
Ideation	53	..	.....	33	..	.....
Affect	..	23	3.02 *	..	23	3.38 *
	76	..	.....	61	..	.....
	..	2	0.35 †	..	13	2.03 †
Behavior	78	..	.....	74	..	.....

* Significant at the 0.01 level of confidence.
† Significant at the 0.05 level of confidence.

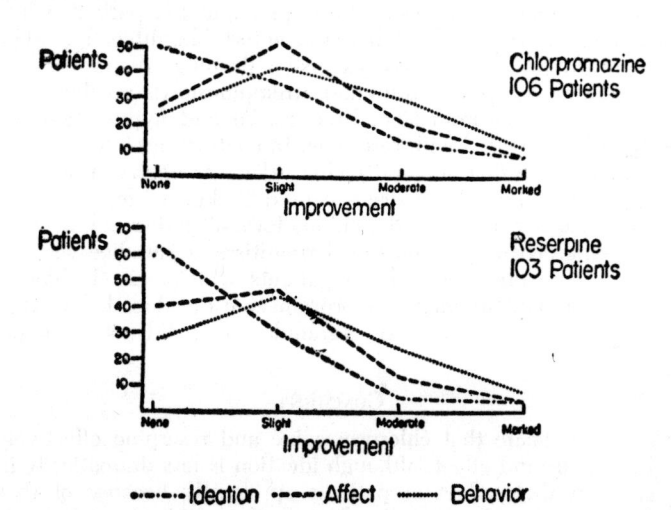

Effects of chlorpromazine and reserpine on ideation, affect, and behavior of patients.

ideationally. The improvement seen in these groups of patients was largely in the range of from none to moderate. The number of patients who showed marked improvement was not impressive. For example, behaviorally, in the chlorpromazine group, 22% were not improved, 39% were slightly improved, 28% were moderately improved, and only 11% showed marked improvement. Behaviorally, in the group treated with reserpine, 26% showed no improvement, 43% showed slight improvement, 23% showed moderate improvement, and only 8% showed marked improvement.

Although the number of patients treated in some of the diagnostic categories, as shown in Table 3, is too small to permit statistical evaluation of results, it was our general clinical impression that improvement in ideation, affect, and behavior was most dramatic in those patients who suffered with the manic phase of manic-depressive psychosis. These patients consistently showed uniform improvement in all three spheres of personality functioning. Depressed patients, on the other hand, showed little to no improvement ideationally or affectively. Some patients with agitated depression, however, showed a slight behavioral improvement. Behavior and affect improved in the restless, agitated, and excited patients regardless of the underlying type of personality disturbance. In other words, the agitated behavior that was observed in patients with schizophrenic reactions, organic reactions (particularly chronic brain syndrome associated with senility), and drug withdrawal states was helped by chlorpromazine and reserpine. The neurotic reactions (obsessive-compulsive and anxiety reactions) and the depressive reactions, as previously mentioned, were altered least by these medicaments.

The incidence of side-reactioins and toxic effects for each drug is shown in Table 5 for 123 patients who received reserpine and 137 patients who received chlorpromazine. Reserpine caused more uncomfortable, subjective side-reactions such as nasal stuffiness, epistaxis, excessive flushing, diaphoresis, chilliness, fatigue, weakness, excessive drowsiness, tremulousness, myalgia, ataxia, and diarrhea, than did chlorpromazine. Bradycardia and hypotension were more frequent in patients treated with reserpine. In contrast, an interesting syndrome of hypertension, hyperthermia, and tachycardia was observed only in patients receiving chlorpromazine. Both drugs caused Parkinsonism, nausea, vomiting, vivid bizarre dreams, pruritus, and a unique form of periorbital, facial, pretibial, and pedal edema. Toxic symptoms of dermatitis and jaundice with or without hepatomegaly were observed only in patients who received chlorpromazine. Thirteen (9.5%) patients taking chlorpromazine developed dermatitis, and 7 patients (5%) developed jaundice. Agranulocytosis did not occur in any patients.

Comment

Our results indicate that chlorpromazine and reserpine effectively modify disturbed behavior and affect, although ideation is less dramatically improved. The drugs exert their effect in patients apparently because of their ability to produce a unique calming and sedative effect without narcosis. The exact site or mode of action of these drugs on the central nervous system is not known. To date, most of the studies made to determine the site or mode of action have utilized reserpine. According to the earlier studies of Bein and others, reserpine acts directly on central autonomic substrates, possibly in the hypothalamus. It was believed that it caused a depression of the central sympathetic functions. Certain clinical phenomena, however, that have been observed in patients receiving these drugs, such as convulsions and Parkinsonism, would seem to indicate that their action might be at a level higher than the hypothalamus. Weiskrantz and Wilson recently reported that the behavior of monkeys with surgical ablation of the amygdaloid nucleus was similar to the behavior observed in monkeys treated with reserpine. These investigators have extended their studies further and have found that a lesion that destroys the cortex of the posterior orbital portion of the frontal lobe and the anteromedial aspect of the temporal lobe, including the amygdaloid nucleus, produces behavior in monkeys that is indistinguishable from that seen in monkeys treated with reserpine. It is known that these portions of the phylogenetically older cerebral cortex do have intimate connections with the hypothalamus and lower centers concerned with the regulation of emotions and behavior.

Because of the rather specific action that these drugs have upon these areas of the brain, they seem to produce an effect similar to that seen in patients with lobotomy. Some have described this effect as a peculiar insulation of the patient against incoming stressful stimuli from the environment. From the psychodynamic standpoint, such an insulating effect is important. Stressful stimuli arising from within or from without the individual usually evoke anxiety, and each individual handles his anxieties according to previously learned ideational and behavioral responses. If the emotionally upset patient can be guarded against incoming stressful stimuli that potentially can further upset the homeostasis of his internal environment, he will be better able to mobilize his previously learned defenses and coping mechanisms in order to handle more efficiently the anxiety or affect evoked by the forces that threaten him from within and from without.

It is unlikely that drug therapy alone could ever totally eliminate all factors of stress that act upon the individual or that drug therapy alone could so alter the individual's responsiveness to stress that anxiety and its physiological concomitants would be forever vanquished. The dynamics and etiology of emotional illness cannot be reduced to such simple terms. However, the advent of these new drugs that seem to have specific regulatory actions on autonomic functions has opened up a whole new field of investigation into the nature, cause, treatment, and management of emotional illness.

The drugs have a relatively wide margin of safety even when used for prolonged periods. Most side-reactions and toxic reactions are reversible and can usually be controlled by temporarily discontinuing use of the drug, by reducing the dose of the drug, or by the use of other medicaments that alleviate the specific symptoms. For example, nasal stuffiness, which is seen so frequently in patients treated with reserpine, is relieved by the use of phenylephrine (Neo-Synephrine) hydrochloride.

Chlorpromazine produces more toxic reactions in patients than does reserpine. Of particular concern to all clinicians is the unusual type of jaundice that has been reported in patients receiving chlorpromazine. The pathogenesis

TABLE 5.—*Incidence of Side-Reactions and Toxic Reactions*

	Reserpine Patients (Total 123)	Chlorpromazine Patients (Total 137)
Nasal stuffiness	34	2
Epistaxis	3	0
Hypotension	39	20
Hypertension	0	9
Hyperthermia	0	5
Tachycardia	0	12
Bradycardia	21	5
Excessive flushing	11	0
Diaphoresis	2	0
Dizziness	7	7
Chilliness	4	0
Fatigue, weakness	12	3
Syncope	2	1
Blurred vision	0	2
Excessive drowsiness	22	17
Tremulousness	19	1
Myalgia	4	0
Ataxia	7	0
Parkinsonism	2	1
Dry mouth	0	2
Heartburn	0	2
Nausea	7	10
Vomiting	3	7
Diarrhea	9	1
Exacerbation of peptic ulcer	0	1
Edema	9	7
Vivid dreams	3	3
Pruritus	2	2
Dermatitis	0	13
Jaundice	0	7
Hepatomegaly	0	3

of such jaundice is obscure. There is no definite evidence of hepatocellular damage revealed by clinical laboratory findings or by histological examination. Apparently the bile pools in the canaliculi of the central zones. Laboratory findings are usually those associated with extrahepatic biliary obstruction, that is, elevation in the values for the icteric index and serum bilirubin and alkaline phosphatase. We found that chlorpromazine gave elevated, false-positive values for icteric index determinations. We also observed that a group of patients who received chlorpromazine placebo medication had elevated values for icteric index. It was concluded that the yellow dye in the coating of the chlorpromazine tablet was responsible for the elevation of these values. Accordingly, a modification of the method for determination of the icteric index was devised that corrected adequately the false-positive values and thus made this test a more reliable index of subclinical or impending jaundice in patients receiving chlorpromazine.

SUMMARY AND CONCLUSIONS

In the treatment of a group of patients in a private psychiatric hospital, chlorpromazine and reserpine were found to be effective in causing significant behavioral and affective improvement in psychiatric patients. However, in the group of predominantly psychotic patients studied, ideation was less significantly and dramatically improved. Although a significant number of these patients showed improvement behaviorally, the degree of improvement was only slight to moderate. Long-range or lasting improvements in patients receiving these drugs are yet to be evaluated. Chlorpromazine and reserpine are similar in their clinical indications and effectiveness. They may be used interchangeably, although such factors as the incidence of side-reaction and of toxic effects and the rapidity of obtaining clinical effect may influence the choice of preference of one drug to the other in individual cases. Of the two drugs, reserpine is less toxic, but it causes more uncomfortable side-reactions in patients than does chlorpromazine. In most instances, toxic effects or side-reactions can be controlled by merely reducing the dosage. Where rapid drug effect is desired, chlorpromazine is the drug of choice. Chlorpromazine and reserpine are valuable adjuvants to the armamentarium of the practicing psychiatrist, particularly for the control of destructive, disturbed, agitated, and hyperactive behavior, regardless of the underlying etiology. The psychiatric conditions for which these drugs were found to be of clinical use, in descending order, are: (1) manic-depressive psychosis, manic phase; (2) agitated states, particularly those associated with organic brain disease; (3) schizophrenic reaction; (4) depressive reaction; and (5) neurotic reaction.

Addendum

Since the time of writing we have had some experience with the use of Deserpidine, a new alkaloid from Rauwolfia canescens. Deserpidine differs chemically from reserpine in the lack of a methoxyl group in ring A. The effect of this new alkaloid was studied with a group of six patients whose response to reserpine had already been well established. There was no observable difference in the effect of Deserpidine as compared with that of reserpine from a clinical standpoint.

CHLORPROMAZINE AND RESERPINE

Francis N. Waldrop, M.D., and F. Regis Riesenman, M.D.
St. Elizabeths Hospital, Washington, D. C.

RESERPINE

Francis N. Waldrop, M.D.

The use of reserpine in the treatment of mentally ill patients was introduced in St. Elizabeths Hospital a little more than a year ago. Since that time approximately 700 patients have been administered this drug for a period of at least 1 month. As a rule, patients were selected, not by their psychiatric diagnosis, but on the symptomatic criteria that they were agitated, destructive, assaultive, noisy, combative, and overactive. Most of the patients selected on this basis suffered from psychotic illnesses, and most had been sick for a period of several years, the range extending from a month or less to more than 20 years. Contraindications to treatment included the history or presence of a gastrointestinal bleeding disorder, particularly peptic ulcer, malignant hypertension, and the presence of pronounced depressive features in the psychiatric picture.

In a majority of the patients the medication was given orally from the first; however, in uncooperative and resistive patients the medication was begun by intramuscular injections. The average beginning dosage, by either oral or parenteral route, was from 2 to 2.5 mg. daily. For a period ranging from 1 to 3 weeks this dosage was gradually built up to a maximum of from 5 to 10 mg. daily. In most instances patients were maintained on the maximum dosage level, barring serious side-reactions, until a tranquilizing effect was achieved or until it was thought that they showed no promise of response. In some instances the maximum dosage of up to 10 mg. daily was maintained for a period of 6 to 8 months before sufficient improvement occurred to warrant reduction of dosage. With those patients who showed a marked diminution in their overactivity, anger, and agitation, or who developed severe Parkinsonian symptoms, the dosage was reduced more promptly. The maintenance dosage, once the tranquilizing effect has been achieved, has varied widely from patient to patient and must be adjusted individually in most cases. Maintenance dosages in this group of patients have varied from 0.5 mg. daily to 9 or 10 mg. daily, with an average of 2 mg. daily.

Because of the variability with which the drug has been used from service to service within the Hospital, it is difficult to assess in a precise way just what have been the effects of treatment with reserpine. In general, about 13 per cent (91) of the total 700 patients failed to show any favorable response after a full month of treatment. This group included a considerable number of patients who have been hospitalized for a period of more than 5 years and who show advanced symptoms of profound mental illness. In many of these instances the patient's illness had apparently reached a sort of stabilization over a long period. It would appear that the longer a patient has been ill, the longer he must receive reserpine and the higher the dosage must be in order to achieve a favorable response. It is not unlikely that a portion of those patients who failed to respond even after 1 to 3 months would eventually have shown a favorable reaction had the drug been continued over a longer period and/or a higher dosage used.

In approximately 62 per cent of patients (or 435) a conspicuous and favorable response was noted in that they became more tractable, placid, cooperative, less tense and active, and quieter. Although these patients showed a definite tranquilizing effect with regard to some of their more obvious symptoms, examination still revealed a persistent underlying core of illness, as indicated by persistent hallucinations, delusions, confusion, disorientation, and faulty emotional responses. Many of the patients in this group are still under treatment, and it is possible that they will eventually show more improvement.

About 25 per cent of the patients treated (or 174) have definitely shown more than a mere tranquilizing effect. The patients in this group have not only become quieter, more cooperative, and less tense and anxious, but have also shown a gradual diminution in abnormal content; i.e., hallucinated voices have gradually receded and in many instances entirely disappeared, bizarre delusions have gradually faded away, and the patients have taken a progressive interest in the real world about them, have been able to deal more constructively with their real problems and able to participate effectively in some sort of rehabilitation program. Nearly all of the patients in this group have suffered from schizophrenia of one variety or another. Patients with organic brain disease, such as those suffering from paresis, cerebral arteriosclerosis, cortical atrophy, and related difficulties, have almost uniformly shown marked improvement in the superimposed psychologic aspects of their difficulties (including agitation, noisiness, overactivity, destructiveness), although they continue to show the deficit symptoms (i.e., memory and intellectual defects) to be expected in the brain-damaged individual.

About 10 per cent (or 75) of the patients who have received reserpine have shown sufficient improvement to date to be discharged or placed on extended visit (these are included in the 25 per cent who have shown more than a tranquilizing response), but the number involved is too small as yet, and the time period too brief, to regard this figure as having any final validity. Even without many discharges so far, a considerable number of patients receiving the drug have enjoyed benefits short of "recovery"— benefits which are extremely difficult to quantitate. Further, while it is believed that reserpine has certainly played a part in the improvement shown by these patients, it would be premature at this time to attribute the beneficial changes exclusively to reserpine.

It is expected that the percentages in the above categories will shift considerably as more patients receive the drug for longer periods and as our criteria for selecting patients for this treatment improve. Some patients who at this time have been treated only 1 to 2 months and have thus far shown little or no response may well progress in the course of the next 3 or 4 months to a point warranting their classification as markedly improved. It also seems quite likely that a number who have already shown a definite amelioration in their symptoms will be favorably considered for visit or discharge in the near future.

In general, when a patient has shown sufficient improvement to be considered for visit or discharge from the hospital, reserpine has first been discontinued. It has not been customary, except on one service, to continue the patient on the drug after he has been placed on extended visit or discharged. As our experience with this form of treatment increases, however, we may find it feasible to discharge or place on visit patients who have a favorable social situation on the outside and who will require an indefinite maintenance dosage of reserpine for control of their more disruptive symptoms (just as epileptic patients may require indefinite use of anticonvulsants).

About 40 per cent of the patients who have received the drug for at least 1 month and in whom the treatment has been terminated after a favorable response have shown a partial or complete relapse to their previously disturbed state. No consistent pattern has yet emerged which enables us to predict reliably which patients are likely to relapse in a relatively short period and which are not. A few patients, after a favorable response and termination of the drug, have maintained their improvement for as long as 6 months and are still doing well.

A great deal more work will be needed before we can begin to talk meaningfully about how long a patient should be kept on a maintenance dose, which patients are likely to relapse, and how soon, and which patients will be able to dispense with the drug altogether after a favorable response. We are really just entering this area of experience, and it is not yet possible to draw any valid conclusions. In general, our practice so far has been the following: After a patient has shown a favorable response the dosage is gradually reduced to successive maintenance levels over a period of 1 to 3 months. If the patient continues to do well even on minimal doses, the drug is terminated. As a general rule, relapse occurs 1 to 2 weeks after the drug is discontinued. In most instances the patients who relapse are then restarted on the drug, their symptoms are again brought under control, and the lowest possible maintenance dose is individually arrived at.

With regard to side-reactions and complications of reserpine treatment, 7 per cent (or 50) were discontinued because of somatic side-reactions. It is interesting to note that by far the greater number of serious side-reactions occurred in women and that in no instance, other than geriatric patients, did a precipitous fall in blood pressure develop. Exclusive of the geriatric group, 4 patients died while receiving reserpine, but these deaths were not necessarily the result of reserpine administration. In 4 per cent (or 31 patients) reserpine treatment was discontinued because of psychiatric complications, nearly always the appearance of depression or a toxic confusional state. Parkinsonian symptoms have rarely required discontinuance of the drug, although in many instances it has been necessary to reduce the dosage slightly. Parkinsonian symptoms appear almost uniformly if the drug is given in high dosage and for a long period, and they seem to represent a normal pharmacologic action of the drug.

In summary, our experiences with reserpine justify a cautious optimism with regard to its effect on the hospitalized, mentally ill patient who is overactive, tense, angry, combative, destructive, and assaultive. About two-thirds of such patients can be helped to the extent that these difficult symptoms are significantly reduced, thus rendering the patient more comfortable, more cooperative, and more amenable to other forms of treatment. In about one-fourth of the patients treated with the drug the beneficial effect appears to have transcended a mere tranquilizing response, and patients have shown significant improvement with regard to their abnormal mental content.

Finally, I should like to point out that there appears little justification as yet for regarding reserpine as a definitive or curative treatment for any form of mental illness. Unquestionably, a great deal enters into the treatment response of a mentally ill patient other than the purely pharmacologic effect of the drug. At this time reserpine appears to be of great value within the mental hospital as an adjunctive form of therapy which facilitates a patient's participation in a broader treatment program, including individual and group psychotherapy, occupational therapy, and vocational rehabilitation.

Chlorpromazine

F. Regis Riesenman, M.D.

Chlorpromazine, or Thorazine, therapy was instituted on the Women's Receiving Service of Saint Elizabeths Hospital on July 19, 1954. As of November 1, 1955, 280 patients have been treated with Thorazine on Women's Receiving Service and a total of over 1,000 in the Hospital as a whole.

Criteria for selection of patients were based mainly on the behavior of the patients. The most excited and disturbed, hyperactive, assaultive, combative, angry, noisy and confused patients were selected, irrespective of diagnosis. Later, a smaller group of patients was considered from the standpoint of diagnostic categories in order to have a well represented group that would enable us more fully to evaluate the efficacy of the drug in a comparative sense.

The therapeutic regimen, in general, was as follows:

The drug was administered in gradually increasing doses, starting with 50 mg. intramuscularly on the first day, increasing by 50 mg. each day until 150 mg. a day was reached. The 150 mg. a day was given in divided doses intramuscularly until the patient was controlled and cooperative. The drug was then given by mouth, 100 mg. 3 times a day. From this point on the dosage of the drug was individualized for each patient, both with respect to total dosage and to duration of treatment. The physiologic effects of the drug included a drop in blood pressure, varying from 10 to 40 mm. systolic and 10 to 20 mm. diastolic. There was distinct pallor in a number of patients. Most of the patients were drowsy during the first 7 to 10 days. Some of them complained of constipation, stuffiness of the nose, and dryness of the throat. The average daily dose for acute patients was 400 mg. and for the chronic patients, 600 mg. The maintenance dosage varied from 50 mg. to 300 mg., with an average of approximately 150 mg. The average duration of treatment was 2 to 3 months for acute cases and 3 to 5 months for chronic cases.

The complications with Thorazine were as follows:

Eleven patients developed jaundice, 17 a Parkinsonian syndrome, 9 dermatitis, 1 hyperthermia, 1 hypothermia, and 2 muscular dystonia. All these complications forced the discontinuance of the drug except for 6 patients with dermatitis. We no longer discontinue the drug in the Parkinsonian states but give Cogentin.

The drug was effective in achieving control and management in 95 per cent of the patients. This meant that they became quieter, cooperative, cared for their own needs, and no longer required seclusion. There was failure, however, to show any favorable response beyond that point in one-third, and another one-third showed mild to moderate improvement; the remaining one-third were markedly improved or underwent complete remission, and these patients have either been discharged or are at present on trial visit.

By far the most favorable response was found in the noisy, overactive, angry, combative and assaultive type of patient. Patients with a lot of anxiety, tension, and concern likewise showed favorable response. The patients showing the poorest response to the drug were mainly the depressives and the retarded, passive, dependent type of schizophrenics. Patients who showed an attitude of indifference or lack of concern, and more or less accepted their illness with complacency, likewise responded poorly.

Some specific characteristics of the drug which are worthy of mention are as follows:

The drug is not habit-forming. Patients may develop a tolerance to the drug if the administration of the drug is not properly regulated, both with respect to dosage and to time. The drug is practically a specific as a tranquilizer, without penalizing the intellectual and perceptional senses and inducing a hypnotic effect or clouding of consciousness, as other sedatives do. It is important to maintain control of the patient at all times, since once control is lost it may be difficult to regain. Although the *modus operandi* is not known, it apparently facilitates repressive mechanisms in the paranoid schizophrenics and creates a feeling of emotional indifference in many patients, so that patients appear to be no longer concerned with their problems and the anxiety is relieved. In this respect, it acts as a chemical lobotomy.

Maintenance doses of the drug are required in practically all cases of paranoid schizophrenic and manic-depressive manic patients. This is good insurance against a relapse. In many patients the maximum degree of responsiveness to the drug may not be obtained or achieved until 1 to 3 months after the termination of the drug, or after cutting the drug to a maintenance dosage. This is the so-called therapeutic lag that is quite characteristic in many cases.

Some 10 per cent of the patients complain of peculiar feelings and somatic disturbances. They are variously described as feelings of depersonalization or somatic disorientation; a feeling of strangeness, peculiar feelings, being out of contact, a feeling of being driven or being restless, anxious and tense; a feeling as if the mind were detached from the body, and a feeling of lethargy and weakness. Some describe their feelings as walking on crushed ice or ice cubes, a feeling as if they were suspended in space or dangling in mid-air.

Some of them complain that they are unable to get into a comfortable position, irrespective of whether they are sitting, standing or lying. Others feel that they are the living dead and act more or less like zombies.

When the drug has achieved maximum therapeutic benefit, the patients describe their feelings as follows: "I have a feeling of peace of mind, a feeling of inner contentment, a feeling of complete confidence in myself."

Thus, Thorazine appears to be practically a specific in the control and management of very disturbed patients. Most of the patients receiving the drug are made more accessible, amenable, and receptive to psychotherapy, as well as to other forms of therapy available in an institutional setting. There is a better morale on the ward. The ward climate undergoes a remarkable transition. Wards become quiet, seclusion is reduced to a minimum, and relatively few injuries occur. The patients seem relaxed, agreeable, pleasant and cooperative. Privileges are accepted and responsibilities assumed. There is considerable interest and enthusiasm shown by the patients in the various activities in which they participate. Interpersonal relationships are improved. Ward personnel are more effectively utilized, and their efforts are channelized and directed toward more constructive goals.

In conclusion, it appears that Thorazine has a definite place and value in the therapeutic armamentarium of mental illness, and as such becomes a valuable aid or adjunct to psychotherapy. The full impact of chemotherapy in psychiatry (the era of pills for mental ills) with respect to its over-all potentialities and efficiency cannot be properly evaluated at this time. The drug, having passed the "acid test" in the experimental and empirical phase, is faced with a third and more important phase, namely, the test of time. We still must view it in a speculative manner and with certain reservations. The integration of chemotherapy and psychotherapy will be a task of psychiatry in the future.

EFFECT OF CHLORPROMAZINE AND RESERPINE ON BUDGETS OF MENTAL HOSPITALS

Werner Tuteur, M.D..
Clinical Director, Elgin State Hospital, Elgin, Illinois

During April of 1956 the chief engineer (James Bryan) of Elgin State Hospital submitted an unsolicited report announcing that repair work at a particular cottage (Hawley) had considerably decreased for a number of months. Being unaware of psychiatric treatment methods, the engineer asked for an explanation.

At this particular cottage (present population: 231), female patients for years had been combative, destructive, and incontinent, and plumbers had been hard pressed to unclog and repair toilets, sewers and drains which patients had stuffed with paraphernalia. Also, carpenters had to be called frequently to repair screens and furniture, and glaziers had been busy repairing windows.

This report tries to give in detail the effect of tranquilizing drugs, through improved patient behavior, on equipment and other aspects of the budget on this particular cottage. The paper covers 3 half-year periods:: January 1, 1954, to June 30, 1954, when chlorpromazine and reserpine had not yet been used at this hospital; January 1, 1955, to June 30, 1955, during which period these drugs were introduced; January 1, 1956, to June 30, 1956, when their effect could be generally felt. Inasmuch as during these 3 periods no other treatment was employed and since it is unlikely that the large number of improved patients represents spontaneous remissions, it may be assumed that the improvement was the result of these drugs.

The clinical improvement, number of patients treated, discharge and return rates of the latter at Hawley Cottage will not be discussed here. Chlorpromazine and reserpine were started at Hawley Cottage during February 1955.

Because of patients' less destructive behavior, there had been a gradual decrease in the cost of maintaining equipment on the ward, such as repairs of toilets, floor drains, showers, windows, screens and furniture (Table 1).

During the first half of 1954, $791.10 had been spent on wages necessitated by the upkeep of the ward; $656.01 were spent for the same purpose during the first half of 1955, and only $290.50 were expended for this purpose during the first half of 1956.

Table 2 gives evaluations of a different kind about Hawley Cottage between January 1, 1956, and June 30, 1956. During this preiod 257 patients were treated. Twenty-five of these were discharged. A number of them are presently

TABLE 1
Comparisons of Expenditures on Skilled Crafts at Hawley Cottage by 3 Half-year Periods
(Wages are Based on Local Union Scales of 1954, 1955, and 1956, respectively.)

Category	1-1-54 to 6-30-54 Hours spent	Wages spent	1-1-55 to 6-30-55 Hours spent	Wages spent	1-1-56 to 6-30-56 Hours spent	Wages spent
Carpenters	31 @ $2.85	$ 88.35	29 @ $3.00	$ 87.00	8 @ $3.15	$ 25.20
Glaziers	31 @ 2.55	79.05	27.5 @ 2.65	72.88	11 @ 2.80	30.80
Plumbers	198 @ 3.15	623.70	157.5 @ 3.15	496.13	70 @ 3.35	234.50
Total	260	$791.10	214.0	$656.01	89	$290.50
Savings	...	.....	Over period 1-1-54 to 6-30-54	135.00	Over period 1-1-55 to 6-30-55	$365.51
					Over period 1-1-54 to 6-30-54	$500.60

Only repairs performed on the ward proper are considered in this survey. The hours express time spent on the ward by craftsmen. Note the decrease in working hours during the first half year of 1955, when tranquilizing drugs were being introduced. By June 30, 1956, when these drugs were in full use, savings in crafts became remarkable, in spite of an increase in union wages during 1955 and 1956.

TABLE 2
Evaluations for Hawley Cottage Covering Period 1-1-56 to 6-30-56

Patients treated	257
Patients discharged	25
Patients returned	5
Total patient days saved by their absence from 1-1-56 to 6-30-56	2,050
Illinois patient day rate	$ 2.20
Amount saved by fewer patient days	$4,510.00
Savings in cost of labor (from Table 1)	$ 500.60
Total	$5,010.60
Amount spent on chlorpromazine and reserpine 1-1-56 to 6-30-56, on 257 patients under treatment during this period	$4,701.82
Total spent on drugs in special chlorpromazine-reserpine clinic on patients discharged from Hawley Cottage between 1-1-56 and 6-30-56	$ 446.55
Total	$5,148.37

Savings clearly offset the major part of cost of drugs. Many "hidden" savings are not tabulated; for example, with the introduction of tranquilizing drugs, the use of sedatives, once administered at this cottage in large amounts, for all practical purposes, was eliminated. Diminished tearing of clothing and bedding, improved health standards decreasing overcrowding of hospital and infirmary units, etc., are other savings difficult to estimate (see text). It may be predicted that the cost of operation of special chlorpromazine-reserpine clinics will be very low in the long run.

gainfully employed. Of these 25, five returned.[1] Other items of gain during this period through use of the new drug therapy are noted in the table. It should be noted that there was clinical improvement of 70% of the patients. There was also diminished tearing of clothing, bedding, mattresses, rubber sheets and blankets and diminishing destruction of shoes. There was a decrease of injuries to employees, resulting in turn in decrease of service-connected sick leave. Health standards increased by the abatement of incontinence and less destruction of plumbing. This resulted in less overcrowding of infirmaries and hospital facilities, where patients by necessity had to be transferred frequently for temporary illness caused by poor hygienic conditions in this cottage. Such savings are difficult to express in dollars and cents (See also legend of Table 2).

One may argue that the savings in cost of labor on this cottage represent "hidden savings," since they do not result in the actual diminution of the labor force. This is certainly true, but skilled labor may thus be used more profitably in other areas of the institution. It is noteworthy that no additional personnel was employed to dispense medication to these 257 patients.

A word regarding the $446.55 spent on tranquilizing drugs for the 25 patients after their discharge from the institution during period from January 1, 1956, to June 30, 1956: A special chlorpromazine-reserpine clinic functions at the hospital at no additional cost, except for drugs dispensed, to prevent patients from relapsing and returning. This amount would support 20 patients for about 10 days in the institution. It may be predicted that any savings will be felt most in the operation of such clinics, the cost of which seems to be very low. Evidence seems to indicate that a majority of patients need these drugs for an indefinite period to avoid relapse.

SUMMARY

Chlorpromazine and reserpine, as a result of their tranquilizing action, have a considerable effect on the budget of mental institutions. Repair work, performed by highly paid union labor, decreases considerably. While savings in skilled labor can be demonstrated, this becomes more difficult when clinical improvement, rehabilitation and happiness of human beings is under consideration, the last likewise applying to families and friends. The evaluations tabulated must not, however, be compared with a profit and loss statement. Clinical improvement of any illness is well worth the effort in human and personal investment, and certainly the money involved. It appears that the cost of maintenance of special chlorpromazine-reserpine clinics to prevent once-disturbed patients from relapsing and returning will be low in the long run.

---

[1] After the introduction of tranquilizing drugs during the first half of 1955 patients began to leave by July 22, 1955. As of this writing, October 18, 1956, a total of 56 patients have been discharged from Hawley, 11 of whom have returned.

CHLORPROMAZINE ALONE AND WITH RESERPINE
Use in the Treatment of Mental Diseases

Leo E. Hollister, M.D., Kenneth P. Jones, M.D., Bernard Brownfield, M.D., and Franklin Johnson, M.D.
Veterans Administration Hospital, Palo Alto, California

Two drugs of great promise in psychiatry recently appeared almost simultaneously. Chlorpromazine, a synthetic drug of the phenothiazine group, was initially introduced as a potentiating agent for anesthetic agents. Reserpine, a pure alkaloid of Rauwolfia serpentina, was produced primarily as a treatment for hypertension. Both drugs, although of different origin and chemical structures, have similar effects on the nervous system and on patients with mental disorders.

In the short span of its use in psychiatry, numerous favorable reports have appeared on the use of chlorpromazine. Little has been written about the combined use of reserpine and chlorpromazine. This study is an assessment of the usefulness of chlorpromazine, alone and combined with reserpine, in psychiatric treatment.

METHOD OF STUDY

Chlorpromazine was used alone in 68 psychiatric patients and in combination with reserpine in 32 patients. The psychiatric diagnoses of patients treated with the single drug were chronic schizophrenic reaction in 50, personality disorder in three, psychotic depressive reaction in one, and various organic psychoses in 14. All the patients treated with the combined drugs had chronic schizophrenic reactions.

The 82 patients with chronic schizophrenic reactions ranged in age from 18 to 77 years; the median age was 34 years. Duration of illness varied between six months and 35 years. Forty-three of these patients had been ill for nine years or more. Sixty-six patients had received some somatic therapy before. Twelve had been treated with bilateral prefrontal leukotomy. The 14 patients with organic psychosis ranged in age from 57 to 80 years. Ten patients had chronic brain syndromes due to senile or arteriosclerotic brain disease, two were syphilitic, one was epileptic and one suffered from the effects of trauma.

Initial trials of treatment utilized the double-blind technique. In all patients except those with organic psychoses, treatment was initiated on a medical treatment ward. Forty patients, most of them schizophrenic, were treated with chlorpromazine or placebos. The dose used was 150 mg. intramuscularly for three to four days followed by oral doses of 100 to 400 mg. daily. Twenty-six patients, all schizophrenic, were treated with a combination of chlorpromazine and reserpine or identical placebos. Two dosage schedules were used: (1) Seven days of parenteral therapy with 50 mg. of chlorpromazine and 5 mg. of reserpine daily followed by oral doses of 200 mg. of chlorpromazine and 3 mg. of reserpine daily; (2) seven days of parenteral therapy with 100 mg. of chlorpromazine and 2.5 mg. of reserpine daily followed by oral doses of 300 mg. of chlorpromazine and 2 mg. of reserpine daily.

After treatment was under way, patients were returned to their usual wards. A preliminary evaluation was made by each patient's psychiatrist during the third week of the trial. Patients who had received active medication were continued on treatment, a flexible dosage schedule being used. Patients who had received placebos were started on the same schedules of active medication. Twenty-eight patients with organic psychosis were treated with a daily dose of 75 mg. orally of chlorpromazine or identical placebos. At the end of 40 days of treatment, an evaluation was made.

Longer term evaluations were made of patients after they had been on treatment with chlorpromazine alone for two to eight months. Most of these patients were started on parenteral doses of chlorpromazine followed by oral maintenance doses of 100 to 800 mg. daily. Only seven patients in this series received a daily dose of more than 500 mg. of the drug. In the case of patients receiving the combined drugs, an evaluation was made at the end of three to four months of treatment. Seventeen patients received the dosage schedule using higher doses of reserpine, while 15 patients received one using higher doses of chlorpromazine. Fifteen patients were not maintained on the combination for the entire course, but were switched to maintenance doses of one drug or the other. In all cases, the reason for this change was the development of some complication of treatment.

All evaluations were made by the psychiatrist familiar with the patient prior to treatment. In general, patients were considered to have shown slight improvement if they were appreciably less disturbed, required less sedation, seclusion or restraint, or could be moved to a ward with less severely ill patients. Criteria for the classification *moderate improvement* were: (a) No further requirement of seclusion or restraint and a markedly diminished need for other forms of sedation, (b) improvement in behavior which permitted the patient to participate in activities programs or group and individual psychotherapy, and (c) social improvement which made possible the granting of ground privileges or passes from the hospital for the first time. *Marked improvement* implied that the patient had made a great change according to the criteria listed above and that he was being considered for release from the hospital. The patients with organic psychosis were evaluated only in terms of whether the drug was satisfactory in controlling aberrant behavior.

Results

The results of the double-blind studies in patients with chronic schizophrenic reactions are summarized in Table 1. The number of patients who improved on active medication was convincingly greater than the number who improved on placebos. Judging solely by the proportion of patients who improved in each group, it might be concluded that the combined drugs were

TABLE 1.—*Results of double-blind studies on 66 patients with schizophrenic reactions treated with Chlorpromazine and combinations of Chlorpromazine and Reserpine*

Treated with	Improved	Unimproved	Worse	Total
Chlorpromazine	13	11	0	24
Placebo	3	15	0	18
Chlorpromazine-reserpine combination	9	6	2	17
Placebo	1	6	0	7

at least as effective as chlorpromazine alone. However, the degree of improvement was frequently greater in the patients who received chlorpromazine alone. Two patients became temporarily worse when the combined drugs were used. A few other patients were so profoundly affected when the combination was used that it became obvious that they had received active medication rather than placebos. However, the evaluations made on these patients were as objective as possible.

The results of longer treatment of patients with chronic schizophrenic reactions are summarized in Table 2. Fifty-six per cent of patients treated with

TABLE 2.—*Results of treatment of 82 patients with schizophrenic reactions with Chlorpromazine and combinations of Chlorpromazine and Reserpine*

	Chlorpromazine Alone	Chlorpromazine-Reserpine Combination	Total
Unimproved	8	6	14
Slightly improved	14	16	30
Moderately improved	19	8	27
Markedly improved	9	2	11
Total	50	32	82
Total with moderate or marked improvement	28 (56%)	10 (31%)	

chlorpromazine alone showed moderate or pronounced improvement. Only 31 per cent of patients treated with the combined drugs showed similar degrees of improvement. Although patients treated with the combined drugs were not treated for as long a period, the dose of drug they received, on the basis of expected additive effect, was greater.

Thirteen of the 82 schizophrenic patients were allowed to leave the hospital for the first time on trial visits or leaves of absence. Others approached this degree of improvement. Only one of the 82 patients required treatment with electroconvulsive therapy along with the drug. Five of the 12 patients who had not responded to bilateral prefrontal leukotomy were moderately or considerably improved by the drugs.

Those schizophrenic patients who showed moderate or pronounced improvement were usually better than they had been at any time since their illness began. Often the change in patients was dramatic, both in the rapidity of onset and in the degree. However, in some patients improvement took a more gradual course. Delusions and hallucinations diminished considerably. Mute and apathetic patients often began to speak appropriately. Severely disorganized speech gradually became more coherent. A few patients seemed to have amnesia for their illness, expressing astonishment upon hearing how long they had been hospitalized. The changes in physical appearance were also noteworthy. Nutrition was improved, dress became neater, and social amenities were restored. Most of these patients, who had previously spurned any psychiatric treatment, appeared now to be able to participate fruitfully in it.

The results of treatment of patients with organic psychosis using a daily dose of 75 mg. of chlorpromazine orally were not striking. Six of 15 patients who received active medication improved. However, three of 13 patients who received placebos improved. It was decided that a higher dose of the drug would be needed to treat patients in this group effectively. Seven of 14 patients who were then treated with a daily dose of 150 to 200 mg. of chlorpromazine showed satisfactory improvement. In general, the degree of disability shown by these patients was not greatly changed by this dose of the drug. In these older patients, higher doses of the drug were sometimes not well tolerated.

The results of treatment were disappointing in three patients with personality disorders and one patient with a psychotic depressive reaction. None of these patients was helped. Two of the patients with personality disorders became depressed from the drug. The patient with a psychotic depressive reaction was made worse, having disturbing hallucinations.

Complications of treatment occurred with considerably greater frequency in patients who received combined treatment than in those who received

TABLE 3.—Complications of treatment of 100 psychiatric patients with Chlorpromazine and combinations of Chlorpromazine and Reserpine

Complications	Chlorpromazine Alone 68 Patients	Chlorpromazine-Reserpine Combinations 32 Patients
Parkinson syndrome	4	9
Excitements	0	7
Convulsions	3*	3
Jaundice	2	1
Reactivation of peptic ulcer	2	0
Skin eruption	0	1
Syncope	1	0

*One patient had previous seizures.

chlorpromazine alone (Table 3). The frequent appearance of the Parkinson syndrome, excited states and convulsions is noteworthy in this group. Often two of these complications occurred simultaneously in the same patient, suggesting that all of them were related to the same toxic effect on the central nervous system. Among patients treated with chlorpromazine alone, these toxic effects occurred only when daily doses of 400 mg. or more of the drug were used. All of these side-effects were completely reversible by temporary interruption of treatment or by reduction in dosage.

The appearance of jaundice was not related to the dose of drug used. This complication occurred within nine to twenty-four days after treatment was begun. Two patients had prodromal symptoms of fever, gastrointestinal disturbances and malaise. Characteristic laboratory abnormalities were elevation of serum bilirubin, alkaline phosphatase, cholesterol and phospholipids. Only one patient had a laboratory sign of parenchymatous jaundice. In his case the result of a cephalin flocculation test was positive. Biopsy of the liver in this patient gave evidence of bile stasis and cellular infiltration around the biliary radicles. The longest duration of jaundice was three weeks, while in one patient jaundice disappeared in 48 hours. This latter patient had had viral hepatitis four years earlier and at that time jaundice had lasted for several weeks. (One patient, not in this series, has been successfully maintained on treatment with chlorpromazine after two brief episodes of jaundice.)

Other complications of treatment were infrequent. Skin eruptions occurred with less frequency than was anticipated. On the other hand, one patient with numerous infected lesions from compulsive scratching became completely free of lesions after treatment. Another patient with psoriasis was improved. Two patients with reactivation of peptic ulcers were continued on treatment by the addition of an ulcer regimen. Two patients died while under treatment, but in neither instance could the death be related to the drug. One patient drowned; the other had a ruptured abdominal aneurysm.

Comment

The effectiveness of chlorpromazine in psychiatric treatment cannot be doubted. Especially encouraging is the frequent amelioration of psychotic symptoms in patients with chronic schizophrenic reactions. In the present series 56 per cent of such patients were moderately or greatly improved by this drug. In a series reported elsewhere, 54 per cent of such patients treated with reserpine in combined parenteral and oral doses showed similar degrees of improvement. Thus, in the authors' experience, both drugs have been equally effective in this most difficult group of patients. It should be emphasized that it is the practice of the authors to continue other forms of treatment while the patients are treated with drugs. Thus, these results represent more than the effects of the drugs alone.

The combination of chlorpromazine with reserpine does not seem to offer any advantage over the use of either drug alone. At lower levels of dosage, no advantage from the use of combined drugs as opposed to use of reserpine alone was noted. In larger doses, use of combined drugs enhanced the toxic effects, particularly those affecting the central nervous system. Quite possibly there exists a middle range of dosage where the combination can be used effectively. However, whether the combination is superior to equivalent doses of either drug alone is questionable.

There seems to be little indication for the use of chlorpromazine in patients with personality disorders or psychotic depressive reactions. In the latter patients, the authors agree with other investigators that electroconvulsive therapy is the treatment of choice. While behavioral aberrations can be controlled in some patients with organic psychosis, there is little reason to believe that this drug can rehabilitate patients with advanced degrees of organic change.

Since the wide use of reserpine and chlorpromazine was begun at the Veterans Administration Hospital, Palo Alto, no patient has been subjected to leukotomy. The use of electroconvulsive therapy in the treatment of schizophrenic patients has diminished to the vanishing point. There is every reason to believe that the drugs are better than either of the other somatic therapies. The fact that almost half of a group of patients in whom leukotomy did not help obtained significant improvement from drug treatment tends to confirm this conclusion. On the other hand, more effective use of psychotherapy for schizophrenic patients now seems to be possible.

The importance of jaundice as a complication of chlorpromazine therapy seems to have been exaggerated. The incidence of 3 per cent in this series is higher than the over-all incidence of 0.9 per cent reported in 3,533 psychiatric patients who were treated with the drug. In any case, the risk does not seem to be greater than the experience here reported would indicate. Furthermore, the jaundice is of mild degree and short duration. It resembles most of the jaundice produced by methyltestosterone. As yet, there is no reason to believe that permanent hepatic damage ensues from this complication.

The production of the Parkinson syndrome by either chlorpromazine or reserpine, and particularly by the combined drugs, is a matter not to be treated lightly. All the evidence to date indicates that this syndrome represents a toxic effect of these drugs. With the usual remedy for toxic effects, diminution of dosage, this phenomenon disappears. To continue treatment in the face of this syndrome may be courting disaster. There is a point at which physiologic effects may become pathologic changes. Until more is known about the implications of this complication, the utmost of prudence is indicated.

RESERPINE IN THE TREATMENT OF DISTURBED ADOLESCENTS

George T. Nicolaou, M.D., and Nathan S. Kline, M.D.
Rockland State Hospital, Orangeburg, N. Y.

INTRODUCTION

In the evaluation of any drug, there are certain questions which must be answered. (1) Does it have therapeutic application? (2) In what conditions is it most effective? (3) Does it have direct "curative" properties, or does it merely serve to repress or alleviate symptoms? (4) Does the drug have undesirable, annoying, or dangerous side effects? (5) What is the optimal dosage? (6) What is the most effective technique and procedure of administration?

The recent introduction of reserpine, the alkaloid of the Rauwolfia plant, as a drug which may be of use in the treatment of psychiatric conditions has given rise to a series of investigations. At Rockland State Hospital the program of investigation is attempting to answer the aforementioned questions in respect to this medication. The original paper by Kline demonstrated that the drug did have effective sedative properties in chronically disturbed adult mental hospital patients. In the dosage used in this experiment (1 mg. daily by mouth), there was no real indication that the drug did more than reduce anxiety, agitation, and excited assaultive behavior. Subsequently, much larger doses of intramuscular preparations were given to determine if this technique of administration would act as a therapeutic agent capable of influencing the course of the disease itself. As a part of this general investigation, research was extended to include a group of disturbed hospitalized male adolescents ranging between 11 and 15 years of age. The following pages report the results of the use of reserpine in this type of patient.

PHASE ONE

Subjects

The diagnostic categories in psychiatry do not always allow for clear-cut placement of a specific patient in a particular group. In child psychiatry, this problem is even greater and more accentuated, both because of the recent concepts of childhood schizophrenia and the varieties of "normal" adolescent behavior which are not too well known or clearly defined. An effort was made, therefore, to select "typical" cases. In *Group I*, 12 adolescents were selected who demonstrated all the classical symptoms (regression, withdrawal, distortion of reality, and disturbances in thinking and affect) associated with the diagnosis of schizophrenia. These patients had all been sick a minimum of five years, with onset of definite psychotic symptoms between the ages of two-and-a-half and six years of age.

Group II consists of 12 patients who were judged to be the most excited, over-active, aggressive, and restless members of the adolescent population, and generally characterized as uncooperative and abusive. The "regressed" schizophrenic patients were excluded from this group even though some of them displayed this type of behavior. Two boys who had been diagnosed as childhood schizophrenics were included, but neither displayed the degree of "regression" or the overt psychotic symptomatology of the Group I patients.

Group III was composed of 15 patients who were selected with criteria of little or no overt aggressiveness, excitability, and restlessness. They were generally characterized as cooperative and comfortable patients. Three of this group carried the diagnosis of childhood schizophrenia, but none showed the classical signs described under Group I.

Controls

Except for a small group of patients whose release was imminent, the remaining 39 patients of the adolescent service were used as controls. This group was made up of primary behavioral and characterological disorders, except for a few non-regressed schizophrenics. They differ from Group II, because they represent the mode rather than the extremes of the overactive-to-comfortable spectrum.

Experimental Design

The following tests were administered to each subject and control wherever possible.
1. Routine leucocyte count
2. Blood pressure
3. Pulse
4. Body weight
5. Wittenborn anxiety scale as modified for children
6. Wechsler-Bellevue sub-tests (digit span, digit symbol, object assembly)
7. Rating scales of overt behavior
   a. comfortable-overactive
   b. cooperative-uncooperative

Two routine leucocyte counts were done on both controls and test subjects before medication was started. This was repeated at two-week intervals throughout the test period.

The Wittenborn anxiety scale as modified for children was administered before and after medication to all test subjects except those in the regressed schizophrenic group. This test could not be reliably evaluated in the latter group because of the severe thinking disorder that most of them displayed. The sub-tests (digit span, digit symbols, and object assembly) of the Wechsler-Bellevue Form I are generally considered the most sensitive to anxiety states. These tests, which can be quantified easily for a comparable analysis, were administered before and after medication to all subjects except those in the regressed schizophrenic group (who were not considered capable of adequately responding to the material).

The rating scale for overt behavior consisted of the subjective evaluation of ten raters, each submitting the rating independently. The rating team was made up of ward personnel, teachers, athletic instructors, occupational therapists, and two psychiatrists, all of whom were well acquainted with each subject and maintained almost daily contact with them throughout the experiment. Each rater was asked to evaluate the subject's behavior based on his over-all contacts before and after medication. Needless to say behavior is a very difficult factor to evaluate. In order to simplify the problem, as well as to make it suitable for comparable analysis, behavior was categorized into the two gross qualities of *cooperativeness* and *comfortableness*. Thus each subject was rated first as to whether he was generally comfortable or overactive. Then, on a different day, he was rated as to whether he was generally cooperative or uncooperative.

Dosage and Regime

The test subjects were given 1.0 mg. of reserpine orally every day for ten weeks, and during this same period the control subjects received a placebo tablet. Both tablets were identical in size and appearance, and the routine of administration was standardized for all subjects. The patients were all advised that they were receiving a vitamin tablet, and, since nearly every patient was receiving this same medication, no one questioned the need or motive. Although the ward personnel were aware of the nature of the experiment, they were not advised as to which of the patients were test subjects and which were controls. Furthermore, several containers were used on each ward, each with a different code name, to reduce the chance of guessing the identity of the test groups. The personnel involved in rating various patients were also subject to the same conditions described above, thus reducing the chance of biased opinions.

Results

1. *Leucocyte Count.* There was no significant change in the leucocyte counts in response to reserpine at the dosages used in this experiment. The variations in cell count were within normal limits, and were comparable to the differences noted in the control group.

2. *Blood Pressure.* Blood pressures prior to medication were all within normal limits for this age group, and ranged from 95/58 to 125/78. All groups showed an average decrease after medication. The data in respect to average changes are presented in Table I.

Each of the individual test subjects on reserpine showed a consistent drop in blood pressure. This decrease ranged from −2.0 mm to −41.0 mm in the systolic pressure and −1.0 mm to −29.0 mm in the diastolic pressure. In contrast, the changes in the control group ranged from +15 mm to −16 mm in systolic, and +8 mm to −16 mm in diastolic pressure. Despite careful investigation, no relationship could be found between changes in blood pressure (or pulse) and either clinical improvement or other test results.

3. *Pulse.* There was no significant alteration in the pulse that could be ascribed to the medication. These data are summarized in Table II.

4. *Body Weight.* During the test period, the control group showed less of a

TABLE I: Blood Pressure Changes

	Controls	Group I	Group II	Group III
Systolic	—4.1 mm	—13.8 mm	—13.1 mm	—8.3 mm
Diastolic	—4.6 mm	—10.5 mm	—14.3 mm	—8.2 mm

TABLE II: Pulse Rate

	Controls Range	Controls Average	Test Subjects Range	Test Subjects Average
Pre-test	70 to 100	87.5	74 to 100	88.0
Post-test	74 to 100	84.1	74 to 98	84.2

TABLE III: Body Weight Changes

	Controls	Test Subjects
Range	—10 lbs. to +14 lbs.	—2 lbs. to +20 lbs.
Average	+2.4 lbs.	+6.8 lbs.

weight gain than did the test subjects. See Table III for summary of data.

5. *Wittenborn Scale.* Answers to the specific items of this scale were assigned weighted scores in order to facilitate comparable analysis. The analysis was based on the comparison of the sum of the weighted scores. An increase in the sum represented an increase in conscious appreciation of anxiety as it applied to the specific items of the scale. Conversely, a lower score represented a decrease in conscious appreciation of anxiety. These data are summarized in Table IV.

6. *Wechsler-Bellevue Sub-Test.* The individual performances on the various sub-tests were quantified, and the sums were compared. An increase in sum represented an increase in performance, and presumably a decrease in anxiety. Conversely, a decrease in the sum was associated with an increase in anxiety. Results are presented in Table V.

7. *Comfortable-Uncomfortable Ratings.* By this rating, the patient was judged to be either comfortable or overactive as a predominant behavioral pattern. Thus, each rating of comfortableness was interpreted as a corresponding decrease in the overactivity, and vice versa. A differential change of under 20% for an individual was not considered significant, and was reported as "no change."

No patients in Group III (Table VI) became more comfortable, because these patients were selected as already being the most comfortable on the ward.

8. *Cooperative-Uncooperative Ratings.* Each subject was rated as being either cooperative or uncooperative, and, as in the case of the comfortable-uncomfortable ratings, the subject was categorized on the basis of the predominant pattern. Thus, each rating of cooperativeness represents a corresponding decrease in uncooperativeness, and vice versa. Here again a differ-

TABLE IV: Change in Anxiety as Measured by the Wittenborn Scale

	Controls %	Group I	Group II %	Group III %
Increase	44	not testable	58	64
Unchanged	16		9	15
Decrease	40		33	21

TABLE V: Wechsler-Bellevue Sub-Test Changes
(Indicating appreciation of anxiety)

	Controls %	Group I	Group II %	Group III %
Increase	40	not testable	64	58
Unchanged	30		36	26
Decrease	30		0	16

TABLE VI: Comfortable-Uncomfortable Rating Scale

	Controls %	Group I %	Group II %	Group III %
More comfortable	50	17	59	0
No change	30	50	33	74
Less comfortable	20	33	8	26

TABLE VII: Cooperativeness-Uncooperativeness Rating Scale

	Controls %	Group I %	Group II %	Group III %
Increased cooperativeness	13	33	41	10
No change	65	59	50	79
Decreased cooperativeness	22	8	9	11

ential change under 20% for an individual was not considered significant, and was evaluated as "no change." See Table VII for results.

As a group, the test patients became much more cooperative following medication. The failure of Group III to reflect this increase was again because the group was selected as the most cooperative to begin with, and there was consequently little room for improvement.

Complications

There were no serious adverse clinical manifestations that could be attributed to reserpine at the dosages used in this experiment. A few of the patients complained of mild nasal congestion during the initial 2 weeks, but this condition was self-limiting; it disappeared after several days with or without treatment. Varying degrees of drowsiness was also noted in 10 of the test subjects. This effect tended to be less prominent after the first month of medication. It usually occurred in the late afternoon, and lasted from 1 to 2 hours, occasionally leading to short naps. In most instances, this side effect could be avoided by giving the medication during the evening hours.

Summary and Conclusions of Phase One

The over-all results of Phase One of this experiment were far from conclusive, although some encouraging features were noteworthy. At the dosages given, there were no adverse physical complications. The decrease in blood pressure, although significant, did not reach levels which were considered dangerous. The pulse levels were not remarkably altered. There were no significant changes in the leucocyte counts. The body weight tended to increase over and above the normal growth patterns for this age group. The Wittenborn anxiety scale seemed to indicate that as a group the patients under medication showed an increase in conscious appreciation of anxiety. Similarly, the Wechsler-Bellevue sub-test also showed that as a group the patients on reserpine showed an increase in anxiety.

In evaluating the comfortable and cooperative ratings, the test groups cannot be compared to the control group, nor with each other, but only with themselves (pre- and post-medication), since the degree of overactivity and cooperativeness was a predetermined criteria for selection; the controls represent the mode, and Groups II and III the opposite extremes of the overactive-to-comfortable spectrum. The results of these ratings, however, suggest that where overactivity and/or uncooperativeness are the predominant patterns, this behavior is significantly altered; these patients became more comfortable and cooperative.

Phase Two

The results in Phase One were sufficiently encouraging to suggest that with larger doses, and particularly with the use of the intramuscular preparation, even more benefit might be obtained. This assumption was further justified by the results on adults reported by Barsa and Kline. Because of the need for individual regulation of dosage, and also because we felt that the activity of the drug had already been demonstrated in Phase One with minimal dosage, the more formal type of control was not included. Since the patients were well known to the psychiatrists, it was deemed sufficient to use clinical evaluations.

Subjects

Twenty-five patients from the Adolescent Service were selected and divided into two groups. *Group A* consisted of 11 patients ranging between the ages of 11 and 14, all of whom showed classical signs of schizophrenia. All had been overtly psychotic for at least five years. Ten patients from this group had been receiving 1 mg. of reserpine orally for over two months. The other patient was a recent admission and had never received reserpine. *Group B* consisted of 14 patients between the ages of 11 to 15 who were considered the most overactive, aggressive, and disturbed youngsters of the service, but who did not show any overt schizophrenic manifestations. Of this group, 10 patients had received 1 mg. of oral reserpine for 10 weeks previously. However, in all cases, 1 to 2 months transpired before they were given the second course of medication. The other four patients had never taken reserpine before.

Dosage and Administration

Initially all patients were given five parenteral injections over a period of five days, starting with 2.5 mg. daily for three days, then 5.0 mg. for the following two days. At the time of the initial injection, they were also started on 2.0 mg. of oral reserpine. One month after the last injection an initial clinical evaluation was made, and all patients who did not show a sustained improvement were given a second course of parenteral medication. There were 15 patients (8 from Group A and 7 from Group B) who had the second course. This consisted of 18 injections given over a period of 3 weeks as follows: 2.5 mg. daily for four days, 5.0 mg. for 10 days, and 7.5 mg. for four days. The oral medication was continued throughout the parenteral course, and during the subsequent two months. The oral dose at this time was increased to 5.0 mg. daily in all cases not showing a sustained improvement after the second parenteral course. Two months after the last injection, all oral medication was discontinued.

Complications

All patients showed from moderate to marked psychomotor retardation while taking parenteral reserpine. Lethargy and drowsiness usually occurred within 1 to 2 hours, and in most instances persisted for 4 to 6 hours. As the dosage increased, this side effect became more prominent, and naps of 1 to 3 hours during the day were not uncommon. Mild attacks of nausea and diarrhea occurred in three cases, but ordinarily these symptoms subsided before specific medication was necessary.

One case, after the third injection, suddenly developed generalized muscular rigidity with opisthotonus and oculogyric crisis. This condition lasted for about two hours, then gradually subsided during the following hour. He was discontinued from the parenteral form, but continued on the oral preparation without further reaction for several months following this episode.

A Parkinson-like syndrome was observed in one case after the eighth injection. The patient showed cog-wheel rigidity, shuffling gait, pill-rolling tremor, drooling, and thick speech. When this developed, the parenteral injections were discontinued. All symptoms disappeared within 24 hours. One month later this same patient was given another course consisting of 18 injections, with larger doses than he had previously received, without any complications.

Results

1. *Schizophrenics.* The observation period varied from two to three months. All patients showed improvement in behavior while on parenteral medication. This was particularly noticeable in cases where overactivity, agitation, and bizarre behavior were prominent. In most instances, however, this improvement was not maintained after intramuscular medication was discontinued, even though patients continued to receive oral reserpine. Only three patients continued to show improvement, remaining comfortable, cooperative, quiet, relaxed, with reduction of bizarre stereotyped behavior. The remaining patients reverted to their previous behavior patterns, usually within two to four days after the last parenteral injection.

Qualitatively, different psychic activity was also observed while the patients were receiving the parenteral medication. The very regressed, out-of-contact cases, became more alert, more responsive, and showed increasing interest in the activities around them. With the exception of one case, however, these changes were not maintained after the parenteral injections were discontinued, even though they were on oral maintenance doses varying between 2 and 5 mg. per day. One case prior to the treatment was delusional, hallucinated, very withdrawn, apathetic, and disinterested. During the course of treatment, he became more alert and interested in the ward activities. The delusional and hallucinatory formations subsided, and he refers to them now as "imaginations." His improvement has been maintained for over four months, the last of which was without medication of any sort.

2. *Non-Schizophrenics.* While receiving parenteral medication, all fourteen patients showed varying degrees of improvement in behavior. Generally they were relaxed, comfortable, cooperative, receptive, and showed greater control of impulsive activity. However, four cases did not maintain the improvement after the parenteral injections were discontinued, even though they were receiving 2 to 5 mg. orally. The remaining 10 patients continued to show progressive improvement while on the oral maintenance dose of 2 to 5 mg. daily.

The final evaluation was made one month after the medication was discontinued. At the time, eight patients were considered improved and since then either have been discharged or are ready for release as suitable placements become available. Two patients have gradually begun to revert to previous aggressive behavior patterns, becoming agitated, overactive, and demanding. These data are summarized in Table VIII.

TABLE VIII: RESULTS OF RESERPINE THERAPY

	No. Cases	On Combined Oral and i.m. Improved	On Combined Oral and i.m. Unimproved	On Oral Following Combined Improved	On Oral Following Combined Relapsed	Post-Medication Improved	Post-Medication Relapsed
Schizophrenic	11	11	0	3	8	1	10
Non-Schizophrenic	14	14	0	10	4	8*	6

* Ready for discharge.

The same patients who showed a sustained improvement in behavior also demonstrated significant changes in their mental status. Overt hostility and aggressive attitudes, which characterized these patients before treatment, were no longer the prominent features. They seemed to reach out and seek interpersonal relationships. Invariably they showed a desire to relate and to enter into cooperative activity. There was a greater willingness to talk about their problems, and to take advice and guidance. Comments such as, "I feel content and happy inside and don't feel like fighting anymore," were not uncommon. One of the patients appraised his status rather appropriately in the following manner, "I know I have improved and want to go home, but I'd rather stay longer to help myself more, go to school, and make up my grades, before I go home for good." Another youngster expressed himself as follows, "Before, I felt bad all the time, so I would fight a lot; now I feel good, and don't have to fight."

The above quotations are but a few examples to illustrate the qualitative changes in psychic activity. Considering that these patients constituted the most difficult problems in the service, both from a therapeutic and management view, these changes are significant. In all the cases which showed sustained improvement, the one common feature was their readiness to acknowledge that they had problems; furthermore, that these problems and their own activity are what culminated in the need for hospitalization.

Although the Rorschach test was not included as a routine in the experimental design, four patients from Group B who showed sustained improvement were recent admissions, and a Rorschach protocol prior to medication was available as part of the admission routine. Two months after the parenteral medication was discontinued they were retested and the protocols compared.

Although the pre- and post-medication protocols for the four patients were in many respects similar, several changes are noteworthy. First of all, there was consistency in the changes in all subjects; they gave somewhat greater number of human responses and substantially fewer animal movement responses. Three of the four patients gave a comparatively greater proportion of responses in which form was the sole determinant. The results suggest that the group as a whole became less impulsive and less spontaneous, but more objective and detached in their appraisal of the environment.

This diminution of impulsivity and spontaneity might well stem from an increase in anxiety. It could also reflect greater striving for self-control, which would stem from an increased need to adapt to and be accepted by the group. The increase in human movement responses definitely suggests greater striving toward forming interpersonal relationships. The changes of the Rorschach protocols in this limited study parallel the clinical observations.

Discussion

The patients who did not maintain any significant improvement were more disorganized, and the emotional integration was considered to be at a lower level prior to the onset of illness, in contrast to the patients who improved. It would seem that the response of these patients who did not improve was more like the reaction seen in the schizophrenic group, who by and large showed marked disorganization and, in most instances, had little if any emotional integration prior to onset of illness. This would obviously imply that the level of emotional integration prior to illness is a very important factor in the success or failure of reserpine therapy. This, of course, is a well founded principle, and its importance and prominence has been demonstrated in all forms of therapy.

The pharmacological effects of reserpine can be easily studied physiologically, and ultimately it would seem that the complete story of this action will be understood. The psychological changes which occur, either as a by-product or direct action, are not as easy to study. What we see clinically is the end product of an intricate psycho-physiological process. During the peak of the pharmacological response, emotional lability was a frequent occurrence. At these times the patients were noted to be very sensitive, often crying without apparent cause, frequently seeking adult contact as though they were reaching for support, and constantly asking for reassurance. Associated with this activity was marked diminution, and in some cases a complete collapse, of the hostile and aggressive defenses.

This seems to suggest that the over-all pharmacological effect tends to "cut through," or in some way alter, the psychological defenses. Since the primary function of the psychological defenses is to allay anxiety, any failure of, or threat to, the defensive structure of the organism is associated with an increase in perception of anxiety. The results from the first phase of this experiment suggest that there was a tendency toward an increase in the conscious perception of anxiety. In addition, the clinical observation and the limited Rorschach studies all tend to support the contention that the psychological defenses are qualitatively altered. This cutting through, or altering, the defenses sets the stage for corrective emotional experiences through interpersonal activity. Once this has been accomplished, the outcome depends on the integrative abilities of the organism and the individual psychotherapeutic needs. Obviously no drug can provide capacities which are lacking; however, it seems that the over-all effects of reserpine do provide the opportunity for existing innate reparative abilities to function effectively within the context of constructive psychotherapy. Aside from the sedative effects and the apparently specific action on psychomotor activity, reserpine is a useful implement in psychotherapy, and to this extent it deserves a definite place in our therapeutic armamentarium in the management of disturbed adolescents. It is our impression that the most effective point of application in this type of patient will be prior to hospitalization, since it is highly probable that admission would not have been necessary if reserpine had been used early enough. This seems particularly true in those cases where aggressive "acting out" characterized the social behavior precipitating institutionalization.

THE USE OF RESERPINE (SERPASIL) IN THREE HUNDRED AND FIFTY NEUROPSYCHIATRIC CASES

Veronica M. Pennington, M.D.,
Mississippi State Hospital, Whitfield, Mississippi

Three hundred and fifty of our most disturbed female patients were given reserpine by mouth, intramuscularly, and intravenously for a period of two weeks to six months. Some continue to take the medication now in the eighth month. Many more have gone home, and are continuing to take it there. Early in the experiment, reserpine was discontinued on some of this group, because our supply has always been limited, and given only where it seemed to do the most good. In the light of our experience since then I would discontinue it on none, because I believe that, in proper dosage, given for the proper length of time, every patient would show some betterment. In some cases no change was noted for as long as three months, and then there was a remarkable degree of improvement.

Method

The 350 patients were selected from four cottages housing a total of 451 females. Patients were classified in fourteen different categories. All but a few whose physical health contraindicated it had received electroshock therapy, and many had had insulin therapy; about five had had lobotomies. Many had from 150 to 500 shock treatments with temporary, but marked, improvement. Requiring this type of treatment meant they could not return to their homes, and remained wards of the state. Some were continually in a confused and clouded state because of excessive shock; when treatments were lessened, they became assaultive and noisy.

The age range was from twenty to eighty; average age was forty-five and a half years. The duration of their psychoses was from two to fifty years; the average psychotic years was sixteen. The total psychotic years was 5,600.

Daily order sheets were put on each cottage and required changes each day, increasing and decreasing the dosage according to the individual needs of the patient. Individual charts were kept giving the condition of the patient before reserpine, and daily thereafter. The amount and kind (by mouth, intramuscular, intravenous), time given, by whom, and physical and mental reactions were charted. Initial blood pressures were taken; weight charts were kept as well as sleep records.

Psychological testing was given before and after reserpine in sixteen cases, and after the reserpine had apparently reached its peak, in fifty-six cases.

Lack of personnel limited our work in this field, but we have begun an intensive study of 100 cases which will be reported later. James Sartin, the psychologist cooperating in this work, feels the results of the psychological testing must be evaluated cautiously, since only a small sample of patients, 9%, was used. In this pilot study, 37.9% were essentially normal, 6.2% were greatly improved, 25% were improved, 32% were classified as "no change" after reserpine. No significant group differences were found.

Psychiatric testing was done daily by personal interview with each patient. Reports from supervisors, psychiatric aides, occupational workers, letters from patients, and dictaphone recordings of the patient's own story about the effects of the alkaloid on them were utilized. Improvements noted by relatives and employers who had formerly known the patient were incorporated.

Three routes of administering reserpine were used: by mouth, intramuscularly, and intravenously. For those patients who refused the drug, the parenteral route was used. Intravenous injections were used for booster effects in the acutely disturbed, who had not been taking the alkaloid long enough for sufficient effect. When given intravenously, the quieting could be noted within an hour. As high as fifteen mg. were given in the twenty-four hour period by the intravenous route.

At first 2.5 mg., parenterally, was given as the arbitrary dose, but by the third month we saw the necessity of increasing the beginning dosage to one whole ampule of five mg. daily; or, by the mouth dosage, to 4 mg. in the morning and 4 in the afternoon. This was then decreased according to the effect on the patient.

Some patients were given an occasional shock treatment for immediate quieting effect.

Twenty-five controls on two wards, making a total of fifty, and five at another time, were given a placebo. At the end of six months the reserpine was stopped on all but fifty; however, the charts were continued daily on all. This retrospect view of the effects of reserpine has proven valuable and enlightening.

When a patient improved sufficiently to be given a leave of absence, the correspondent was written and asked to come for him. Many were contacted while they were visiting the patient and asked to take him home. Others noted the marked improvement and requested a leave.

The correspondent was given two mimeographed prescriptions for 300 one-milligram tablets of reserpine (Serpasil) and requested to purchase the medicine before leaving Jackson so there would be no discontinuance of the medication.

A mimeographed slip with instructions for the patient to take the medicine regularly and to see the family physician every two weeks for a check-up was signed and given each correspondent. Many of the family doctors wrote inquiring what type of examination was wanted; our reply gave them the indications for increasing or decreasing the dosage. Patients were encouraged to write the physician or make appointments for an interview when adjustments of dosage could be made and psychotherapy given.

When patients were returned from a leave of absence in exacerbation, an attempt was made to find out if they had continued taking reserpine while away from the hospital. All but a few cases had neglected taking it. The others required a larger dose.

Findings

In the six month period of this experiment, 42.8% of those taking reserpine were returned to their homes. Many more were ready to return, but their relatives, especially husbands, would not come for them, so alienated had they become by long absence. Twenty percent of this 42.8% were returned to the hospital; all but a few of the returnees had discontinued taking the medication while on leave.

It took from four to eleven days, in some cases three months, for improvement to be noticed. At first medications were discontinued on all but a few of these patients showing no betterment after two weeks. Those few who continued to take it in spite of no betterment improved so greatly by the third month that those for whom the treatment was formerly discontinued were again given the alkaloid.

This improvement was shown by clarity of thinking, coherence, orientation, improved rapport with associates, cleanliness, application to gainful occupation, interest in life, diminishing expression of delusional trends and hallucinatory experiences, pride in self, responsiveness, and quiet, peaceful living. The greatest improvement was shown in the field of personal relationship, conformity to normal standards of behavior, being en rapport with their fellow men.

Improvement has been so gradual in some that it was imperceptible from day to day, but when reserpine was discontinued on a large group after six months, these patients regressed to their former disturbed pattern. The improvement they had made could easily be seen in retrospect. When the drug was resumed, they again made a comparable improvement.

I will categorize the benefits and side effects of reserpine by systems.

The Digestive System

Those catatonics and idiots who have to be fed developed hyperphagia, and gained greatly in weight on reserpine. Many patients with chronic anorexia, who had never been normal in weight, ate ravenously and gained many pounds. Those patients who had always been constipated, particularly the seniles and arteriosclerotic cases, had thorough and regular evacuations with reserpine. One and four-tenths percent of the cases had occasional diarrhea, entirely controlled by reducing the reserpine dosage and giving bismuth. Ptyalism was one of the first symptoms of overdosage, and occurred in 3.8% of the cases.

Eye, Ear, Nose and Throat

Miosis was a frequent early symptom, but did not impair gross vision. Oedema caused by water retention caused nasal stuffiness in .58% of this group. Partial blocking of the eustachian tube caused slight difficulty in hearing and a heavy feeling in the chest with an asthmatic feeling; this was due to the same cause. These were produced by dosages of from 10 to 13 mg. daily. This oedema substantiates the hypothesis that reserpine acts on the hypothalamus, affecting the antidiuretic substance.

Genito Urinary System

Premenstrual tension and dysmenorrhea were definitely relieved in this group. Robert Greenblatt found that premenstrual oedema was considerably worsened, although the tension was lessened by reserpine. This again could be evidence that the antidiuretic substance of the hypothalamus is affected by reserpine in its water metabolism function. The estrous cycle appeared to be unaffected. Urine analyses done on the high dosage cases were normal.

Skin and Musculature

Psychophysiologic skin reactions were remarkably affected. One patient's entire chest, back, upper arms, and neck showed a generalized eczematoid rash for years; this cleared up in two weeks as her mental condition improved. At the beginning of the medication, particularly when large doses were given, 1.1% complained of cramp-like pains in the lower extremities and one complained of the same condition in her arms. The pains were very moderate and stopped with reduction of dosage. Difficulty in walking occurred in 2.9%; this was alleviated in all cases when reserpine was decreased.

Nervous System

Miosis has been mentioned. The return to mental normality, the marked improvement in chronic patients whose psychoses had existed from 2 to 50 years, with 42.8% returned to their homes, marks the psychic good done by reserpine. Overdosage produced in .88% a Parkinsonian-like tremor of the upper extremities with interosseous position of the hand and fingers, the "pill-rolling" movement with accompanying mask-like facies. The festinating gait was not observed, possibly because the overdosage was discontinued as soon as the palsy was noted. This syndrome disappeared when the medication was discontinued, and returned when overdosage was resumed. One and one-tenth percent of the group had convulsive seizures. These were not known epileptics, but were all of the schizophrenic, catatonic type that are known to show conspicuous motor behavior including grand mal attacks. All had had many shock treatments, which in our experience predisposes to convulsive seizures in some cases. Therefore, the percentage given above cannot be attributed to reserpine alone. Nightmares occurred in .29%, and the dreams were like alcoholic hallucinations.

Circulatory System

The pulse rate was reduced in almost every case, but only to a beneficial degree. Blood pressure in the hypertensive was brought back to normal, with a reduction or elimination of dizziness, headaches, and other symptoms of hypertension. Normal and low blood pressures were not affected to a marked degree. Psychophysiologic cardiovascular reactions were greatly benefited. On high dosage, .88% had one syncopal attack with no recurrence after reduction. Blood pressures taken some little time after the attack were not abnormally low.

GENERAL

Patients whose assaultiveness was held in partial abeyance by electroshock therapy were completely relieved by reserpine; our so-called "back halls" and "disturbed wards" became quiet and less untidy. Patients began to participate in occupational therapy work and outside activities. Our hydrotherapy section went into disuse. Accidents were rare. We have used no restraint for two years on our so-called violent ward accommodating 128 patients. The first year is accounted for by electroshock therapy, and the second by Serpasil. Only two or three patients are secluded for a portion of a day.

Patients with irritating and antagonistic character traits, who have been shunted from one ward to the other, were transformed remarkably into likeable, helpful friends. Patients who for years refused to lift a hand became avid workers. The sleep charts showed marked improvement, and practically all patients were pleased with their uninterrupted hours of rest. The wards became quiet, and the usual restlessness was markedly reduced.

Some patients who had to be kept in a clouded state with electroshock therapy to prevent assaultiveness and self-injury became clear and oriented with reserpine.

Forty-two and seven-tenths percent of the group were cases of schizophrenic reaction, catatonic. Of these, 2.8% were restored and 5% greatly improved. All improved to a degree.

Fourteen and one-tenth percent were schizophrenic reaction, paranoid type. Of this classification, 31.1% were restored and 33.7% were greatly improved. All were benefitted.

Twenty-four and seven-tenths percent were schizophrenic reaction, hebephrenic type. Of these, 10.8% were restored, and 33.7% greatly improved. Only a few of this group seemed not to have benefitted, but these will be given a longer trial on the alkaloid.

Twenty-nine hundredths percent were involutional psychotic reaction type, characterized by somatic preoccupation and agitation. These improved, but none recovered.

Chronic brain syndrome, associated with circulatory disturbance with cerebral arteriosclerosis, constituted 3.5%. Of these, 26.3% were restored mentally and improved physically; 26.3% were greatly improved mentally and helped physically. Since some cases in this category improved spontaneously, the exact part played by Serpasil cannot be determined.

Fifty-eight one-hundredths percent of the group were cases of chronic brain syndrome associated with disturbance of nutrition, senile brain disease, and presenile brain disease. In these, only a slight improvement was noted; they were less restless and less noisy.

Chronic brain syndrome associated with convulsive disorder with psychotic reaction constituted 2.6% of the group. Of these, 22.2% were restored in their behavioral pattern and the number of their seizures was reduced. When the alkaloid was discontinued, the number of seizures spurted upward. These patients were also receiving Dilantin and one quarter grain of phenobarbital all through the experiment. We did not keep graphs of seizures before reserpine, but have done so since. Individual slips for the purpose of reporting seizures were used. The epileptic personality was definitely improved.

Huntington's chorea case constituted .58% of the cases, and all were improved mentally. Their athetoid movements were definitely decreased. Deglutition was improved.

The 5.6% of mentally deficient, moderate to severe cases, showed 26.3% greatly improved in conduct, alertness, ability to care for themselves, and physical betterment.

Two and six-tenths percent showed chronic brain syndrome associated with central nervous syphilis (meningoencephalitic type). These showed improvement in conduct and gained in weight.

Twenty-nine hundredths percent cases exhibited chronic brain syndrome associated with congenital spastic paraplegia. The recovery rate was 100% from their psychoses and great improvement physically, facilitating their getting about. Side effects presented no difficulty since they could be controlled or eliminated as the examiner desired. Some of the extremely assaultive patients were kept in a relaxed, drowsy condition for several weeks to prevent aggressive acts. During this time, they were easily roused for eating and care as well as for exercise; many times during the day they walked about of their own volition. This was a great improvement over the clouded state produced by shock therapy.

Freis noted depressive symptoms in four out of five cases who were taking a maximum of 2 mg. of reserpine daily. He suggests that .25 mg. be the upper limit in dosage. This complication has not been noted in our group, but lethargy and placidity have been noted.

Conclusions

Three hundred and fifty neuropsychiatric patients, ages 20 to 80, with a 2 to 50 years duration of their psychoses, were given varying amounts of reserpine, from ½ mg. to 16 mg. by mouth, intramuscularly, and intravenously, according to their individual needs for a period of from two weeks to six months. Some continue to take the medication now in the eighth month. Observation and charting has continued for two months after the alkaloid was discontinued to test its lasting effects.

Physical improvement in general health, appetite, sleep, weight, evacuation, and blood pressures of the hypertensive was noted.

Twenty-three and two-tenths percent assaultive, eneuritic, denudative, noisy, coprophagic patients, and those showing stupor, mutism, negativism, waxy flexibility, disorientation, confusion, delusional trends, hallucinatory experiences, and apparent regression have been restored to normal life; 35.2% have been greatly improved. This makes irreversible regression doubtful.

Forty-two and eight-tenths percent of this group have been returned to their homes. Of this percentage, 20% have returned to the hospital, but all except a few of these had discontinued the use of reserpine.

Those remaining in the hospital are greatly improved or bettered to a degree.

Side effects were minimal and none serious; all were dosage controlled and reproduced several times by manipulation of the amount given. Feeding, seclusion, accidents due to assaultiveness, and noise have been eliminated by reserpine. Continued use for a period of eight months did not make increase in dosage necessary, once the maintenance dose was arrived at. Electroshock therapy has been reduced from 217 to 23 weekly, and, with bigger supplies of reserpine, probably can be discontinued.

DRUG THERAPY—CLINICAL AND OPERATIONAL EFFECTS
Changes in the Mental Hospital Resulting from the Addition of Chlorpromazine to the Total Therapeutic Program

Benjamin Pollack, M.D.
Assistant Director, Rochester State Hospital, Rochester, New York

The first concern of psychiatry is, of course, the welfare of the mentally ill; the value of any psychiatric treatment is best measured by its effect on the patient. The efficacy of chlorpromazine hydrochloride (Thorazine) has been discussed by numerous investigators whose clinical results have appeared, and are appearing, in a lengthy and still growing list of articles. These articles deal primarily with the changes the drug causes in the behavior and mental state of patients.

At the Rochester State Hospital (a 4,000 bed mental hospital) it has been obvious that the extensive use of chlorpromazine causes changes not only in those to whom the drug is given, but also in those who give it. Since June, 1954—when chlorpromazine treatment was first begun at Rochester—profound changes have occurred in the administrative routine of the hospital, the morale and duties of the hospital personnel, and in the attitude of the surrounding community.

Some of the significant changes are subtle ones, but others are quite apparent. Recently, selected personnel of the Rochester State Hospital were asked to prepare written reports which mentioned and discussed the changes they thought particularly noteworthy. The author then evaluated these reports and provided additional observations.

The main purpose of this article is to present a summary of the information thus gathered. Because these far-reaching changes arose from the addition of the tranquilizing drug to the total therapeutic program, a brief report is included of the clinical results obtained by chlorpromazine therapy on 900 patients treated over the period extending from June, 1954, to August, 1955. This report supplements previously published studies on the drug. By September, 1957, over 5,000 patients had been treated with Thorazine.

CLINICAL RESULTS

Chlorpromazine is no cure-all. It is most effective when combined with all the other psychiatric tools we have. Its primary effect is to change behavior by altering the patient's sensitivity to his emotions, to his delusions and to his environment. Excited, restless patients become quiet and well-behaved. Either rapidly or slowly after this change in behavior there often occurs an improvement in the patient's thought content, and in his manner and degree of response.

In our hospital, over 5,000 patients have been treated with chlorpromazine: the behavior of 66% of these patients has improved significantly, and 41% of them have demonstrated considerable improvement in their mental condition. In evaluating this therapy, it is important to distinguish between improvement in behavior and actual improvement in the mental condition (Table 1).

Although the addition of drugs to the total treatment program of the chronic schizophrenic may be less immediately dramatic compared to the results obtained in acute cases, the following table shows that the effects on behavior are still gratifying and that fair results are produced in the long-term treatment of the psychosis. (See Table 1A).

TABLE 1

Results of chlorpromazine treatment, as of August 1955, on 900 patients of various psychiatric diagnoses

	Behavior	Psychosis
Recovered	14%	6%
Markedly Improved	30%	15%
Much Improved	22%	20%
Improved	16%	12%
Unimproved	18%	47%

TABLE 1A

Percentage of 285 schizophrenic patients improved in behavior or in psychosis after treatment with chlorpromazine, according to duration of illness

Duration of illness	Behavior Improved	Psychosis Improved
Under 1 year	86%	71%
1 to 5 years	71%	49%
5 years and over	67%	29%

Table 2 demonstrates the diagnostic classification of 248 patients who were released from the hospital and who at one time or another had received chlorpromazine in addition to other therapeutic aids. Eighty-five percent (211) of this group were patients who had originally been treated in the hospital with this drug; 15% (37) were treated only on convalescent leave after they had left the hospital, and a relapse was threatened. Of the 211 patients who had been treated in the hospital, 66% (138) continued their treatment outside the hospital; 24% (51) discontinued treatment, and the treatment status of 10% (22) is unknown.

CHANGES IN THERAPY

Perhaps the most striking change in therapy caused by chlorpromazine is the greatly reduced need for giving electroshock treatments. Because chlorpromazine is either superior or equal to electroshock for most patients, the number of EST's has been reduced about 60 to 90%. Shock therapy is now used chiefly in treating resistive depressions and other psychoses, and then it is often combined with chlorpromazine. Insulin and psychosurgery are

TABLE 2
Study of 248 * patients released from hospital

	TOTAL		TREATED IN HOSPITAL & OUTSIDE		TREATED IN HOSPITAL ONLY		TREATED ON CONVALES. CARE ONLY		TREATMENT STATUS UNKNOWN	
	No.	Percent	No.	Percent	No.	Percent	No.	Percent	No.	Percent
TOTAL	248	100.0	138	55.6	51	20.6	37	14.9	22	8.9
Diagnosis:										
Schizophrenia	134	100.0	74	55.2	29	21.6	19	14.2	12	9.0
Psychoneurosis	20	100.0	14	70.0	3	15.0	2	10.0	1	5.0
Involutional Psychosis	29	100.0	16	55.2	4	13.8	8	27.6	1	3.4
Drug Psychosis	3	100.0	2	66.7	1	33.3	0	0	0	0
Manic Depressive	37	100.0	19	51.4	9	24.3	5	13.5	4	10.8
Psychosis CAS & Senile	12	100.0	7	58.3	2	16.7	2	16.7	1	8.3
Psych. With Psych. Pers.	3	100.0	2	66.7	0	0	1	33.3	0	0
Alcohol Psychosis	7	100.0	2	28.6	2	28.6	0	0	3	42.8
Undiagnosed	3	100.0	2	66.7	1	33.3	0	0	0	0

* Includes 21 patients (8.5%) returned to Hospital.

rarely used. The greater alertness and receptiveness of chlorpromazine-treated patients are reflected in the greatly increased participation in occupational and recreational therapy. For example, in 1954 only 15 of 54 patients were able to attend a disturbed ward picnic; in 1955, 49 out of 51 were able to attend. The quality of occupational therapy projects has improved considerably, and lengthier and more difficult projects have been initiated than were heretofore possible.

Chlorpromazine has also been effective in reducing the amount of restraint and seclusion necessary. In an early study of 87 patients who had required almost constant restraint and seclusion for from 5 to 20 years, we found that 43 of them could be kept out of restraint all the time. Daytime restraint has been all but eliminated on acute wards. The restraint that is now used is applied for brief periods without the necessity of the prolonged restraint previously invoked. (Much of this restraint is used only with bed-ridden patients for facilitation of medical and surgical care.) A striking change has been noted on the infirmary wards where restless, irritable, suspicious or resistive elderly patients have become quieter and better behaved so that the need for supervision has been reduced.

When patients are more receptive and cooperative, they are also more demanding of other activities to occupy their waking hours. Nurses must rack their brains to provide these activities. More extensive and more varied programs are needed. The use of the drug imposes the need for more medical examinations in order to make frequent checks on the patients' response, and to make the individual dose adjustments required. There is also a greater need for more intensive and more frequent psychotherapeutic measures.

It must be emphasized that drug therapy for mental illness is an addition to and not a substitution for other forms of treatment. In depressions electroshock is often much superior and more rapid in its results, particularly when combined with drug therapy which may decrease very much the number of such treatments required. It certainly does not replace psychotherapy or psychoanalysis, but it can produce a more rapid transference and in this manner facilitate the treatment of patients who become more receptive and communicative and willing to undertake treatment.

Changes in Environment

Because acute wards are now quieter, and the patients more manageable, it is no longer necessary for patients to "graduate" from one ward to another; they are often treated in, and discharged from, the ward to which they were admitted. The changes in the patients' behavior, the tremendous decrease in destruction, are evidenced in the many chairs, sofas, television sets, drapes, pictures, and other useful or decorative furnishings that are now common in the formerly rather barren and sparsely furnished areas of previously acutely disturbed wards.

Perhaps the most important environmental change is one which is difficult to describe, the more "medical" atmosphere now surrounding the function and appearance of the hospital. Many patients and their relatives regard shock therapies, wet packs, and restraint as punishment rather than therapy. Treatment with medication seems a more normal procedure, and one which implies that mental illness is an ordinary disease which can be treated in the same manner as other diseases.

To take full advantage of the opportunity a more "normal" milieu offers, it is necessary to provide more facilities for the patients' comfort, with more outlets for their increased initiative.

Changes in Release and Admission Rates

Some patients who formerly remained in the hospital because of the need for maintenance EST can now be treated with chlorpromazine at home. Others who had failed to respond to other treatments have improved enough to leave the hospital. More patients are being released, and the demand for hospital beds may possibly lessen in the future. Some patients who apply for voluntary admission can be adequately treated as outpatients.

A study of 150 discharged patients (Table 3) demonstrated that the relapse rate in chlorpromazine-treated patients was about 5%; in patients who did not receive the drug it was about 30%. This becomes quite significant when it is noted that 57% of the group of released patients had been sick 2 to 5 years or longer.

These figures indicate in a rather striking fashion the need for long-term continued drug therapy in patients suffering from chronic psychoses, particularly the paranoid and catatonic form of schizophrenia.

More patients are treated as outpatients; each must be seen often. The problems of their general medical management, and of placing them in homes and jobs have made the administration of the outpatient department much more complicated and time-consuming.

Changes in Personnel

One of the by-products of drug therapy which should be stressed is the stimulus given to the ward personnel in the treatment of patients. It has been

TABLE 3

Study of 150 * patients on convalescent care who were given chlorpromazine in the hospital and/or on convalescent care

	NUMBER PATIENTS	PERCENTAGE
TOTAL....................................	150	100.0
Treated in hospital and continued while on convalescent care.........................	68	45.0
Treated on convalescent care only	43	29.0
Treated in hospital and discontinued while on convalescent care.........................	39	26.0

Number of patients returned to hospital

	TOTAL	NUMBER RETURNED	PERCENTAGE
Patients taking chlorpromazine outside hospital	111	6	5.0
Patients not taking chlorpromazine outside hospital	39	11	30.0

* Duration of Psychosis: 1 year 21%; 1-2 years 22%; 2-5 years 26%; 5+ years 31%.

our finding that our ward personnel are extremely enthusiastic about this medication. Various expressions have been used by such personnel: "The ward seems quiet." "There appear to be no annoyances on the ward." "The work seems more interesting because the patients can talk and react as individuals." This stimulation of the personnel plays an important role in the individual treatment afforded by them to the patients, and has awakened interest in therapy in the ward physicians, attendants and nurses. There is increasing emphasis on therapy rather than on mere custody.

This increased enthusiasm has to be properly channelled. An educational program must be set up to teach the practice of basic psychotherapeutic techniques, the aims and methods of the new treatment, and the complications which may occur. Stress is placed upon the need for the inclusion of all in a clinical therapeutic team in which each person plays an important role.

Changes in the Community

The community gives evidence of the new hope and optimism which have arisen since the advent of drug therapy. Relatives visit the patients more frequently. Physicians in general practice are more cooperative, and more willing to refer patients for hospital, outpatient, or office psychiatric treatment. Some physicians who are not psychiatrists use chlorpromazine to treat mild cases of mental illness. Legislators have shown a greater concern with the problems of mental illness now that more positive and easily administered therapy is available. The interest of journalists, church, and civic groups has increased. Families led to expect quicker more permanent results, are more critical and demanding; they often insist on drug therapy for unsuitable patients. Physicians must be advised on the selection, course of action and complications of drug therapy. There is an increasing need for more facilities and rehabilitative aids to take care of patients who could attempt outside adjustments but who cannot get care in the usual family situation.

Conclusions

It is important to remember that chlorpromazine is no "cure-all;" it is one step in the total therapy of the patient. It makes the patient more accessible to psychotherapy, and to a "total push" program in which recreational and occupational therapy, habit training, social acclimatization and competition play vital roles. As its use becomes more widespread, the changes it produces will become more strikingly evident; the problems it creates, more demanding of solution.

USE OF A CHLORPROMAZINE-DEXTRO-AMPHETAMINE COMBINATION IN ANXIETY NEUROSES

Thomas M. Hart, M.D.

Chlorpromazine and dextro-amphetamine sulfate, a depressant and a stimulant of the central nervous system, respectively, have become familiar chemotherapeutic agents in the practice of many physicians, but generally have been administered separately. The action of chlorpromazine on higher neural centers in the general area of the diencephalon provides alleviation of anxiety, tension, agitation, and apprehension. This "tranquilization" contrasts with the stimulation of dextro-amphetamine, which also acts on the higher centers of the brain, and increases central activity. Frequently, different symptoms of the same disorders have been treated with one of these two agents. Since "associated" or secondary depression and fatigue often complicate neurotic disturbances, a combination of the two drugs seemed to promise advantages over the use of chlorpromazine alone. Some practitioners have recently reported adding small quantities of dextro-amphetamine to the regimens of patients already receiving chlorpromazine. A combination of these two agents is now available in 5/1 chlorpromazine-dextro-amphetamine ratio in two strengths: 25 mg./5 mg. and 10 mg./2 mg.

Both drugs have been used in treating neurotic states and in acute and chronic alcoholism. The selective central nervous system action of chlorpromazine provides detached calm without suppression of mental faculties. The stimulation of dextro-amphetamine increases psychomotor activity, counteracts depression, and lessens the sense of fatigue. These drugs have been used in treating acute and chronic alcoholism. Both drugs have been administered to counteract incoherence and inco-ordination and to abort beginning tremors. In many cases chlorpromazine controls emesis, lessens anorexia, and enables the patient to take liquids; whereas, dextro-amphetamine exerts an antagonism to the depressive effects of alcohol. Concomitant actions of the two drugs appeared a desirable therapeutic approach in a variety of conditions seen in office patients.

MATERIAL AND METHOD

Experience with both drugs in general practice suggested anxiety neuroses, as well as alcoholism, as conditions in which the combination could reasonably be expected to prove effective. It was administered, accordingly, to 24 patients: 18 anxious neurotics, four alcoholics, one arteriosclerotic with early senility, and one patient with migraine. These patients were not responding to the usual sedatives. Their general complaints included constant fatigue, insomnia, cancerphobia, chest and back pains, and dysmenorrhea. Personal factors underlying these complaints included the familiar ones met in office practice—overwork, loss of job, combat nerves, prolonged engagement, marital disharmony, and guilt associated with mongolism in an unwanted child. Four cases were considered to be primarily alcoholism, but sporadic alcoholism was a symptom in some of the other neuroses. Somatic conditions existing concurrently with the neuroses included symptoms of menopause, anemia, and rheumatoid arthritis.

The patients ranged in age from 19 to 76, although most were between 30 and 60. Distribution between the sexes was about equal. The 25 mg./5 mg. chlorpromazine-dextro-amphetamine combination was administered three times daily to 18 patients, four times daily to six patients. A few patients were started on the 10 mg./2 mg. strength, but their dosage was later increased. Duration of treatment varied from five days to 120 days—except for a few patients continued on the medication beyond that time. Most patients were treated for periods of from ten to 60 days.

Results

The combination produced excellent response (full relief of symptoms) in 14 patients (58 per cent) and good response (approximately 75 per cent) in six patients (25 per cent). It produced poor response (slight or no relief) in four patients (17 per cent). Chlorpromazine-dextro-amphetamine relieved or considerably reduced the anxieties and apprehensions of the neurotics. Their tense, worried outlooks gave way to calm, more confident adjustments to their situations. Patients receiving the combination showed increased energy and renewed interest in their activities. This effect may well have been produced by the dextro-amphetamine. The combinations exerted a definite antiemetic effect, quieted psychomotor agitations, and controlled delirium tremens in alcoholics. It also counteracted the depression and other unpleasant symptoms of withdrawal, cleared consciousness, and relieved the need for a morning drink which so many of these patients experience. The alcoholics exhibited restored vigor and improved mood, effects frequently seen from use of dextro-amphetamine. In the patient suffering from migraine, the combination brought about complete relief of symptoms, but these returned when the medication was withdrawn. The patient with arteriosclerosis and early senility showed no improvement, and the combination was withdrawn.

Side effects included two reactions of overstimulation, jitteriness and insomnia, apparently due to the dextro-amphetamine. These two patients, who had poor responses, were placed on chlorpromazine alone, one with a good response, the other with a poor response. One patient whose response was generally good experienced moderate drowsiness on the 5/1 ratio. A higher proportion of dextro-amphetamine was included in his regimen. One patient had moderate genito-urinary complaints (urinary frequency and urgency) and moderate anorexia.

H. H., 76, a male, suffering from anxiety neurosis and cerebral arteriosclerosis, was placed on t.i.d. dosage of 25 mg./5 mg. combination. He lived at home with his wife and their seven daughters, all of whom were over

35 years of age, three of whom were divorced, and four of whom were unmarried. With this background, his extreme agitation and nervousness were quite understandable, but had been refractory to other sedatives. His response to the combination was good. He improved considerably in his adjustment to his situation and has remained calm on continued medication.

J. G., 49, a male, was suffering from a situational neurosis following birth to his wife of a mongoloid child. Since his wife was relatively advanced in life for pregnancy, neither spouse had wanted a child. Feelings of guilt increased the strain of adjustment to the child's condition. The patient's extreme nervousness was refractory to other medication, but his response was excellent.

G. C., 49, a male, had been a chronic alcoholic for 15 years, despite a successful legal practice. He had taken as much as seven ounces of triple bromides in a single day in nearly successful efforts at suicide. He was placed on q.i.d. dosage of 25 mg./5 mg. His response to the combination—his only medication—was dramatic and was rated excellent. With a significantly improved outlook, he became able to meet his problems, and he lost his desire to drink.

Discussion

The results in this trial indicate that use of the combination of chlorpromazine and dextro-amphetamine offers a definite benefit. The stimulation of dextro-amphetamine seemed to aid the neurotics, as well as the alcoholics, in their readjustments. Many neurotics appear to aggravate their conditions and increase the severity of their symptoms by excessive introspection and brooding. In their inactivity they multiply the number and extent of their real and imagined problems. Assigning the effects observed in these patients to one or the other agent in the combination is uncertain at best and is complicated by the fact that both drugs produce some similar effects in these conditions. The combination relieved anxiety and agitation, as chlorpromazine alone often does, and brightened the outlook of the patients and made them alert, as dextro-amphetamine alone often does. Perhaps through the latter agent, the combination gave them an optimistic approach to life for the first time in weeks or months. It restored their attention spans and increased their capacity for work. At the same time it stimulated them to enjoyable, purposeful activity, which was very important to them, since it eliminated or reduced their time for brooding over the multiplicity of their problems. Chlorpromazine-dextro-amphetamine exerted an unique effect on the alcoholics in this study; it relieved their desire to drink, and, in addition, it restored them to their normal life patterns with satisfying rapidity. The alcoholic experiencing withdrawal symptoms frequently faces a void. He must compensate in his daily routine not only for the loss of exhilaration, but also for the time formerly spent in his compulsive pleasure. The combination controlled psychomotor agitations and emesis, restored appetite, and relieved the sense of void and replaced it with increased energy, which prompted a return to activities and interests long-neglected.

The combination was effective both in short-term situational neuroses and in neuropsychiatric disturbances that had continued for periods of months or years. Patients experiencing temporary disturbances were carried through such periods until the source of disruption had been removed or they had adjusted to new life circumstances. Patients suffering neurotic disturbances of longer duration, as well as psychotic episodes in some cases, showed good to excellent responses on chlorpromazine-dextro-amphetamine, although many of these conditions had been refractory to other agents. Vague fears and agitations, along with more definite ones like cancerphobia, disappeared. Sleep and appetite returned to normal. Alleviation of symptoms and return of confidence permitted return to work or to a full schedule of duties in most cases where performance of duty had been seriously interrupted. The alcoholics were benefited in the same ways in confronting the problems which caused their conditions. In addition, they largely escaped the craving or unconscious substitutions familiar in withdrawal.

Summary

1. A combination of chlorpromazine and dextro-amphetamine was administered to 24 patients, chiefly anxious neurotics and alcoholics, in office practice.

2. After some initial treatment with 10 mg./2 mg. chlorpromazine-dextro-amphetamine tablets, all patients received 25 mg./5 mg. tablets. Dosage was t.i.d. in 18 patients, q.i.d. in six patients.

3. Results were excellent in 14 patients (58 per cent), good in six (25 per cent), and poor in four (17 per cent). The few side effects encountered in this series consisted of moderate genito-urinary complaints in one patient, moderate anorexia in one, moderate drowsiness in one, and overstimulation, presumably by dextro-amphetamine, in two.

4. The combination provided relief from anxiety and apprehension in neurotics and controlled psychomotor agitations, emesis, and delirium tremens in alcoholics. Patients in both groups showed increased energy and renewed interest in their activities.

5. In the combination, the chlorpromazine component appeared to calm the neurotics and to alleviate the withdrawal symptoms of the alcoholics. The dextro-amphetamine component appeared to reduce the inactivity and brooding of the neurotics and to restore vigor and relieve the sense of void in alcoholics.

CLINICAL STUDY OF PROCLORPERAZINE, A NEW TRANQUILIZER FOR THE TREATMENT OF NONHOSPITALIZED PSYCHONEUROTIC PATIENTS

Thomas J. Vischer, M.D.
Associate Professor of Medicine, Hahnemann Medical College and Hospital, Philadelphia, Pennsylvania

Not only for the psychiatrist but also for practitioners of almost every other aspect of medicine, tranquilizing drugs have taken on great importance. The stress-laden situations of modern life, the paucity of trained psychiatrists and the cost and length of most standard psychiatric treatments have invited acceptance of virtually any drug that promises to permit mentally ill patients relatively normal, useful lives.

Acceptance of the tranquilizing drugs, however, must be based more upon experience than promises. To be sure, many investigators have reported their experience with certain of the tranquilizers—particularly their effect in psychotic and nearly psychotic patients. For example papers on chlorpromazine or reserpine in the treatment of severely disturbed patients have certainly not been lacking. On the other hand there is a dearth of published data on tranquilizing drugs for nonhospitalized patients suffering from the milder mental and emotional disturbances. It is not difficult, of course, to see why this should be so: the response of such patients to treatment—unlike that of psychotic patients—is rarely dramatic. The changes in behavior or in the way patients feel are frequently so subtle as to go unnoticed by the physician, who must almost always depend on the patient's often unreliable reports.

It was with these thoughts in mind that I welcomed an opportunity to evaluate, in a preliminary way, my experience with proclorperazine in the treatment of 38 patients. Previous studies on 215 patients by a group of investigators seemed to indicate that proclorperazine—like chlorpromazine, a phenothiazine derivative—was well suited for the treatment of the mental and emotional disturbances commonly seen in everyday practice. These investigators reported good or excellent results in 76 per cent of the patients treated. Moreover, the drug was found to act rapidly, and in the recommended low dosage (usually 10 to 30 mg. a day) to have few side effects.

METHOD

The patients included in this series are fairly representative of those seen daily by the practicing physician. The average age of these 11 males and 27 females was fifty-seven and a half years. Sixteen had primary vascular disease:

hypertension; arteriosclerotic heart disease; cerebrovascular accidents; and thrombotic episodes. Others suffered from migraine headaches, chronic alcoholism, rheumatoid arthritis and involutional melancholia. Two were postoperative recovery cases. All these patients exhibited considerable psychoneurotic overlay, which had made previous treatment difficult and, to the patient, comparatively ineffective. Some were long-standing cases of involutional and senile depression. Several chronically complained of all varieties of psychosomatic illness—headaches, vertigo, visual disturbances, palpitation, profuse sweating, anorexia and other minor gastrointestinal disturbances.

In general, patients were placed on a regimen of 5 mg. of proclorperazine, given orally three or four times daily. The average duration of treatment was four and eight-tenths weeks.

Results

In all cases proclorperazine was prescribed for psychoneurotic symptoms, including anxiety, depression, nervousness, confusion, tension and emotional instability. The clinical results show that after treatment 21 patients were totally free of such symptoms and obtained a better response than they had to any previous medication. Confusion and depression disappeared dramatically, and primary complaints became less important to them as they became far more relaxed, less nervous and less tense. Many were able to return to work or had renewed interest in their surroundings and hobbies. Sixteen patients achieved partial relief, and only 1—with a twelve-year case of involutional melancholia with several psychiatric hospitalizations—showed only slight improvement. Five patients experienced side effects—mild drowsiness that cleared after the initial phase of medication or rather the dosage had been readjusted to the individual patient's requirements. The administration of proclorperazine made concomitant use of large doses of sedatives unnecessary. For example, several patients had received up to 0.06 gm. (1 gr.) of phenobarbital three times daily. Proclorperazine made these doses superfluous.

Discussion

Admittedly, this is a relatively small group from which to draw highly accurate conclusions. Yet when, as a result of proclorperazine therapy, over 90 per cent of these 38 patients experienced relief from psychoneurotic symptoms, the usefulness of the drug cannot be denied. Placebo response, although it must exist to some extent, can probably be ruled out as a major factor, since most of the patients had not responded to previous treatment with a variety of drugs that usually produce a subjective response.

The results in this study indicate that proclorperazine is a highly effective drug for the treatment of patients in everyday practice who suffer from psychic stress alone or accompanied by physical complaints. More extensive investigations will prove this drug a valuable addition to the therapeutic tools available to the practicing physician.

Case Reports

The following cases are typical of the gratifying results seen with this new compound:

J. M., a 43-year-old woman, complained for over ten years of lumbosacral pain caused by progressive bilateral sacroiliac arthritic changes and marginal lipping, spurring and some condensation of the lumber spine. A severe involutional melancholia included extreme nervousness, depression, tension and periods of hysterical agitation. Treatment for several years with unusually large doses of hypnotics and sedatives, as well as protein injections, afforded her little relief. Proclorperazine, 20 mg. daily, was prescribed, and within five days there was total symptomatic relief, such that all day and night sedation was eliminated. After twelve days she complained of slight drowsiness, which disappeared when her dosage was cut to 15 mg. daily. After two months she has continued to be completely free of symptoms—with no more pelvic pain, depression, tension or nervousness—and she no longer requires concomitant medication. Her mental and emotional outlook is better than it has been for many years, and she takes renewed interest in her daily contacts and in her home life, which she had neglected for many years.

H. M., a 62-year-old male, had a three-year history of bouts of extreme agitation and depression that included crying spells and voluntary tremors, for which a psychiatrist prescribed electroshock treatments in 1952. His history also included coronary infarctions in 1935 and 1953, and an operation for a ruptured appendix in 1942. Up to one grain of phenobarbital, four times daily, as well as heavy doses of hypnotics at bedtime, had been necessary for over two years to provide temporary control of his depression and agitation. Rauwolfia compounds served to increase his depression. Proclorperazine was prescribed, 20 mg. daily, with theobromine. After ten weeks of treatment his mental outlook is greatly improved; he is no longer depressed, nor has there been any recurrence of the tremors. He has taken up golf and is making plans for returning to work.

M.C., a 54-year-old woman, had a 14-year history of involutional melancholia, with extreme nervousness, constipation and gastric distress. Previous therapy with large doses of tranquilizing agents was only partially successful. On two occasions she has been hospitalized to receive electroshock therapy, with partial improvement continuing for as long as two months. During recent exacerbation proclorperazine considerably relieved her mental depression, constipation and distention for about three weeks. The dosage was increased to 40 mg. daily but was decreased to the original 15 mg. per day when she experienced some drowsiness. Under proclorperazine therapy she was far less nervous, showed decreased aggression and became calm. However, her depression has returned and she has been hospitalized for the third time.

B.C., a 60-year-old practical nurse, had been extremely nervous and depressed for many years. Barbiturate sedation, and urinary antispasmodics for dysuria and frequency, had given only temporary relief. A vaginal repair, for cystocele and rectocele, partially decreased her dysuria and frequency. One week's therapy with chlorpromazine was effective in further reducing her nervous agitation, depression, dysuria and frequency. Three weeks after taking proclorperazine, 20 mg. daily, her symptoms disappeared and she remarked: "I feel much better, and there is a relaxation inside."

G.H., a 76-year-old woman, had a ten-year history of essential hypertension, complicated by extreme nervousness and tremors. In 1950 a mastectomy was performed for carcinoma of the breast, and she received large doses of testosterone. Theobromine was administered for hypertension. The rauwolfia compounds were unsuccessful in relieving her depression and lethargy; instead, they made her move markedly depressed—a finding borne out by recent publications attributing depression to rauwolfia therapy. After less than three weeks of treatment with proclorperazine, 15 mg. daily, she no longer had any tremors, was substantially less nervous and reported: "Doctor, I feel like doing and going."

F.C., a 46-year-old salesman, had a ten-year history of anxiety, tension, nervousness, and idiopathic colitis that was controlled by small doses of opium derivatives and pectin. For four years he had been subjected to the intense pruritus of intermittent attacks of erythema multiforme. In addition he had been treated with Luminal, Metamucil and phenobarbital. He was given proclorperazine, 15 mg. daily, to be taken with methylcellulose. Four days of therapy with proclorperazine provided complete relief of the colitis, and the erythema multiforme did not return. After six weeks of therapy he has no complaints—no nervousness or irritability. For the first time in ten years he is symptom free and has recently been praised by his company for his improved sales record.

W.R., an 80-year-old woman, had a 30-year history of psychoneurosis, which included nervousness, depression, anxiety, anorexia, post-prandial nausea and abdominal distention. For 20 years there has been a gradual development of arteriosclerotic heart disease, general arteriosclerosis and paroxysmal atrial fibrillation, complicated by precordial pain that was relieved by tetranitrate. For many years she had received one-quarter grain of phenobarbital, three times daily, for her psychoneurotic distress with no apparent improvement in emotional outlook. After 17 days of treatment with proclorperazine, 15 mg. daily, she was totally free of symptoms. On the 43rd day of treatment, after she had complained of slight drowsiness, the dosage was reduced to 5 mg. per day. The drowsiness disappeared, and ten days later she continued to be symptom free. Her emotional improvement has been marked and there is no longer any gastric distress, depression or anxiety. Moreover, procloperazine evidently has relieved the tension that was partially responsible for the precordial pain, for she no longer requires tetranitrate. On her last visit she remarked: "I am going out by myself for the first time in years."

Summary and Conclusions

Proclorperazine, a recently developed analogue of chlorpromazine, shows great promise in the treatment of the mild mental and emotional disturbances commonly seen in everyday practice and treated on an ambulatory basis. It is particularly valuable for the many cases in which psychoneurotic symptoms make treatment of the primary disease less effective.

In this preliminary clinical study 21 of 38 mildly disturbed patients seen in general practice were afforded total symptomatic relief, and 16 were partially relieved. In 1 case proclorperazine produced little improvement, but this was a long-standing case of involutional melancholia, relieved temporarily only by electroshock therapy. The complete absence of side effects, except mild drowsiness, was most gratifying. In most cases patients treated with proclorperazine showed prompt and marked improvement in emotional outlook.

Laboratory studies of 36 of these patients who have been treated continuously with proclorperazine for periods of up to eleven months showed no significant pathologic change in liver function as expressed through the serum bilirubin, cephalin flocculation and serum alkaline phosphatase. A complete blood count (including sedimentation rate and hematocrit), fasting blood sugar, blood urea nitrogen, cholesterol and urinalysis all remained within normal limits throughout the study.

THE USE OF AZACYCLONOL AND PIPRADROL IN GENERAL PRACTICE

Thomas G. Allin, Jr., M.D., and Raymond C. Pogge, M.D.

A number of new compounds have recently been developed for the treatment of nervous and mental diseases. Most of the original clinical research was conducted by neurologists and psychiatrists, but the practical applications of these drugs in the field of general practice are probably even greater. Two of the drugs most likely to be confused with one another are pipradrol (Mera-

FIG. 1. Pipradrol (Meratran).

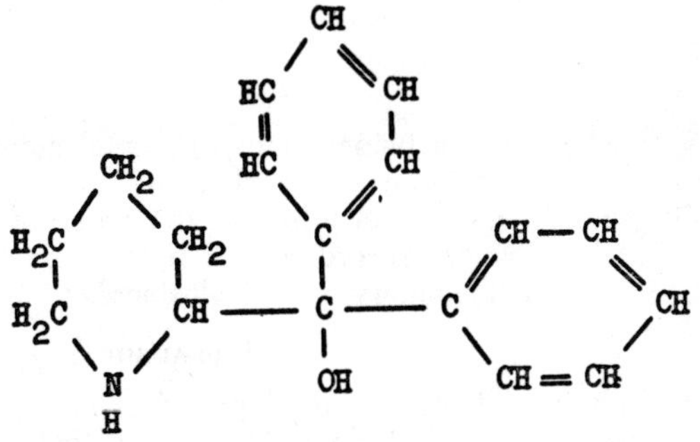

tran) and azacyclonol (Frenquel). These two compounds are isomers of each other. The structures are usually represented as shown in figures 1 and 2.

It appears that these two compounds both influence that portion of the brain concerned with the function of alerting. Varying with the activity of the septal area or the reticulodiencephalic-activating system, the person may be very alert, moderately wide awake, drowsy, asleep, or psychotically out of contact with his surroundings. Therefore, the various diseases in which pipradrol or azacyclonol is indicated are, in general, psychosomatic disorders. However, the effect of these two compounds on the alerting system of the brain is different and, in some respects, somewhat the opposite.

Pipradrol stimulates the alerting mechanism of the brain, but it differs from the amphetamine group of compounds in that it is not a sympathomimetic amine and it has virtually no effect on the peripheral nervous or cardiovascular systems. In contrast to pipradrol, azacyclonol is neither a stimulant nor a depressant of the normally functioning alerting system. When the alerting system of the brain is functioning normally, it is difficult to demonstrate any pharmacologic effect of

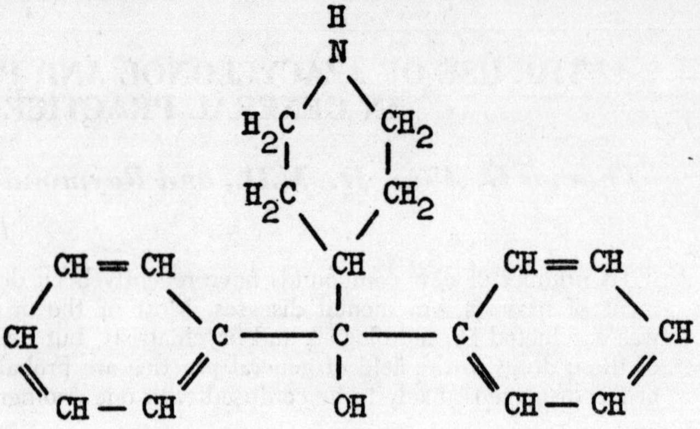

Fig. 2. Azacyclonol (Frenquel).

azacyclonol in human beings or experimental animals. But when this alerting system is behaving in an abnormal manner, as a result either of experimental conditions or of spontaneous disease, the action of azacyclonol appears to correct this abnormality. Accordingly, it is an anticonfusion drug, sometimes described as antihallucinatory or antidelusional.

Pipradrol

The pharmacologic effects of pipradrol in experimental animals were described by Brown and Werner. They found that it produces a measurable increase in coordinated and purposeful activity. This effect is grossly similar to that which can be produced by suitable doses of amphetamine. However, there are important differences. Of great significance is the absence of a period of depression following the period of pipradrol stimulation. This period of depression following amphetamine is believed to reflect in experimental animals something comparable to the letdown that occurs after a period of amphetamine stimulation in human beings. In addition to this absence of afterdepression, it was noted that pipradrol does not possess the sympathomimetic and pressor effects that are characteristic of amphetamine.

Fabing *et al.* conducted exploratory studies with pipradrol in human beings, in the belief that a central stimulant that has properties demonstrated in experimental animals to be different from those of other stimulants should behave differently in clinical practice. In the private practice of neurology and psychiatry, Fabing found that pipradrol has interesting clinical applications. These uses have since been extended into the field of general practice, in which pipradrol is useful in a number of common conditions.

The Use of Pipradrol in Medical Practice. The most important use for pipradrol is in the symptomatic treatment of emotional fatigue which usually occurs as a manifestation of a mild reactive depression. There are no characteristic physical findings in such cases, but the patients usually complain of fatigue, and it becomes apparent from their history that they are unhappy and discouraged. Even the slightest task or decision requires too much effort. In relatively severe cases, the patient feels quite unworthy and expresses a pathetic sort of helplessness.

Social and economic readjustments associated with premature retirements and fear of aging are common causes of mild reactive depressions in elderly patients. The geriatric indications for pipradrol were first described by Pomeranze. In patients of this type, relatively small doses of the drug (2 mg./day by mouth) are more successful than the usual dose of 6 mg./day commonly employed in other adult patients. At the low dosage level the patient is not consciously stimulated and may even feel that the doctor is not using an effective medication. This is best illustrated by the usual remark of the patient who states that the pills did not help and that it was unfortunate that he was a poor subject for the medicine, since he stopped feeling tired or unhappy shortly after his visit to the doctor. Because of the subtle nature of the action of pipradrol in geriatric patients, objective measurements were made of a number of psychic and psychomotor functions, employing the usual double-blind method, in which neither the test subject nor the tester knew which patients were receiving pipradrol during one test period and the placebo during another. It was found that there are three measurable objective changes in which the performance of a group of normal men with an average age of 79 years were better during the period of pipradrol administration. The difference was statistically significant. These three methods depend on the ability of the subject to estimate an arbitrary period of time in which the error was about 35 per cent less during the pipradrol period than during the placebo period; strength of handgrip; and size of drawing of the human figure. The size of drawing of the human figure is a very interesting reflection of the subject's outlook on life. In optimistic persons who are well adjusted and content, the tendency is to draw larger figures than are drawn by persons who are pessimistic and withdrawn. The figures drawn during the pipradrol test period were bigger than those drawn during the placebo test period, and as with the tests of time estimation and hand strength, the difference was statistically significant.

Obstetric Use of Pipradrol: Obstetric patients are often subject to emotional fatigue and mild depression. The symptoms may occur before or after delivery, and pipradrol is equally effective during both periods.

Use of Pipradrol as an Adjunct in the Dietary Treatment of Obesity. The use of pipradrol as an adjunct to the dietary treatment of obesity is potentially confusing, since the drug does not inhibit appetite. However, in a double-blind study it was found that obese patients are able to follow their diet better when receiving pipradrol than when receiving a placebo. This is reflected in a greater loss of weight. The difference is statistically significant.

Several explanations for this phenomenon have been proposed. One is that fatigue is a common result of caloric, and especially protein, limitation and that this is overcome by pipradrol, so that the patient is not tempted, instinctively or intentionally, to consume added food to overcome the sense of fatigue.

Another explanation that has been suggested is that overeating is frequently the psychologic result of a depression; it ceases to express the patient's emotional upset after pipradrol has corrected the depression.

Pediatric Uses of Pipradrol. There are two conditions occurring in children in which the general practitioner will find pipradrol useful. The first is in the group of behavioral disturbances in which the child is unable to live at peace with his environment and family, or in which he does poorly in school despite normal intellect. In cases of this type the pipradrol dosage varies from 1 mg. to 3 mg. daily, and improved behavior can be expected in about one half of the children. In a few cases, behavior may become worse. The action of pipradrol in these children is, therefore, similar to that of amphetamine, but the advantage of pipradrol rests in the virtual freedom from insomnia and anorexia commonly produced by amphetamine.

The second childhood disorder that is frequently helped by pipradrol is enuresis. The dose is 1 mg. to 3 mg., and the drug is best administered late in the day or at bedtime. The aim is to give enough pipradrol to diminish the depth of sleep without preventing it. This varies from patient to patient, and it is therefore best to start with 1 mg. at bedtime, increasing the dose gradually until the desired response is obtained.

Use of Pipradrol in Chronic Disease. Emotional fatigue and mild depression are often associated with chronic disease and the convalescent period. In particular, patients with cancer and various neurologic disabilities are understandably discouraged and unhappy. Pipradrol has been extremely helpful in improving the outlook of such patients, although it can hardly be expected to have any effect on the course of the disease.

Use of Pipradrol in Alcoholism. There are many causes of alcoholism. In those cases where the patient drinks as a reaction to a depression, pipradrol is extremely useful. It is, however, necessary to determine the cause of the drinking before the successful use of pipradrol can be predicted.

Drug-Induced Sedation. In addition to the fatigue and depression that can accompany almost any organic disease, there may occur sedation or drowsiness as a side effect of drugs. The most obvious examples are reserpine, the anticonvulsants, chlorpromazine, meprobamate, and the antihistamines. In patients who become drowsy or depressed from these drugs, pipradrol can be administered concurrently; it overcomes the drowsiness without interfering with the antihypertensive properties of reserpine or the anticonvulsant properties of drugs like diphenylhydantoin.

Neurologic and Psychiatric Uses of Pipradrol. Only occasionally will the general practitioner use pipradrol for the treatment of neurologic and psychiatric disorders. Somewhat larger doses than are recommended in the treatment of emotional fatigue and mild depression are frequently helpful in controlling narcolepsy, blepharospasm, and torticollis. In the psychiatric field pipradrol is of limited value since the stimulation usually increases the pre-existing psychotic behavior. Ordinarily, this is undesirable. In psychotic depressions large doses of pipradrol occasionally produce dramatic results, but in general, electroshock treatment is preferable.

Side Effects of Pipradrol. In clinical dosage, pipradrol is virtually free from side effects. The early signs of moderate overdosage are nausea, vomiting, and insomnia.

A case of gross overdosage with subsequent recovery has recently been described. A young adult patient with suicidal intent took a single dose of 250 mg. of pipradrol (125 times the recommended single dose and more than 40 times the recommended daily dose). The patient of course was kept awake, and when first seen, appeared to be suffering from a reaction similar to chorea. She complained of apprehension and severe abdominal pain. Sodium Amytal, administered by mouth in repeated doses of 300 mg., did not influence the overstimulation caused by pipradrol. Symptoms were terminated by intravenous[1] Sodium Amytal in a dosage of 250 mg. Thereafter, recovery was uneventful; and liver and kidney function tests, as well as blood counts and urinalyses, revealed no toxic effects from the very unpleasant experience associated with such gross overstimulation. The patient is said to have indicated that in her next suicidal attempt she would employ a more pleasant drug!

Summary of Pipradrol Dosage and Indications. Pipradrol is administered by mouth. The tablets contain 1 mg.; the daily dose in children varies from 1 mg. to 3 mg./day. In adults, the usual dose is 6 mg./day although many patients respond favorably to 3 mg.; in geriatric patients the dose is 2 mg. given early in the day.

Medical indications are emotional fatigue and depression, for example as seen in geriatric patients, in obstetric patients, in the obese, in the chronically ill, in alcoholics, and in those who are depressed or sedated as a result of drugs.

AZACYCLONOL

The pharmacologic effects of azacyclonol in experimental animals were described by Brown *et al.* in March 1955. The characteristic stimulation produced by pipradrol in experimental animals can be inhibited partially by premedication with azacyclonol. With azacyclonol alone, there is a slight but measurable and statistically significant decrease in spontaneous activity of experimental animals. Fabing *et al.* and Himwich *et al.*, working independently, established that the characteristic action of azacyclonol in human beings is to correct hallucinatory and delusional disturbances. This occurs in some but not in all patients.

Importance of Antihallucinatory Drugs in General Practice. The three outstanding indications of azacyclonol are, of course, schizophrenia, toxic psychoses such as alcoholic hallucinosis, and postoperative confusion and delirium. Although, theoretically, patients with these illnesses should be referred to specialists of treatment, all three problems are of importance to the general practitioner and will increase in importance as more and more patients are discharged from mental hospitals to be controlled by maintenance doses of the various new drugs, one of which is azacyclonol. The use of all of these new drugs is, therefore, of tremendous potential interest to the general practitioner.

Use of Azacyclonol in Schizophrenia. In schizophrenia, the primary defect is the inability of the patient to distinguish between the reality of his perceptions

---

[1] Barbiturates employed intravenously in treating gross overdosage should be used cautiously and symptomatically.

and conceptions that refer to the objective world around him and the basic unreality of the hallucinations and delusions through which he gains his knowledge of his autistic or psychotic world. As a result of responding in the objective world to his interpretation of his psychotic world, his behavior becomes inappropriate and psychotic. A drug that terminates hallucinatory and delusional activity interrupts the patient's contact with his dream world, leaving him only the surrounding objective world of reality. This can be accomplished with oral maintenance doses of 20 mg. of azacyclonol, three times a day over prolonged periods, in a substantial number of the schizophrenic patients who are treated within four or five years of the onset of their disease. In patients who have been sick for a longer time, azacyclonol is occasionally effective, but the results are not so encouraging. However, many patients even of this type will be returned from mental hospitals to their community on maintenance doses of azacyclonol. In some cases a better effect will be obtained by adding one or more of the other drugs that have tranquilizing or antianxiety properties. All of these released patients will require medical supervision after they return to their community, partly to ensure that they continue to take their medication and partly to make certain that their behavior is sufficiently well controlled by the medication to permit social and economic rehabilitation.

Use of Azacyclonol in Alcoholic Hallucinosis. One of the most dramatic conditions responding to intravenous doses of 100 mg. of azacyclonol is alcoholic hallucinosis. Patients suffering from this condition continue to see and hear things that are not there, even after they stop drinking. In almost all cases, these peculiar manifestations vanish within a few hours after the intravenous administration of a single dose of 100 mg. of azacyclonol. In some cases a maintenance dose of 20 mg., given by mouth three times a day, is desirable. There is evidence that continued administration of azacyclonol may relieve some patients of their desire for further drinking. This may possibly be the result of an antiobsessive or anticompulsive effect of azacyclonol in those alcoholics who suffer from compulsive drinking. Against this suggested explanation is the observation that, in general, the results of azacyclonol therapy have been rather disappointing in the treatment of most obsessive-compulsive states. Such patients usually do better following lobotomy than they do on azacyclonol therapy.

Use of Azacyclonol in Postoperative Confusion and Delirium. Postoperative confusion and delirium occur fairly commonly, especially in elderly patients who have undergone urologic surgery. The condition manifests itself usually on about the third postoperative day and is characterized by acute hallucinations and delusions. The patient may think, for example, that the container with parenteral fluids by which he is being fed intravenously actually contains snakes that are being infused into his circulation. To this he will naturally respond by hurling the bottle against the wall and ripping the needle out of his vein. Such reactions usually respond within an hour to the intravenous injection of 100 mg. of azacyclonol. The drug usually has to be repeated at intervals of eight hours for a period of several days. Oral maintenance dosage has not been explored fully since patients of this type generally recover after relatively few days, and the period during which they are treated is one in which parenteral fluids are usually being administered. It is convenient to add the parenteral solution of azacyclonol to the saline or dextrose infusion.

Dosage and Administration of Azacyclonol. The oral maintenance dose of azacyclonol is 20 mg. three times a day. Initially this can be supplemented with intravenous azacyclonol given concurrently in a dosage of 100 mg. every eight hours for periods of up to several weeks if necessary. The intravenous route need not be employed; it serves merely to accelerate the response to oral azacyclonol which otherwise might be delayed in some cases as much as several weeks. A response has occurred, at least in 1 case, within an hour following the administration of the first 20 mg. tablet.

Side Effects of Azacyclonol. In the clinical dosage, azacyclonol appears to be virtually free from side effects. There is a suggestion that in nonpsychotic patients there may be a slight sense of stimulation. Overdosage in psychotic patients seems to be free from side effects.

Summary of Azacyclonol Dosage and Indications. Azacyclonol is indicated in the symptomatic treatment of hallucinations and delusions associated with schizophrenia, alcoholism, and the postoperative state. Despite the use of a wide variety of doses by various investigators, it appears that 20 mg. by mouth three times daily may be adequate for maintenance therapy. Azacyclonol can be administered parenterally early in the course of treatment, in which case it is given intravenously in a dosage of 100 mg. every eight hours. Concurrent administration of intravenous and oral azacyclonol is frequently helpful early in the course of treatment of schizophrenia. In patients in whom hallucinations are associated with alcoholism and the postoperative period, it is not always necessary to employ the oral maintenance dose. Many patients of this type respond favorably to a relatively small number of intravenous injections.

FRENQUEL

Richard C. Proctor, M.D., and Theodore Odland, M.D.
Bowman Gray School of Medicine, Winston-Salem, North Carolina

Our study of the effect of Frenquel in psychotic patients stems from our earlier observance of Meratran and from the work of Howard D. Fabing of Cincinnati in noting the ability of Frenquel to block the development of LSD-25 psychosis. Brown and Werner found that Meratran differed significantly from other central nervous system stimulants, such as the amphetamines. No cardiovascular pressor reactions, no appetite loss, and little disturbance in nocturnal sleep have been observed with this compound, which is useful therapeutically in mild depressive states as well as in narcolepsy and certain selected motor tic syndromes. Himwich and his associates state that Meratran is not a sympathomimetic drug, and they demonstrated that a certain reticular substance of the rabbit brain is stimulated by the compound, followed by cortical stimulation. Heath at Tulane found that Meratran had a unique ability to cause rapid high voltage activity in the septal area of the monkey electrographically.

Because Meratran appeared to act centrally without observable concomitant effects on the automatic nervous system and because its site of action appeared to be in the upper brain stem tegmentum, it was felt that other compounds of similar clinical configuration might also be of value as therapeutic agents in disorders of the central nervous system. Frenquel is the first of this group of isomers of Meratran to be so utilized.

Frenquel is the gamma-isomer of Meratran. The NH radical is moved from the 2-position to the 4-position in the piperidyl ring in the synthesis of this benzhydrol compound.

Brown has found that Frenquel is different from the parent compound neuropharmacologically. It is not a central excitant but rather, is an antagonist of central stimulation produced by other agents. The early studies of Fabing in Cincinnati stimulated us to try the drug clinically. Their first experiments were with healthy graduate students. LSD-25 was ingested to produce a typical psychotic state characterized by hallucinations and delusions. After this initial part of the study the students were started on the blocking agent orally for a week before the LSD-25 was given. When it was ingested, no hallucinations or delusions took place. Similar experiments were carried out on house officers, with similar results, utilizing LSD-25 to produce the psychoses. In addition to this, mescaline-produced psychoses have been blocked by Frenquel. One subject was cleared of the symptoms in a matter of minutes by the intravenous administration of Frenquel.

Our studies have been carried out directly on psychotic patients, both in and out of a hospital setting. We attempted no blind experiments, since we believe that suggestion on the part of the physician would have little effect on an acutely disturbed psychotic patient. The patients were not told of the use of a new therapeutic agent. Those who were able to comprehend were simply told: "This is something we want to try to see whether it will help you."

The majority of patients were given complete blood counts, urinalyses, thymol turbidity tests, and blood urea nitrogen studies prior to the beginning of therapy. Some of the patients who have been treated recently have not had these studies, and, of course, patients who were suffering from alcoholic hallucinosis were not tested prior to therapy.

Methods and Results

We have attempted to utilize the medication on patients who symptomatically showed hallucinations of any type, as well as delusions. Unless these symptoms were present, the treatment was not attempted. The studies were carried out in three groups of patients. One group consisted of 27 patients in a hospital for chronic disorders, giving little more than custodial care and, more recently, reserpine, to the patients. Ten of this group were eliminated from the study because of grossly abnormal laboratory studies. This concerned the administrators of the hospital more than the investigators. The remaining 17 were started on Frenquel, 20 mg. three times a day orally. The results have been poor, as we anticipated. Five of the 17 showed improvement in the symptoms, three marked and two mild. Of the patients who showed the most improvement, two were suffering from marked mental deficiency, with hallucinations and delusions, and the other was suffering from schizophrenia. The remaining 12 patients who showed no improvement ranged from those suffering from epileptic deterioration to others suffering from cerebral arteriosclerosis, all having some type of organic psychotic process. Diagnostically, the breakdown was: five with mental deficiency, five with chronic brain syndromes, one with epileptic deterioration, and one with an obsessive-compulsive state, nymphomania, and cerebral arteriosclerosis.

The second group of patients has been treated at Graylyn. This is a 45-bed intensive treatment center operated by the Department of Psychiatry and Neurology of the Bowman Gray School of Medicine. These patients represented in the main more acute psychotic states prior to the onset of deterioration, though some of the latter were included. Here the results in several patients have been gratifying. Again, the same laboratory studies were carried out as in the previous group, though here no patients had to be eliminated because of untoward laboratory results. A total of 35 patients have been under treatment to date. One patient was eliminated from the study because it appeared that after a few days her "paranoid delusions" concerning her husband's infidelity were not delusional but rather, factual. Patients were started in 20 mg. of Frenquel four times a day, orally, although later, in some, the dosage was changed but without influencing the response. The results revealed 20 patients with marked improvement in their symptoms; six with moderate improvement, and eight with little or no improvement. In the latter group, those who showed little or no improvement, three represented chronic brain syndromes. One suffered from Pick's disease, two from cerebral arteriosclerosis, and two from an exacerbation of previously diagnosed schizophrenia. The patients in the group who showed moderate improvement, or six out of the 34, represented the following diagnostic categories: one, schizophrenia of nine years' duration; one, chronic brain syndrome, and four, depressive reactions with delusions and hallucinations. Moderate improvement indicates that there was a decrease in the delusions and hallucinations of the patient but not complete elimination of them.

In the last group, labeled "marked improvement," the following diagnostic categories were represented: twelve with schizophrenia; one with chronic brain syndrome; one, depressive reaction in a schizoid individual; two, acute unclassified psychotic episode; and four cases of involutional depression. In this group of 20 patients, there was complete alleviation of all hallucinations and delusions except in the patient who had a chronic brain syndrome. She lost her hallucinations completely, but the delusions have persisted, though minimally. These patients ordinarily would have received some form of somatic therapy for their illness. Naturally, with these patients, psychotherapy has been much easier to carry out because of the absence of post-shock confusion, and rapport has been much easier to establish.

The last group of patients comprised 20 with acute toxic hallucinosis. Nineteen had acute alcoholic hallucinosis, and one had hallucinations resulting from bromide intoxication. These patients were seen in the emergency rooms of the two hospitals in Winston-Salem and a few by local internists on home calls. The results obtained in this group of patients have been amazing. In all but three of the patients suffering from delirium tremens there was complete alleviation of symptoms within a matter of hours. The dosage utilized varied a great deal. Frenquel was given intravenously in doses ranging from 20 mg. to 100 mg. initially. Where lower doses were given, they had to be repeated before complete response was obtained. In some patients the response occurred within thirty minutes, while in others it took three to four hours before maximal results were obtained. The one patient with bromidism responded initially to a dose of 100 mg. intravenously, but within six hours the hallucinations returned. When oral medication was given, the patient again responded within four hours.

Case I: Miss "H," a 22-year-old single white female school teacher, was admitted to Graylyn on April 20, 1955, in an acutely disturbed and psychotic state. Her history revealed that she was well until April 14, six days prior to her admission. She experienced a sudden onset of talking in a bizarre fashion, incessant giggling, ideas of reference, delusions and hallucinations. By April 16, two days after onset of the illness, she developed the idea that she should get married, that she was pregnant, and, later on, that she was "having a baby." Her examination mentally at the time of admission showed her to be disarrayed, intermittently clutching her abdomen and stating that she was having labor pains. There was overproduction, incoherence, and rambling in her speech. She developed the delusion that she had had intercourse with

God and was going to have the son of God. She responded to auditory hallucinations and occasionally to visual hallucinations. She was confined to a disturbed room, and a diagnosis of acute schizophrenic reaction was made. She was given 25 mg. of Frenquel intravenously at the time of admission and was started on Frenquel 20 mg. three times a day orally. On the second hospital day, she was smearing feces all over her body and continued to be agitated and bizarre. In an effort to control this, we started her on Thorazine, 25 mg. intramuscularly every six hours. On the third hospital day, this was increased to 50 mg. every six hours. She continued to be somewhat hostile and belligerent but was an easier management problem. Three days later she developed a hyperventilation syndrome and some muscular twitching. All medication except Frenquel was discontinued. Serum chloride, carbon dioxide, total protein, and A.G. ratio were all within normal limits. By April 28, or the eighth hospital day, she was in fairly good contact. She was able to discuss her confusion, expressing some ambivalence about whether or not she had been "off the beam." Her improvement continued. On April 28, she was also started on light doses of insulin to improve her appetite, on which she has continued up until the present time. By the eighth hospital day, she was able to be moved out of the disturbed section, and she has continued to improve since that time. As stated, the insulin has been given in light dosage without any evidence of coma, but the Frenquel has been continued at 20 mg. three times a day. She now shows no evidence of her bizarre ideation, her delusional patterns, or her hallucinations. Psychotherapy has been continued with a satisfying response.

Case II: "John D.," a 46-year-old married white male, was seen in the emergency room of a local Winston-Salem hospital. His family gave a history of his being an alcoholic for twenty years; and he had consumed a fifth of whiskey a day for a week prior to admission. He was acutely intoxicated, disturbed, and had auditory and visual hallucinations. He complained that airplanes were in the room swooping at him and he continually tried to avoid them. He was disoriented as to time and place. He was given Frenquel, 100 mg. intravenously, and within thirty minutes he was calm, oriented, and no longer disturbed. He asked, "What happened to the planes? I thought they were all in the room. Was my mind playing tricks on me?" He was hospitalized for 4 days for massive vitamin therapy, sedation, and general medical care, but there was no recurrence of his delusions or hallucinations.

Case III: "Joseph C.," a 39-year-old married white male, was seen at home because of an acute alcoholic hallucinosis. He had been an alcoholic for several years and the week prior to being seen, had consumed large amounts of whiskey. He was confused, disoriented, and complained of seeing animals in the room in the form of spiders, snakes, and rats. He was given 50 mg. of Frenquel intravenously, and within thirty minutes the delusions and hallucinations disappeared. Three hours later, the physician was called to return to the home because of a recurrence of the original symptoms. A second 50 mg. was given intravenously, and again the symptoms disappeared shortly. His family was instructed about giving him fluids, vitamins and sedation, and the original symptoms did not recur.

Conclusions

Frenquel offers a new neuropharmacologic approach to certain acute psychotic states where delusions and hallucinations have been the primary symptoms. In certain selected cases, early results have been encouraging. In patients whose psychoses are associated with organic brain deterioration or chronic brain syndromes, the results have been poor, but we feel that the medication can safely be utilized for a trial of therapy in these patients. We are unable to explain why Frenquel is beneficial in some patients with organic psychoses and not in others. The most encouraging results have been in the treatment of acute toxic hallucinosis, where all but 3 of the patients were relieved of their symptoms within a few hours.

We offer this report only as a preliminary one. Further and more intensive studies are being carried out by us. Follow-up studies must be done in these patients before long-term evaluation of the drug can be presented.

AZACYCLONOL (FRENQUEL) IN THE TREATMENT OF CHRONIC SCHIZOPHRENICS

Joseph A. Barsa, M.D., and Nathan S. Kline, M.D.
Rockland State Hospital, Orangeburg, N. Y.

Azacyclonol has been found to antagonize the effects of certain hallucinogenic drugs. For this reason it was decided to investigate its use in chronic schizophrenics whose delusions and hallucinations were quite marked. A group of 60 female schizophrenic patients, 23-69 years of age, was chosen for this study. They had been continuously hospitalized from 2 to 24 years, although only 8 patients had been in the hospital for less than 5 years; 31 were diagnosed as catatonic, 17 as paranoid, 4 hebephrenic, and 8 mixed type.

The patients were divided into 2 groups of 30; one was given 40 mg. azacyclonol twice a day, and the other group received 200 mg. twice a day. At the end of 6 weeks the patients' improvement was related. In the low dosage group 1 was slightly improved, 24 showed no improvement, and 5 seemed worse. Of those on the higher dosage, 1 was slightly improved, 27 were unimproved, and 2 seemed worse. No toxic reactions or unpleasant side-effects were noted.

Since the results of treatment with azacyclonol alone were disappointing, it was decided to study the effects of azacyclonol with small doses of reserpine and chlorpromazine. Therefore, 30 of the above patients (15 receiving low dosage of azacyclonol and 15 receiving high dosage) were given, in addition, 3 mg. reserpine daily; the remaining 30 patients received 25 mg. chlorpromazine twice a day as well as azacyclonol. At the end of 6 weeks of the combined medication, the patients were again rated as to their improvement. Of those on azacyclonol and reserpine, 4 were moderately improved, 4 slightly improved, and 22 unimproved. Of those on azacyclonol and chlorpromazine, 4 were slightly improved, 24 unimproved, and 2 were worse.

It was then decided to compare the effects of azacyclonol with the results obtained with large doses of chlorpromazine in the same group of patients. The 60 patients, therefore, had all medication discontinued for 1 month. They were then treated with chlorpromazine alone in dosages ranging from 200 to 1,400 mgs. a day. Their improvement at the end of 3 months was as follows: 5 markedly improved, that is, either discharged or ready for discharge, 24 moderately improved, 19 slightly improved, and 12 unimproved.

From this study we conclude that azacyclonol either alone or in combination with small doses of reserpine or chlorpromazine is ineffective in the treatment of chronic schizophrenic patients. These same patients, when later treated with chlorpromazine alone in large doses, showed considerably greater improvement in their mental state.

THE EFFECT OF MERATRAN ON TWENTY-FIVE INSTITUTIONALIZED MENTAL PATIENTS

J. W. Schut, M.D., and H. E. Himwich, M.D.

Meratran is a new drug with potentialities for use in the fields of psychiatry and internal medicine. Brown and Werner examined its pharmacological properties in animals and concluded that it was a stimulant of the central nervous system. They stated also that its effect was not limited to the cerebral cortex, but that it acted upon subcortical mechanisms as well. Rinaldi and Himwich found that Meratran stimulates the subcortical area which is the source of the alerting, arousal, or awakening reaction. This effect will be elaborated below. Though Meratran is a stimulant and therefore resembles amphetamine in some of its actions, it does not belong to the group of sympathomimetic drugs, for it does not characteristically evoke the overactivity of the sympathetic nervous system characterized by dilated pupils, sweating, fast heart rate, and increased blood pressure. Meratran has also been used in a large number of patients with various psychiatric and neurologic diagnoses by Fabing, Hawkins and Moulton, and they found it was particularly useful in depressions, whether of endogenous or reactive origin. It appeared from these data that Meratran merited a further trial in certain psychiatric disorders characterized by depression and inactivity.

Twenty-five patients with varying psychiatric diagnoses, all having chronic courses, were selected from the hospital population, because they exhibited depressive features, regression, or were feeding problems (see Table 1 for diagnoses). Prior to the administration of Meratran each patient had a physical, psychiatric, and neurologic examination. Several of the patients had organic brain disease as a basis for their psychosis as indicated by the association of positive neurologic findings. The duration of the observations was 7 months and included four 6-week periods and one 3-week placebo period (see Table 2). These patients were divided into 2 arbitrary groups. While one group was taking Meratran the other received placebo, except for the third 3-week period when all patients were on placebo. This was a "double-blind" study, neither the patients nor the investigators were aware of the group receiving the actual medication until the completion of the study.

The clinical evaluations comprised not only abnormal behavior such as the effects of Meratran on delusions and anxiety, but also sleeping, eating, tidiness, activity, and other aspects of adjustment, both to ward and hospital activities. We were particularly concerned in ascertaining whether the patients became greater or lesser problems to the attendants. As an aid in assessing any changes

TABLE 1
Diagnoses of Patient Sample

Name	Age	Sex	Comitment Date	Diagnosis
V. A.	57	F	9-24-21	Schizophrenia, hebephrenic type
I. B.	60	F	6-16-49	Involutional psychosis with paranoid trends
J. B.	69	F	4-6-48	Psychoneurosis, mixed type
S. C.	79	M	3-21-51	Senile psychosis with simple deterioration
M. D.	63	F	10-23-49	Involutional melancholia
R. D.	52	F	1-5-27	Schizophrenia, hebephrenic type
H. F.	63	F	10-23-50	Schizophrenia, paranoid type
T. H.	50	F	5-10-47	Schizophrenia, paranoid type
L. R.	74	M	3-21-49	Psychosis with cerebral arteriosclerosis
J. S.	62	M	6-13-18	Schizophrenia, hebephrenic type
R. T.	44	M	1-2-46	Schizophrenia, hebephrenic type
M. M.	50	M	6-21-28	Schizophrenia, hebephrenic type
D. B.	38	F	6-16-49	Schizophrenia, undetermined type
E. B.	57	F	10-18-41	Schizophrenia, hebephrenic type
E. B.	60	M	6-21-17	Schizophrenia, hebephrenic type
W. F.	50	M	6-18-36	Schizophrenia, hebephrenic type
J. L.	72	M	1-10-24	Schizophrenia, hebephrenic type
R. L.	39	M	3-25-37	Schizophrenia, hebephrenic type
M. M.	51	F	2-1-51	Schizophrenia, hebephrenic with neurosyphilis
O. M.	59	F	3-11-37	Schizophrenia, paranoid type
P. P.	54	F	5-7-48	Schizophrenia, mixed type
J. R.	60	M	2-3-16	Schizophrenia, simple type
A. S.	58	F	1-15-50	Anxiety neurosis
M. S.	65	F	6-24-31	Schizophrenia, catatonic type
M. S.	67	M	10-7-48	Psychosis with cerebral arteriosclerosis
R. W.	51	F	5-16-28	Schizophrenia, paranoid type

a standardized set of questions was devised. When the daily rounds were made the patients were asked these questions which included their reactions to the hospital and to the routine of the ward. The attendants were also questioned in regard to the patients' behavior, their adjustment to care and ward management, and whether they became more or less disturbed. At the end of each 3-week period the remarks of the attendants were transcribed and formed part

TABLE 2

Plan of Experiment and Duration of Administration of Placebo (P) or the Meratran (M)

(Meratran, in one dose of 2.5 mg, was given daily during the first and second 6-week period. Placebo was administered to all patients during the third period. The dose of Meratran was increased to 5 mg daily in 2 divided doses, during the fourth and fifth periods.)

Experimental Periods	Duration in weeks	Group I	Group II
1	6	P	M
2	6	M	P
3	3	P	P
4	6	M	P
5	6	P	M

of the basis for the clinical evaluation of the drug. We recorded our impressions of each patient after compilation of data: whether unchanged, improved, or made worse.

The influence of Meratran on the cardiovascular system was assessed in several ways. Besides preliminary observations of blood pressure and heart rate, 15 additional determinations of these functions were performed on each patient during the 7-month period of observation. Record of the time of day and its relationship to the time of administration of the drug was kept in most instances. Weekly weight records were obtained.

Results

It is realized that the various effects of the treatment are not necessarily independent of each other, nevertheless for clarity of description the different effects will be presented separately. These included changes in activity, communication, mood, interest, hospital adaption, delusions, anxiety, sleep, heart rate, blood pressure, eating, and appetite.

Activity.—An increase of activity was noted in 14 of 25 patients. Whether abnormal or normal this heightened activity was consistent. Activity was exhibited as useful work on the ward, increased participation in O.T. and R.T. On the other hand, such abnormal manifestations as pacing were accentuated.

Communication.—In 3 of the patients who were most blocked, salutary results were observed. Two patients with schizophrenia, who were particularly non-communicative, were dramatically benefited on the larger dose of Meratran. In the other patient, who had been blocked for many years, this feature disappeared entirely, but at the same time delusions were activated. In general, it may be said that patients became more talkative on Meratran.

Mood.—Here again the global action of Meratran to intensify the type of behavior present was observed. Two patients with manic features were further stimulated while 13 patients with depressive features were relieved of this symptom to greater or lesser degrees. When there was a proper channel for the activity evoked by Meratran, any anxiety and nervousness became less obvious.

Interest.—Fifteen patients on Meratran were happier and their field of interest widened. Such improvement appeared especially in depressed patients; it was also an encouraging sign in schizophrenics without delusions and with restriction of interest. Those regressed patients who showed improvement were more interested in themselves, in other individuals as well as in outside activities.

Hospital Adaptation.—The regressed patients presented less of a problem in ward adjustment. Our schizophrenic patients with long hospital histories and severe deterioration are included in this group. They tended to cooperate more in purposeful ward activities. Dressing habits, tidiness, and general appearance improved. Many of the improvements observed on the ward may be regarded as secondary to the increase of interest. Similarly the changes to the worse in hospital adaptations were secondary to activation of delusions and/or anxiety.

Delusions.—In general, it may be said that patients with delusions experienced activation while on Meratran. This applies to 6 of our patients, one of whom with paranoid delusions became hostile and combative. As a rule the activation of the delusions disappeared abruptly when the medicine was discontinued.

Anxiety.—In 6 patients exhibiting anxiety Meratran increased the severity of their symptoms. This intensification was noted especially in those patients in whom this abnormal activity was present originally; in these instances Meratran served to stimulate it.

Appetite.—The effect of Meratran on appetite was not important and in most cases was secondary to changes in behavior. When improvement was extended to appetite the food intake was usually increased, but when delusions were activated appetite was poor. However, patients on Meratran might lose 2 or 3 pounds during the first few days of the treatment before their weight became stabilized.

Sleep.—Sleep was not altered except in 2 patients with heightened abnormal activity and activation of delusions resulting in insomnia. In general, however, except for this complication, the effects on sleep were not significant. When the medication was given in 2 doses, the second followed the noontime lunch period which might have prevented it from interfering with sleep.

Heart Rate.—In one case the medication was discontinued because of tachycardia. Small doses of phenobarbital would bring the elevated heart rate back to normal in a short time.

Discussion

Prior to the controlled, "double-blind" study, 12 depressed patients, most of whom presented various problems in ward adjustment, were selected for securing preliminary data. The impressions derived from this pilot study were encouraging. It was seen from early observations that the depressed patients became less so and were more active; other patients became less regressed and exhibited improved ward adjustment. For that reason a new investigation was set up with 25 chronic psychotic institutionalized patients with different diagnoses. These patients were chosen because of depressive or regressive symptoms.

It may be said in general that these earlier pilot impressions were confirmed and also extended. In regard to patients with depressive features it was observed that activity was increased and mood elevated. In our group of 25 patients, there were 7 with the diagnosis of hebephrenic schizophrenia who improved. All of these had a restriction of interest and were inactive. It is therefore logical to state that if this psychosis is associated with depressive features the patient may benefit by the use of Meratran. One of our patients who improved more than any other had a diagnosis of involutional psychosis. This same increased activity, however, when applied to patients with delusions and anxiety worsened their clinical situation. Certain types of schizophrenia did not improve, especially the paranoid and the hebephrenic types associated with delusional systems. Three disturbed patients with a diagnosis of cerebral arteriosclerosis also failed to improve. Thus the indications and the contraindications are clear cut. Retarded and depressed patients without delusions or anxiety are 2 groups that may derive benefit from this drug. Another practical result is better ward adjustment in the most deteriorated patients so that they became less of a problem in regard to ward care. This applies especially to the long hospitalized schizophrenics who revealed an improvement in cooperativeness.

The effects on sleep were unimportant except in the patients whose condition was aggravated by the drug and who exhibited insomnia. On appetite, too, the changes may be regarded as secondary rather than primary as appetite changed with the condition of the patient. On the other hand, the small loss of weight which was frequently an initial feature may have been due to the increased activity of the patients. In most instances the effects on the heart were negligible. Meratran is not a sympathomimetic drug, but tachycardia was observed in one patient. What sensitized this patient's heart to the drug is unknown.

The degree of change often correlated with the magnitude of the dosage. Some patients improved with 2.5 mg. and others with 5 mg. Still others who exhibited no increased activity might have done so with even larger doses but such an increase was excluded from our "double-blind" study because we wished to control the dosage factor. By the same token ill effects appeared in some patients with 2.5 mg. and in others with 5 mg. while still others exhibited only good effects at all dosage levels. Thus it is important to individualize the treatment of each patient.

The durations of the various effects were not the same. The increased activity often extended into the placebo period as did the increased interest and lessening of retardation, possibly because of new-built habits. The same prolongation did not apply to the activation of delusions except in one instance. There also seemed to be other short-lived results, such as a feeling of well being, alleviation of fatigue, and alertness, most marked soon after the drug was given.

Finally as regards the mechanism of action of Meratran: as indicated in animal experiments, Meratran affects cortical and subcortical functions. Evidence has recently been obtained for a mechanism that can explain some of the pharmacological actions of this drug, such as increased activity, improved attention and interest, alleviation of depression, as well as activation of delusions and anxiety. When the various cortical and subcortical structures of the rabbit brain were studied, with the aid of the EEG apparatus, it was observed that the subcortical area, responsible for the alerting reaction, was stimulated by Meratran. This area in turn transmitted the stimulation to the cortex as the electrocorticogram lost its characteristic regular resting pattern and assumed the faster frequencies and lower amplitudes characteristic of the alerting response. Such changes to a more alert status may furnish part of the basis for the altered behavior induced by Meratran.

Summary

A study was conducted on 25 institutionalized psychotic patients with chronic courses, selected because of their depressive and/or regressive symptoms.

Meratran was found to be a central nervous system stimulant useful in the field of psychiatry and with certain indications and contraindications: (1) indications: (a) schizophrenics without delusions having restriction of interest and activity and with depressant features, (b) psycho-motor retardation and/or blocking of communication, (c) long-term hospitalized schizophrenics with severe deterioration; (2) contraindications: (a) patients with delusions, (b) patients with anxiety, (c) disturbed patients with cerebral arteriosclerosis.

CLINICAL STUDIES ON α-(2-PIPERIDYL) BENZHYDROL HYDROCHLORIDE, A NEW ANTIDEPRESSANT DRUG

Howard D. Fabing, M.D., J. Robert Hawkins, M.D., and James A. L. Moulton, M.D.

The purpose of this study was to determine the clinical usefulness of a new antidepressant drug, Meratran, in ambulatory patients and to select clinical indications for further study. This report summarizes our data on the first 131 patients although more recent experience has included 320 cases.

PHARMACOLOGIC STUDIES

Selection of this compound for clinical trial was based on the experimental work of Brown and Werner. This compound has the following formula:

It differs from other known central stimulants in both chemical structure and pharmacologic activity. The acute LD_{50} dose of the compound was found to be 30 ± 1.6 mg./Kg. when given intravenously at the rate of 20 mg. per minute in rats. In the same animals the acute LD_{50} dose was 180 ± 22 mg./Kg. orally. By the subcutaneous route, also in rats, the LD_{50} dose was 240 ± 51 mg./Kg. In rabbits the intravenous acute LD_{50} dose given at the rate of 20 mg. per minute was 15 ± 1.8 mg./Kg. These LD_{50} doses, weight for weight, are apt-

TABLE 1

COMPARATIVE ACUTE LD_{50} VALUES AND STANDARD ERRORS ESTIMATED BY THE METHOD OF MILLER AND TAINTER (1944)

Compound	Rabbits Intravenous (20 mg./min.) mg./Kg.	Rats Oral mg./Kg.	Rats Subcutaneous mg./Kg.	Rats Intravenous (20 mg./min.) mg./Kg.
Meratran hydrochloride	15 ± 1.8	180 ± 22	240 ± 51	30 ± 1.6
dl-amphetamine sulphate	10 ± 1.6	70 ± 6.5	67 ± 7	30 ± 1.8

parently lower than those for dl-amphetamine sulphate (see Table 1).

Doses that are quite small in relation to the LD_{50} dose induce prolonged periods of purposeful hyperactivity in experimental animals. Hyperactivity increases as the dose is increased in rats. Dogs also experience increased activity on small doses but remain or tend to become friendly and to eat readily. Larger doses in both rats and dogs frequently cause forced circling movements. Convulsions do not occur until the LD_{50} dose of this compound is reached. After the period of hyperactivity or after convulsion no depression of central activity is noted. In rabbits 1/3 to one LD_{50} dose of this compound given intravenously arouses animals completely from light barbiturate depression and is capable of waking rabbits from deep barbiturate depression. The compound is not capable of acting as an antidote against lethal barbiturate depression in the rabbit. Doses of the compound which cause hyperactivity in the experimental animal have little or no effect on blood pressure, pulse rate, and respiration.

Consideration of these findings indicated to us that the compound appeared to have central stimulating action without overt convulsant action in laboratory animals. There appeared to be a wide margin of safety between the dose producing manifestations of central stimulation and the lethal dose. Furthermore, the increased activity in experimental animals appeared well-organized with small doses, and not to be associated with irritability and hostility, since the animals could be handled and petted and fed throughout the test period. Because of these attributes it was decided to conduct therapeutic trials with this compound.

Selection of Cases

Private patients with a variety of neuropsychiatric conditions were treated with varying doses of Meratran orally, usually starting with 1.0 mg. or 2.5 mg. tablets 2 or 3 times daily until a response was observed.

The first patients tested were 2 middle-aged women who were suffering from narcolepsy of long standing. It was found that these patients could tolerate this compound in doses from 20 to 100 mg. daily without observable side effects and with salutary clinical response.

Reasoning by analogy that drugs of the amphetamine series, which are effective in the treatment of narcolepsy, are also of therapeutic value in depressive states, patients with this type of mood disorder were studied next.

Impressive results were seen in 30 of the first 34 cases of reactive depression and in 17 of 27 cases of endogenous depression of mild to moderate severity. Agitated depressive states did not respond favorably, and seemed to be made worse in some instances by the use of the compound. Among the most heartening observations in depressed patients were that nocturnal sleep and appetite were usually unaffected in therapeutically effective doses and that cardiovascular pressor reactions did not occur. Blood pressure and pulse rate observations failed to reveal any trend toward increase in either of these physiologic functions, nor did the patients complain of subjective sensations of tachycardia, flushing, or pounding sensations in either the chest or the head.

On occasion the response of patients with reactive depression was sudden and dramatic. The case of a 31-year-old stenographer is illustrative:

This girl became engaged to a grocer some 15 years her senior and realized a month later that the engagement was not a good match. She is a person given to intellectual pursuits, and enjoys reading, music, and other cultural activities. Her fiance's whole life was concerned with his storekeeping activities and not much else and he threw all the burden of decision-making on her. When she broke the engagement she had difficulty in facing friends, in meeting social situations and in making an adjustment to the change.

On consultation she complained of being forgetful, apprehensive, restless, and bored. She spoke of occipital headaches, moderate sleep disturbance, a feeling of depression but not of suicidal degree, marked difficulty in concentration, and of diffuse anxiety symptoms such as cardiac palpitation, tremulous feelings in the abdomen, and a general feeling of muscular tension.

After it was determined that the physical and neurological examinations were normal she was placed on Meratran, 2.5 mg. twice daily.

This patient was an intelligent girl and a good objective reporter. When she left the office after her first visit she was discouraged at the thought that another doctor had given her another pill. She took the first tablet at 4:00 p.m. that day and noted a salutary response after her evening meal. She stated, "I felt like a completely different person. I no longer felt bored and restless, but my reaction was the reverse of that; I felt a surge of ambition." She slept well that night, better than she had been sleeping previously; on waking next morning she felt well. She happened to be on vacation at the time and had not been taking any interest in things around her home. On this day she reported that her activity and her interest picked up but that she had some palpitation and "nervous feeling" on her second day. This cleared up after 3 or 4 days. She remained on vacation for one week and returned to her office. She stated, "My self-confidence was completely restored. If someone mentioned my engagement, it was just one of those things. I had no qualms of conscience; I went back with a buoyant feeling. I would say my efficiency was better, more from the fact that I could concentrate and had more interest. Before that it was just routine, but now I had more interest, and naturally I turned out better work." Shortly thereafter she sought increased responsibility and she received an increase in salary.

Medication was continued in this case from June 30 to August 15, some 6 weeks. By that time she was completely adjusted to her broken engagement, her active depression had lifted, and the medication was dropped. She summarized her response as follows:

"If I had come to talk to you and if you had said, 'You had better get hold of yourself: this is your problem and you will have to face it,' I do not think it would have been of much benefit, because another doctor had said, 'you should just get out and forget.' It is easy to say, but not easy to do, and I do not think I could have done it without the medication, although I would have made the effort. As I told you, I could not concentrate, even to reading a book, and I do not think I could have done it without the medication. I was in such a state that I did not care what anyone would have said, it would not have helped. It took the medication to do it."

Illustrative of the favorable response of a patient with endogenous depression is the following:

A 64-year-old retired public official was seen in his fourth depression of psychotic proportions. He was suicidal and was urging his wife to enter into a suicide pact with him. He had been given electroshock therapy by another physician for his previous attack and refused to undergo it again. Meratran was given in desperation. After the dosage was graduated upward until a level of 25 mg. per day was reached, this man emerged from his psychotic depression and became well. One gets the impression that the medication certainly helped him over a serious phase of a depressive reaction. His previous attacks had always been of relatively short duration, and there may have been a factor of natural remission in this case, but both the patient and his wife insisted that the turn came abruptly when a level of 15 mg. per day was reached and improved when it was carried higher.

The patient became very dependent upon this medication and refused to withdraw it. After maintaining himself at 25 mg. per day for approximately 6 weeks, while traveling to a meeting in another city he left his tablets in a motel along the way. He became panicky as he had to read a paper the next day. Despite this he was able to read his paper, was able to extemporize during a discussion period, and to think clearly. He was tense that evening, but attended a banquet and sat at the speakers' table. He got through the evening without difficulty. On the following day he returned home and resumed his medication. Despite his reluctance the drug was slowly withdrawn. He spent his vacation at the Grand Tenton National Park and greatly enjoyed it. Some 6 months after medication was begun he had tapered off from its use entirely and has maintained good health for the ensuing 8 months.

In retrospect, there is little doubt that this medication had a salutary effect in his case and that if he had been willing do to so, he could have dropped his medication much sooner than he did.

The compound has been employed in other types of neuropsychiatric illnesses with varying results. The response in patients with ambulatory schizophrenia was discouraging, and that in a small group with pseudoneurotic schizophrenia, little better. It was hoped that patients with neurasthenic reactions would benefit by use of this drug, but such was not the case. Patients with presenile dementia, presumably Alzheimer's Disease, were in most cases not benefited. Neither the motor nor psychic manifestations were helped in 5 cases of Huntington's chorea. Patients with psychoses associated with cerebral arteriosclerosis were not helped if involvement was severe. Three upset paranoid patients were not improved. Seriously incapacitated obsessive-compulsive patients were made worse, if anything, by the medication.

Patients with anxiety reactions, in which there was no depressive element, often experienced an increase of anxiety symptoms on this medication. However, if depressive features were present, the response was often good, and on a few occasions excellent, but we concluded that this medication was contraindicated in the control of anxiety symptoms when they were present in pure culture.

There is a small but significant group of epileptics who become depressed and tense when their seizures are controlled by anticonvulsant drugs. These patients are always a puzzle therapeutically. This drug, when added to anticonvulsants, has helped 4 patients of this type in a gratifying way. There is another group of epileptics who become drowsy and dull when effective doses of hydantoin drugs are administered. Meratran, administered in small doses along with the hydantoins, will often circumvent this side reaction.

Preliminary observations suggest that this compound may open a new avenue for the treatment of certain tics, a group of conditions which provide a stubborn challenge for most therapists. We have been fascinated by our observations of an elderly lady who had a severe blepharospasm of 4 years' duration.

Spasm of her orbicularis oculi muscle bilaterally was so severe that she was almost totally incapacited by her almost constantly closed eyes. She was covered with bruises caused by repeatedly bumping into doors and furniture in her home. She was a proud woman yearning for independence, but because of her inability to keep house, she had reluctantly put herself in her daughter's care. When her daily dose of this compound was raised to 15 mg. daily for one month she proudly entered the office exhibiting a quilt she had sewed together. She had not picked up a needle during the previous 4 years. Although tic movements of her periocular muscles are still discernible to a small degree, she is now making pin money by addressing envelopes for a mailing company in her home. Before the medication was used she was unable to write.

Two other cases of blepharospasm and one of spasmodic torticollis have been under observation a short time and these patients also appear improved. The neurophysiologic implications of this therapy in tic cases are challenging, to say the least. Parenthetically, our observations do not indicate at this time Parkinsonian syndromes are affected favorably.

Dosage

It makes no difference whether the medication is given before or after meals. A pleasant clinical observation is that we have encountered no case of anorexia in the entire series of 320 cases; appetite is unaffected, and often improved as depressive symptoms abate. Occasional patients complain that they are too alert at bedtime, and our usual advice in such cases has been to drop the evening dose. This has been necessary in only one each of 37 reactive depressions and 34 psychotic depressions.

On the usual dose, 2.5 mg. 3 times a day, anxiety symptoms developed in 3 cases among the reactive depressions, and in 5 cases among the 34 endogenous ones. This incidence of anxiety reactions is significantly high to suggest that in office practice an initial dose of 1.0 mg. t.i.d. should be tried for approximately one week, and that if no somatic anxiety reaction occurs, and if the therapeutic results are not adequate at that level, the dose may be advanced to 2.5 mg. t.i.d. Further alteration in dosage is dependent upon the response of the individual patient, and upon the skill of the physician. Total dosage of 15, 20, and 25 mg. daily has been employed on occasion in response to therapeutic demand. In no case has there been any clinically observed alteration in pulse, respiration, or blood pressure at these levels. As was pointed out earlier, one severe narcoleptic patient has taken an average of 100 mg. daily for more than a year. Thorough studies of cardiovascular responses, liver function tests, blood counts, and urinalyses have remained normal throughout that time.

General rules on dosage can be outlined graphically. The depressive reactions merge imperceptibly from one category to the next in relation to severity. This is portrayed best by the spectrum (Fig. 1). The mildly depressed should receive quite small doses whereas the seriously depressed may require many times more. Overdosage at any level may initiate uncomfortable tension symptoms. It is necessary to maintain dosage below this critical level in all cases.

A case of overdosage deserves brief mention.

A 2½-year-old child weighing 25 pounds swallowed 15 mg. of her grandfather's medication at about 10:00 a.m. An hour later the grandparents noted that the child was excited and emitted a continuous stream of vocal expression and that she ran from room to room in frenzied activity. At lunchtime she ate voraciously and quickly. After lunch she resumed her hyperactivity and it was noted that she brushed her hands across her forehead alternately in a stereotyped way, as though brushing her hair out of her eyes. At 6:00 p.m. she again ate greedily. She was put to bed at 7:00 p.m. and was asleep an hour later. She awakened at 5:00 a.m., still voluble vocally, but her motor hyperactivity was now confined to the brushing movements of the hands against her forehead. She ate breakfast hurriedly, and it was then that the grandparents decided to bring her to the hospital. There it was noted that her blood pressure was 180/120 and the pulse was 160 plus. The child was frightened and crying, and it was thought that her emotional state might have occasioned her cardiovascular reaction. The stereotyped hand movements stopped when an object was placed in her hands, but resumed when it was removed. Sodium amytal, grains I, was given intramuscularly. She slept for 3 hours. Although somewhat tense, she was definitely quieter on waking, and was permitted to return home. The stereotypy returned from 7:00 to 9:00 p.m., when she fell asleep. On awaking the following morning she was full recovered. Her pulse and blood pressure returned to normal levels.

Discussion

Clinical trial discloses that Meratran is an effective central stimulant. It is closest in its action to drugs of the amphetamine series. This conclusion is predicated upon the similar therapeutic action of these compounds in depressive reactions and narcolepsy. Marked differences are noted, however. Foremost is the failure of the newer medications to affect the appetite and cardiovascular responses. Furthermore, insomnia almost never occurs when the compound is administered in proper dosage. Anxiety symptoms occur, but with lesser frequency and less unpleasantness subjectively than with amphetamines. The management of patients at the office level is in our experience easier with this compound than with the amphetamines because of these less troublesome side reactions.

Preliminary observations indicate that the range of usefulness of this compound in office psychiatry is roughly the same as that of the amphetamines, namely, the depressions of less severe type, when anxiety or agitation are not major symptoms. In other psychiatric disorders it is not therapeutically effective. We are also encouraged by indications that it may be of therapeutic value in selected cases of tic movements as well as in narcolepsy, and as an adjunct in the management of selected cases of epilepsy.

Conclusions

1. The pharmacology of a new antidepressant drug, Meratran, is reviewed briefly.
2. Clinical trial in 320 cases disclosed that the therapeutic indications of this compound are roughly similar to those of the amphetamines.
3. Reactive depressions responded effectively in 90% of our relatively small series.
4. Endogenous depressions responded favorably in 65% of our cases.
5. The drug has proved valuable in office practice because the appetite loss and the cardiovascular pressor reactions sometimes observed after the administration of the amphetamines are not encountered. In addition, the drug seldom interferes with nocturnal sleep, and when it produces anxiety side reactions these are less severe and less disturbing subjectively than those encountered with the amphetamines.
6. When anxiety or agitation comprise a sizable proportion of the clinical picture the drug should be used with caution.
7. Preliminary observations indicate that the drug may have therapeutic usefulness, in addition to the depressive states, in some of the tics, in narcolepsy, and as an adjunct in the management of certain epileptics.
8. Effective dosage ranges (except in narcolepsy) vary between 3.0 and 25.0 mg. daily.
9. Wider clinical trial of this compound appears justified.

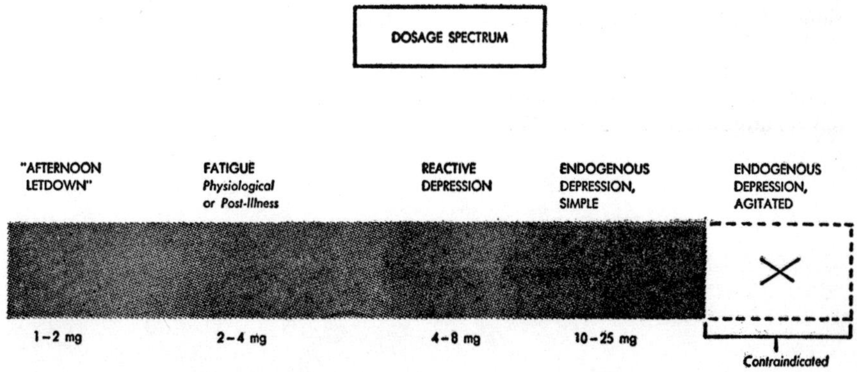

Fig. 1.

Discussion

PAUL H. HOCH, M.D., (New York City).—Up to the present we have used the drug, MRE-108 (DOL) on 21 schizophrenic patients with different symptomatologies. Several of them showed depression. It was also used in 5 cases of depression of which 3 were manic-depressive depressed and 2 involutional depressions. There were no reactive depressions in our series. The DOL was used orally on these patients in doses of from 1 to 25 mgm. per day. Doses above 2½ mgm. per day were given in divided amounts, b.i.d. and t.i.d. Placebos indistinguishable from the drug were alternated with DOL in periods varying from one day to 2 weeks. In the schizophrenic patients there were no significant objective differences in effects between drug and placebo with doses below 10 mgm. In some patients there was an increase in tension and motor activity, but it was small and therefore difficult to evaluate. In doses of 10 mgm. and above per day a marked change was noted between the drug and the placebo. All patients frequently mentioned restlessness, insomnia, and tension. All but one complained of poor appetite. There was objective increase in motoractivity, tension, and affective lability in all but 2 patients. All patients receiving the higher doses complained of diffuse tension and discomfort. None felt improved. Many felt more anxious, confused, and complained of an increase in various symptoms, especially rumination, depressive and aggressive manifestations. The effects of the higher doses of DOL seemed to last one day after the drug was discontinued. In one patient the medication was discontinued after 3 days because of his extreme anxiety reaction. There were no other sequaelae. We were impressed by the amphetamine-like side effects of the drug such as anorexia, insomnia, diffuse increase of tension, and restlessness, but with little or no euphorizing effect in these schizophrenic patients. Two of the depressed patients showed a temporary improvement with the drug for about a week. After this, however, the mental status returned to the same level. In the other depressed patients there was no change in their mental condition. All these patients received 2½ mgm. t.i.d. When this dose was increased to 15 mgm. daily, the same amphetamine-like effect became manifest as described in the schizophrenic patients, but without producing any improvement in the mental condition.

We feel that the drug needs further investigation especially before claims can be substantiated that it is very effective in depressed patients and that it has no amphetamine-like action.

MEPROBAMATE: ITS PHARMACOLOGIC PROPERTIES AND CLINICAL USES

F. M. Berger, M.D.

The recently introduced drugs, called ataraxics, that are used to alleviate certain symptoms of neuroses and psychoses can be divided into two broad classes. The first group, which has chlorpromazine and the Rauwolfia alkaloids as its most important representatives, is characterized by its important effects on the autonomic nervous system. The other, represented by meprobamate, acts on the central nervous system only, without affecting autonomic functions. The present article describes briefly how meprobamate was developed, summarizes its pharmacologic actions, and outlines the clinical results that it has produced.

The Development of Meprobamate. The parent substance from which meprobamate was developed is mephenesin. Chemically, mephenesin is 3-o-toloxy-1, 2-propanediol. It was introduced in 1946 as a muscle relaxant and is widely used in a variety of conditions where muscle spasm is a factor.

The greatest disadvantage of mephenesin is its short duration of action. After it was established that the evanescent action of the drug was due to the oxidation of mephenesin in the body to B-o-toloxy-lactic acid, which is physiologically inactive, various related compounds were prepared in which blockage of the hydroxyl groups by various radicals made this method of detoxification inoperative. Unexpectedly, mephenesin carbamate and other related o-toloxypropyl carbamates did not possess a longer duration of action than mephenesin. Meanwhile, it was also shown that certain 2, 2-disubstituted-1, 3-propanediols, while possessing pharmacologic properties similar to those of mephenesin, had in addition a particularly intense action at supraspinal levels. The dicarbamate derivatives of these compounds were long acting, although most of the substances had only a low order of activity. Among these, 2-methyl-2-n-propyl-1,3-propanediol dicarbamate, to which the generic name "meprobamate" was assigned, was unusual in possessing both pronounced muscle-relaxant and potent anticonvulsant properties and in exerting a marked taming effect on monkeys.

The Chemistry of Meprobamate. The compound was discovered in the Wallace Laboratories in 1950. It is a white crystalline powder of characteristic bitter taste, melting without decomposition at 105 to 106 C. The solubility of Meprobamate in water is low but it can readily be dissolved in most organic solvents. Meprobamate is stable in dilute acid and alkali and is not broken down at hydrogen ion concentrations occurring in gastric or intestinal juices.

The structural formula of the drug is as follows:

$$NH_2-CO-O-CH_2-\underset{\underset{CH_2-CH_2-CH_3}{|}}{\overset{\overset{CH_3}{|}}{C}}-CH_2-O-CO-NH_2$$

It is remarkable that a compound of such simple chemical structure should have such well-defined pharmacologic action. Meprobamate is one of the very few simple aliphatic compounds used in medicine, and its low toxicity may be the result of this simple structure. All other tranquilizers and central nervous system depressants possess in their molecules either ring structures (chlorpromazine, reserpine, azacyclonol, the barbiturates, methyprylon, glutethimide) or unsaturated linkages (methylparafynol, ethinamate, ethchlorvynol). The absence of a ring structure in the meprobamate molecule helps to explain the absence of habit-forming and addictive properties of the drug. The low incidence of side effects observed with meprobamate may be related to the absence of the highly reactive unsaturated linkages.

Pharmacologic Properties. Meprobamate has three pharmacologic properties of unusual interest; they are muscle-relaxant action, anticonvulsant action, and a taming effect best observed in monkeys.

The muscle-relaxant action is similar to that of mephenesin but of greater potency and longer duration. Only voluntary skeletal muscles are affected. The diaphragm is relatively insensitive to the action of meprobamate, and for this reason, respiration remains unimpaired even after administration of extremely large doses of the drug. Meprobamate is much more effective in reducing muscle spasm than normal proprioceptive muscle tension. Small doses will remove spasm and tremor experimentally produced by strychnine, neostigmine, and tetanus toxin, while much larger amounts are required to decrease normal muscle tension.

Meprobamate has a strong anticonvulsant action and is particularly effective in protecting animals from convulsions and deaths caused by toxic doses of pentylenetetrazole. It possesses a very wide margin of safety. In mice, less than one tenth of a lethal dose of meprobamate protects from a lethal dose of pentylenetetrazole. Meprobamate is also very effective in protecting animals from death caused by strychnine. The antagonistic action of meprobamate against these chemical convulsants is superior to that of many barbiturates, mephenesin, and trimethadione because it is apparent in doses that given by themselves do not have sedative effects and do not affect the animals in any way. Meprobamate also effectively modifies electroshock seizures in animals.

Meprobamate produces characteristic behavior changes that can best be observed in monkeys. After a suitable dose of meprobamate, the animals lose their fear, hostility, and aggressiveness and become tame and friendly. Appetite is unimpaired and full interest in the environment retained. The behavior of the meprobamate-treated animals differs strikingly from that displayed by monkeys receiving reserpine or chlorpromazine. After reserpine the animals, while tame and unaggressive, are listless and catatonic. Monkeys receiving chlorpromazine also lose interest in their surroundings but remain suspicious and capable of attacking when handled or prodded.

The Site and Mode of Action. Meprobamate has a marked blocking action on interneurons. This action can be demonstrated at the level of the spinal cord by showing that the knee jerk, which has a reflex arc with no interneurons, is not affected by the drug, while the flexor reflex and the crossed extensor reflex, which have one or more interneurons interposed between the afferent and efferent arcs, are decreased or abolished.

The most striking property of meprobamate is its selective action on the thalamus. Electrical recordings taken from the thalamus show that meprobamate in low doses causes marked synchronization of activity which manifests itself by a slowing of frequency and a marked increase of voltage. The pattern is quite different from the spindling seen after barbiturate administration. Simultaneous recordings taken from the cerebral cortex and other subcortical structures are not affected in any way. Leads taken from the hypothalamus and the limbic area also remain unchanged. After larger doses, an increase in voltage in certain subcortical structures, particularly the caudate nucleus, also becomes apparent. Extremely large doses are required to produce changes in the cortical pattern.

The selective action of meprobamate on the thalamus is a unique property of the drug. Other ataraxics, such as chlorpromazine and reserpine, do not cause such changes. It is of interest to speculate about the possible connections between selective changes in the thalamus and the effectiveness of the drug in psychoneurotic conditions. It may well be that one of the physiologic expressions of psychoneurosis consists of reverberation of discharges in the complicated interneuronal system of the thalamus. It is possible that the thalamic interneurons are especially sensitive to the action of meprobamate and that the blockage of some of these interneurons in the thalamus produces a synchronizing and normalizing effect on this structure.

Meprobamate does not seem to affect the autonomic nervous system. It does not change the responses of animals to acetylcholine, epinephrine, or histamine. In this respect the drug differs greatly from other ataraxics, which have potent adrenolytic, atropine-like, and antihistaminic action.

Toxicity. The acute toxicity of meprobamate in animals is very low. For instance, in mice the intraperitoneal administration of 800 mg./kg. is required to produce death in 50 per cent of the animals. This figure indicates that meprobamate is about four or five times less toxic than most barbiturates. The chronic toxicity of the drug is also unusually low. Animals tolerate 1 per cent of the drug in their diet during their whole life span, and this does not significantly reduce their growth rate, resistance to infections or other unfavorable environmental stimuli, or fertility.

The low toxicity of the drug is further attested by the results in human beings who have taken large numbers of tablets in suicidal attempts. Five such cases have come to my notice. After 20 to 50 tablets, these patients became somnolent, but all recovered spontaneously within 48 hours and suffered no aftereffects. The use of analeptics other than hot coffee was not required.

Fate in the Body. The results available up to the present indicate that approximately 10 per cent of the drug is excreted in the urine unchanged. The bulk of the remaining 90 per cent of the drug is apparently excreted as a conjugate with glucuronic acid. We have not succeeded in isolating the expected hydrolytic or oxidation breakdown products of meprobamate in the urine. A simple test to determine blood levels of meprobamate is not at present available.

Clinical Uses

Every new drug passes through three stages before its clinical usefulness is established. During the first stage, it receives enthusiastic and often uncritical acceptance for a variety of conditions. Meprobamate appears at present to be in this stage. During the second phase, a reversal of judgment frequently occurs and the value of the drug is doubted by many. Eventually, during the last phase, the true clinical value of the product is established.

The numerous reports evaluating meprobamate in the treatment of anxiety and tension states and other manifestations of psychoneurosis, such as sleeplessness and tension headaches, suggest by their consensus of opinion that the drug may have real merit in the treatment of these conditions. The value of meprobamate as a muscle relaxant in rheumatic conditions also appears widely recognized. Clinical trials relating to the possible usefulness of the drug in the treatment of psychoses and of certain forms of epilepsy are in progress, but definite conclusions have not yet been reached.

The Psychoneuroses

The psychoneuroses constitute an ill defined disease entity that can manifest itself by a variety of symptoms. Instead of following a formal classification system, it appears preferable to discuss the effects of meprobamate under the diagnostic headings widely used by physicians.

Anxiety and Tension States. Meprobamate has been found uniformly successful by all investigators using the drug in these conditions. It has been reported of assistance in controlling the irrational fears and vague sense of dread characteristic of the anxiety state, in relaxing the associated bodily tensions, in lessening irritability, and in improving the ability to concentrate. Unsociable patients again became able to take part in the life of the community. Many lost their morbid preoccupation with their symptoms and were able to resume the efficient pursuit of their careers. Patients also became much more accessible to psychotherapy. The drug increased their confidence in the physician and often enabled them to loosen their emotional defenses.

The incidence of improvements and recoveries described by various authors varies between 70 per cent and 95 per cent of cases. Improvement in the patient's condition, as a rule, could be observed within the first few days of treatment. Almost immediate results could be seen in treatment of agitation in anxiety states. With some patients, treatment had to be continued for three to four months before full improvement could be obtained.

The favorable results obtained with meprobamate appear to be objectively demonstrable and not due to suggestion. Selling found that patients given placebos after a period of meprobamate treatment complained about the return of their symptoms in every case. Hollister *et al.*, using a double-blind technique, had no difficulty in differentiating between true and placebo effects. Of 17 patients, 11 improved only after meprobamate, whereas only 3 improved after placebo alone. In 3 instances improvements were noted after both the placebo and meprobamate. Dickel *et al.* devised an electromyographic test to measure ability to relax muscle tension. They found that meprobamate produced a definitely increased ability to relax on command and a marked improvement in the patient's general coordination. These changes were correlated with the improvements in emotional response observed in the same patients.

Meprobamate appears to be more effective for the treatment of anxiety and tension than barbiturates or mephenesin. Borrus obtained excellent results in 67 patients with anxiety reactions who had previously failed to respond to barbiturates and mephenesin. Similar results were reported by Lemere and Selling. Hollister *et al.*, using a double-blind technique, found meprobamate of a similar effectiveness in relieving symptoms of anxiety reactions as reserpine and as the alseroxylon fraction of Rauwolfia. Phenobarbital proved much less effective than meprobamate or reserpine in this study. Hollister concluded that meprobamate, because of its effectiveness and lack of side reactions, was the most generally useful medication in the treatment of anxious patients.

Osinski studied a group of 113 hospital outpatients suffering from anxiety reactions, many of them having proved refractory to previous treatment with barbiturates or to a combination of barbiturates and other ataraxics. There were 40 patients who had been unresponsive to such previous treatment, and of these 70 per cent showed good or very good response to meprobamate.

Lemere compared chlorpromazine and reserpine with meprobamate. In his experience, the results with chlorpromazine and reserpine in office practice were much less spectacular than those reported following use of these drugs with severely disturbed patients in state hospitals. Lemere considers meprobamate, which he used in over 250 patients in his general psychiatric practice, to be the drug of choice for the relief of tension and anxiety.

Tension Headaches. In tense and anxious people, adverse life situations often give rise to sustained contractions of the posterior muscles of the head and neck which secondarily produce pain in the head, neck, and shoulders. This most common type of headache, sometimes also called psychosomatic or nuchal headache, is in reality only a manifestation of psychoneurosis in which the symptom of headache predominates. For this reason, the effectiveness of meprobamate in this condition is not unexpected. The drug may be of particular value in this condition not only because of its action on psychoneurotic symptoms, but also because of its relaxant action on skeletal muscles.

Selling observed that the most dramatic reports of recovery in patients given meprobamate came from cases where tension headache was the chief complaint. Of 27 patients with this complaint, 23 either recovered or reported sufficient improvement so that they were no longer concerned with this symptom. Meprobamate has also been found of value in the treatment of vascular headache. The drug can be administered to hypertensives with safety because it does not affect the blood pressure. The effect of meprobamate on migraine has not been studied.

Patients receiving electroshock treatment usually develop headache within an hour following treatment. Thal reported that the administration of a single tablet of meprobamate one hour prior to giving the electroshock prevented the occurrence of the headache in every instance. (In this study, 120 female psychotic patients were observed.)

Insomnia. All sedatives and hypnotics when administered to human beings in appropriate clinical dosage produce a characteristic sleep pattern in the electroencephalogram. Meprobamate, in common with other ataraxics such as chlorpromazine and reserpine, does not produce such changes. Sleep patterns after meprobamate have not been observed even after administration of large doses to human beings. (A healthy male subject of 31 years took 8 tablets within one hour; there were no changes in his electroencephalogram.) Thus, it would be incorrect to call meprobamate a hypnotic. This observation notwithstanding, the drug has been found of considerable value for the induction of sleep, probably through relaxing the anxieties and tensions that prevent its natural onset.

Sleep following meprobamate differs in several respects from that following the administration of barbiturates. After barbiturates, unconsciousness sets in suddenly. After meprobamate, on the other hand, the patient is able to lie quietly without worrying until he drifts into sleep. Patients can be readily wakened. Sleep is usually dreamless and restful and is not followed by a "dopey" feeling on awakening.

Selling found it possible to produce sleep with meprobamate in every case except in patients suffering from true psychotic depression, and was able to discontinue entirely the use of barbiturates or similar somnifacients in his practice. While meprobamate proved of particular value in enabling the patient to fall asleep, many patients awakening early in the morning were enabled to return to sleep by taking a supplementary dose of meprobamate during the night.

Mulinos *et al.* evaluated meprobamate in 26 hospital patients all of whom had previously been taking a hypnotic (usually pentobarbital). They found that 87 per cent slept well after meprobamate as compared with 46 per cent after a placebo. In another study, Mulinos *et al.*, using meprobamate with 106 hospitalized patients, also reported it to be an effective hypnotic. Under placebo, only 7 per cent of his patients slept well, whereas 64 per cent did so under meprobamate. Doses as large as 1 gm. (2½ tablets) taken at night caused no hang-over or other aftereffects.

Lasagna, in a double-blind study carried out on 46 chronically ill hospitalized patients troubled with insomnia, compared meprobamate with four hypnotics. He found that meprobamate had about the same order of hypnotic effectiveness as phenobarbital, both as to time of onset and duration of effect. He also observed that a dose of 800 mg. was not appreciably more effective than one of 400 mg. except that the duration of sleep was usually somewhat increased at the higher dose.

Grinker and Borrus have both observed that when meprobamate is used as a tranquilizer during the day, patients so treated will often require no additional sedative to produce sleep at night. This effect was noted particularly in agitated patients suffering from anxiety states and depression.

Lemere feels that meprobamate is the drug of choice in the treatment of insomnia in ambulatory office patients. Alcoholics in the withdrawal phase have also been reported as obtaining restful sleep after meprobamate. In this respect, meprobamate appeared far superior to barbiturates and other types of hypnotic drugs.

Alcoholism. In the treatment of alcoholism, meprobamate helps to control withdrawal symptoms during the sobering-up phase. After withdrawal has been accomplished, the drug facilitates adjustment to life without alcohol. It has not been found to be habit forming.

The persistence of anxiety, tension, and insomnia in alcoholics even after they have abstained from alcoholic beverages for considerable periods of time makes the frequency of relapses understandable. In these patients, meprobamate alleviates tension, restlessness, and insomnia and appears in these respects much superior to barbiturates and other hypnotics.

Thimann found meprobamate to be a safe, rapid, and effective sedative for the subacute stage of withdrawal from alcohol. Severely intoxicated subjects were initially treated with paraldehyde or chloral hydrate during the acute stage, and were transferred to meprobamate only one or two days after admission. In cases of mild intoxication, meprobamate could be administered immediately upon admission. O'Hollaren also believes that meprobamate is of little value in the severely intoxicated patient and that the usefulness of the drug lies chiefly in enabling the patient to control his tenseness and irritability during abstinence from alcoholic beverages. In the control of tremor, meprobamate proved very effective and definitely superior to mephenesin.

Fox evaluated meprobamate as well as a number of other drugs in acutely intoxicated patients admitted to a private hospital. Meprobamate used alone and in low dosage did not control violently agitated patients. In larger doses (about 2 tablets four times a day), and particularly when given in conjunction with small doses of chlorpromazine, meprobamate produced results that were much superior to those obtained with any other therapeutic regimen previously tried. Patients so treated commented that they felt better at the termination of treatment, and their period of hospitalization could be shortened. Barbiturates were not needed during the withdrawal period.

Psychosomatic Symptoms. Meprobamate has proved of value in a variety of conditions of psychosomatic origin.

PAIN. Gastric pain of psychosomatic origin responded well to meprobamate, but pain due to ulcer was not relieved. Kessler and Barnard found meprobamate useful in the control of somatic pain accompanying neoplastic disease. It is unlikely that the drug could have affected the threshold to pain perception directly, as pharmacologic tests in animals did not show the drug to have an analgesic action. However, it is possible that by lessening the patient's anxiety, meprobamate may have increased his tolerance to pain.

NEURODERMATITIS. Selling and others reported that meprobamate cleared up skin rashes of psychosomatic origin. Sokoloff found the drug of considerable value as an adjunct in the treatment of idiopathic anogenital pruritus.

MENSTRUAL STRESS. In some women, symptoms of anxiety and tension appear only shortly before and during their menstrual periods. In these patients, meprobamate is often of great value in reducing irritability, pressure, headache, and general discomfort. Pennington and Dixon also reported on the value of meprobamate in premenstrual tension and dysmenorrhea.

Behavior Problems. Selling reported on 10 tense and restless children who presented behavior problems. Of these, 7 benefited by meprobamate treatment. The drug helped them to quiet down and to concentrate better. In Perlstein's series of 29 very serious behavior problems (including 7 psychotics), only 7 showed benefit from meprobamate.

PSYCHOSES

Up to the present, the result of only one study relating to the value of meprobamate in hospitalized psychotic patients has become available. Pennington, at the Mississippi State Hospital, compared the effectiveness of meprobamate, reserpine, chlorpromazine, azacyclonol, pipradrol hydrochloride, and whole root Rauwolfia in 1250 patients in a study extending over 18 months. Most of the patients were schizophrenics. According to her report, the results obtained with meprobamate were quite similar to those obtained by her and other investigators with chlorpromazine and reserpine. About 3 per cent of the patients were completely rehabilitated. Improvement was marked in an additional 29 per cent, and moderate in 50 per cent of the patients. The remaining 18 per cent were not influenced.

To achieve these results, higher dosage than that used in the treatment of psychoneuroses was needed. A few patients required as many as 12 tablets twice daily. Most received about 3 to 4 tablets daily. Under this regimen, sleep was improved, appetite increased, and psychotic delusional trends were often dispelled. Some belligerent patients who formerly had required several shock treatments a month for control became calm and could be kept with other patients while taking the drug.

Borrus and Selling evaluated meprobamate in a few ambulatory schizophrenics who were making marginal adjustments. Of 12 of these patients, 6 showed some improvement, mainly of better social adjustment, after meprobamate.

Manic-depressives and hypomanics who were obviously disturbed but not committably psychotic were also favorably affected by meprobamate. There are usually difficulties in getting these patients to take the medication because they do not believe themselves to be sick. Many of them were able to keep out of trouble as long as they took the drug.

Available evidence does not indicate that meprobamate is of value with patients suffering from psychotic depression. Because of the suicidal tendencies of these patients, it is of great importance to keep them under close supervision and to differentiate their condition from that presented by the anxiety reactions. Such a diagnosis is often difficult to make.

Several investigators have reported that reserpine sometimes causes depression and suicidal tendencies in certain subjects. Meprobamate has not been known to elicit suicidal tendencies, nor to aggravate these tendencies when present.

Electroshock treatment is no contraindication to the administration of meprobamate. Selling observed that meprobamate is often of value for the control of postshock confusion. Thal, in a well controlled study of 120 psychotic patients, observed the effect of meprobamate premedication on electroshock treatment. One 400 mg. tablet was given one hour before electroshock. Under premedication, the patients were less apprehensive, experienced less postshock confusion, and regained full consciousness more rapidly than patients not receiving the drug. Postshock headache did not occur. The convulsive response to electroshock itself was only slightly altered. The tonic phase was perhaps slightly less intense in onset, while the duration of the clonic phase was slightly shortened.

Epilepsy

The strong anticonvulsive action of meprobamate in animals made the evaluation of the drug in various forms of epilepsy of great interest.

Meprobamate appears to be of no value in the treatment of grand mal. Thirty-one cases not responding to other anticonvulsants were treated during an eight month period with up to 8 tablets of meprobamate per day. The drug proved ineffective. Perlstein found that meprobamate, like trimethadione and other anticonvulsants useful in petit mal, sometimes precipitated grand mal spells in patients subject to both grand mal and petit mal spells.

Perlstein stated that meprobamate is of considerable value in the treatment of idiopathic petit mal seizures. Although not as effective as trimethadione, it seemed to be at least as effective as paramethadione and all other anti-petit mal drugs. It has the advantage over trimethadione and paramethadione in being relatively non-toxic. The drug appeared markedly more effective in idiopathic petit mal seizures, where 83 per cent (of 18 cases) were benefited, than in organic petit mal, where only 22 per cent (of 53 cases) were helped. Livingston reported favorable results in some cases of minor motor (akinetic and massive myoclonic) seizures in children who as a rule were also mentally retarded.

Muscle Spasm

Meprobamate shows a muscle-relaxant action on skeletal muscle similar to that of mephenesin but of greater intensity and longer duration. For this reason, one would expect the drug to be of value in conditions where muscle spasm is a factor, such as in various rheumatic conditions, poliomyelitis, spasticity due to upper motor neuron lesions, cerebral palsy, and related conditions.

Chronic Rheumatic Conditions. Smith evaluated meprobamate in over 100 cases of chronic rheumatic conditions. He found that fibrositic symptoms were greatly improved in those cases where muscle spasm predominated. Some of the conditions successfully treated with meprobamate were: rheumatoid spondylitis, cervical myositis (wry neck), and acute and chronic low back strain. The drug was found completely ineffective in true rheumatoid arthritis.

Eisenberg and Neviaser evaluated meprobamate in 107 patients presenting a wide variety of conditions involving muscle spasm, pain and tenderness, restriction of motion, and spinal tilt. About 90 per cent of the patients were significantly improved, 65 per cent showing marked improvement or complete recovery. Relief was greatest in acute and chronic low back strain, cervical myositis, and various osteoarthritic conditions. Symptoms caused by ruptured intervertebral discs and by postoperative conditions appeared to respond less well to treatment. The authors concluded that meprobamate is in all respects greatly superior to mephenesin. They believe that it is the best muscle relaxant available for the symptomatic treatment of acute and chronic low back strain, cervical myositis, and certain osteoarthritic conditions.

Cerebral Palsy. Schesinger evaluated the effect of meprobamate on 39 patients, all of whom took the drug for well over a year. He reports an enhancement of motor effort and reduction of involuntary movements of a greater degree than with any other drug including all the mephenesin analogues. Meprobamate dampens activity sufficiently to allow corrective therapy and motor training. Its use appears particularly worth while in the athetoid and dyskinetic patients.

In Perlstein's series, meprobamate showed some effectiveness in 10 of 44 patients suffering from cerebral palsy. The most responsive cases were the athetoids where three marked and five moderate responses were obtained among 26 cases. Patients with pyramidal tract involvement were not often helped. These results have, in general, been confirmed by Baird. Gillette observed a very definite reduction of tension in both spastic and athetoid patients. This change was not referable to better emotional control as most of these patients were too young to present emotional problems. About three days after treatment was instituted, the application of braces became easier, speech improved, movement could be carried out with greater speed and ease, and the involuntary movements decreased.

Various Neurologic Conditions. Occasional cases of hemiplegia and paraplegia have shown a decrease in flexor spasm, but clinically useful improvement is obtained in only a few cases. Painful muscle spasm in acute poliomyelitis has been effectively relieved with meprobamate without producing any respiratory embarrassment. Multiple sclerosis and Parkinsonism have proved unresponsive to meprobamate treatment. In many of these patients, however, meprobamate produced restful sleep.

Dosage and Side Effects

The dosage used by most investigators is one or two 400 mg. tablets three times a day. For sleep, 2 tablets about 30 minutes before retiring are usually taken. With seriously disturbed psychotics, much larger doses may be required. Extensive clinical investigations have shown meprobamate to be a drug of extremely low toxicity. Patients receiving 1 or 2 Gm. of meprobamate daily for over 12 months showed no evidence of systemic toxicity. A few patients, given up to 4 Gm. per day, and followed for six months, also showed no evidence of toxic effect. Blood dyscrasias, urinary changes, or liver damage attributable to its use have not been observed.

The only side effect reported with any frequency is drowsiness. The incidence of drowsiness appears to vary greatly in the different series reported. It is more likely to occur after 2 tablets three times a day than after 1 tablet three times a day. Perlstein believes that adults are less susceptible to drowsiness at higher doses than children. Some patients who complain of drowsiness when first taking the drug may lose this symptom after continued administration for a week or so. Drowsiness can often be controlled by reducing the dose. If this is undesirable, the concomitant use of amphetamine usually counteracts any drowsiness due to meprobamate administration.

The only serious side effect reported after meprobamate up to the present is allergic reaction. This response develops, as a rule, in patients who have had only one to four doses of meprobamate and have not had previous contact with the drug. In mild reactions of this type, there is an itchy urticarial or erythematous rash, which may be generalized or confined to the groins. More severe cases may also have fever, fainting spells, angioneurotic edema, and bronchial spasm.

Treatment consists of the administration of epinephrine, antihistamines, and possibly also hydrocortisone. Meprobamate should be stopped and no further attempt made to use this medication.

Certain patients have complained of gastric discomfort after taking meprobamate. Because the incidence of this common complaint was noted to be similar after the drug as after a placebo (when a double-blind technique was used), it appears unlikely to be of any consequence.

Summary

Meprobamate is a new tranquilizer with muscle-relaxant properties. It differs from other tranquilizing drugs both in the simplicity of its chemical structure and in its mode of action. Meprobamate has a selective action on the thalamus and a blocking action on spinal interneurons. The drug does not affect autonomic functions.

Meprobamate has proved to be of particular value in anxiety and tension states and in related conditions such as tension headache, sleeplessness, and menstrual stress. The muscle-relaxant properties of the drug are of value in the treatment of cervical myositis, acute and chronic low back strain, various osteoarthritic conditions, and cerebral palsy. The drug has also been used in the treatment of psychotics and in certain cases of petit mal epilepsy, but its value in these conditions has not yet been established.

Side effects with meprobamate occur, rarely. Some patients complain of drowsiness when first put on the drug, but this often passes away in a week or so if the medication is continued. A few cases of allergic skin reactions have occurred, but no cases of blood changes or liver or kidney damage have been reported. The drug appears to be nonaddictive and non-habit forming. It can be used with patients undergoing electroshock treatment and does not precipitate depression.

Addendum

Since the above article was written, much additional work has been done on meprobamate, including a number of important studies of the behavioral effects of the drug on normal humans.

In a controlled study of 50 normal subjects, Marquis *et al.* studied the effects of meprobamate on the skills required for driving. Three tests were given: (1) a test which measured the subject's ability to steer and stop a model car at various speeds using standard automobile controls; (2) a test to determine visual acuity, depth perception and visual balance, and (3) a motor steadiness test. All three tests were given to all subjects with meprobamate alone, with meprobamate in combination with alcohol, and with placebo. The authors concluded that 800 mg. meprobamate produced no effect on the skills required for safe driving, and did not increase the impairment produced by alcohol.

To another group of normal subjects Reitan administered a battery of psychologic tests under standardized and controlled conditions. Subjects were tested for alertness, sustained attention, accuracy of visuomotor coordination, motor speed, speed of reaction and problem solving. Reitan reported that, following 400 mg. meprobamate q.i.d. for six days, no impairment of performance was observed, and that at four times the normal dose, impairment of performance was slight.

Comparisons of the effects of meprobamate, chlorpromazine, pentobarbital, and placebo on human performance of a perceptual-motor task under anxiety-producing conditions were carried out by Holliday *et al.* on 50 normal subjects. Results showed that only the meprobamate group exhibited a continued improvement in performance or continuing capacity for learning over successive trials. The authors concluded that meprobamate tends to abolish the disruptive effects of anxiety on performance and learning as measured in their study, whereas the other drugs tested do not.

TREATMENT OF ANXIETY STATES WITH MEPROBAMATE (MILTOWN)

Walter A. Osinski, M.D.
Department of Psychiatry, Albany Hospital, Albany, N. Y.

In June, 1954, a drug, meprobamate (Miltown), was called to my attention. The drug was discovered and studied pharmacologically by Dr. Frank M. Berger, who was also responsible for developing mephenesin.

Meprobamate is 2-methyl-2-n-propyl-1,3-propanediol dicarbamate. Pharmacologic experiments showed that the drug exerts selective interneuronal blocking action, as does mephenesin. It relaxed skeletal muscle but did not affect monosynaptic reflexes, peripheral nerve, or the myoneural junction. Meprobamate was also reported to be longer acting and more reliable in its results; it did not produce the nausea and vomiting that were often concomitants of therapy with mephenesin. Strikingly different from the effects of mephenesin was a pronounced and long-lasting tranquilizing effect apparent on all animals studied.

Monkeys treated with meprobamate lost their natural fear and hostility and became friendly and amenable to petting and handling. Interestingly, they did not become "dopey" or indifferent to their surroundings, but remained alert and curious and fully retained their appetite. Neuropharmacologic investigations using electroencephalographic recordings showed pronounced influence of the drug on subcortical structures, with greatest slowing and synchronizing of potentials from the thalamus. This tranquilizing action of the drug interested me in testing its possibilities clinically with patients in the Psychiatric Department at Albany Hospital.

Scope of the Study

The patients studied were seen during the period Sept. 15, 1954, to May 1, 1955, and were mostly referred from general practitioners or from medical consultants. All patients studied showed extraordinary anxiety, tension, or "nervousness" either as the only complaint or as important among other complaints. Within the limits of this criterion of selection, all patients who came during the period of the study were included, regardless of the diagnosis and regardless of whether the illness was acute or chronic.

Patients who required hospitalization were not accepted, and the psychotics who were included were borderline and ambulatory. One hundred and thirteen patients were treated with meprobamate during this study.

Procedure. Patients were given a psychiatric interview on admission and were seen at intervals of one week, and later of two weeks, as progress permitted. Psychotherapy was in all cases minimal. Patients who did not show good results from meprobamate treatment in a reasonable period of time—usually two to three weeks—were transferred to other treatment. All patients, however, whatever the duration of treatment, have been included in the analysis of results.

Dosage. The standard dosage used was one 400 mg. tablet three times a day. A few patients received an additional tablet before going to sleep at night. In occasional instances the dosage was reduced to one tablet twice a day when this appeared adequate as a maintenance dosage.

Standards of Evaluation. Two criteria were used in evaluating the results of treatment with meprobamate: (1) the extent of relief from presenting symptoms and (2) the degree of improvement in social and work adjustment. The following definitions were followed in assigning final ratings: Very good improvement—Substantial to complete relief of symptoms with good social and work adjustment. Good improvement—Considerable relief of symptoms with significant improvement in social and work adjustment. Some improvement—Some relief of symptoms but no improvement in social or work adjustment. No improvement—Negligible or no response to treatment with meprobamate.

TABLE I
Response to Meprobamate Treatment of 113 Psychiatric Patients

Diagnosis	Total cases	Very good	Good	Some	None	% Very good or good	% Some improvement
Psychoneurosis							
Anxiety state	52	15	26	8	3	79	94
Phobic	4		2	1	1		
Obsessive-compulsive	6	1		4	1		
Conversion reaction	6			2	4		
Other	19	2	11	2	4	68	79
Personality disorder							
Alcoholic addiction	7	4	2		1		
Barbiturate addiction	2	2					
Manic-depressive	7	2	2	2	1		
Schizophrenia	4		1	3			
Involutional depression	2			2			
Various	4	2	1		1		
Total	113	28	45	24	16	65	86

RESULTS

Table 1 shows the conditions in which meprobamate was used and the results obtained. In patients classified as being in anxiety states, anxiety, "nervousness," and tension were the sole or clearly dominant presenting symptoms. The psychoneurotic conditions classified under "other" did not fit into any of the other categories and presented mixed symptoms such as anxiety and depression or other more complicated neurotic patterns.

The results shown in table 1 indicate that meprobamate has a definite effectiveness in anxiety states. In other disturbed conditions the drug appears of value in proportion to the components of anxiety and tension that are present. These results confirm closely the observations of Borrus and Selling. Meprobamate was also of considerable value in the treatment of alcoholism and of barbiturate addiction.

The manic-depressives were treated with meprobamate only after prior treatment of the depression by electroconvulsive therapy. The results reported, therefore, describe the degree to which postelectroshock confusion and tension were relieved in these conditions. The schizophrenic group consisted of 1 acute paranoid, 2 acute unclassified, and 1 chronic undifferentiated. The 1 case showing a good response was in the acute unclassified category. The group listed as "various" consisted of 2 cases of cerebral arteriosclerosis and 2 of posttraumatic encephalopathy, all with anxiety. The completely unresponsive case was one of cerebral arteriosclerosis.

The following cases illustrate the manner in which symptoms of tension and anxiety were overcome by the use of meprobamate.

Case 1. This 33 year old white woman gave a history of always having been somewhat nervous, even as a child. Both her parents were considered to be excitable people, but there was no evidence of mental illness. She made an uneventful adjustment in high school, and after graduation obtained a job as a secretary.

During the five years prior to her coming to the psychiatrist she had noticed fatigability and poor appetite and on occasion developed headaches. During the three months before her visit she began to complain of tension feelings in the back of the neck, occasionally experienced dizzy spells, and was aware of nervousness, particularly under pressure. About this time she was not only quite active on her job but was making preparations for her marriage. Although she did not express any concern about her contemplated marriage and did not believe herself to be unduly upset, she was quite disturbed about her symptoms, namely, fatigability, tension feelings in the neck, and feeling somewhat sluggish.

Psychiatric interview failed to reveal any significant pathology. However, during the interview she appeared quite tense and restless and displayed increased heart rate and perspiration. The mere discussion of the various factors that might be contributing to her present state of affairs did not bring about any change in her symptomatology. She was evaluated by a general practitioner who considered that she might be suffering from a hypothyroid state, but this was not substantiated by clinical tests.

She was started on phenobarbital, ¼ gr. four times a day, without significant change. She was then started on meprobamate, one tablet three times a day, and within one week was free from her acute tension symptoms. She began to sleep soundly. Her general feeling of apprehension and concern over her physical status quickly disappeared. When interviewed two weeks later she told the examiner that she did not feel it was necessary to continue the medication any longer. When medication was discontinued, she continued to get along uneventfully. She married and is now pregnant and does not display any evidence of the symptoms that were evident at the time of her first interview.

Case 2. This 31 year old white man was apparently well until about three years before coming to treatment, at which time he began to notice nervousness, inability to concentrate, and periodic episodes of depression. These symptoms occurred at a time when he was attending a religious school and was having considerable difficulty in accepting his intended role as a clergyman. Although he was passing his subjects satisfactorily and was being praised for his accomplishments, he remained very uncomfortable. In spite of these symptoms, he continued to pursue his objective. One day while attending classes he suddenly fainted. He was taken to a physician who evaluated him from a physical standpoint and made a tentative diagnosis of idiopathic epilepsy. He was placed on diphenyldantoin and phenobarbital but his symptoms continued. He had at least four more spells and finally had to leave the school.

After returning home he obtained a job as a clerk but soon found considerable difficulty in relating himself to people, particularly his superiors. His tension symptoms began to mount. He became irritable and found it difficult to concentrate on his work. At this time he consulted a psychiatrist. He was quite dejected over the fact that he had lost almost six years of his life in study, and he considered himself a failure. Psychotherapy gradually resulted in the disappearance of his depressive symptoms but he continued to remain quite tense.

He was started on amobarbital sodium, 1 gr. three times a day, and on this regimen noted only moderate improvement. He was then placed on 50 mg. of chlorpromazine four times a day and his symptoms became much more intense. After one week this drug was discontinued and he was then placed on meprobamate, 400 mg. three times a day. After one week he told the psychiatrist that for the first time in approximately four years he had experienced the best relief of his symptoms.

He is now working on his job, is married, and is getting along uneventfully. He has noted that it is necessary for him to continue taking 400 mg. of meprobamate three times a day. Whenever he stops the medication his symptoms return to a moderate degree. He has continued to get along on the drug without formal psychiatric treatment.

Combined Therapy. In 21 cases other drugs were used in conjunction with meprobamate. In table II the therapeutic response obtained after administration of meprobamate with other drugs is analyzed and the results are compared with those obtained after meprobamate only. Meprobamate was given in combination with amobarbital sodium in 11 of the cases of anxiety reactions, 3 of the cases of the "other" psychoneuroses, and 1 of the cases of cerebral arteriosclerosis. The combined treatment accounted for four of the very good and seven of the good responses in the anxiety reactions, one very good and two good reactions in the "other" psychoneuroses, and the one very good result in allaying anxiety in cerebral arteriosclerosis. Meprobamate was used with amphetamine in 4 cases, resulting in one very good and one good response in the group of anxiety reactions, one complete failure of response in a case of

TABLE II
Meprobamate Used with Other Drugs

Medications used	Total cases	%	No of cases Very good	Good	Some	None	% Very good or good	% Some benefit
Meprobamate alone	92	81.4	21	33	23	15	58.9	83.7
Meprobamate with amobarbital sodium	15	13.3	6	9			100.0	100.0
Meprobamate with other drugs	6	5.3	1	3	1	1	66.6	83.3
Total	113	100.0	28	45	24	16	64.6	85.8

alcoholism, and a good response in 1 of the depressives and 1 of the cases of post-traumatic encephalopathy. One phobic patient who had previously been receiving chlorpromazine received meprobamate in addition, but with continuing minimal effect.

An interesting observation was that in the course of this study, certain patients who did not respond to either amobarbital sodium alone or meprobamate alone showed a striking response to a combination of the two drugs when 0.1 Gm. of amobarbital sodium was given with 400 mg. of meprobamate. While the small number of cases treated with a combination of meprobamate and other drugs included in this study are insufficient to permit generalizations, they do seem to indicate that further experimentation might prove rewarding.

Duration of Treatment. Of the 73 cases that showed good to very good results, 65 per cent were on meprobamate treatment from one week to three months (14 from 6 to 30 days, 21 from 31 to 60 days, and 13 from 61 to 90 days). The remaining 22 cases in this group took meprobamate for from three to seven months, mostly on maintenance doses to sustain the good results achieved earlier.

Side Effects. Of the 113 patients treated with meprobamate, 6 at first complained of sleepiness. This effect wore off with time in all cases. Ten patients reported that they were troubled by dizziness, as a result of which 7 were transferred to other medication. Other side effects were not reported.

Previous Therapy. To compare the results obtained with meprobamate with those obtained under previous therapy, table III was compiled, those cases without previous therapy being omitted.

Other drugs used concomitantly with amobarbital sodium were chlorpromazine, chlorpromazine and reserpine together, estrogen, bromide, and nicotinic acid. The last of these combinations was the only one to show any response. Other drugs used with electroconvulsive therapy were chlorpromazine (5 cases with some response, 2 with poor response), dextroamphetamine (1 case, good response), estrogen (1 case), Tuinal and amphetamine (1 case), and amobarbital sodium with chlorpromazine (1 case), all with poor response.

In this group of 94 cases suffering from a variety of psychiatric conditions, 93 per cent proved refractory to a number of widely used drugs. Sixty per cent

TABLE III
Comparison of Results of Meprobamate and Previous Therapy

No. of cases	Drug or treatment	Previous therapy Response Good	Some	Poor	Meprobamate therapy Response Very good	Good	Some	None
44	Amobarbital sodium	1	2	41	13	21	6	4
8	Amobarbital sodium with other drugs		1	7	2	2	3	1
3	Phenobarbital			3		3		
1	Reserpine			1	1			
6	Electroconvulsive therapy	3	2	1		2	4	
21	Electroconvulsive therapy with amobarbital sodium	1	5	15	3	8	4	6
11	Electroconvulsive therapy with other drugs	1	4	6	1	4	4	2
94	Total	6	14	74	20	40	21	13

of these refractory cases showed a good or very good response to meprobamate therapy. The results appear even more striking when the comparison is limited to those cases suffering from anxiety reactions. Of 40 cases suffering from anxiety states that proved refractory to previous treatment, 70 per cent showed a good or very good response to meprobamate therapy.

Some of the cases mentioned in table III that were refractory to previous therapy but responded to meprobamate treatment required the joint administration of two drugs for optimum results. Thus, four of the very good responses and 10 good responses were from meprobamate combined with amobarbital sodium, and one very good and three good responses from meprobamate combined with dextroamphetamine. One case did not respond to the joint administration of meprobamate and dextroamphetamine, and another case showed only minimal improvement from meprobamate and chlorpromazine.

DISCUSSION

A number of excellent drugs have become available recently for the treatment of the emotionally disturbed. Probably greatest attention has been directed to chlorpromazine, a potent drug developed in France and widely used in Europe and in this country in neuropsychiatric states. Its particular value is with severe psychotics. In milder cases, however, the possible occurrence of serious side effects must be weighed against the therapeutic benefits.

Reserpine, the other most widely used tranquilizer, is fundamentally a hypotensive agent. Patients on reserpine therapy often pass through a stage of excitation during the first two or three weeks of treatment which may be distressing to both the patient and his relatives. Others may become listless and depressed. Meprobamate, which differs from both reserpine and chlorpromazine in chemical structure, does not have a specific effect on blood pressure, does not cause listlessness, agitation, or depression, and so far has not caused serious side effects. While experience with this new drug is not yet of long standing, indications suggest that in the treatment of anxiety states, meprobamate is just as effective as chlorpromazine or reserpine, and has the additional advantage of being safer and better tolerated.

The tranquilizers used previously have a definite influence on the autonomic regulatory mechanism of the body. Meprobamate does not seem to affect this mechanism, thus making it possible to achieve therapeutic results without disturbing the delicately adjusted autonomic equilibrium of the body. The good therapeutic results obtained with meprobamate in cases that proved refractory to treatment with a number of conventional remedies suggest that meprobamate has a mode of action that differs from that of chlorpromazine, reserpine, and the barbiturates.

SUMMARY AND CONCLUSIONS

Meprobamate was administered to 113 ambulatory patients treated at the Psychiatric Department of Albany Hospital. Meprobamate showed definite effectiveness in psychoneurotic anxiety states, and appeared to have a selective action in conditions in which anxiety and tension are prominent factors. A large number of cases that had proved unresponsive to various other forms of treatment including reserpine and chlorpromazine responded well to therapy with meprobamate.

The combination of meprobamate with amobarbital sodium in certain cases seemed to be of greater value than either drug given alone. A few patients reported drowsiness or dizziness, the former subsiding spontaneously upon continued administration. Other side effects were not reported. While meprobamate appears at least as effective as other tranquilizers, it seems to be safer and better tolerated and has the added advantage that it does not affect the autonomic functions of the body.

MEPROBAMATE IN ANXIETY REACTIONS INVOLVING DEPRESSION

Abraham Ruchwarger, M.D.
St. Elizabeths Hospital, Washington, D. C.

Because the treatment of depression has not been wholly satisfactory, and because good results have been reported in certain cases following the use of meprobamate, I considered the possibility that reported results might be improved with higher dosage, and my experience has proved favorable.

I have used the drug in private psychiatric practice with 70 patients, mostly from the middle and lower-middle income groups, who were generally unable to afford long-term psychiatric therapy. Included were 10 with severe neurotic depressions. Of these, 3 were reactive depressions with anxiety components, and 7 were primarily anxiety reactions but with pronounced depressive tendencies of suicidal intensity. The depressions were mostly acute and usually accompanied by insomnia.

These patients received 10 400-mg. meprobamate tablets a day, 2 just before or immediately upon rising, 2 after each meal, and 2 before retiring. The early morning dose was found to be important since it followed a refreshing night's sleep and inhibited the initial formation of the day's depression.

All patients received psychotherapy. One of the great benefits of meprobamate was that it enabled patients who before taking the drug had been too depressed to talk, to do so. Often their relief and gratitude were so great that they were eager to cooperate further in treatment.

Of the 10 patients with depressions treated with meprobamate 7 showed good results and 3 fair. The patients with chronic cases were more resistant than those with short histories. Nearly all patients were able to sleep well with the drug.

The following case histories are illustrative of the patients who were benefited by meprobamate.

ILLUSTRATIVE CASES

Case 1. A 29-year-old married woman with 2 children was compelled because of her husband's occupation to move frequently. Her friendships were constantly disrupted, and she felt rootless and was unable to adjust to her feeling of isolation. She was suicidal and when first seen was in a complete catatonic stupor. She had been given chlorpromazine without help by a doctor in another city. On a regimen of 10 400-mg. meprobamate tablets a day she emerged from her depression, was able to sleep well, and became accessible to psychotherapy. Under continued meprobamate therapy the improvement in her mood also lasted and she made an adequate adaptation to her difficult life situation.

Case 2. A man aged 69, living alone, had been retired against his will and had been completely unable to cope with his changed status. His life seemed meaningless, and he felt worthless. Panic had overtaken him, and he was on the verge of a breakdown. He could not take a bus or go out on the street alone. He did not associate with anyone. He was agitated, talked aloud to himself, and banged his head against the wall. I was called in by his landlord when he attempted to commit suicide. On meprobamate he improved greatly. His agitation and his panic subsided. He joined a club, is able to travel about the city alone, and is taking a trip to Florida by himself.

Case 3. An old man aged 72, who had come from a foreign country to live with his 2 children, found himself unable to adjust to the new environment. He felt lonely and depressed and was unable to sleep even with sedatives. When brought to me he was suicidal. On the standard meprobamate dose of 2 tablets 5 times a day he quieted and began to sleep regularly. He developed a more philosophic attitude. He went to school and studied English. He even got himself a part-time job. This patient would normally have been considered a case for shock treatment, but his improvement on meprobamate has been sustained without relapse.

Case 4. A woman aged 50 developed a severe psycho-neurosis with anxiety, depression and somatic symptoms. She was referred to me in the psychiatric department of the hospital where she was being treated for colitis and diarrhea. She had received shock treatment some years previously and had undergone psychoanalysis without help. On release from the hospital she became restless and agitated and was unable to sleep. She locked herself in her room and cried constantly. She lost her job and was without work for 6 months. When she returned for treatment I placed her on the usual dose of meprobamate. From the beginning her anxiety and tension subsided greatly, and she was cooperative in psychotherapy. After 3 weeks her mood had improved sufficiently to permit interest in trying to obtain a job again. Although previously she had been unable to concentrate even on reading the newspaper, she now took a secretarial course and got good marks. She felt that she had to fortify herself with meprobamate just before her job interview, but she reported that she felt completely relaxed when it happened, and she succeeded in getting the job.

Case 5. A man aged 47, married, with a grown daughter, was a severe psychoneurotic of long standing with acute anxiety and suicidal tendencies. For 18 months he had been in a mental hospital where his brother also was a patient. He had had at least 60 shock treatments. Upon release he had been unable to secure a job for 3 years. Shortly before he came to see me he had found one that gave him satisfaction and paid him relatively well. At the same time his daughter married, which also made him happy. Then to his bewilderment and panic, just as everything appeared to be going fine, he started to break down again. He went into a suicidal depression, could not sleep, cried, and was terrified that he would lose his job. He was placed on the standard meprobamate regimen and after just a few days improved so much that his wife telephoned to say that she felt she had to express her gratitude as well as that of her husband. When he returned to see me he was much more relaxed and was able to talk freely. He has maintained his improvement.

Case 6. A woman aged 27, married, with 1 child, had had an acute schizophrenic episode of about 2 weeks' duration with hallucinations, ideas of reference, and feelings of persecution. She neglected everything and roamed about the house at night. Although it seemed impossible to help her without hospital treatment, the husband asked, because he had no one to take care of the child, to see if one of the new drugs would not make it possible to keep his wife at home. After 2 meprobamate tablets this patient slept for the first time in 2 weeks. She also got breakfast for the first time, made the beds, and cleaned the house. Her husband stated that her delusions seemed to be gone. After she had been on 10 tablets a day for 2 days I saw her again. She was a little sleepy but was mentally clear and lucid. No delusions were present. She asked, "What was wrong with me?" After 3 more days the drowsiness passed, and in 10 days she was fine. Her agitation and floor-pacing were gone. She said she felt "slowed down." In a few more days she felt so like her old self that she cut down the dosage of meprobamate on her own initiative. This, however, brought a return of her delusions, and the full dose had to be resumed. After 3 sessions of psychotherapy it did not seem necessary to continue treatment other than meprobamate. This patient would certainly have had to be kept in a mental hospital without meprobamate treatment.

In the treatment of depression meprobamate appears to be of greatest benefit in cases associated with tension and anxiety. At the higher dose levels used, even serious depressions proved responsive to treatment.

In addition, meprobamate has the great advantage of being virtually free of side-effects. This fact has been noted by all previous investigators of the drug. Toxic side-effects were not observed from extended use of meprobamate at doses of 4 Gm. per day. Those patients who required the higher doses of the drug for therapeutic effect were also able to tolerate them without undue sleepiness. Some patients did become somewhat drowsy for several days, but this condition was never incapacitating and soon subsided.

I am also able to confirm Lemere's observation that, unlike reserpine, meprobamate does not aggravate depression where it already exists or precipitate it in patients being treated for other conditions.

In severely depressed patients it is important to sustain the dose of 2 400-mg. tablets 5 times a day for an adequate period and not to attempt to reduce it as soon as good results are obtained. Premature reduction of the dose will almost always result in relapse and is frightening to the patient. Since toxic effects did not accompany the uses of the drug, I consider it safe to continue at the known effective dose for a period adequate to enable the patient, with psychotherapy if possible, to work out a more satisfactory emotional adjustment.

Summary

Meprobamate in doses of 2 tablets 5 times a day proved an effective treatment for neurotic depression. Best results were achieved in acute cases associated with anxiety and tension. However, even severe and suicidal patients proved responsive, including several who would have required hospitalization or electroshock treatment without the drug. Nearly all patients slept better and became more cooperative in psychotherapy. No toxic effects or side-reactions were observed with meprobamate other than transient drowsiness in a few patients. The drug did not increase depression. It proved important to avoid premature reduction of the effective dose in order to prevent recurrence of symptoms.

CLINICAL STUDY OF A NEW TRANQUILIZING DRUG
Use of Miltown

Lowell S. Selling, M.D., Ph.D., Dr.P.H.

Anxiety neuroses or tension states occur so frequently that there is a real need for rapid therapy to relieve the patient and enable him to recover. Attempts to find a useful drug are being made constantly, and among the most promising of these drugs are the propanediol derivatives developed by Berger. Studies of mephenesin suggested that tension states and other psychoneurotic conditions could be alleviated, but the drug was not consistent in its activity. The second propanediol derivative to appear was 2,2-diethyl-1,3-propanediol, which showed much more promise. Although it was consistent in its control of tension states, its duration of action was too short. The most recent compound of this type, Miltown (2-methyl-2-*n*-propyl-1,3-propanediol dicarbamate), is the subject of the present study. The pharmacology of Miltown was described by Berger. The drug has a selective blocking action on interneurons. It produces relaxation of skeletal muscles without affecting respiration and other vital functions and also has important effects on the brain.

Material and Methods

The present study was made on 187 patients who came into my office between Jan. 15, 1953, and April 1, 1954. All were examined physically, by the referring physician, by a medical consultant, or by myself. If any patient showed signs of an organic neurological disorder, or any other physical ailment, either during the physical examination or in the laboratory tests, he was eliminated from the study. Patients who were clearly psychotic were also excluded, although some are included here who were felt to be on the borderline between an anxiety neurosis and a psychotic depression. If the depressed patient did not respond to Miltown in one week, he was treated in some other manner; however, any patient who received Miltown as part of his treatment is tabulated. There was no separate group of control patients, but some of the patients taking Miltown later received placebos for control observations.

Miltown was supplied in 400 mg. tablets. The usual dose was one tablet after each meal and one at bedtime. During the study reported here, 54,100 tablets were dispensed. The largest amount of drug consumed by a single patient, over a period of more than 15 months, was 860 gm. The maximum daily dose was eight tablets for a 105 lb. (47.6 kg.) patient who was in a tension state. The dose was reduced after three weeks. Most patients were maintained on a standard dose of Miltown: one tablet (400 mg.) after each meal and one at bedtime. As soon as possible the dose was reduced, and finally the drug was withdrawn. All patients had regular sessions of psychotherapy in addition to treatment with the drug. Usually there were three sessions a week for the first two weeks and two a week for the next two. Then the appointments were stretched out until a maximum interval of six weeks was reached. Soon after this, both drug therapy and psychotherapy could usually be discontinued.

Results of Miltown Treatment in Psychiatric Patients

Diagnosis	No. of Patients	Recovered	Improved	Not Improved	Improved or Recovered, %
Tension state	43	17	24	2	95
Anxiety state	29	10	17	2	90
Alcoholism	10	5	4	1	90
Behavior problems, children	10	1	6	3	70
Conversion hysteria	19	6	6	7	60
Involutional depression	16	6	7	3	80
Situational depression	7	3	2	2	..
Psychasthenia	4	0	3	1	..
Postelectroshock confusion	13	9	3	1	90
Organic confusion	9	2	5	2	..
Paranoid psychosis	4	2	2	0	..
Psychotic personality	5	0	1	4	..
Manic-depressive psychosis, manic state	4	2	2	0	..
Manic-depressive psychosis, depressed state	6	0	3	3	..
Schizophrenia	5	0	1	4	..
Other diagnoses	3	1	2	0	..
Total	187	64	88	35	..

RESULTS

The diagnoses and results of treatment are summarized in the table. The following remarks will clarify some of the terms used in the table. The patients in a tension state were those who complained primarily of feeling "tight." They frequently said, "I get so tight and my muscles are so taut that I can't sleep." Very frequently, they had a headache that they located at the base of the skull. These patients had a minimum of fear or anxiety. In the anxiety state group are those who have very obvious symptoms of anxiety psychoneurosis. Alcoholism, as used in 10 cases here, applies to persons who came to the psychiatrist while they were drinking. The children with behavior problems were all restless and tense. Most patients with involutional depression who are listed here were primarily depressed rather than tense and had a great deal of difficulty in standing the heat. I use the term psychasthenia to refer particularly to the obsessive-compulsive-ruminative type of psychoneurotic. These patients complained primarily of ideas that kept forcing themselves back into their consciousness and of actions they had to perform in order to remain comfortable. The patients with paranoid states who are listed were nonpsychotic with fairly intact personalities and had some mild delusions, usually of infidelity.

It appears that Miltown was of considerable value in anxiety and tension states. Related psychoneurotic conditions, such as behavior problems and conversion hysteria, were also favorably influenced. In alcoholism, Miltown helped to avoid serious withdrawal symptoms and assisted in keeping alcoholics sober after withdrawal was completed. In frank psychoses, the results are not so favorable but may merit additional studies. It is interesting to note how patients with various types of symptoms responded to treatment with Miltown. These results are summarized below.

Headache.—The most dramatic reports of recovery or improvement in the patients who were given Miltown came in those cases where the patient's chief complaint was tension headache. The tension headaches are characterized by being located at the base of the skull and usually were linked up with a feeling of tension or a feeling of being "keyed up." Of 27 patients with this complaint, 23 either recovered or reported sufficient improvement so that they were not concerned with this symptom.

Tension, Anxiety, and Fear.—Miltown was of considerable value in relieving tension. Of 86 patients complaining of this symptom, all but 7 showed marked improvement. The tension state was usually relieved in three to four months. The average office patient had great difficulty in distinguishing between anxiety and fear. I have not differentiated but rather have included both symptoms to show the value of this therapy in such cases. Ninety per cent of the patients showed improvement with therapy.

Depressive and Manic Symptoms.—Patients who coupled the complaint of depression with vague fears and a feeling of tension and anxiety usually derived benefit from Miltown, but those who were suffering from a psychotic depression did not markedly improve. There were 14 patients who had to have electroshock treatments after Miltown had been tried, with unsatisfactory results. One other problem faced by the psychiatrist in office practice has been the control of hypomanics who were obviously disturbed but were not committably psychotic. Four patients had obvious manic symptoms. This number is insufficient to justify a dogmatic statement, but, in all four patients, treatment with Miltown made it possible for the family to keep the patient at his daily occupation in such a way as to cause a minimum of trouble or comment by fellow workers. The manic symptoms recurred almost immediately when use of Miltown was discontinued.

Menstrual Stress and Psychosomatic Symptoms.— Five patients with menstrual stress, so called because their tension was limited only to the time of their period, stated that while taking Miltown the stress diminished markedly until they were symptom-free and were discharged. Psychosomatic pain, which was found in 23 patients with stomach distress, and peripheral pain, found in 2 patients, responded to Miltown in the majority of cases. In three patients with neurodermatitis who were treated with Miltown, the condition cleared within a reasonable time (from one month to six weeks).

Sleep.—It was apparent at the start of this study that poor sleeping behavior was easily corrected. Since receiving my first shipment of Miltown for clinical trial in January, 1953, I have not needed to use a barbiturate or similar somnifacient. By adjusting the dose of Miltown, it has been possible to produce sleep in every patient except in those suffering from a true psychotic depression. Twenty-one patients who were recovering from electroshock treatment had considerable difficulty in going to sleep without medication for a period of from two to four weeks. In each of those patients, a single Miltown tablet helped to bring on sleep, and the nightmares that so often occur on discontinuance of electroshock treatments were not usually noted. Dreams almost never occurred with Miltown. When Miltown was used to replace other soporifics when dreams were the source of complaint, the dream disappeared. An interesting feature of therapy with Miltown is the lack of drowsiness during the morning when the medicament has been administered the previous night.

Miltown as an Adjunct to Psychotherapy.—The psychotherapist has patients with whom he cannot achieve rapport. It was found that all patients became more responsive to suggestion, to hypnosis, and to free association (conversational or discursive) therapy. Several patients who had emotional blocking in early psychotherapy sessions responded adequately after taking Miltown. The feeling of ease and relaxation that Miltown brought about very definitely increased the patient's confidence in the physician and broke down his emotional defenses.

Comparison of Miltown with Phenobarbital and Placebos.—I have records of 19 of the patients treated with Miltown who had taken phenobarbital before coming to me for treatment. None of these patients preferred phenobarbital to Miltown. Two patients were given phenobarbital instead of Miltown because they complained of sleepiness while taking Miltown, but, in short time, they asked for a restoration of Miltown administration. Placebos identical with Miltown in all but taste were given to 16 patients who had been receiving Miltown. Before the end of a week, all of them complained so much about the return of their symptoms that they had to be returned to Miltown therapy immediately. Miltown is not habit forming in the pharmacological sense, and tolerance did not develop. Most of my patients discontinued taking Miltown without difficulty and usually of their own volition. Long-time users did not require increased doses to get the Miltown effect but spontaneously were able to cut down the dosage.

Duration of Treatment.—Patients were treated for periods of time ranging from less than a month to more than eight months. Most of these are considered to have recovered, but 12 patients have remained in the same condition, although the dose of Miltown has been cut to one tablet a day and is probably providing only psychological support. In about half the patients, withdrawal from Miltown could be effected within a week. In the other half, careful and gradual withdrawal was necessary, and, toward the end, placebos were sometimes substituted.

Adverse Reactions.—Only three patients were truly allergic to Miltown. The first had two fainting spells and a temperature of 102 F. two and a half hours after administration of two tablets. He was given 150 mg. of tripelennamine (Pyribenzamine) orally every four hours, but it took two days for his temperature to go down and for edema to disappear. He was not given any more Miltown. Urticaria developed in the second patient after four days of treatment with Miltown. She was given 50 mg. of diphenhydramine (Benadryl) hydrochloride with each dose of Miltown, which controlled the urticaria. An angioneurotic edema developed in the third patient after Miltown had been taken for six days. The edema cleared up in one day after discontinuance of Miltown. Five patients complained of gastric discomfort after taking Miltown. One woman weighing 107 lb. (48.5 kg.), who was suffering from anxiety neurosis, took 20 mg. of Miltown over a period of 24 hours. When seen, she was markedly sleepy and her pulse rate had slowed to about 40 per minute. She was kept awake by keeping her moving and by administering hot coffee over a period of two hours. Later she was allowed to go to sleep, and she awoke after 10 hours. A male patient hoarded a supply of Miltown and probably ingested about 100 tablets (40 mg.) within 24 hours. He suffered no serious adverse effects. From these examples, I believe that this drug can be considered comparatively nontoxic.

SUMMARY AND CONCLUSIONS

Miltown (2-methyl-2-n-propyl-1,3-propanediol dicarbamate) is a practical, safe, and clinically useful central nervous system depressant. It is not habit forming. Miltown is of most value in the so-called anxiety neurosis syndrome, especially when the primary symptom is tension. Miltown is also useful in keeping alcoholics sober after withdrawal is completed, and it has much value in accomplishing withdrawal with a minimum of discomfort. Favorable results have also been obtained in neurogenic conditions of the skin, in abdominal discomfort, and in several kinds of headache. Miltown is an effective dormifacient and appears to have many advantages over the conventional sedatives except in psychotic patients. It relaxes the patient for natural sleep rather than forcing sleep.

PRELIMINARY STUDY ON THE USE OF HYDROXYZINE IN PSYCHOSOMATIC AFFECTIONS

Luis Farah, M.D..
Hospital Civil de Guadalajara, Jalisco, Mexico

The physician is often consulted by patients whose illnesses are caused or further complicated by emotional stress. Effective management of these disorders cannot begin until the stress-producing stimuli are removed or the threshold of tolerance to the stimuli has been raised to a level where reactions are within normal limits and peace of mind is restored.

The ideal corrective measure, from the standpoints of economy and expediency, would be removal of the stress-producing stimuli. The medical literature records many instances where rapid remission of peptic ulcer, for example, has occurred after patients had changed occupations, had taken vacations long overdue, or had solved familial problems. The number of these fortunate individuals is low, percentagewise; the vast majority of troubled patients are forced to live with their stimuli, either by the pressure of circumstance or because a clear delineation of these stimuli is obscured by interlocking complexity. Thus, the physician is faced with two alternatives (1) he can guide his patients to the development of a philosophic attitude toward the stimuli, as they are recognized, by psychotherapy, or (2) he can insulate his patients against the stimuli by drug therapy. The latter alternative is the easiest, quickest, and safest approach.

Choice of a drug to induce emotional calm should proceed according to the following criteria: (1) it should produce a therapeutic response rapidly, (2) it should be effective in the majority of cases, (3) it should not produce addiction, (4) toxicity should be minimal in the therapeutic range, (5) incidence of secondary effects should be low, (6) tolerance (resistance) should not develop with continued use of the drug, (7) it should be suitable for inpatient and outpatient therapy, and (8) it should not dull the senses, decrease perception, or interfere with mental acuity. Investigation of the drug hydroxyzine (Atarax) was conducted on the basis of these criteria.

CHEMISTRY

Hydroxyzine is designated chemically as 1-(p-chlorobenzhydryl)-4-[-2-(2-hydroxyethoxy)ethyl] diethylenediamine. The hydroxyzine contained in the Atarax tablets and Atarax syrup used in this study was the dihydrochloride salt, the structural formula for which appears in figure 1.

The chemical structure of hydroxyzine indicates that it is related to a group

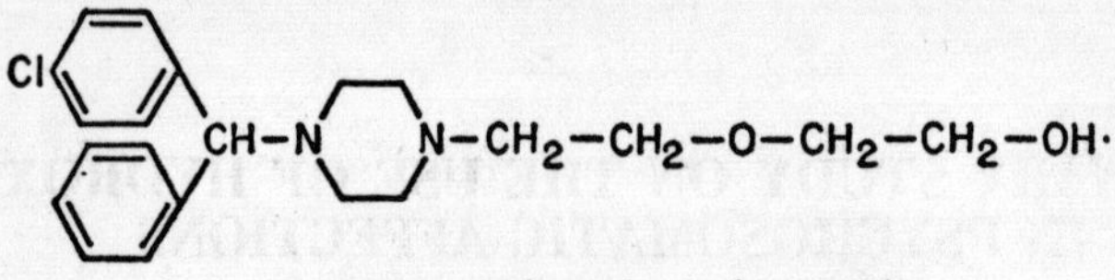

FIG. 1. Hydroxyzine hydrochloride

of antihistaminic susbstances identical with respect to their basic benzhydryl and piperazine configurations. Synthesis of hydroxyzine has created special pharmacodynamic properties that differentiate it from preparations of similar structure. Pharmacologic studies have shown that it has remarkable sedative properties, an effect that points to its possible usefulness as an ataraxic drug. The sedation produced by hydroxyzine, slightly different in character and much greater in intensity than that found as a common side effect of antihistaminic drugs, thus becomes a basis for all the drug's therapeutic indications. On the other hand, its antagonistic effect on histamine has aroused very little interest.

Pharmacologic Study on Animals

A simple examination of the behavior of animals subjected to the action of hydroxyzine was sufficient for an evaluation of its basic pharmacodynamic action.

Rats treated with hydroxyzine became quiet within a short time, their movements became slower and steadier, they assumed the most suitable position for undisturbed repose, and maintained this posture as long as they were left undisturbed. However, as soon as they felt some threat from the outside, they immediately fled from the danger, without loss of their customary agility and alertness.

Acute toxicity tests on 50 rats showed that the LD_{50} of intravenously administered hydroxyzine was 70 mg./Kg. A 1 per cent solution, pH 5, injected within one minute into the saphena vein, caused agitation among the animals; however, with a dose of 30 mg./Kg., this symptom was not observed. In acute oral toxicity tests on 50 rats, the maximum dose tolerated was 850 mg./Kg.; the average, 690 mg./Kg.

In chronic toxicity tests among rats, 5 animals withstood daily injections of 10 mg./Kg. for 30 days without mortality. Oral administration of 100 mg./Kg. in 5 rats produced no mortality over 30 days; 4 out of 5 rats withstood daily feedings of 200 mg./Kg. over a period of 30 days.

Clinical Methods

Hydroxyzine was administered by the oral route only. Coated tablets containing 25 mg. of hydroxyzine dihydrochloride or a syrup containing 2 mg./cc. was administered in daily dosages that varied, according to the patient, from 25 to 100 mg. Selection of the individual dose required adjustment to the proper degree of sedation, since the individual requirement did not seem to depend on the age, sex, or body weight of the patient. As an illustration, an initial daily dose of 25 mg. was reduced to 10 mg. for proper sedation of a robust adult weighing 198 lb., whereas in a 5 year old child, the same initial dose was raised to 100 mg. for proper sedation, without any untoward effect. In general, the hypermotive and restless patients with animated movements were given large doses without experiencing troublesome incidents. As the hyperactivity decreased, the dosage was gradually adjusted downward to a maintenance dose. On the other hand, patients with less severe symptoms were given small doses initially that were then increased as required to reach the therapeutic level, or decreased to an even lower level if somnolence or depression developed.

Hydroxyzine was administered to a group of 96 patients: 54 male and 42 female. Ages ranged from 2 to 93 years, and the duration of treatment varied from one week to two and one-half months. Patients were selected in several different categories of psychic and somatic disorders in order to determine the areas of psychosomatic medicine in which hydroxyzine would be most useful. In the group of patients with psychic manifestations, the drug was used in states of anguish and anxiety, in psychogenic insomnia, in infantile neuroses, and in states of senile excitation. Somatic manifestations were represented by circulatory, respiratory, and digestive disorders, as well as menopausal disorders, muscular aches and pains, and pruritis. Separation of these two broad classifications was not clear-cut. Most patients with manifestations of anxiety also complained of organic disorders; therefore, classification of the disorders was based on the one that appeared to be most prominent.

Six normal persons, serving as controls, received hydroxyzine in high enough doses and for a sufficient number of days to determine the normal physiologic effects of the drug.

Clinical Results

The clinical results of this preliminary study are presented in table I. In view of the wide variety of clinical types represented and the shortness of the observation period, the over-all results shown in the table may be somewhat misleading. In spite of these limitations, the table may be useful as a check list of areas in psychosomatic medicine where hydroxyzine may be therapeutically beneficial.

A brief summary of some clinical cases assigned to the various groups may serve as a key to the clinical results with hydroxyzine.

Psychic Manifestations. Patients suffering from crises of anguish due to emotional shock generally responded favorably to the treatment; the same was true of patients with anxiety neuroses of long duration.

For example, 1 patient, after being subjected to a reducing cure that caused him to lose about 30 lb., underwent an intense episode of anxiety neurosis, accompanied by great restlessness and constant excitation. Psychotherapy combined with hypnotic sedatives did not yield the anticipated results. Hydroxyzine quieted the patient from the very first day, his insomnia disappeared, and shortly afterward the pathologic manifestations ceased completely.

In a group of children and older persons, the response was satisfactory. It is interesting to note that tolerance to the drug was excellent, even in cases

TABLE I
Therapeutic Results with Hydroxyzine

	No. of cases	Satisfactory	Average	Inadequate
1. *Psychic manifestations*				
Temporary anguish neuroses	9	6	2	1
Permanent states of anxiety	12	7	3	2
Infantile neuroses	5	5		
Senile excitation	7	7		
	33	25	5	3
Somatic manifestations				
Circulatory				
Neurocirculatory asthenia	14	7	4	3
Tachycardia	5	3	1	1
Psychogenic arterial hypertension	2	2		
	21	12	5	4
Respiratory				
Bronchial asthma	4			4
Vasomotor rhinitis	1	1		
	5	1	0	4
Digestive				
Spasm of the esophagus	2	1	1	
Duodenal ulcer	2	2		
Peptic pseudo-ulcer	3	3		
Nervous dyspepsia	7	4	2	1
Mucous colitis	6	4	1	1
	20	14	4	2
Endocrine				
Menopausal disorders	9	6	2	1
Cutaneous				
Generalized pruritus	1		1	
Pruritus vulvae	2	2		
	3	2	1	0
Miscellaneous				
Feeling of unbalance	2	2		
Muscular aches and pains	2	1	1	
Facial tics	1	1		
	5	4	1	0
Total	96	64	18	14

where the patients were given relatively large doses. An explanation for this phenomenon was the great emotional tension present in these patients at both extremes of the age scale.

Circulatory Manifestations. Although nearly all the patients suffering from anguish and anxiety complained of palpitations and of an oppression around the heart, classification in this group extends only to those patients who indicated circulatory disturbances as the principal reason for their consultation.

One patient suffered from frequent attacks of paroxysmal tachycardia as the result of emotional irritation. Normal heart rhythm was restored with hydroxyzine, and the tachycardia did not recur during the two months in which he continued treatment.

An episode of psychogenic hypertension manifested itself in the case of the director of an institution when he was informed of the theft of a million pesos.[1] His arterial pressure rose to 220/110 mm., while for three days, excitation, anguish, and insomnia prevented him from taking any action in the matter. With 50 mg. of hydroxyzine, however, insomnia and anguish disappeared and he was able to act in a balanced and moderate manner. His blood pressure returned to normal within a few days after institution of treatment with the drug.

Respiratory Disorders. Hydroxyzine proved to be completely ineffective in 4 adult asthmatic patients. Its only usefulness in this connection was in modifying the insomnia and palpitations that were experienced as the result of adrenaline injections.

Digestive Disorders. A woman of 40 years was suffering from extensive dilatation of the esophagus and regurgitations as a result of spasm of the cardia, without detectable organic lesion. She had been treated previously by dilatations and hypnotic sedatives, but without favorable result. Upon daily administration of 75 to 100 mg. of hydroxyzine, the regurgitations began to disappear and she was thus able to swallow and retain nearly all foods. At the end of five weeks, her weight had increased by 7.7 lb. A new roentgen-ray study revealed a slight improvement, which was not in accordance with the patient's impression of being practically cured. This occurred at the time a new anxiety crisis set in, resulting in reappearance of the symptoms, although in diminished intensity. When treatment was resumed, the manifestations were brought under control.

A patient suffering from a duodenal ulcer that had been detected by roentgenogram was placed on the usual diet with antacids for a period of two months, but the epigastric pains persisted despite this treatment. At the time, the patient experienced great vexations and emotional problems that had to be solved. Upon treatment with 75 mg. of hydroxyzine per day, the epigastralgia as well as the hyperacidity disappeared.

Satisfactory results were also observed in other patients exhibiting a similar clinical syndrome and in whom the gastric ulcer was no longer apparent at the time of the follow-up roentgen-ray examination.

The most interesting results in this group of diseases of the digestive ap-

---

[1] U. S. equivalent: $80,000.

paratus were undoubtedly those obtained in a number of cases of chronic mucous colitis, which showed very pronounced improvement with hydroxyzine treatment, after having undergone various previous examinations and treatments with no previous improvement.

Menopausal Disorder. On a number of occasions, the effectiveness of the product was demonstrated in circulatory and nervous disorders connected with the female climacteric, i.e., when used in conjunction with hormone treatment.

Pruritis. A young girl of 18, shortly before her scheduled marriage, was afflicted with intense pruritus vulvae, with eczematous lesions aggravated by scratching. Cortisone derivatives produced poor results. Administration of hydroxyzine caused the pruritus to disappear within one hour, and the effect lasted for eight hours, at first, and then for six hours on the following days. Administration of the product at this interval was continued for two weeks, and the patient recovered without suffering a subsequent relapse.

Miscellaneous Symptoms. Included under this heading are 2 patients with nervous conditions who experienced a feeling of unbalance or nausea and in whom good results were obtained with this product.

For a period of two years, an extremely nervous patient had insistently complained of a pain in the back and in the nape, as if due to muscular rheumatism. Hydroxyzine was tried for two months, and the symptoms disappeared without further relapse, although they were replaced by other psychosomatic manifestations when treatment was interrupted.

The case of a 5 year old child with a facial tic is interesting because of the perfect tolerance of the drug in relation to the patient's weight. With a dose of 25 mg., the child's restlessness only increased and the tic did not begin to disappear until a dose of 100 mg. was used, without resulting in any observable prolongation of sleep or decrease in play activity.

Toxicity. No manifestations of toxicity were noted during the period of

TABLE II

Side Effects Reported by Patients in This Study*
(In Descending Order of Frequency)

Description	Occurrence
1. Increased intestinal peristalsis	Frequent
2. Mild rhinorrhea	Occasional
3. Increase in appetite, weight gain	Infrequent
4. Unsteadiness	5
5. Muscular weakness	3
6. Temporary constipation	2
7. Flatulence, tympanism	1

* In patients reporting side effects, these secondary effects usually were multiple; hence, two or more of the above effects may be covered by 1 patient's report.

observation with the doses used. The effects described in table II must be attributed to the product's physiologic effects rather than to any toxic phenomena. None of the patients developed euphoria; on the contrary, it was noted that they were better able to judge reality at its true value, and there is therefore no reason to expect that the product may cause a mania in any condition.

Discussion

The most constant effect exhibited by hydroxyzine was neurosedation, a state for which Delay et al. have proposed the term "neurolepsy." This state is characterized by diminished nervous and psychic tension, followed by tranquillity and peace of mind. Hydroxyzine, unlike such drugs as the barbiturates, bromides, and chloral hydrate, produces a calming effect without hypnosis. The sequence of events in this new pharmacologic activity is neurosedation first, followed by release from muscular tension; as tension vanishes, normal sleep is made possible. These three steps in the action of hydroxyzine will be discussed separately.

Sedation. Of the 96 patients observed, 95 confirmed the sedative effect. In only 1 patient was there an occurrence of excitation, the reverse of the usual reaction. This was the case of a nurse who exhibited excitation, arterial hypotension, and tachycardia one-half hour after taking the first 25 mg. dose. In hyperemotive patients presenting symptoms of anguish and anxiety, the drug produced a more favorable state of calm and tranquillity than any drug previously used. The patients did not lose interest in their customary activities but lost only their exaggerated response to external stimuli, and they were able to appraise the importance of these factors with serenity.

The intellectual state of the patients underwent no change, as demonstrated by the fact that 4 patients used their free time playing chess, dominoes, and cards—stating that they had won their respective games more easily under the effect of hydroxyzine because they played with greater self-assurance, forgetting their affective, financial, and professional preoccupations. On the other hand, in healthy persons to whom the product was administered and in many patients who were not suffering from excitation but rather from psychic depression, the feeling experienced as a result of sedation was annoying and disagreeable.

Relaxation of Muscle Tone. A sensation of asthenia or lassitude resulting from the relaxation of muscle tone, in the most widely varying degrees of intensity, was spontaneously referred to by half of the patients treated. Some of them declared that, although they felt the strength of their muscles had remained intact, they required a definite amount of mental effort in order to execute movements.

Others stated that their eyelids felt heavy and that they had a feeling of weakness in the facial muscles. Some experienced paresthesia, which they compared to the feeling of little drops of cold water or to mild itching. The foregoing sensations were described as pleasurable.

In 2 patients, the relaxation was observed objectively by the fall of the upper eyelids and by the absence of facial expression, denoting mild muscular asthenia. When the patients voluntarily closed their eyes, the lids could be lifted easily with the finger, in accordance with the method described by

Thevenard. The antinicotinic effect of hydroxyzine was noted by some of the patients who were habitual users of tobacco, this as a result of the muscular hypotonia, which neutralized the increase in muscle tone due to the nicotine.

Induction of Sleep. As a direct consequence of the effects referred to above, i.e., calmness and muscular relaxation, sleep set in more easily to the extent that the patient was relaxed in bed and sheltered from the effects of noises and external excitations.

When the doses used were higher than those required by the patient's nervous tension, diurnal somnolence set in, indicating a need for reducing the dosage and, occasionally, for interrupting the treatment. The sleep induced by hydroxyzine was generally nocturnal and similar to physiologic sleep, slightly prolonged in time. Dreams and nightmares decreased in a satisfactory proportion of cases. The drug's effect on insomnia of psychic origin was generally greater than that produced by barbiturates. Night terrors ceased entirely in the case of 2 children, and somnambulism vanished in that of another. The principal characteristic of the sleep induced by hydroxyzine was its complete reversibility and the fact that the patients awoke as easily as they usually did.

The pharmacologic effects of hydroxyzine as clinically demonstrated in its three components, i.e., sedation, relaxation of muscle tone, and induction of sleep, seemed to be more intense at the start of treatment and to grow weaker on successive days, as if there were some acquired tolerance on the part of the organism. The serenity persisted, however, with continuing treatment.

It would be useful to know, from the anatomic point of view, the site at which hydroxyzine exerts its effect. This point of the drug's action should be studied experimentally in connection with another product, chlorpromazine, which exerts a similar effect on the central nervous system. Hiebel *et al.* succeeded in localizing the site of action of chlorpromazine in the reticular formations of the brain stem.

Recent physiologic research has shown that control of the states of wakefulness and sleep, control of neuromuscular tone, and also control of the tone of the sympathetic nervous system are dependent on the electrical activity of the reticula. If we extend these data to hydroxyzine, in view of its pharmacologic similarity to chlorpromazine, we might conclude that hydroxyzine also depresses the activity of the said reticular functions, thereby accounting for the effects, mentioned above, that are put to good use in the treatment of psychosomatic diseases.

Mechanism of the Psychosomatic Manifestations. The nerve centers are in constant communication with the deep organs by means of the nerve fibers, which are traversed by the emotional impulses. Emotions of all kinds, regardless of whether they originate in the external world in the form of physiologic or psychic traumas, or whether they are generated in the inner world by memories or by the imagination, are consciously picked up by the cerebral cortex. The energy contained in these emotions is derived in the form of nervous impulses descending, through separate stages, from the cortex to the peripheral endings of the sympathetic nervous system that penetrate into the visceral tissues.

The persistent increase in cortical dynamism causes the appearance of conditioned reflexes, compelling the neurons to unite with each other in different ways in order to form new, more easily traversable pathways, along which the emotional excitations preferably travel. When the nervous impulses are transmitted with ordinary frequency and via appropriate fibers, the functions of the organs stimulated are physiologic. But when the excitations reach the viscera with excessive frequency and are received by nervous pathways of recent formation, the functional alteration is manifested by the morbid symptoms of psychosomatic affections.

With overly intense and repeated excitations, structural changes make their appearance in the tissues, and the disease, which was functional at the outset, is transformed into an organic disorder. Conversely, when the nervous impulses are deficient and travel at a reduced frequency—as the result of a reduction in cortical dynamism—pathologic symptoms of a functional nature likewise make their appearance.

Most synthetic antihistaminic substances block the passage of nervous stimulations. Hydroxyzine, by virtue of its chemical formula, belongs to this group and is useful only in the treatment of affections involving an increase in emotional tension. It has no effect where the psychosomatic manifestations are the result of psychic depression; the latter conditions call rather for treatment with a stimulant.

Treatment of the above diseases may be approached from the psychologic point of view; an attempt is made, through the use of psychotherapy or such physiologic means as stimulants and depressors of the nervous system, to modify the activity of the cerebral cortex.

Nearly all drugs that act on the nervous system occasionally produce inverse reactions that are the opposite of the ordinary reactions, and for this reason it is advisable to watch closely patients being treated with hydroxyzine.

Comparison of Hydroxyzine with Chlorpromazine and Reserpine. In the course of treatment, administration of hydroxyzine was alternated, in some patients, with that of another neuroleptic agent, thus making possible the following comparisons: (1) Chlorpromazine increased dreams and nightmares, it altered the number of pulsations by increasing or decreasing them, and it produced orthostatic hypotension. (2) From the point of view of the digestive apparatus, dryness of the mouth and a decrease in intestinal peristalsis were noted with chlorpromazine. However, chlorpromazine had other effects, such as blocking the vomiting and hiccup reflexes and other desirable properties, specific to this substance. (3) In equal doses, the neurosedative effect of hydroxyzine was superior to that of chlorpromazine; clinically, hydroxyzine caused no disturbance in the regulatory mechanisms of circulation and, in general, did not exhibit the sympathetic action of chlorpromazine. (4) Reserpine was likewise free of any sympathetic action but its absorption was very slow and it accumulated in the organism. It had a pronounced hypotensive effect and led to bradycardia. Sedation was more inconstant than with hydroxyzine.

Conclusions

An effort should be made to isolate the factors affecting the satisfactory tolerance of hydroxyzine. Two factors probably are involved: emotional tension and individual sensitivity.

The first of these factors seems to be basic, since it was observed in the present series of cases that: (1) the majority of the restless and agitated patients—with increased emotional tone—tolerated hydroxyzine satisfactorily and that the psychosomatic symptoms improved; (2) in a group of healthy persons whose emotional tone was normal, the sedative effect of hydroxyzine was described as disagreeable; (3) the patients suffering from psychic depression derived no benefit from the treatment and exhibited troublesome reactions.

In order to determine whether hydroxyzine therapy would be useful, it is necessary to judge the degree of intensity of the nervous and psychic tension, keeping in mind the fact that all cases showing improvement—even though apparently involving very dissimilar diseases—can be reduced to a common denominator, i.e., hyperemotivity. Selection of the cases to be treated depends on clinical and paraclinical study, and on an examination of the patient's personality.

The most constant pharmacologic effects of hydroxyzine are neurosedation, induction of sleep, and muscular relaxation; the best therapeutic results are observed in conditions accompanied by nervous excitation, insomnia, and muscular hypertonia. The first two symptoms can be ascertained by questioning the patient; since the increase in muscle tone is closely related to affective tone, it can be revealed in the movements, positions, and attitudes of the patient.

Hydroxyzine seemed to satisfy all the criteria of an ideal ataraxic drug for use in nonpsychotic hyperemotivity and tension: that is, (1) it produced the desired therapeutic response rapidly; (2) it was effective in sedation of the majority of patients (94 out of 95); (3) continued use did not seem to create dependence on the drug; (4) toxicity was negligible; (5) side effects were minimal; (6) resistance to the drug did not develop (although the period of study was rather short); (7) it was suitable for outpatient and hospital use; and (8) it had no deleterious effect on the senses or on mental acuity. Last, hydroxyzine can be used as a kind of pharmacologic test for measuring the degree of emotional tension.

SUMMARY

1. Hydroxyzine (Atarax) favorably modified psychosomatic manifestations when they were caused by an increase in emotional tension. In states of excitation, anxiety neuroses, and corticovisceral conditions, the therapeutic results obtained were often much more favorable than those produced by other therapies.

2. Two other drugs, chlorpromazine and reserpine, exerted the same basic action as hydroxyzine, i.e., conservation of the state of consciousness with concomitant nervous sedation. Among the patients to whom these drugs were administered alternately, many exhibited more satisfactory results with hydroxyzine. However, chlorpromazine and reserpine are important in other clinical applications where hydroxyzine is ineffective.

3. The effect of hypnotic sedatives in moderate doses is irregular and inconstant. In strong doses, such as those used for sleep cures in psychosomatic medicine, there is danger of intoxication and the treatment cannot be prolonged for more than two to three weeks. With hydroxyzine, on the other hand, a

neuroleptic treatment can be safely carried on for several months, since the drug is extremely low in toxicity and gives results that are comparable and sometimes superior to those obtained with other drugs.

4. If hydroxyzine treatment is interrupted after a short period of one or two months, manifestations of the disease reappear with less intensity. It may therefore be hoped that its administration for a sufficiently long period will be able to restore functional regularity in some patients.

5. The dosage of hydroxyzine must be adjusted initially in order to find the proper level of effectiveness. Variations in the patient's feelings and emotional tone necessitate such adjustments, which are deducible from observation of the patients during the course of treatment.

6. For control of nonpsychotic hyperemotivity and tension, hydroxyzine appears to be the drug of choice.

A CLINICAL TRIAL OF BENACTYZINE HYDROCHLORIDE ("SUAVITIL") AS A PHYSICAL RELAXANT

Anthony Coady, M.B., M.R.C.P.,
Senior Medical Registrar, Royal Northern Hospital; Lately Medical Registrar, Chase Farm Hospital, Enfield

and Eric C. O. Jewesbury, D.M., M.R.C.P., D.P.M.,
Neurologist, Royal Northern, North Middlesex, Chase Farm, and Luton and Dunstable Hospitals

A new drug has recently been introduced into this country for use in states characterized by emotional and physical tension. This drug, benactyzine hydrochloride ("suavitil"), is the hydrochloride of 2-dithylaminoethyl benzilate. It is a member of the group of anticholinergic substances, and experimental work in Denmark suggests that it produces a state of emotional and physical relaxation without drowsiness. For convenience its name in this paper is shortened to benactyzine.

Previous Observations

Jacobsen and Sonne (1955) found that benactyzine, injected subcutaneously into rats, abolished states of tension previously induced by certain conditioned and unconditioned stimuli. When the rats were expecting a mild electric shock they tended to remain immobile in a characteristic attitude with arched backs, stiff legs, and raised tails. After the administration of benactyzine, not only did the rats become relaxed in their attitude but they also resumed normal activity, as if there was diminished anticipation of the coming stimulus.

Jacobsen and Skaarup considered benactyzine to be the most effective of a series of anticholinergic compounds in modifying or abolishing signs of stress induced by "conflict-situations" in cats. Some effect was also seen after alcohol, but scopolamine and chlorpromazine showed no effect by the technique employed.

The effect of the drug on the responses of the human autonomic system to emotional stimuli was next investigated (Jacobsen *et al.*, 1955a, 1955b). In general, the responses (as shown by changes of pulse and respiration rate and of skin temperature and resistance) were less pronounced when the subject was under the influence of benactyzine, given orally, than without premedication or on control tablets.

Jensen (1955), in a clinical trial of the drug on a group of 110 neurotics, reported a beneficial effect in 75% of the cases. Both Jensen (1955) and I.

Munkvad (1955, personal communication) found that the patients who are likely to respond most favourably to benactyzine are those with persistent anxiety or tension, especially when associated with preoccupation or rumination.

The general pharmacological effects of the drug have been reviewed by Jacobsen (1955), who emphasizes its low toxicity, lack of hypnotic effect, and the fact that no tendency to addiction has been observed in about 600 patients treated. He states that in normal human subjects doses of 4 to 6 mg. produce a feeling of relaxation of the voluntary muscles and a blockage of the spontaneous thought stream. Side-effects such as dizziness and ataxia were also noted.

Purpose and Methods of Present Investigation

The present paper concerns 80 patients who, with only four exceptions, regularly attended the neurological outpatient clinics at three hospitals (the Royal Northern, Chase Farm, and Luton and Dunstable) where we together observed them. Our main purpose was to investigate the possible effect of benactyzine in producing muscular relaxation both in purely organic types of rigidity and spasm, and in cases where underlying psychogenic factors might also be present. The latter included such conditions as facial tic, writers' cramp, and spasmodic torticollis. A few case of intractable pain (unexplained facial pain and postherpetic neuralgia) where an obsessional factor was believed to be present were also studied. The diagnostic classification of the patients is given in Table I.

Table I.—*Diagnosis and Therapeutic Response to Benactyzine of 80 Patients*

Diagnosis	No. of Cases	Improvement with Benactyzine, not with Control	Improvement with Control, not with Benactyzine	Equal or Almost Equal Improvement with Benactyzine and Control	No Improvement with Benactyzine or Control	No Improvement with Benactyzine Control not Used	Improvement with Benactyzine Control not Used	Self-contradictory (Though 2 Said No Improvement with Benactyzine)
Disseminated sclerosis (with spasticity)	29	4	1	7	3	9	4	1
Facial tic	11	2	2	2	3			2
Parkinsonism	8	2		2	2	1		1
Facial pain	6	1	2			1		2
Writers' cramp	4	1	1			1		
Spastic dysarthria (cerebral arteriosclerosis)	4				3	1		1
Post-herpetic neuralgia	3	1			1			
Spasmodic torticollis	3		2	1				
Dystrophia myotonica	2					2		
Cerebral thrombosis (hemiparesis)	2			1	1			
Migraine (with tension)	2		1	1	1			
Stutter	1		1					
Primary spastic paraparesis	1							
Muscle spasm after poliomyelitis	1					1		
Friedreich's ataxia	1			1				
Spinal meningioma (with flexor spasms)	1				1			
Myoclonus	1				1			
Totals	80	11	9	15	18	16	4	7

We also wished to observe the incidence and nature of side-effects of benactyzine given to these patients in relatively small doses by mouth. Results were recorded in all of the 80 patients and also in two normal subjects who received gradually increasing oral doses up to 15 mg.

The method employed in 72 of the cases was to give a basic course of 2 mg. of benactyzine three times daily by mouth for two weeks. In a few early instances where tablets (known to us to be benactyzine) given in this way were without any effect, we prolonged the course for a further one or two weeks. In 10 of the cases an additional two weeks' treatment with 3 mg. three times daily was given, and in three cases the dose was increased to 4 mg. three times daily. In eight other cases 4 mg. three times daily for one week (preceded or followed by the same dose of control tablets) was given as an initial dose. The lack of rigidity in dosage schemes was intentional, but we did not find any improvement in therapeutic effect from prolonging or increasing the dosage within these limits. On the other hand, as is described later, the increased incidence of side-effects with 4 mg. led us to use 2 mg. as our standard dose. At the beginning of the investigation and in some later instances benactyzine alone was given to 22 patients, only 4 of whom reported improvements. In certain cases the patients were specially observed for any change in the degree of spasticity or tendency to clonus during the first hour after taking benactyzine in single doses of 2 to 4 mg. Patients were always unaware of any change in the tablets, and in the majority (37) of these cases we ourselves were unaware whether benactyzine or control tablets were being prescribed. The patients were seen by both of us at the end of each fortnight's course—sometimes more often—and their response, if any, assessed on both a subjective and an objective basis. The occurrence of any side-effects from the tablets was noted, but we were careful to avoid asking any leading questions about the possible nature of these effects.

RESULTS OF THERAPEUTIC TRIAL

The results of the investigation of therapeutic effects in the various diagnostic categories are given in Table I. The response of the whole group is summarized in Table II. From these figures it is evident that, so far as improvement

TABLE II.—Summary of Results in 80 Patients

Controlled Series (53 patients):
    26 reported improvement with benactyzine
    24 reported improvement with control tablets

Uncontrolled Series (27 patients):
    4 reported improvement with benactyzine
    18 reported no improvement with benactyzine*
    5 were bad witnesses

* Control tablets were deliberately not used in these cases.

in organic conditions is concerned, benactyzine was without significant effect. Some patients were enthusiastic in their reports of diminished nocturnal spasms and cramps, greater mobility and confidence in walking, and increased general activity, but these effects occurred almost equally, whether the patient was receiving benactyzine or control tablets. No immediate or transient therapeutic effects were observed in the patients who were kept under special observation during the hour following administration of benactyzine. The progress-reports of patients receiving tablets which turned out to be inert provide a telling illustration of the importance of control studies in an investigation of this sort.

Ten patients with disseminated sclerosis reported the disappearance or marked diminution of flexor spasms and jerks of the legs in bed at night. In five of these, improvement persisted either with or without control tablets. One man in particular who had been disturbed by frequent nocturnal jerks of the legs became completely free from them and said that he slept properly for the first time in years. He noted the improvement within two days of taking benactyzine, which he continued for two weeks. The striking feature, however, is that in the subsequent six months he has had no further nocturnal jerks, although taking only occasional control tablets. Some patients with severe nocturnal spasms have not benefited at all from the drug. Thus, in the case of spinal tumor (extradural meningioma) troublesome spasms were unaffected by benactyzine, but almost completely disappeared immediately after successful removal of the tumor.

In another case a persistent liability to painful spasms and cramps in the legs after an old attack of poliomyelitis was unrelieved by doses of 4 mg. of benactyzine, but responded afterwards to quinine.

Although we have not been able to demonstrate any immediate diminution of spasticity or clonus after administration of benactyzine, we cannot entirely exclude the possibility that certain patients may by some indirect means be relieved of troublesome nocturnal cramps and flexor spasms as a results of its use. At least, we feel that further investigation of this point is warranted.

Side-Effects in Patients Treated

No major systemic toxic effects from large doses of benactyzine have been reported in the Scandinavian series, nor have any been observed after the comparatively small doses which we have given. Certain transient effects, mainly of a subjective kind, however, were common. We prefer not to call them toxic, for many of them are clearly the effects claimed as advantageous in the psychiatric studies. Out of 72 patients receiving the standard 2 mg. dosage, 29 (40%) reported such side-effects. All of eight patients receiving a dosage of 4 mg. reported side-effects. Of the 50 patients who received both benactyzine (2 mg. and 4 mg.) and control tablets, 30 (60%) reported subjective effects after the benactyzine and 9 (18%) reported subjective effects after the control tablets. (In 18 of the 50 cases the control tablets were given before the benactyzine, and 4 of these patients reported various symptoms after the controls alone.)

The two groups of side-effects most commonly described by patients were feelings of general apathy or detachment (for example, "everything is too much effort," "lazy," "faraway feelings") and altered sensations in the limbs (for example, hands and feet feel "heavy," "unsteady," or "disjointed"; "as if my legs weren't there"; "knees feel like jelly"; "my feet seem glued to the floor"; "insecure in walking"). These two main groups of symptoms (separately or together) each occurred in 20 patients. Feeling of dizziness were described by 13 patients. The dizziness and strange feelings in the limbs often became pronounced on first standing up. Slight nausea was reported by three patients, throbbing or tingling sensations by three patients, and blurred vision by one patient. One patient experienced micropsia and another described "a horrible frightened feeling." Among individual patients taking 2-mg. doses there was much variation in their susceptibility to the drug. If subjective effects occurred at all, they developed quickly and lasted from a few minutes to about one and a half hours. When the drug was taken immediately after a meal the liability to symptoms was less and their onset was delayed.

EFFECT OF LARGER DOSES IN CONTROL SUBJECTS

Single doses of 2 mg. by mouth before meals were given to several healthy medical observers without hint of the possible effects. Some of these described "slight far-away feelings," a sense of relaxation or detachment amounting sometimes almost to depersonalization, loss of alertness, difficulty in concentrating, and slight hesitancy in speech.

Two medical observers, who were given increasing single doses from 2 mg. up to 15 mg. at a time, noted an ever-increasing degree of thought blockage. When single doses of 7 mg. or more were given, the thought blockage began to show itself by repeated breaks in conversation with such remarks as "I don't know what we were talking about just then"; "I can't remember what I was going to say"; "What did I say?"; or "Have I said that before?" The larger doses resulted in some slowing and slurring of speech and impaired performance of simple mental tests such as serial sevens and Babcock sentence. Such remarks as "I can't be bothered to think or to articulate," "I feel lazy—not drowsy," were made. In each case the subject usually wanted to lie down and shut his eyes, or else gazed remotely into the distance. His thoughts were easily distracted (sometimes by flights of ideas and visual imagery), though full insight and awareness were preserved. There was, however, a striking flatness of affect. Altered sensations in the limbs occurred after small doses —for example, hands felt "heavy," " a long way off," or " on the end of rods," and legs seemed to "sag at the knees." Objective incoordination was not pronounced. Clumsiness in complicated procedures, such as piano-playing, became evident after a dose of 9 mg., but this seemed more related to lack of attention, since simple finger-nose testing and handwriting were unaffected. Slight unsteadiness of gait was observed only after the highest doses.

The effects invariably began about 20 minutes after taking the tablets on an empty stomach. They developed quite suddenly, lasted for about one and a half hours, and then disappeared almost as quickly as they had come. The development of such symptoms suggests that it would be a wise precaution to warn any patients taking regular doses of more than about 4-5 mg. of benactyzine that they should not drive a car while under treatment.

No significant changes in pulse or respiration rate or in blood pressure occurred in the control subjects during the action of the drug. There was no notable pupilary dilation or dryness of the mouth, and no alteration of normal muscle tone or power or of reflexes was observed. Deep and superficial pain sensibility remained unimpaired; indeed, both subjects were acutely aware of discomfort from a tight-fitting cap and hard head-rest used in the prolonged electroencephalogram (E.E.G.) recordings.

E.E.G. FINDINGS

The effect of benactyzine on the E.E.G. of the two control subjects was observed after subcutaneous injection of 5 mg. and 7 mg. respectively. Subsequent symptoms were more intense than when the same dosage was taken by mouth, but their rate of onset and duration were similar. Continuous E.E.G. recordings (kindly arranged by Dr. B. G. Parsons-Smith) showed at first a well-marked stable alpha rhythm in each control subject and in one of them a considerable amount of underlying beta rhythm at 22 c/s. As the usual symp-

Suppression of normal E.E.G. rhythms by benactyzine in two control subjects (electrodes in transverse post-central position). Top: Records from subject A before and 20 minutes after subcutaneous injection of 5 mg. of benactyzine. Bottom: Records from subject B before and about one hour after subcutaneous injection of 7 mg. of benactyzine.

toms began to develop, both the alpha and the beta rhythms became suppressed, and thereafter for prolonged periods the records were quite flat (see Fig.). Random low-voltage 4-c/s waves in both frontal regions occasionally occurred. Short spells of low-voltage alpha rhythm reappeared at times, and this alternating suppression and return of the normal rhythm became more noticeable as the effects of the drug wore off and the normal E.E.G. pattern began to be restored. The same suppression of normal activity in the E.E.G. during this height of the subjective symptoms after subcutaneous injection of benactyzine has been noted but not yet reported in Denmark (G. Hess, 1955, personal communication). No such effect is produced by reserpine, chlorpromazine, or other compounds derived from the antihistamines.

Summary

The possible effect of the new drug benactyzine hydrochloride ("suavitil") in relieving muscular rigidity, spasm, or pain has been investigated in a group of 80 neurological patients.

No effect on muscle tone and no significant relief of symptoms were produced by a two-weeks course of 2 mg. of benactyzine three times daily by mouth.

No temporary reduction of rigidity or of tendency to clonus was observed after individual doses.

Although subjective improvement was reported after benactyzine by many of the patients, similar improvement after inert control tablets was reported by almost exactly the same number.

Some, though not all, patients who had previously been much troubled at night by flexor spasms reported that these had disappeared and that they were now able to sleep well. This possibly indirect effect warrants further investigation.

No systemic toxic effects were observed, but transient, mainly psychological, "side-effects" occurred in 40% of 72 patients who received a dosage of 2 mg. of benactyzine. All eight patients who received 4 mg. showed such side-effects.

These transient symptoms, though they may constitute part of the therapeutic effect in psychiatric cases, seem to us to be a disadvantage in the possible regular use of the drug in other types of case.

With single oral doses of more than about 6 mg. normal control subjects showed increasing thought blockage, impairment of concentration, slowness and clumsiness in carrying out complicated procedures, and a general flatness of affect. Such symptoms developed within about 20 minutes and lasted up to about one and a half hours.

Because of these symptoms it seems to us unwise to allow any patient to drive a car if he is being treated by large doses of benactyzine.

A striking suppression of the normal rhythm of the E.E.G. after administration of benactyzine has been demonstrated.

SUAVITIL IN THE TREATMENT OF PSYCHONEUROSES

Olaf Ostergaard Jensen

Suavitil is the hydrochloride of benzilic acid diethylaminoethylester. It has a peripheral anticholinergic effect and a specific effect on the central nervous system. In normal persons 4-6 mg. induce a peculiar blocking of the spontaneous associations, by one observer described as a maximal absent-mindedness, but the central effect is particularly pronounced when the subjects are exposed to psychic stress. In animal experiments with cats (Jacobsen and Skaarup, 1955) and with rats (Jacobsen and Sonne, 1955) certain stress-induced behaviour patterns are normalized by Suavitil. In human experiments Suavitil abolished or diminished the vegetative responses to emotion (e. g. skin temperature in the face, pulse frequency, etc.) (Jacobsen *et al.*, 1955). Therefore, it was found worth while to submit this compound to a clinical trial. Some clinical, preliminary experiments have been made by Munkvad (1955). Here a more detailed analysis of the clinical effect on psychoneuroses is presented.

The experiment is carried out in the Danish Red Cross Sanatorium, Hald. Some 2000 patients from the whole country are yearly submitted to treatment here, by general practitioners or other hospitals. About a third of these are psychoneurotics.

MATERIAL

In all 110 patients have been treated: 44 males and 66 females. The average age has been 40 years (16-75) for the males and 39 years (15-76) for the females. Most of the patients had been treated in several other hospitals before they were admitted to the sanatorium. 96 of the patients have been treated in the sanatorium, 14 only ambulatory. Ten of the hospitalized patients have continued their medication ambulatorily after discharge.

The Suavitil group is compared with a control group of 110 patients treated during the same period, picked out at random, but so that approximately the same types of patients are represented in both groups.

All patients have been submitted to our usual routine therapy consisting of occupational therapy, physical therapy, and psychotherapy in the form of personal interviews. The patients in the experimental group received no other sedatives than Suavitil (or placebo), while the patients in the control group were given barbiturates (pentothal or phenobarbital, the later often combined with bromides), corresponding to the routine medication used here for psychoneuroses during the past years.

The patients have generally been treated during their total stay in the sanatorium—an average of 70 days. The ambulatory patients were treated during a similar period.

Assessment of the Results

The following terms have been used in the assessment of the results:

"Good effect": Practically all neurotic symptoms have disappeared, and the remaining symptoms are only slightly disturbing. The effect exceeds the average.

"Moderate effect": Important neurotic disturbances have been abolished. Some symptoms remain, but the patients state spontaneously a considerable improvement.

"No effect": Means that the effect is uncertain. Some patients are not necessarily unimproved, but here the result is merely what could be expected according to our experience with patients of this type.

The assessment is based on the patients' own statements and our impression of the patients' willingness to accept a psychotherapeutical explanation and cooperate in the therapy. Moreover, their general behaviour in the wards was observed by the nurses, especially their relations to the daily routine and their fellow patients. The "normal progress" is well known by our experienced personnel. In no cases did the assessments of the different instances disagree.

Results

Table 1 shows the all-over results obtained after three weeks' treatment with

Table 1.
All-over results in the experimental group and in the control group.

Effect	good	moderate	none	total number of pts.
Controls	25 (23%)	28 (25%)	57 (52%)	110
Patients treated with Suavitil	56 (51%)*)	19 (17%)	35 (32%)	110

*) P 0—1 %

varying doses. There is no difference between the reactions of male and female patients. In some cases the effect of Suavitil medication was very striking as shown in the following example of case histories, which also gives an idea of the type of patients treated:

Case A: Married female patient, 28 year old. Psychoneurosis with depressive reaction. She had previously been completely healthy. She married eight years ago, but three years ago her husband suddenly disappeared and joined the Foreign Legion and was sent to the war theatre in Indo-China. He never sent her money, and she had to work in order to support herself and her two children. Her work was some distance from her home, and the whole situation gave her many worries. She was anxious about her husband, whom she still loved in spite of the fact that she despised his lack of responsibility. She reproached herself that she neglected her children. Her many speculations overcame her after all. She felt exhausted and sick and slept badly. Upon admittance to the sanatorium she had completely lost her spirits, was out of balance, irritable, and wept frequently. Somatically, she complained of muscular pain and showed objectively strong muscular tension.

During the first ten days of her stay she was given pentobarbital without improvement. During the following eight days 0.5 mg. Suavitil t.i.d. was without effect. The dose was subsequently increased to 1 mg. t.i.d. Her spirits almost immediately improved, she felt much more able to judge her situation, and her sleep improved. After three weeks' medication the Suavitil tablets were substituted by placebo tablets. Three days after all her former symptoms reappeared, and her thoughts became again chaotic. After ten days she again was given true Suavitil tablets with the effect that she again felt improved, resolved to divorce her husband and move to another town, where she would be able to do more for her children.

Case B: 56-year-old male, married. Psychoneurosis with anxiety reaction and obsessive-compulsive traits. For many years he had worked as a technical supervisor in a big industrial firm, frequently under hard pressure. From time to time he found the personnel difficult to manage. He always wanted perfect work, and when occasionally something went wrong he felt extremely worried. Moreover, as extremely polite conduct always has been an unwritten law in his working place he has had no possibilities of ab-reacting the worries. During the last years he began to doubt his abilities, and he felt anxious and uncertain towards the personnel and with himself. He feared committing suicide. The state developed into considerable depression, he was tired, and ruminated constantly. Prior to his admittance to the sanatorium he was treated with pentobarbital and phenobarbital without effect.

After his admittance he was at once given Suavitil, 1 mg t.i.d. After a few days his behaviour became more natural, and later he subjectively stated that his anxiety was reduced. After twelve days Suavitil was replaced by placebo tablets. His anxiety and compulsive thoughts soon returned, and he was further depressed, because he found his initial progress stopped. Twelve days later he again was given Suavitil, and the symptoms rapidly disappeared. He regained his self-confidence and energy, and felt that he after all was able to manage his job.

Further Analysis of the Material

The longer the disease has lasted the poorer the results seem to be, although

Table 2.
The effect in relation to the duration of the present neurosis.

Result	1 year or less	1-10 years	more than 10 years
Good	14 (64%)	31 (57%)	11 (33%)
Moderate	4 (18%)	5 (10%)	10 (29%)
No	4 (18%)	18 (33%)	13 (38%)
Total	22	54	34

the difference hardly is significant (Table 2). Some patients revealed no psychic trauma in their histories, in others an apparent psychic trauma was found. Some of the latter patients were up against insoluble problems, for example unhappy marriages, which could not be dissolved because of the children, chronic somatic diseases giving a feeling of invalidism among very active patients, frigidity affecting normal sexual intercourse, etc. From Table 3 it can be seen that the effect is considerably less when persistent insoluble

Table 3.
Prognostic factors.

Results	No apparent psychic trauma	Persistent psychic trauma	Persistent insoluble conflicts
Good	7 (46%)	41 (59%)	8 (29%)
Moderate ..	2 (14%)	12 (16%)	8 (29%)
No	6 (40%)	16 (25%)	12 (42%)
Total	15	69	28*)

*) $P = 1-2\%$.

problems are present. No statistical significant differences can be seen between the groups of patients with no psychic trauma and those with psychic traumata, but without "insoluble" problems.

The psychoneurotic disorders with anxiety, neurotic-depressive, and partly with obsessive-compulsive reactions or asthenic reactions seem to be influenced

Table 4.
The effect in the different types of psychoneurotic disorders.

Effect	good	moderate	no	total
Psychoneuroses with:				
Anxiety reaction	5	1	1	6
Obsessive-compulsive reaction	2	3	2	7
Neurotic-depressive reaction	35	5	10	50
Hysterical reaction without anxiety reaction	0	0	4	4
Somatic symptoms*)	1	3	1	5
Asthenic reaction	11	6	11	28
Hypochondrial reaction	1	1	3	5
Endogenous depression	0	1	3	4
Senile dementia	0	0	1	1

*) Myosis, heart troubles, etc. No. cases of gastric ulcer, asthma, etc. have been included in this group.

by Suavitil (Table 4).

All patients were submitted to a psychological examination at their admittance. In about a third of the cases the basic constitution could be determined, and the response of the treatment in the different constitutional factors is seen from Table 5. It is remarkable that psychoneuroses developed in a depressive

Table 5.
Basic factors and their influence on the treatment.

	good	moderate	no	total
Endogenous depressive constitution	4	1	0	5
Character neurosis	3	2	2	7
Psychopathy	4	1	7	12
Low I. Q.	1	0	1	2
Climacterium	6	2	3	11

constitution seem to respond well to the medication in spite of the fact that the endogenous depressions do not react. The figures are small, but the trend is clear. On the other hand, a psychopathic constitution diminishes the chances for a good effect of Suavitil. Among the 12 patients with a psychopathic constitution, 3 had depressive reaction (effect in all cases), 4 asthenic reaction (effect in one case), 3 anxiety reaction (effect in one case), 1 an obsessive-compulsive reaction, and 1 a hysterical reaction.

Placebo Reactions

Placebo tablets have been administered to 40 patients, who responded well or fairly well to the Suavitil medication. The patients, the nurses, and my colleagues were unaware which kind of tablets were given. In one case the beneficial effect of the previous Suavitil medication was maintained, and one patient felt better. The others relapsed, but the improvement was regained when Suavitil was given again.

Effective Doses and Side-Effects

Only a few of the patients reacted to a daily dose of 0.5 mg. t.i.d. With a dose of 1.5 mg. t.i.d. almost the same effect was obtained as after 1 mg. t.i.d. daily, but the higher dose may cause a slight blocking of the thoughts in a few cases.

Only few and insignificant side-effects have been observed. Some patients have complained of a slight dizziness, a slight blocking of the thoughts and an undefined feeling of "queerness." No systemic side-effects have been observed: no icterus, no depression, no Parkinsonism. Complete blood examinations have been made on 50 patients during the whole medication without showing any sign of blood changes. In no cases has Suavitil caused euphoria. Obviously the patients felt better, but this was only a mere restoring of the natural feeling of well-being, and there has never been any tendency to increase the dose.

Effect in Ambulantly Treated Patients

Fourteen patients suffering from types of psychoneuroses in which a good result could be expected were treated ambulantly. A good result was found in 11 cases, and a moderate in 2 cases. All had previously been treated in vain for a longer time by general practitioners with the common sedatives (especially barbiturates) (10 with a neurotic-depressive reaction, 33 with an obsessive-compulsive reaction, and 1 with asthenic symptoms). Ten of the patients treated in the sanatorium continued the medication after they had been discharged with a continued good result.

It is still too early to assess the lasting results of the medication, but the few available observations seem encouraging. One patient started to work after her discharge in a place where difficulties very frequently arise, but she felt calm and unimpressed even in complicated situations and even after she had discontinued the medication for two months. Five other patients have spontaneously discontinued their medication because they felt completely well.

Discussion

In the cases where an effect was obtained the improvement began after a few days' medication. The patients became more open and sociable, more relaxed, and much better fit for psychotherapeutical measures. A few days later the patients felt a subjective effect. One of the patients described it as follows: His former chaotic thinking decreased and was little by little replaced by plan and system. The rumination preventing sleep disappeared and the sleep became normal again. He found his fellow patients more kind and conversable. His spirits rose, but without any tendency to euphoria.

In the good cases all symptoms within the psychoneurotic syndrome disappeared, but the trend to speculate and ruminate seemed to be especially early and favourably influenced. The patients felt that a barrier had been established between them and the external influences, especially the purely practical difficulties. This was not caused by lethargy, but by the feeling from the side of the patients that even their problems had a solution. In this way a vicious circle was broken, a better effect of psycho-therapy obtained, and the whole psychoneurotic complex was dissolved with a subsequent improvement.

However, the barrier can be forced if the external noxious influences are too intense. This is confirmed by the observation in Table 3 that patients with insoluble persistent practical problems are less beneficially influenced by Suavitil.

Summary

110 patients with psychoneuroses have been treated with Suavitil (benzilic acid diethylaminoethylester, hydrochloride)—a new drug with a specific effect on the central nervous system. A beneficial effect was obtained in 75% of the cases, much superior to what could be seen after medication with barbiturates. Especially patients with anxiety reactions, depressive reactions, and obsessive-compulsive reactions responded favourably to the medication.

A NEW DRUG EFFECTIVE ON THE CENTRAL NERVOUS SYSTEM

E. Jacobsen

During recent years, some new compounds have been brought into use in the treatment of psychoneurosis, first chlorpromazine, and reserpine; later more have been added, and a new Danish product has also been brought under clinical trial. Benactyzine (NFN)[1] differs in many respects from the other types of drugs brought into use in neuroses. The compound has been known since 1936 and its peripheral effects are comparatively well known. It is spasmolytic; the anticholinergic effect is about 25% of atropine and especially the mydriatic effect is pronounced. The anti-Ba+ + effect is about 50% of papaverine. Moreover, it is a local anaesthetic and has a quinidine-like effect on the heart 3 times as strong as quinidine itself. However, these peripheral effects have never been utilized clinically except for the mydriatic effect, where a solution for topical use has been marketed.

The toxicity is low, (LD_{50} in rodents is about 100 mg./kg. i. p.). The toxic symptoms in animals are few and uncharacteristic, first appearing after administration of 75% of the average lethal dose. In normal human subjects, doses of 4-6 mg. have very pronounced effects: dizziness, ataxia and a feeling of relaxation of the striated muscles. A subjective feeling of a blocking of the spontaneous thought stream, "a maximal absentmindedness," is very striking. Hallucinations or confusion are never seen, even after high doses. After moderate doses, only a slight or even no decrease of the mental functions is found in psycho-technical tests. Objectively, the a-waves of the EEG disappear during the height of the subjective symptoms after 4-6 mg. subcutaneously.

Small doses of Benactyzine potentiate the anaesthetic effect of Evipan (hexobarbital), a few other barbiturates, and alcohol in mice, and abolishes the Hermann-Straub tail-raising reaction after morphine.

In doses giving no or few objective and subjective effects Benactyzine has a clear influence on the reaction in different stress situations. The behaviour of rats expecting a mild electric shock in the Gellhorn cage is normalized after doses of 1-4 mg./kg. s. c. At the same time the conditioned responses are more frequent and coordinated. The conflict-induced behaviour of cats in experiments with the Masserman technique is also normalized after about 0.2 mg./kg. s. c. In man daily doses of 0.07 mg./kg. perorally during one week were able to

---

[1] Benactyzine (NFN) is the generic name. Registered names in different countries are Suavitil (R) or Parasan (R). Chemically it is the hydrochloride of benzilic acid diethylaminoethylester.

diminish or abolish the autonomic reactions after induced, graduated emotions.

The experiments in rats, cats and man indicate that Benactyzine in doses giving practically no other symptoms is able to increase the emotional threshold for external influences. This effect together with the blocking of the thoughts, which also involves rumination, gives a strong indication for its usefulness in the treatment of psychoneurotics. Preliminary clinical experiments by Munkvad and the more detailed analysis by Ostergaard Jensen and Ostenfeld have confirmed this assumption. A rough estimate indicates that Benactyzine is able to add further 50% to the present therapeutic results in psychoneuroses with anxiety, asthenic, depressive, or obsessive-compulsive reactions. Psychoneuroses with hysterical reaction seem to be unaffected or perhaps even worsened. No effect is seen on endogenous depressions.

The side-effects of Benactyzine are slight and seem only to be due to the atropine-like effect of the drug. Of special importance is that no indication of an addiction to the drug has been noted in the about 600 patients hitherto treated. On the contrary, not a few patients have spontaneously stopped the medication when they felt better.

The mentioned properties of Benactyzine, the thought-blocking effect, and the increase of the emotional threshold supports the self-limiting tendencies of psychoneuroses in the optimal cases, psychotherapy is facilitated and the patients get a better insight in their problems. As also stated with some other new remedies, it takes some time (a few days to some weeks) until an effect is seen. This opens interesting theoretical perspectives. In psychoneuroses, apparently some vicious circulating processes within neuron chains in the central nervous system must be broken and new more healthy pathways opened, before an improvement is seen.

Benactyzine seems to work on a level in the central nervous system different from the other drugs used in psychoneurosis. It does not induce sleep as the barbiturates. It has no effect on the metabolism and body temperature as does chlorpromazine. It has no effect on the normal or pathological blood pressure as reserpine. Chlorpromazine has not the described effect on the stress-induced behaviour in rats and cats, and reserpine only to a slight degree. Unlike reserpine, Benactyzine has no effect on the aggressive tendencies in monkeys, and also in man it mainly seems to work on the effect of conflicts rather than on aggression. Many drugs derived from antihistamines have a depressing effect on the spontaneous activity of rats; this is not seen with Benactyzine. Finally, neither reserpine, chlorpromazine, nor other compounds derived from the antihistaminics have a specific effect on the EEG.

The perspective of possessing a full register of different drugs, acting on different levels of the central nervous system, opens wide possibilities for the pharmaco-therapy of mental diseases. It is to be hoped that the new Danish product may offer a contribution to this important field of the medical science.

MODERN DRUG TREATMENT AND PSYCHOTHERAPY

Alexandra Adler, M.D.
New York University College of Medicine, New York, N. Y.

For the past fifty years, ever since the new methods of psychotherapy were developed, there has been a difference of opinion as to whether additional use of sedatives during psychotherapy is advisable or not. Some have held that the use of drugs might seriously interfere with psychotherapeutic procedures. Members of various contemporary schools of psychotherapy have thought that a patient, if given a sedative, might erroneously believe that the chemical by itself would lead him to recovery and thereby interfere with the desired development of his own inner resources and initiative. Others, on the other hand, stated that if adequate explanations were given, patients would be able to anticipate and avoid such erroneous reactions. It is undoubtedly always the ideal goal to free a patient of the necessity of resorting to sedatives. If, however, planned as a temporary measure to help a patient over acute episodes in the beginning of treatment or later on during an exacerbation of his condition, the use of sedatives has been accepted by many. Within the last few years new chemicals with decided advantages have been offered to the medical profession in the field of psychiatry. These differ from barbiturates, bromides, and other previously used sedatives in that they produce the desired results without inducing sleep. Thus the patient can continue to work, participate in his usual activities, and is approachable by psychotherapy while under sedation.

The new chemicals used during treatment of neuroses differ from those used for psychoses. In neuroses, the meprobamates, widely known as Miltown and Equanil, hydroxyzine in the form of Atarax, and many additional compounds help, in the main, by producing relaxation from tension, often with subsequent lessening of anxiety. For instance, a young woman applied for treatment because, for the past few weeks, she had suffered from such tension and anxiety that she had had to quit a responsible job and had not been able to face having to return to work. The psychodynamics in this case, namely, longstanding rivalry with a successful sister and lack of proper guidance by the parents, were evident and the outcome of psychotherapy seemed promising. Much time and energy, however, would have been lost if the patient really had had to give up a desirable position for which she was well prepared. If it is evident that support through psychotherapy will not be adequate soon enough, as it would have been in this case, a temporary adjustment can now often be achieved comparatively easily with the help of one of the tranquilizing drugs. During the further course of psychotherapy, careful attention has to be given to the reactions, physical and mental, of each individual patient so that adequate dosage, eventual increase, decrease or cessation of drug therapy can be determined.

In the psychoses and, in particular, in schizophrenia, the drugs most often used are, as generally known, chlorpromazine, in the form of Thorazine, and the Rauwolfia derivatives. Their effect is more than mere relaxation: under their influence patients often act as they do after psychosurgery, in particular, after frontal lobotomy, inasmuch as their responses to stimuli of destructive as well as of constructive nature are usually diminished. This results, on the one hand, often in a diminution or complete disappearance of hallucination, delusion, hostility and other forms of unrealistic thinking. This, in turn, may result in a positive response to work, and the patient's interests in human contact may increase. Although schizophrenic patients are usually aware of these welcome changes, they are often even more impressed by certain drawbacks caused by drug therapy which, in turn make them dissatisfied and unhappy: the patients suffer from their inertia, they feel tired, complain of lack of interest in anything and often of a lack of sexual drives. This often causes intense depressions. As with lobotomized patients, they lose the sense of purpose in life and often feel useless. Their newly acquired insight into their psychiatric disability often makes them ponder about whether they are or were psychotic, with resulting unhappiness, whereas before drug therapy they considered themselves sane. Formerly, they often had felt superior to and even contemptuous of their environment. Now they realize that their feelings of superiority had been based on phantasy. They often comment, however, that living in phantasy was more pleasant than realizing their shortcomings. Consequently, the psychiatrist treating the schizophrenic with modern drugs has to be constantly on the alert to the reactions of his patient. He has to find out what can be achieved without the drugs, what psychiatric symptoms are eliminated through drug therapy, whether certain features, such as inertia, depression, blocking, and many others are caused by the underlying schizophrenic process or by the tranquilizers, and whether an increase or a decrease of dosage, respectively, improves the patient's adjustment.

It has become clearer than prior to the introduction of modern drug treatment that the schizophrenic, like any other human being, reacts favorably or unfavorably, respectively, to certain events. If the schizophrenic is well known to the psychiatrist, such reactions can often be correctly anticipated and, if necessary, controlled with an adjustment of dosage. The type of aggravating event is often different from that which may profoundly shock a normal person. For instance, one schizophrenic, on a long-term maintenance dosage of Thorazine, which is always kept as low as possible, may still react with panic and renewed formation of delusions when he feels slighted because he is excluded from a social event in which his relatives or friends take part. Such a situation occurs often because, although even if greatly improved through the medication, schizophrenics still often are not up to the standards of their former friends. On the other hand, actually catastrophic events which concern someone else, such as death of their closest relative or a deadly disease in the family, may leave them unmoved. This shows that a "holistic" approach, based on a thorough knowledge of the patient and his reactions, is needed to control dosage correctly in order to produce the best possible results.

Another impressive observation is that, while under the influence of modern drugs, quantity and quality of some other psychological manifestations change. This is, in particular, true of the dreams and of memories of the past. Whereas before modern drug treatment it was usually possible to interpret also the dreams of schizophrenic patients as an important manifestation of their conflicts, hopes and frustrations, their dreams while under drug treatment have often the character of a toxic delirium and, so far, it sometimes has proven difficult to relate such dreams to the specific personality of the dreamer. Such patients often have dreams of violence and mutilation, perpetrated and suffered by people unknown to them, which frequently hardly add to previous knowledge of the personality of the patients. Could it be that this change in the character of the dreams is related to the attenuation of purposeful thinking and planning of the patient while he is tranquilized? We know that the urge to solve a certain problem is in general at the basis of dreams, which, incidentally, evidently is the reason why the mentally deficient, who are unable to plan, hardly ever dream. This reduction of purpose and planning seems to change the habitual character of the dreamer while, at the same time, hallucinatory components come to the fore which are more often observed under the influence of intoxications, such as, for instance, during a fever delirium.

Memories of past events during the life of the schizophrenic also change while he is under drug treatment and, so far, we have no definite explanation of this phenomenon. Patients will suddenly remember vividly some details of their past which, in my experience, do not date back to the early period of the first years of life, to which commonly greatest importance is attributed when attempting to understand a patient. A woman, for instance, who for many months had been functioning adequately with the help of Thorazine, noticed that she suddenly clearly remembered some clothing that she wore years ago on certain occasions and she kept wondering how such recollections came about. The fact that this woman is particularly clothes-conscious may here be of significance. Another patient suddenly remembered names of places, for instance, night clubs which he had visited many years ago. Could it be that these recollections that keep puzzling patients because of their vividness and colorfulness, may be more related to the pattern of hallucinations, although their content corresponds to reality? Further study will be necessary in order to find out more about the significance of the appearance of vivid recollections of former forgotten material while the patient is under drug treatment.

In favorable cases the drug can finally be completely withdrawn and the schizophrenic patient may use his newly acquired knowledge and insight for a better adjustment. In other cases the drug is used over an indefinite period. Future years will bring important experience about the final adjustment of patients after their release from drug treatment, as well as of those under continued drug treatment. A thorough knowledge of the management and the effects of "psycho-pharmaco-therapy," as this new type of medication has been called, and experience with and interest in the management of the whole personality of the patient are necessary.

Undoubtedly these recent advances in drug treatment of psychiatric conditions represent a promising and fascinating development the importance of which for related fields of the natural sciences and psychology cannot be foreseen as yet. It has given new hope to many who long have been incapacitated and has offered new tools to those trying to help.

PSYCHOTHERAPY AND ATARAXICS
Some Observations on Combined Psychotherapy and Chlorpromazine Therapy

Stanley Lesse, M.D., Sc.D.,
Neurological Institute of the Presbyterian Hospital and the College of Physicians and Surgeons, Columbia University, New York, N. Y.

More than a thousand published reports and hundreds of conferences have weighed the benefits, indications and complications of chlorpromazine in psychiatric patients. This amazing total has appeared in less than four years, for it was only in 1952 that the first reports on 4560 R.P., the research code number by which chlorpromazine was originally designated, appeared in the literature. To my knowledge, aside from a few passing remarks, to the effect that chlorpromazine may "be of aid in psychotherapy," no detailed, serious investigation has been made into the combined use of psychotherapy and chlorpromazine. In this paper, we will present some preliminary observations on this subject gathered in a wide spectrum of psychiatric patients, seen over a period of more than two and one-half years.

METHODOLOGY

During the past two years, the author has used chlorpromazine in more than 250 patients. These were by far the sickest of our patients. Those who were not as ill were managed by psychotherapy alone. All received psychotherapy of various types in conjunction with the drug therapy. In well over 100 cases the psychotherapy was purely supportive in nature in which case persuasive, suggestive, reassuring or directive techniques were applied.

The material for this paper was gathered in the main from a study of 70 patients who were treated with psychoanalytically oriented techniques in combination with chlorpromazine. In 68 patients the therapy can best be described as brief psychoanalytically oriented psychotherapy in which the patient was seen at least two and sometimes, for short periods, three times per week. The treatment period varied from three months to more than six months in this group. The combined ataraxic-psychotherapy technique was also utilized for short intervals in two patients who were undergoing intensive reconstructive psychoanalyses.

The patients ranged in age from 15 to 55 years. Diagnostically they covered a very broad scope of psychiatric illnesses commonly seen in active psychiatric practices. Broadly categorized, 35 patients had psychoneuroses of various subtypes, while the remaining 35 had more malignant psychiatric ailments, namely:

(a) 25 patients were diagnosed as having schizophrenia of various subtypes, (b) 10 were classified as involutional psychoses.

The maximum daily dosages of chlorpromazine ranged from 200 to 800 mgm. per day.

Situations Where Chlorpromazine Was Used

All of the patients with psychoneuroses of various types were treated psychotherapeutically for at least two months before chlorpromazine was utilized as an adjunct therapy. With regard to those having involutional psychoses or schizophrenia, the drug was started as early as the first interview or as late as six months after the beginning of treatment.

Reasons for Using Chlorpromazine in Conjunction with Psychotherapy

Chlorpromazine was used as complementary therapy to psychotherapy for several reasons. In many of the involutional psychotics or schizophrenic patients the degree of anxiety and the bizarreness of symptoms was such, when they were first seen, that they were not amenable to psychotherapy on an out-patient basis and would have required immediate hospitalization where they would have remained for long periods receiving electroshock or other therapies, isolated from society. Chlorpromazine was added in an attempt to decrease the level of anxiety, and secondarily the other symptoms, so that the patients might be capable of cooperating in a psychotherapeutic relationship. The drug was also added during the course of therapy, in some schizophrenic patients, to control rapidly mounting anxiety which might be accompanied by difficulties with reality contact and which, in some instances, threatened to reach panic levels. Prior to the advent of chlorpromazine and some of the other ataraxics, we would have been forced to terminate therapy in these patients and institute electroshock therapy on an ambulatory basis or hospitalize the patient.

Chlorpromazine was utilized also in many psychoneurotic patients and in some pseudoneurotic schizophrenics, who were considered to be good candidates for psychoanalytically oriented psychotherapy, but in whom the degree of anxiety was such that weeks or even months might have been required in an attempt to decrease the level of anxiety to the point where the patients were capable of remaining in or benefiting from dynamically conceived psychotherapeutic techniques. The drug was added here in an attempt to shorten the period necessary to ameliorate the anxiety to levels compatible with office psychotherapy. In several instances the drug was utilized in a few very sick schizophrenics to soften the impact of anxiety laden insights at a time when the patients were "ready to run from therapy." Lastly, the drug was given to a few anxious individuals, who produced very few dreams, in an attempt to stimulate the production of dreams. The rationale for this will be given later.

Some Observations on Combined Therapy

(1) *Chlorpromazine and Transference Relationships*

The use of drugs of any type in conjunction with psychotherapy poses a problem. In the case of chlorpromazine some very interesting situations were encountered. It should be remembered that the drug was utilized only in those patients who revealed marked anxiety. Most of these patients, especially the schizophrenic and involutional depressed groups, approached therapy with pleading expectation. Many patients, who obtained a striking amelioration of tension and anxiety in a matter of days or even a week, showed a rapid and unquestioning gratitude and even an eagerness to relate to the psychiatrist.

It is my impression, from my own experience, that the transference relationships during the early weeks of psychotherapy with a very anxious patient are often tenuous, and that it is usually not until the patient no longer feels he is in constant jeopardy, that a strong positive transference is established.

It was noted, in many instances, that the relationship between psychiatrist and patient, in cases where combined treatment was successful in rapidly decreasing painful tension in a matter of a week or several weeks, was of a nature that often took many months to achieve in extremely anxious patients treated with psychotherapy alone. In many instances this relationship was a very positive one, the patient relating to the therapist in an effort to please him. The therapist became, to some of these patients, "the good father" who could do no wrong. He was looked up to with childlike awe. As the patient spoke about traumatic events of childhood, I did not note much hostility being transferred to me. In other words, any negative transference trends were blunted and minimized in comparison with what might be expected. One patient had a series of dreams in which her father was pictured as a threatening monster, while the therapist was conceived as a protecting, strong, kind individual who either gave battle to the monster or was able to carry the patient to safety.

In general, the affectual impact of the patient's story was blunted, a fact which was deleterious to the patient's gaining emotional insight in some instances.

Another group of patients revealed what may be called "drug transference." This situation occurred only in those patients who obtained a rapid decrease in anxiety and tension. However, instead of forming the complete childlike dependency upon the therapist directly expecting him to perform magic, the therapist became merely the purveyor of a "magic elixir." In connection with this, it should be noted that the public and medical practitioners alike have been subjected to a barrage of advertisements and reports claiming astounding therapeutic success from the use of chlorpromazine in certain types of psychiatric problems. Each patient "knows that the drug was meant for him" and he receives the medication with an aura of positive expectation. In some patients, I am convinced that improvement stems partly and at times wholly from this mass hypnoid suggestion.

Strong, positive transference relationships with this second group did not occur. In contrast to the first group discussed above, the dreams of these patients at times "personified the drug." By that I mean that the drug was symbolized as the protecting parent-like person.

Among those who obtained a rapid amelioration of anxiety there were also some who minimized the severity of their illnesses and as a result some were very evasive and very resistant to any free-association techniques. A few stopped therapy in a matter of weeks. It was obvious that a few remained in therapy mainly to obtain the drug. However, they were afraid, when the therapist suggested that their "local family doctor could carry on the administration of the drug, if that was all they were interested in." They had associated the therapist with the drug, and he was more or less a high priest who had a special knowledge of how best to manage the magic potion.

In those situations where the patient was given chlorpromazine for short periods, after being on psychotherapy alone for a period of several months, situations in which the drug was used as an adjunct treatment to manage a period of extreme anxiety, the transference relationship that had been established during the months of psychotherapy was not affected greatly. There was a more realistic attitude toward the drug and its possible effects. In these patients, though the medication was of help in ameliorating an emotional state which had bordered on panic, no "drug transference" of any marked degree was noted, but rather the benefits were attributed to the therapist's good judgment. In these cases the drug was discontinued as soon as it was felt that the level of anxiety was decreased to levels commensurable with the continuation of dynamically oriented therapy in the office setting. In some patients, as the drug was being withdrawn, there were mild transient expressions of concern that extreme tension might return. Also, there were some who had a series of dreams about food. One adolescent, on the day that the drug was stopped, dreamed of being nursed at the breast.

(2) *Chlorpromazine and Dreams*

I was struck, very early in my experience with chlorpromazine, with the spontaneous comments by many patients that they were "dreaming much more than ever before." I soon found that this statement was verified by most of the patients who evidenced marked anxiety. It did not occur when the drug was given to patients who did not overly demonstrate severe tension states.

The most striking observation, aside from the fact that dreams were being presented in greater numbers, was the finding that the affectual impact of the dream was the first thing to be effected. For example, there were many patients who related nightmares or rage-filled dreams prior to the onset of drug therapy, who after being on chlorpromazine for a brief period, related essentially the same dreams with similar symbols but with the affectual impact blunted considerably. Nightmares lost their terror and rage dreams were denuded of their anger. These same dreams or similar dreams were often reproduced for a number of days before the manifest content of the dreams changed. It appeared, when we considered the psychiatric problem as a whole, that the general level of anxiety or rage was decreased initially to a degree which permitted the affectual pressure behind the dream to decrease, but that there was enough residual anxiety or rage, though not overtly expressed, to stimulate the production of the dream. It was not until the levels of anxiety decreased below a certain threshold, which was unique for each given patient, that the content of the dream changed.

I have observed this phenomenon in several other situations. First, this situation is seen in the later stages of psychoanalyses in which the significantly improved patients may have dreams, which early in therapy would have been accompanied by great terror or rage, and which now are free of great emotional impact. This, in fact, is one of the criteria for improvement.

I have observed similar phenomena in experimental situations. Working with schizophrenic patients who had been given so-called "hallucinogenic drugs" such as mescaline or lysergic acid, we produced some terrifying or rage-filled hallucinations. If these patients were then given intravenous chlorpromazine, some demonstrated that the affect accompanying the hallucination was blunted before the hallucination itself disappeared. I witnessed the same psychophysiological phenomena, during my studies of lobotomies performed under local anesthesia. I found, broadly speaking, that there was a quantitative relationship between the amount of frontal lobe white matter cut and the degree that the patient's anxiety was decreased. I found also that the affectual component of hallucinations was ameliorated before the sensory aberration itself disappeared.

It has been mentioned that some very anxious patients, early in therapy, after obtaining a marked decrease in anxiety as a result of chlorpromazine, developed a very strong childlike dependency on the therapist, which was reflected in their dreams. The physician in these situations was usually pictured as the good, protecting, all-powerful and wise father-like figure. We found that unless this magical expectation was interpreted early in therapy, treatment would become stagnant, the patient expecting everything to come from the psychiatrist.

Early in the course of drug therapy, before the patients' stress was significantly ameliorated, and later, as the drug was being decreased or even shortly after it was stopped, there were frequently dreams of desire in which food symbols were common. One patient had several dreams in which he had a craving for milk. Another patient, an adolescent, about whom I have already related, had dreams of suckling at the breast shortly after chlorpromazine was stopped. In patients such as these, we found that psychotherapy would progress quicker and along a more realistic basis, if the dependency expectations were interpreted. This was often facilitated by the very obvious dream symbols.

(3) *Chlorpromazine and Clinical Symptoms*

If patients are studied in acute experimentally produced stress situations, for example during the use of various stress producing drugs, it can be demonstrated often that as the patient's tension mounts different symptoms will be manifested, the nature and the sequence of these symptoms being unique for each given patient. I have seen this observation confirmed in patients exposed to the stress of operations performed under local anesthesia. These patterns can be seen in office practice, if one is especially attuned to correlating the quantitative degree of anxiety and the various psychiatric symptoms.

The commonest pattern seen in practice is an anxiety state produced by a situation with which the patient cannot cope. This anxiety, in turn, fires off unconscious conflicts and the combination mushrooms into a pan-anxiety state. At some point in this psychophysiological chain of events clinical symptoms such as phobias, obsessive compulsive reactions, hypochondriacal complaints, psychosomatic manifestations, etc., appear either individually or in succession, the exact symptom, group of symptoms and pattern of symptom appearance being individual for a given patient. The symptoms appear to be unconsciously produced as secondary defense mechanisms against the painful anxiety. As the tension mounts, more of these secondary defense mechanisms come into play. If these secondary defense mechanisms fail to decrease the magnitude of the anxiety, the patient's ego defenses are overwhelmed and panic ensues.

With chlorpromazine therapy the opposite process is often seen. One notes that the degree of anxiety quantitatively must be decreased before a symptom or a group of symptoms disappear. This is noted, to be sure, when the patient is treated purely psychotherapeutically, but it can happen faster and more obviously with chlorpromazine. Often there is a delay of days between the time that the anxiety is decreased and the time that the symptom disappears. In this instance the symptom does not plague the patient to the degree that it did before the tension was decreased. The greater the amelioration of anxiety the more symptoms have disappeared. It is my impression that the last symptom to appear as the anxiety was increased was often the first symptom to disappear as the anxiety decreased. This particular observation must be studied further to see whether it can be explained purely by the laws of chance or whether it has significance.

(4) *Chlorpromazine and Depression*

Chlorpromazine has no beneficial effect on depressions which are not accompanied by marked anxiety and is of significant benefit in approximately only 1/3 of those with marked agitation. Some very interesting findings have been observed in the treatment of the agitated depressions. The depression is not ameliorated to any degree until the agitation or anxiety is first diminished. In some of the patients treated with the combined psychotherapy-chlorpromazine technique the anxiety could be decreased so that at first glance the patient seemed to be considerably improved. However, further probing revealed that only the affectual impact was blunted and that the malignant core of the syndrome remained lurking, as it were, beneath the artificial, relative calm. The clinical picture could be even more confused in other patients who obtained partial benefits from the combined technique. Some in this group appeared less anxious and depressed objectively and even denied subjective feelings of depression. However, probing revealed continuation of marked fatigue, lack of initiative, insomnia, anorexia and continuation of the pre-therapeutic hypochondriacal symptoms. This picture can easily lull a physician, particularly a clinician not specifically trained in psychiatry, into a false sense of security, in that he feels that the danger of suicide has been removed. I have in my files several records of patients seen by me in emergency consultation after they had made suicidal attempts while on chlorpromazine. These patients had shown such partial improvements, and a false sense of security permitted a relaxation of the vigil that is necessary with a patient having a severe depression with suicidal preoccupation. When the vigil was relaxed, patients had shown a sudden, precipitous increase in agitation and had made impulsive attempts to destroy themselves.

Severe agitated depressions, with strong suicidal preoccupation, in my opinion, should not be treated in the office with combined psychotherapy and chlorpromazine. Electroshock therapy is still the treatment of choice in this very sizable group of patients.

(5) *Patients' Reactions to the Adverse Effects of Chlorpromazine*

More than 50% of the patients treated with chlorpromazine have some adverse effect from its use. These side effects range from mild fatigue, dryness of the mouth or mild pruritis to marked jaundice or severe Parkinson-like syndromes. Because of the severity of side effects the drug had to be discontinued in one of every eight patients in whom it was used.

Most of these adverse effects occur during the first two weeks of drug therapy. If chlorpromazine is going to have a very beneficial effect on a patient, this benefit too usually begins during the first two weeks. Among those patients who obtained striking benefits from the medication, only to have the drug stopped because of a severe and often alarming side reaction, several interesting observations were made. Two patients manifesting very severe masochistic trends, or if you will, marked retroflexed rage, after going through severe acute influenza-like bouts, appeared clinically much better. The physical suffering they experienced had temporarily satisfied their unconscious demands for punishment.

I found to my surprise that even though the drug had to be withdrawn in some instances or other drugs added to combat the uncomfortable side effects, only two patients ran from therapy. In many instances a measure of improvement was retained and psychotherapy would be continued in the absence of the medication. Several of the sickest patients with severe hypochondriacal mechanisms were made much more tense by the episodes. In several patients, this was graphically illustrated by dreams in which they were caught in catastrophic situations.

In four schizophrenic patients, the drug had a paradoxical reaction in that it markedly increased the severity of the illness. This occurred in patients who required a clear state of awareness at all times in order to retain their contact with reality. The chlorpromazine in these schizophrenics, by causing fatigue or drowsiness, precipitated an active psychotic break necessitating the use of electroshock therapy.

(6) *Chlorpromazine and the Psychotherapist*

Chlorpromazine, when indicated in very anxious patients, should be administered in adequate doses following a brief explanation to the patient as to the reasons for its use and its mode of action. The therapist should do some honest "soul searching" before using the drug. One may find that he may be using the medication as a crutch or as an "easy way out" of a difficult psychotherapeutic situation which could best be handled by "working the problem through." The use of drugs as an adjunct to psychotherapy can readily blind one to his own feelings of inadequacy in the management of a particular situation. With increasing experience in the use of the tranquilizers a therapist's judgment improves as to when the drugs can or cannot be efficaciously utilized.

CONCLUSIONS

Chlorpromazine and the other newer ataraxic drugs bring a new concept of therapy to psychiatry. They work by decreasing the patient's anxiety. There have been some psychotherapists who have commented to the effect that to use drugs in combination with analytically oriented psychotherapy prostitutes the technique. This narrow concept is reminiscent of the intolerance to psychoanalysis present a generation ago. Combined psychotherapy-chlorpromazine therapy is in a research phase. Used properly, it can bring a number of very anxious neurotic and schizophrenic patients, who otherwise would be poor candidates for dynamically oriented psychotherapy, into its scope.

In a significant number of instances combined therapy eliminates the necessity for psychiatric hospitalizations. In properly chosen situations, it can be an effective tool in preventing patients who may mount to extreme anxiety during psychotherapy from withdrawing from treatment in a panic. We have found that combined therapy can effectively shorten the period usually necessary to ameliorate a patient's anxiety to levels at which he feels secure enough to emotionally incorporate the insights that the psychiatrist seeks to impart.

There are limitations and hazards in the combined therapies. Unless the therapist is deft in his management of the situation, an unrealistic dependency relationship can evolve that stifles all attempts to make the patient function on a mature plane. Some patients as soon as their tension is relieved run from therapy.

Combined psychiatric treatment, consisting of analytically oriented psychotherapy and chlorpromazine or others of the so-called ataraxic group, affords the psychotherapist an excellent opportunity to study the relationship between anxiety and the various clinical psychiatric symptoms.

It would appear, when one reviews the current trends in medicine, that progress in psychiatry will depend to a great extent upon the joint, closely integrated efforts of psychotherapists, biochemists and neurophysiologists. This new partnership will require patience, tolerance and intensive cooperation between those active in these various fields of medicine.

Part Three

CLINICAL EXPERIENCE:

(B) IN RELATED CONDITIONS

MILTOWN AS A TRANQUILIZER IN THE TREATMENT OF ALCOHOL ADDICTS

Joseph Thimann, M.D., and Joseph W. Gauthier, M.D.
Washingtonian Hospital, Boston, Massachusetts

Clinical reports on the new drug, Miltown (2-methyl-2-*n*-propyl-1,3-propanediol dicarbamate), have shown it to be an effective tranquilizer in anxiety and tension states. As these conditions are prominent in the postalcoholic state, and because Miltown is related to mephenesin, a drug which has proved of value in the treatment of alcoholics, an investigation of the action of this new drug as an adjuvant to the usual therapy of alcoholism was undertaken.

Like mephenesin, Miltown is an interneuronal blocking agent which relaxes skeletal muscle without affecting peripheral nerve or the myoneural junction. Pharmacological studies showed, however, that Miltown had a duration of action approximately 10 times that of mephenesin. In addition, and unlike the parent compound, Miltown produced a pronounced and long-lasting taming effect on animals without impairment of appetite or alertness. Electroencephalographic records showed marked synchronization of potentials from the diencephalon, and particularly from the thalamus, after the administration of Miltown.

In the present study Miltown was administered to 65 hospitalized alcoholic patients, and to 6 drug addicts, at the Washingtonian Hospital in Boston. Patients were given the drug during the subacute stage, usually immediately following initial detoxification treatment with chloral hydrate, paraldehyde or insulin. In some cases when the acute stage was not very severe Miltown was given immediately upon admission. The aim was to relax the patient during this painful period when tremor, apprehension, guilt feelings, irritability and sleeplessness are at their worst. The usual dosage was two tablets (each containing 400 mg.) three times a day, or every 3 or 4 hours as required.

RESULTS

The results are summarized in Table 1. Of the 65 alcoholic patients, 5 showed what we have called "very good" improvement. The response of these patients to Miltown was striking and prompt. They were substantially relieved of severe anxiety symptoms. Tremors subsided. They slept, ate, and felt well. In 33 additional patients improvement was graded as "good." Their anxieties were appreciably diminished, their mood improved, gross tremor and internal tremulousness were controlled to a substantial degree. These patients also slept well and their appetite improved. An additional 11 patients showed "some"

TABLE 1
Response to Miltown in a Group of Alcoholics and Drug Addicts

	No. of Patients	Very Good	Good	Some	None
Alcoholics	65	5	33	11	16
Drug addicts	6		3		3

improvement. In these the effect of the drug was perceptible but mild; in some, certain symptoms improved while others remained unaffected. In the remaining 16 patients the improvement is recorded as "none." This classification covers those patients with whom the drug was ineffective in the doses given. It also includes those—very frequently seen among alcoholics— who for psychological reasons reject all medications which keep them conscious and thus aware of their problems. They insist upon deep sedation which will "knock them out," with the result that adequate objective trial of a drug such as Miltown cannot be completed. In summary, then, the table shows that 75 per cent of 65 alcoholics treated received some benefit from Miltown during the withdrawal period, including 58 per cent who showed good or very good improvement.

The number of drug addicts treated is, of course, too small for purposes of evaluation. It is interesting to note, however, that the three who showed good response were all addicted to heroin. Of the remaining three, two suffered from a combination of alcohol and drug addiction (one to opiates and one to barbiturates), and the third was addicted solely to barbiturates.

In addition to its administration during hospitalization, Miltown has also been given to patients upon discharge, or during the adjustment period of the semihospitalization plan to help relieve their tensions, to support their effort to live without alcohol, and to encourage return to the therapist for periodic interviews. While statistical evidence of the effect of this supportive therapy cannot yet be presented, clinical observation suggests definitely that Miltown does help patients to keep from drinking and does strengthen their willingness to continue in psychotherapy, thereby definitely improving the prognosis for their rehabilitation. It has been our impression that such support often means the difference between the success and failure of total therapy.

Discussion

The search for effective relaxants as adjuvants in the treatment of alcohol addiction is a continuing one. The problem is to find an agent which will tranquilize the patient without subjecting him to the danger of a new addiction on protracted use. The potent sedatives generally used in the past— paraldehyde, chloral hydrate and the barbiturates—all entail this danger. In more recent years, therefore, a number of nonsedative agents have been tried with a view to evaluating their effectiveness and to defining their place in the total pattern of the treatment of alcoholics. Some general comments about them may now be made.

Relaxants fill the gap between the acute stage of alcohol intoxication with severe central nervous depression and the late postalcoholic stage when the body has adjusted to withdrawal. During the interim period the central nervous system has recovered to the extent that outright sedation is no longer necessary or desirable, yet the patient still urgently needs help in tranquilizing his emotions, controlling tremor and securing the recuperative benefits of sleep. A good relaxant can fulfill this function.

Relaxants also meet an important need in helping the patient to readjust to life outside the hospital where the old pressures of home, job and social life quickly reassert themselves. They sustain the patient's will to abstinence by keeping his anxieties and tensions at a minimum. They also encourage his periodic return to the therapist and lessen his resistance to psychotherapy. The fact, in itself, that the therapist "gives" him something to calm him and to support his effort persuades the patient that the therapist cares for him, and this strengthens the transference. His prognosis for recovery is thus on all scores improved.

Our study showed that Miltown fulfilled the functions of a good relaxant. It has in addition a number of characteristics which specially recommend it as an adjuvant in alcoholism, and particularly for prolonged use. Outstanding among these advantages is the fact that Miltown does not appear to disturb autonomic functions. Apparently it does not cause gastrointestinal disturbance, or lower blood pressure, or increase the development of cardiac disease if the patient resumes drinking. Very important also is the fact that Miltown does not seem to increase depressive reactions in patients already in danger of being overwhelmed by their own feelings of guilt and failure.

Conclusions

It was our experience that Miltown is an efficient tranquilizer, without side reactions or aftereffects. It proved a useful adjuvant in the treatment of addiction to alcohol and drugs, especially during the subacute, withdrawal period. It afforded definite relief from anxiety, agitation, sleeplessness and tremor in many cases. It has also helped alcoholic patients to keep from drinking by relieving their tensions after returning to their old environment, and by strengthening their willingness to return to the therapist for his continuing help. Miltown was found to be essentially nontoxic and apparently its continued use did not result in habituation or addiction. Of special importance is the fact that Miltown does not appear to affect autonomic balance—which in alcoholics is often unstable—adversely. Neither does it entail the danger of increasing depression.

THE USE OF CHLORPROMAZINE HYDROCHLORIDE IN THE TREATMENT OF BARBITURATE ADDICTION WITH ACUTE WITHDRAWAL SYNDROME

William Brooks, M.D., Lawrence Deutsch, M.D., and Robert Dickes, M.D.,
State University of New York, College of Medicine, New York, N. Y.

The steady increase in barbiturate addiction during recent years is a serious medical problem. Acute barbiturate intoxication ranks highest among admissions to general hospitals for acute poisonings, and barbiturates are now the most popular suicidal agents. Barbiturate addiction only recently has been recognized as a clinical entity. In 1949 it was shown experimentally that following the regular administration of large amounts of barbiturates, tolerance and well-defined abstinence changes developed quite consistently. It was formerly believed that barbiturates did not cause addiction, but rather habituation, and that abrupt withdrawal produced no symptoms except craving for the drug. Isbell *et al.* have stated that addiction to barbiturates is not only real, but more undesirable than addiction to any of the opiates. In chronic barbiturate addiction, abstinence is in fact more dangerous to life than is abstinence from morphine, in morphine addiction. The treatment of barbiturate addiction is difficult, and management of the withdrawal syndrome is lengthy and necessitates constant care.

A case is presented wherein chlorpromazine hydrochloride (Thorazine) was used in the treatment of chronic barbiturate intoxication, exhibiting the acute withdrawal syndrome. Contrary to customary treatment, barbiturates were abruptly withdrawn on admission to the hospital.

The patient, a 39-year-old, white housewife, was a known barbiturate addict for many years. She was admitted to the Kings County Hospital on September 29, 1954, with severe nausea, vomiting, abdominal cramps, weakness, and insomnia of one and one-half days' duration. At the time of admission she had not taken drugs for 16 hours.

The present illness began over 10 years ago, when the patient sought help for nervousness. Phenobarbital was prescribed. Shortly thereafter she began to take secretly increasingly large doses of various barbiturates. She finally averaged 2 to 3 grams daily. Hospitalized voluntarily in 1950, in a state mental hospital, where barbiturates were withdrawn gradually, the patient was discharged in 60 days, and soon thereafter was ingesting her usual amount of barbiturates. Paraldehyde was taken, rarely, when barbiturates were unavailable.

In 1952, the patient was admitted to the Kings County Hospital because of severe nausea, vomiting and tremulousness. At the time of admission she had been ingesting as much as 4.0 grams amobarbital sodium daily. Barbiturates were gradually withdrawn over a 31-day period. Shortly after discharge the patient was again taking 3.0 grams of amobarbital sodium daily.

During the same year she was again admitted to a state mental hospital on a voluntary basis. This admission lasted 4 months, and as usual barbiturates were withdrawn gradually. She also received 15 electroshock treatments. The patient said that she felt somewhat better following these, though somewhat confused and amnesic. Shortly after discharge from the state hospital, the patient was once again taking as much as 4.0 grams of the drug daily.

On September 1, 1954, she again presented herself at the Kings County Hospital because of nausea, vomiting, and severe depression. She was treated over a 14-day period, during which the barbiturates were gradually withdrawn. As usual, following discharge, the drug intake was resumed.

On September 29, 1954, two weeks after discharge, the patient again presented herself for admission. She had been without drugs for 16 hours and complained of nausea, vomiting, abdominal cramps, weakness, and insomnia. Physical examination revealed a very apprehensive, well-nourished and developed woman, who was sitting up in bed, vomiting and retching almost continually. Her lips and tongue were dry. She exhibited coarse tremors of the hands and fasciculations of the muscles of her extremities were evident. Her reflexes in general were hyperactive but equal. The remainder of the physical examination was within normal limits.

Course

During the first day the patient tolerated nothing by mouth and intravenous infusions were given to restore fluid and eletrolyte balance. Thorazine, 25 mg., was given intramuscularly at 6-hour intervals; and 8 c.c. of paraldehyde was given intramuscularly at 4-hour intervals. The vomiting and retching diminished in frequency and ceased in 18 hours. The patient appeared less apprehensive and much improved, though insomnia persisted.

Thorazine, 50 mg. 3 times a day, was given orally on the second and third days. Paraldehyde was reduced to 4 c.c. intramuscularly, at 4-hour intervals. The patient was much more relaxed and comfortable. However, coarse tremors and twitchings of various muscle groups were occasionally noted.

Thorazine was increased to 50 mg. 4 times daily, on the fourth and fifth days. Oral paraldehyde, 3 c.c. every 6 hours, was administered. The patient appeared calm and remarkably improved. There was return of her appetite and she tolerated well a 2,000-calorie, high protein, multi-vitamin supplemented diet. The coarse tremors decreased and muscular twitchings were infrequent. The patient still complained of insomnia.

Paraldehyde was discontinued on the sixth day and Thorazine was increased to 50 mg. every 4 hours. Considerable improvement was noted in the patient's physical and emotional status. She became cheerful for the first time since admission, applied cosmetics, listened to the radio and was ambulatory.

From the seventh to the thirteenth day, she was maintained on Thorazine,

50 mg. every 4 hours. The patient continued to improve. She became stronger, developed a feeling of well-being, and was able to sleep better by the ninth day.

On the thirteenth day, Thorazine was drastically reduced to 20 mg. every 4 hours, without producing any untoward effects. Improvement continued to an uneventful recovery. Thorazine was discontinued on the fifteenth day, and the patient was discharged from the hospital on the following day.

Patient was seen one month after leaving the hospital, and as yet had not resumed drug intake. She had gained weight and stated that she felt well.

She was seen again 3 months after discharge. She stated that she had not taken any sedation, and had no need to do so. Her only complaint was occasional insomnia.

Discussion

Isbell et al. presented a study which emphasized that sudden withdrawal of barbiturates or reduction to 20%-50% of the accustomed dose, is followed by a clear-cut withdrawal syndrome. This syndrome is characterized by weakness, apprehension, anxiety, slight fever, anorexia, nausea, vomiting, tremors, disturbance in the cardiovascular adjustment on standing, insomnia, convulsions, and psychosis. Convulsive seizures occurring during barbiturate withdrawal have been observed quite commonly at the United States Public Health Service Hospitals at Lexington, Kentucky, and Fort Worth, Texas. Hewitt reported 12 cases in which a toxic psychosis occurred during barbiturate withdrawal. Curran discussed the effects of barbiturates on emotional processes and occurrence of psychosis with barbiturate intoxication. Any combination of the above-mentioned symptoms may occur with drug withdrawal. Recovery from chronic barbiturate intoxication, and from the withdrawal syndrome, when it occurs, is usually complete and without permanent residual damage. At present, treatment of barbiturate addiction consists of withdrawing the drug slowly, perhaps over a period of a month. Some observers give an adequate dosage of a narcotic drug during the gradual withdrawal of the barbiturate in order to avoid the danger attendant on the concomitant abstinence. Isbell et al. report that unless the patient becomes psychotic, the acute withdrawal symptoms gradually disappear after 2 or 3 weeks.

The use of Thorazine made it possible to immediately withdraw barbiturates and to effect a rapid amelioration of symptoms. Consequently, the hospital stay was considerably shortened.

It is our feeling that the improvement noted was due to the effects of Thorazine and that paraldehyde was unnecessary. Significant doses of paraldehyde were given only during the first 96 hours. Paraldehyde was discontinued on the fifth day and it alone would in no way constitute adequate treatment for this withdrawal syndrome.

Summary

A patient with barbiturate addiction and the acute withdrawal syndrome was treated successfully with Thorazine. We feel this drug warrants further clinical investigation in the treatment of drug addiction.

USE OF CHLORPROMAZINE IN THE WITHDRAWAL OF ADDICTING DRUGS

Charles E. Friedgood, M.D., and Charles B. Ripstein, M.D.
Coney Island Hospital, Brooklyn, New York

The abrupt withdrawal of addicting drugs gives rise to well defined symptoms, including restlessness, nausea, emesis, insomnia and perspiration. Many of these effects, as Himmelsbach has pointed out, are manifestations of disturbances that are autonomic in origin. His findings and those of others indicate that the use of opiates, by upsetting homeostatic equilibrium, calls into play autonomic compensatory action, which then becomes a hyper-reaction requiring these drugs to preserve the quasi equilibrium. Consequently, withholding opiates from addicts temporarily produces an autonomic imbalance that results in the manifestations of the abstinence syndrome.

Investigators in Europe have reported that a new phenothiazine derivative, chlorpromazine, blocks or appreciably inhibits irritative neuroendocrine reactions. Their findings, therefore, led us to investigate whether chlorpromazine would alleviate the symptoms of opiate and barbiturate withdrawal.

MATERIAL

The clinical characteristics of 8 patients withdrawn from addicting drugs are presented in Table 1. The patients, 5 men and 3 women, ranged in age

TABLE 1. *Clinical Characteristics of 8 Patients Withdrawn from Addicting Drugs with Chlorpromazine.*

PATIENT	SEX	AGE	DRUG	DOSAGE	DURATION OF ADDICTION	COMMENT
		yr.		mg./day	yr.	
G.K.	M	26	Pentobarbital	900	4	Borderline schizophrenia; insoluble marital troubles.
V.O.	F	34	Demerol	400	2	Functional abdominal pain
K.C.	F	50	Morphine	120	2	Functional abdominal pain
A.S.	M	42	Morphine	90	½	"Renal colic"
A.L.	M	46	Demerol	600	5	Chronic peptic ulcer
C.M.	M	36	Morphine	120	1	Exaggerated complaints from latent duodenal ulcer
M.R.	M	55	Morphine	300	3	Cancer of rectum; perineal resection; colostomy; involutional depression.
R.F.	F	53	Morphine	180	1½	Cancer of breast; radical mastectomy with metastases; fracture of hip.

from twenty-six to fifty-five years. Five were addicted to morphine, 2 to Demerol, and 1 to pentobarbital. The duration of addiction ranged from six months to five years. Of the 8 patients only 2 had required drugs for control of pain. Five others complained of pain, but physical examination revealed no basis for their complaints. The remaining patient, a barbiturate addict, was a borderline schizophrenic whose marital troubles bothered him considerably. According to Rayport these patients would be classified as medical addicts since they first received the drug from a physician.

REGIMEN

All opiates and barbiturates were abruptly and completely withdrawn, and chlorpromazine therapy instituted. Five patients were initially given a single 50-mg. dose intravenously and a 100-mg. dose intramuscularly. Four hours later, and every four hours thereafter for the next two or three days, they were maintained on 100-mg. doses, administered intramuscularly. Intravenous infusions of fluids and vitamins were given concurrently. After the third day the patients were placed on oral medication, usually 50 mg. four times daily, and fed on a high-calorie diet supplemented with vitamins. Two patients were initially given the drug (100 mg.) intramuscularly instead of intravenously, and continued on this dose every four hours for five days before oral medication, 50 mg. three times daily, was substituted. The barbiturate addict was started on 50 mg. intravenously and 100 mg. orally, and subsequently maintained on oral medication, 50 mg. three times daily.

All patients were followed with liver-function studies—determination of cholesterol esterification, bromsulfalein retention, alkaline phosphatase, thymol turbidity, cephalin flocculation and serum albumin-globulin ratio—before, during and after chlorpromazine therapy. In addition electroencephalographic and electrocardiographic tracings were taken as well as daily intermittent checks on vital signs. When discharged from the hospital, patients were usually maintained on chlorpromazine, 25 to 50 mg. orally three times daily. They were re-examined weekly, and, if necessary, their dosage was adjusted. All continued the therapy for at least a month on an outpatient basis before the drug was discontinued.

RESULTS

None of the patients withdrawn from addicting drugs with chlorpromazine experienced the phenomena that constitute the abstinence syndrome. Most patients, when chlorpromazine was first started, slept for intervals as long as twelve hours, but could be roused by gentle shaking or prodding. All were kept in bed while they were on parenteral medication so that postural hypotension, which sometimes follows the administration of chlorpromazine, would not occur. Seventy-two hours after the withdrawal of the addicting drug the dosage of chlorpromazine was gradually reduced, and oral feedings were started. Unlike the addicts experiencing withdrawal symptoms, who have anorexia, these patients ate well. No nausea, vomiting or diarrhea occurred. On a dose of 50 mg., given orally four times daily, most patients were, at first, lethargic and seemingly indifferent to their surroundings. Their attitude might be better characterized as lack of responsiveness because they certainly were aware of what was going on around them. Psychomotor excitement was greatly inhibited. Only the barbiturate addict reported feeling jumpy and gave signs of agitation. Otherwise, no problems of restlessness, agitation or insomnia were encountered. Of particular interest was the fact that none of the patients craved or demanded addicting drugs. As therapy was continued, the psychomotor-sedative effect of chlorpromazine diminished and the patient became moderately alert. In contrast to the restiveness and hostility often seen in addicts during withdrawal, these patients were relaxed, calm and co-operative.

The 4 patients with functional complaints reported relief of their pains, and commented that they felt less tense than usual. It would, of course, be pointless to withdraw narcotics from patients with chronic intractable pain without first relieving their pain. In this series 2 so-called medical addicts were successfully withdrawn from opiates. The first, who suffered from chronic peptic ulcer, remained on chlorpromazine for seven days, being fed parenterally and prepared for surgery. On the eighth day a subtotal gastrectomy was performed, and recovery was uneventful. Postoperatively, he was comfortably maintained on chlorpromazine, 100 mg., given intramuscularly every four hours, in combination with Sodium Amytal, 450 mg. intramuscularly at bedtime, and was discharged twelve days later. The other, a woman with cancer of the breast and widespread bone metastases, was admitted to the hospital because of a pathologic fracture of the hip. Morphine, 30 mg. every hour, failed to relieve the pain. On chlorpromazine she became quiet, and her complaints ceased. After being withdrawn from morphine, this woman has for the past eight months been maintained on chlorpromazine 25 mg., given orally three times daily, and despite the fact that x-ray examinations show that the lesions present before her withdrawal are still present she has required only occasional non-narcotic analgesics for the occasional pains.

Of the 2 remaining patients, both of whom had apparent emotional disturbances, 1 had become addicted while receiving morphine to relieve pain after an abdominoperineal resection, which left him with a colostomy, and the other had become addicted by surreptitiously taking pentobarbital to relieve his tension. The patient with cancer never adjusted himself to the colostomy, became depressed and continually complained of abdominal pain in the region where the incision had been made. Morphine, 30 mg. every two or three hours, failed to relieve the pain. After withdrawal, however, the patient ceased to demand opiates, gained weight, regained his spirits and gradually became adjusted to taking care of himself. The patient who had been addicted to pentobarbital is a borderline schizophrenic with much anxiety and tension that was first related to his being in the service and later to his marital problems. Although his family reports that the patient is improved, his prognosis is doubtful.

Laboratory studies have given no evidence of liver dysfunction or blood dyscrasia in this series. Lethargy, dry mouth and constipation were reported by patients when they took the drug on an outpatient basis.

Since withdrawal plays a relatively minor role in the treatment of addiction, it is recommended that all patients continue to receive psychiatric guidance. Five of the patients in this series have been followed for more than six months, and 3 for three months, and none give any indication that they are presently using addicting drugs.

Discussion

During the withdrawal period addicts treated with chlorpromazine can abruptly and completely discontinue the other drugs with little or no discomfort. This is contrary to the belief that any method of withdrawal that does not use some opiate may result in death of the patient. Restlessness, agitation and insomnia seldom occurred; no nausea, vomiting or diarrhea resulted. Our findings, though preliminary, indicate that chlorpromazine offers many advantages over methadon substitution and morphine withdrawal in the treatment of opiate addicts. Since only one barbiturate addict was observed in this series, no general conclusion can be made regarding the effectiveness of chlorpromazine in managing barbiturate addiction. Results in this patient, however, indicate that the drug is probably of value.

Since chlorpromazine augments the action of narcotics and barbiturates it should be used cautiously in persons who are suspected of recently using these agents.

There are several possible reasons why chlorpromazine is effective in managing the opiate-abstinence syndrome. The first, which has already been cited, deals with the findings of French investigators, notably Laborit *et al.*, that the drug depresses the central and autonomic nervous system. When given in sufficient doses, it has a lobotomylike effect in that patients are relaxed, emotionally indifferent, quiet and immobile. Several investigators have reported cure of morphine addiction by prefrontal lobotomy performed to relieve intractable pain. A second possible reason for the usefulness of chlorpromazine in withdrawal of narcotics stems from its potent antiemetic action. Friend and Cummins and Moyer and his co-workers have reported extensively on this use of the drug. Their results have shown that chlorpromazine relieves nausea and vomiting caused by morphine, methadon, Demerol and codeine.

Summary

A new drug, chlorpromazine, that depresses the automatic nervous system, was evaluated in the treatment of the symptoms of opiate withdrawal, since such symptoms seem related to autonomic hyper-reaction. None of the 8 addicts treated, including 1 barbiturate addict, experienced the phenomena that constitute the abstinence syndrome. They slept most of the time during the first three days of treatment. Afterward, dosage was reduced, and oral feedings begun. No nausea, vomiting or diarrhea was noted. Psychomotor excitement was greatly inhibited. No problems of restlessness, agitation or insomnia occurred, although the barbiturate addict reported feeling irritable. In contrast to the restlessness and hostility often seen in addicts during withdrawal, the patients in this series were relaxed, calm and co-operative. Our findings are believed to indicate that chlorpromazine warrants further study in the treatment of withdrawal symptoms from opiate and barbiturate addiction.

THE USE OF CHLORPROMAZINE IN THE TREATMENT OF ACUTE ALCOHOLISM

Salomon N. Albert, M.D., Edward L. Rea, M.D., Cecil A. Duverney, M.D., James Shea, M.D., and Joseph F. Fazekas, M.D.
District of Columbia General Hospital, Washington, D. C.

Delirium tremens and psychomotor agitation are frequent complications of acute alcoholism, and their treatment at the present time consists for the most part of good symptomatic therapy. Perhaps the most difficult problem encountered in the management of such disturbances is the selection of an appropriate agent to control the manifestations of central nervous system excitation. Practically all available sedatives and central relaxants have been found to be either only partially effective, or to produce such intense depression that the patient is entirely dependent on the medical and nursing staffs to maintain his vital functions. Another objection to heavy sedation is that frequently on awakening the patient exhibits signs of excitation or release either from the alcohol ingested, or from the sedative prescribed or from both. The ideal agent would be one that would relieve the patient of his excitation without causing too much depression or subsequent release, and which would permit him to help in his own management. The latter is particularly important in a hospital ward where many such patients are managed at one time.

Chlorpromazine has been used successfully in the management of disturbed psychiatric patients. Sanguineti and Laricchia and Sizaret and Salomon have reported good results with the drug in 12 subjects with delirium tremens.

In this preliminary report we are presenting our experiences with this drug in 64 patients admitted to the alcoholic ward of the District of Columbia General Hospital, 21 with delirium tremens and the remainder with psychomotor agitation. In addition to the above disturbances, many presented complications commonly associated with chronic alcoholism, i.e., malnutrition, dehydration, avitaminosis, and cirrhosis. In order to evaluate the efficacy of the drug the usually prescribed adjuvants, such as vitamins, insulin and myanesin, as well as various sedatives and anticonvulsants, were withheld. The only immediate therapy consisted of fluids and chlorpromazine. The drug was given intravenously, intramuscularly, and orally.

RESULTS

Effects of Intravenous Administration. In 16 patients chlorpromazine was given in doses from 100 to 200 mg. intravenously in 250 to 500 c.c. of 5% glucose in either water or saline. This solution was administered within a period of approximately 30 minutes, and after about 15 minutes from the time of the beginning of the intravenous administration, most patients were asleep. The first noticeable effect of the drug was tachycardia. Mental and muscular relaxation were next noted, and the patient would then drop off to sleep, usually before 100 mg. had been administered. Varying degrees of hypotension were observed but never to below critical levels with the patient in the horizontal position. The sleep pattern of these subjects could best be described as natural sleep; i.e., they could be aroused with very little stimulation, and on awakening, patients without delirium tremens were well oriented and cooperative. Sleep persisted for 3 to 5 hours, and during this period the patients could be awakened to eat, drink, or go to the bathroom, after which they would immediately go back to sleep. One patient became excited after being given 50 mg. but fell asleep after 100 mg. had been administered. When the effects of the drug wore off, it was either discontinued or again given either intravenously, intramuscularly, or orally, as indicated by the condition of the patient.

Effects of Intramuscular Administration. The difficulties attendant upon the administration of fluids in the disturbed patient are generally recognized, particularly when large numbers must be cared for at one time. Chlorpromazine may be given intramuscularly, but because of its irritant effect it must be injected into deep muscle tissue. To date we have treated 28 patients with chlorpromazine given intramuscularly in doses from 100 to 150 mg. In some of these patients the injection was repeated within 6 to 8 hours when required. Except for the delay in onset of action (approximately 1 hour), the effects of the drug intramuscularly are essentially similar to those following intravenous administration. Acute hypotension has not been encountered in patients given the drug intramuscularly. Once the patients are asleep, intravenous fluids may be administered without the usual difficulties. At the present time we have discontinued the intravenous use of chlorpromazine because of the satisfactory results obtained by its intramuscular and oral administration and because fluids may be ingested in adequate amounts while under the influence of the drug.

Effects of Oral Administration. The drug has been given orally to practically all patients in this study in doses of from 100 to 200 mg. Oral administration has been resorted to when the patients showed only a moderate degree of excitation on admission or following intravenous or intramuscular medication. When given orally, approximately 60 to 75 minutes are required for the drug to become effective. Acute hypotension has not been noted following oral administration.

Discussion

Many of our patients were chronic alcoholics, and their reaction to the drug may be of interest, since most of them have previously received either barbiturates, paraldehyde, or both. The impressions of the patients were very favorable, and probably most important was the comment that "you are not nervous after you come out of it the way you are with paraldehyde."

It is our present opinion that the time required to overcome the excitatory state is neither shortened nor prolonged by chlorpromazine. The course of therapy required varied from 1 to 4 days. In no instance was there intense central nervous system depression attendant with its use, nor was there any evidence of synergism with the alcohol that may have been present. There were no fatalities in the present series of cases.

Chlorpromazine is recognized as a potent antiemetic, a property that appears to have considerable value in the management of subjects with acute alcoholism. Many of our patients complained of vomiting prior to admission, but in only 1 patient was vomiting associated with the use of chlorpromazine. As previously indicated, all other subjects had no difficulty in retaining food or fluids.

Convulsions are frequently observed in patients with acute alcoholism, and it may be significant that convulsions did not occur in the present series of cases.[1] Courvoisier has reported that chlorpromazine has mild anticonvulsant properties.

As previously indicated, the mean arterial pressure may occasionally fall following the intravenous administration of the drug. As long as the patients are maintained in a horizontal position the hypotensive action of the drug should not be any cause for concern if given as outlined above. Orthostatic hypotension with syncope has been encountered on 2 occasions when the patients either sat up or were ambulatory. The blood pressure returned to normal when the patient was placed in the horizontal position.

Chlorpromazine is reported to act synergistically with aliphatic narcotics. We have not found it necessary in this series of patients to use either paraldehyde or barbiturates in conjunction with chlorpromazine. If one desires to use combinations of drugs, it would be advisable to reduce significantly the dose if either barbiturates or paraldehyde are given along with the chlorpromazine.

Much work has been done on the pharmacologic properties of chlorpromazine; however, there is little information regarding its mechanism of action on the central nervous system. The evidence to date would suggest that chlorpromazine may have a blocking effect on the diencephalon. Its multiplicity of actions, the induction of sleep, hypothermia, hypotension, and its antiemetic effect all suggest hypothalamic action.

Summary

Chlorpromazine has been used in the management of over 64 subjects with acute alcoholism, 21 with delirium tremens and the remainder with psychomotor agitation. It was found to be highly effective in controlling the acute mental and physical aberrations associated with these states, the drug inducing a sleeplike state from which the patient could be easily aroused to take required nourishment and fluids. The time required to recover from the excitatory phase does not seem to be influenced by the drug; however, it appears that it possesses definite advantages over the sedatives usually employed.

---

[1] Since this report we have seen convulsions in 3 patients receiving chlorpromazine.

USE OF CHLORPROMAZINE IN CHRONIC ALCOHOLICS

James F. Cummins, M.D.,
Assistant in Medicine, Peter Bent Brigham Hospital, and Research Fellow in Medicine, Harvard Medical School,

and Dale G. Friend, M.D.,
Senior Associate in Medicine, Peter Bent Brigham Hospital, and Associate in Medicine, Harvard Medical School

One of the pressing problems in the treatment of any alcoholic is the adequate control of the withdrawal symptoms of tremulousness, excitement, and agitation accompanying any present day therapy. In utilizing disulfram therapy, it is necessary that the patient be without alcohol for a period of 6 days prior to the initial administration of this drug, if a disulfram reaction is to be avoided. This period of sobriety has been a hazard for many of those embarking upon the disulfram program because no medication previously available would control the psychomotor agitations as effectively as "one more drink."

It is a common experience among those who treat patients with disulfram that after varying periods of sobriety patients will often stop taking the drug and go on a planned "bender." Usually after several days of debauchery, these people want to quit drinking but are unable to do so because of the nagging and craving for alcohol. Moreover, they are very fearful of the symptoms of tremulousness, excitement, and agitation attendant to any "drying out" procedure mandatory before reinstitution of the disulfram program.

Psychomotor agitation is a phenomenon frequently observed in patients following moderate or severe inebriation. This can be most distressing, not only to the patient himself, but to the family, the doctor, and hospital ward personnel, because of the inability to control this agitation adequately. These symptoms may vary with the individuals, depending on the length and severity of the intoxication.

Withdrawal symptoms may take the form of any one of the following patterns; boisterousness, bravado, profanity, incoherent speech, clumsiness, sadness, elation, tremulousness to a point where the patient may not be able to sit quietly, insomnia, changes in personality, hallucinations, marked fear, and sometimes frank psychotic episodes. Patients may become combative and abusive to others around them, or so violent as to require commitment for psychiatric care for their own protection, as well as that of personnel. Others may exhibit profound automatism. Death from acute intoxication is a real possibility. The agitation gradually decreases over a period of days until the only complaint the patient has is a sensation of "butterflies or crawling things in the stomach." Meanwhile, the patient has experienced an emotionally distressful period. Sedation with paraldehyde, barbiturates, and chloral hydrate has been used in the past to control this excitement. Usually, these drugs have proved only moderately successful in the average case, and in delirium tremens or severe psychomotor agitation have been woefully inadequate. In our experience, none of the commonly employed measures such as hydration with 10% dextrose and water, insulin, ACTH, Cortisone, adrenal cortical extract, or thiamine has been of outstanding value in combatting postalcoholic psychomotor agitation.

During the past year, we have studied the antiemetic drug chlorpromazine and found it to be effective in preventing nausea and vomiting produced by a wide variety of drugs and clinical conditions. Since it is well known that nausea and vomiting are commonly produced by the ingestion of disulfram in the presence of alcohol, we decided to evaluate the effectiveness of chlorpromazine in suppressing these symptoms. In addition to its antiemetic effect, it has been observed that this compound also exhibited a mild sedative effect and has many of the properties of the antihistamine compounds such as diphenhydramine. It was felt this feature might prove somewhat useful in reducing the psychomotor excitement. While this study was in progress, we had the opportunity of conversing with Dr. Martensen-Larsen, who has treated a number of acute and chronic alcoholics with disulfram, diphenhydramine (Benadryl), and sodium chloride. He noted some suppression of nausea and vomiting with this regimen.

Material and Methods

We have treated a total of 60 patients suffering with acute or chronic alcoholism, incipient and frank delirium tremens who presented themselves to the emergency ward or alcoholic clinic for help. Each person was given a complete physical examination, including electrocardiogram when possible, prior to the institution of any therapy. About half of the patients treated had previously been followed in the alcoholic clinic and results of extensive work-ups, including chest roentgenograms, electrocardiograms, routine laboratory examinations, bromsulfalein tests, and psychometric examinations were available.

Irrespective of the quantity of liquor consumed, patients were given simultaneously 100 mg. of chlorpromazine and 500 mg. of disulfram, by mouth, within 6 hours, chlorpromazine 50 mg. was repeated. Twenty-four hours later, 500 mg. disulfram and 50 mg. chlorpromazine were administered. Forty-eight hours following initial therapy, 500 mg. of disulfram and 25 mg. of chlorpromazine were given. Thereafter, for one week 500 mg. of disulfram was administered daily. The dosage of disulfram was then adjusted to the patient tolerance, usually 0.25 or 0.5 gm. daily. If the patient was vomiting, 50 mg. of chlorpromazine was given intramuscularly and, with suppression of the vomiting, oral medication was begun according to the above schedule, except that the first oral dose was 50 mg. rather than 100 mg. chlorpromazine. In addition to the above therapy, in the more severely dehydrated patient some attempt was made to overcome this by intravenous dextrose and water.

Initially, patients were observed for 24 to 48 hours on the emergency ward. However, since no untoward effects were noted in these cases of frank delirium tremens, the medication schedule was carefully taught to a responsible person, wife or friend, who accompanied the patient, and the entire program was carried out on an outpatient basis.

Results

It was immediately apparent that chlorpromazine was effective in suppressing the nausea and vomiting produced by the disulfram-alcohol reaction. Of much greater interest, however, was the effect of this drug combination in preventing the usual post-alcoholic psychomotor agitation accompanying withdrawal. Within an hour or so most patients tended to become drowsy, quite calm, and some actually went to sleep. The sleep was described as refreshing and usually the most restful these persons had been able to obtain in weeks. This sleep period usually lasted 10 to 12 hours. Most patients had to be awakened for the repeat dose of chlorpromazine. Within 24 hours, patients were hungry, and they were able to take solid foods. Some tremulousness was still apparent at the end of this 24 hour period, but restful sleep could be secured at any time during the entire withdrawal period. Patients in several instances were able to return to work within 72 hours without having experienced the "jitters," tremulousness, or "butterfly" sensation so common during the withdrawal stage.

Controls were studied using chlorpromazine alone. Patients who had been drinking for a period of days were given chlorpromazine in a schedule as described above. In addition, a series of 6 patients were given chlorpromazine intramuscularly in similar amounts to avoid any possible absorption failure. In none of these patients were results as satisfactory as with the combination of drugs. Patients would continue to drink. The agitation was, at best, only partly relieved, and in only 2 cases were the patients able to sleep.

Controls using disulfram alone were not tested for it is known that disulfram administered in the presence of alcohol produces a severe physiological and psychological series of reactions. The nausea and vomiting attendant with this drug combination is the basis of conditioned reflex therapy.

Nausea and vomiting are variously reported to accompany disulframethanol reaction in 60% to 85% of cases treated. On the other hand, there are some persons who do not get a disulfram reaction with small amounts of drug and liquor, but, at best, these comprise only 1% to 2% of patients. We feel that the number of patients in this series is sufficiently large to eliminate this possibility. However, 2 patients who were being treated on an ambulatory basis for acute and chronic alcoholism, and incipient delirium tremens omitted the chlorpromazine prescribed, taking only the disulfram as outlined above. Both of these patients on consuming 0.5 gm. disulfram experienced a mild disulfram reaction. Neither stopped drinking and again took 0.5 gm. disulfram the next morning. Following a total dose of 1.0 gm. within 12 hours, a more severe form of disulframethanol reaction developed. Nausea and vomiting, agitation, tremulousness, flushing of facies, and palpitation were noted. Chlorpromazine was administered to these individuals, 100 mg. intramuscularly, with prompt disappearance of symptoms. The mild hypotensive episode in one of these patients disappeared soon after intramuscular injection.

Conclusions

1. We have presented a method for treating chronic alcoholics which eliminates the need to wait for "drying out" prior to the administration of disulfram.

2. Disulfram and chlorpromazine, when administered together in adequate dosage to the inebriated alcoholic, produce a tranquilized state more effectively than with any current method of sedation.

3. No untoward side effects have been noted in the treatment of these 60 alcoholic patients. Nausea, vomiting, and hypotensive episodes have not been noted in our experience with this combination of drugs.

4. Chronic alcoholics treated in the described manner do not suffer with the usual postalcoholic psychomotor agitation.

MEPROBAMATE (MILTOWN) AS ADJUNCT IN TREATMENT OF ANOGENITAL PRURITUS

Oscar J. Sokoloff, M.D.

Recently published studies of a new tranquilizing drug called meprobamate (Miltown) reported very encouraging results with psychiatric patients, particularly with those suffering from anxiety and tension states. The drug (chemically 2-methyl-2-n-propyl-1,3-propanediol dicarbamate) was reported to possess muscle-relaxant properties similar to those of mephenesin but of much longer duration, as well as unusual tranquilizing properties apparently related to a specific effect on the activity of the thalamus. All investigators described the drug as extremely low in toxicity and devoid of important side-effects.

Because certain dermatological syndromes have so frequently appeared closely bound up with emotional factors, the use of sedatives as an adjunct to therapy has become widespread in these conditions. Until recent years the barbiturates were most commonly used. Their usefulness, however, was limited by the fact that they dulled the sensorium and entailed the possibility of addiction. More recently chlorpromazine and reserpine have been used with success as antipruritic agents. While good results have been obtained, both drugs have produced numerous side-effects. Reserpine has been reported as giving rise to nasal congestion, depression, weakness, and nausea. Chlorpromazine has in some cases resulted in a general "malaise," sleepiness, heaviness of the head and limbs, vertigo, digestive disturbances, and jaundice. Because of the possibility of such reactions, Tilley has recommended that administration of the latter drug in dermatological conditions be limited to hospitalized patients who can be kept under careful supervision.

The present study was undertaken to assess the value of the new drug meprobamate as a possible adjuvant for the treatment of pruritus in private dermatological practice. As a beginning it seemed wise to limit the study to idiopathic pruritus ani and pruritus vulvae, both for practical reasons (they are among the commonest complaints in everyday practice) and for reasons of therapeutic rationale. It was our feeling, based on clinical experience, that emotional factors played an important role in the etiology of idiopathic pruritus ani and pruritus vulvae, and formed a very strong component of its persistence. It was our thought, therefore, that a tranquilizing drug might be almost clearly indicated in such a condition.

PATIENT SELECTION

All patients with presenting symptoms of anogenital pruritus were carefully screened by history, rectal examination, culture examination for fungi, and clinical observation. Where a specific diagnosis could be made, such as seborrheic dermatitis, contact eczema, psoriasis, tinea, intertrigo, or other complicating pathology, these patients were excluded from the study. Only those cases which were considered idiopathic in origin were selected for trial.

The resulting group consisted of 29 patients, 18 male and 11 female, ranging in age from 18 to 55 years. All cases were chronic, of three months to two years' duration.

METHOD

All patients under study were placed on a cleansing routine. They were told to cleanse with cold cream after stool, to pat dry after bathing or showering, and to apply 1% hydrocortisone (Hydrocortone) ointment when there was an urge to scratch.

The patients were then treated in three groups. The first containing five patients, was treated with x-ray locally, 1/8 skin unit dose unfiltered, and with 1% hydrocortisone ointment applied locally. In addition, these patients were given phenobarbital ½ grain (30 mg.) t.i.d. The second group, consisting of 14 patients, received the same x-ray and hydrocortisone treatment, but instead of phenobarbital, received meprobamate 400 mg. q.i.d. The third group, of 10 patients, received only x-ray and hydrocortisone, without sedation of any kind.

Results from Use of Phenobarbital, Meprobamate, and No Sedation with Twenty-Nine Cases of Pruritus Ani and Pruritus Vulvae

	Total Cases	Improved*	Failure
Phenobarbital	5	5	
Meprobamate	14	14	
No sedation	10	7	3†
Total	29	26	3†

* Pruritus controlled for duration of time the patient was under treatment.

† All cases subsequently controlled after Miltown was added to the treatment.

RESULTS

Results of the study are summarized in the Table.

In the group receiving x-ray, hydrocortisone, and phenobarbital, itching was controlled in all cases. However, patients complained of dullness and sleepiness, and did not like to use the sedative on the job because it interfered with their work.

In the group receiving x-ray, hydrocortisone, and meprobamate the pruritus was also controlled in all cases. With this drug, however, patients remained alert and physically active and were able to perform normally on their jobs. Three of the patients did experience an initial period of drowsiness which, however, wore off, and was never severe enough to interfere with their work. No other side-effects were reported.

In the group of 10 patients receiving x-ray, hydrocortisone, and no sedation there were three failures, all of which responded when meprobamate was added to the treatment.

Comment

That a close relationship should exist between pruritus and certain dermatological conditions might be expected from the fact that embryologically nerve tissue and skin are both formed from the ectoderm. Attempts to throw light on the functional nature of this relationship have taken many forms. One approach has been to try to relate certain kinds of skin conditions to "character types." Other approaches have been psychoanalytically oriented, or have attempted to relate the results of psychiatric study to those resulting from neurological and physiological investigations.

The average dermatologist in private practice is not equipped to make expert judgments among these various views. I can only express my firm personal conviction, as a result of extensive clinical observations, that at least in the cases of idiopathic pruritus ani and pruritus vulvae there does exist a strong relationship between the itching and certain conflicts, fears, or problem situations in the patient's life.

The onset of the pruritus usually appears associated with two events. First, careful questioning almost always reveals that there was some predisposing experience in the medical history which may have directed the patient's attention, consciously or unconsciously, to the affected area. In some cases there may have been constipation, in others diarrhea (possibly following antibiotic medication); in some there may have been a fungus infection or other pathology. In any case, the predisposing condition has usually ceased to exist.

Then, at a later time, some emotionally charged event precipitates the pruritus which becomes localized in the area of previous excitation. The event may be situational, such as a decisive examination, or a promotion to a new and demanding job which the patient fears to be beyond his capacities. Or it may represent the aggravation of unsolved family-related personality conflicts of long standing. In any case, the event is always disturbing and fraught with tensions and anxiety.

Once started, the pruritus perpetuates itself as the patient substitutes for the painful emotions which he does not know how to control the pleasurable and often sensually tinged gratification derived from scratching.

This close relationship between symptom and emotional state should, I believe, determine the kind of therapy to be used in pruritus ani and vulvae. In my experience, the patient finds greatest relief when he is treated, within the limitations of dermatological practice, in an essentially psychiatric sense. The patient is hardly ever aware that his emotional problems are in any way related to his skin condition. The doctor must, therefore, take sufficient time to talk to the patient at some length and, by showing interest and patience, draw him out about his personal life as well as about his symptoms. Careful questioning will usually bring the disturbing factors to light, together with their tie to the onset of the pruritus. When this relationship can be demonstrated to the patient, it in itself brings great relief, for the condition is now no longer entirely incomprehensible to him, and thus less frightening. As a result, he will more readily accept the suggestion that his recovery is related to modification of some of his personal attitudes and conflicts, and he may be willing to exert greater effort toward this end.

At the same time, treatment must also be directed toward giving symptomatic relief as quickly as possible. Patients are therefore given x-ray and hydrocortisone to subdue the itching locally and are instructed in ways of avoiding further local irritation.

The place of a tranquilizer such as meprobamate in this regimen is to help bring the patient's anxieties and tensions under control more rapidly than would otherwise be possible. In many cases control could not be achieved at all, without psychiatric help, unless such a tranquilizer were used.

Meprobamate has an effect on the patient which is unlike what I have seen following administration of any other drug. Not only does the patient lose his tensions; he also seems to loses his fears and his panicky sense of urgency about his problems. He feels, "This too shall pass," and is able to deal with difficult situations with a serenity he has often never known before. At the same time, the patient never describes himself as feeling detached or "insulated" by the drug. He remains completely in control of his faculties, both mental and physical, and his responsiveness to other persons is characteristically improved. This enhanced cooperativeness is of great value in the doctor-patient relationship.

Summary and Conclusions

A study was undertaken to evaluate the effectiveness of meprobamate (Miltown) as a tranquilizer in idiopathic anogenital pruritus. Two comparable groups of patients were used as controls, one receiving phenobarbital as a sedative and the other receiving no sedation. Results showed that a number of patients were unable to bring the itching under control when no sedation was employed. Patients given phenobarbital were relieved of itching, but suffered from unpleasant feelings of "dopiness" and dullness of perception, often to the extent that work was impeded. In patients receiving meprobamate, on the other hand, remission of the pruritus occurred without impairment of physical activity or mental alertness, and without side-reactions of any kind.

Meprobamate is an effective addition to conventional dermatological therapy. Although the present study was limited to an evaluation of the drug's effectiveness in pruritus ani and pruritus vulvae, it will almost certainly be found to have value also in other dermatological conditions where the history reveals underlying components of anxiety or tension. Alopecia areata, atopic eczema, and linchen planus are particularly suggested for further study.

USE OF TRANQUILIZERS IN DISEASES OF THE SKIN

Paul LeVan, M.D., and Edwin T. Wright, M.D.

Within the past two years the use of tranquilizers in dermatology has become increasingly frequent. The administration of these drugs in inflammatory dermatosis has stemmed not so much from consistent effectiveness in treatment as from the great need for an agent to reduce anxiety, nervous tension, emotional stress and pruritus. The role played by these factors in the pathogenesis and course of many of the inflammatory diseases of the skin has been adequately emphasized by Sternberg, Obermayer, Sulzberger, Rein and others.

Agents previously used to diminish the effect of psychic and emotional factors included barbiturates, chloral hydrate, bromides and the antihistamine drugs. They were unsatisfactory for the most part because of side reactions, habit formation, development of tolerance, and because sometimes they did not bring about relaxation of the patient. Hence, when chlorpromazine and reserpine became available they were given enthusiastic and wide-spread trial.

Some 274 patients with inflammatory conditions such as atopic dermatitis, neurodermatitis, eczematoid dermatitis, lichen planus, psoriasis and pruritus ani et vulvae were treated at the University of California Medical Center at Los Angeles and at the Veterans Administration Center Hospital with either chlorpromazine or reserpine. The observations of clinical response were varied and confusing. Therapeutic results ranged from excellent to poor. The degree of tranquilization varied greatly from patient to patient, and in a number of subjects agitation rather than a tranquilizing effect was observed. Similarly, the control of pruritus was extremely variable and while diminution of this symptom was observed, total abolition was seldom achieved without adjunctive therapy. In many instances, evidence of tranquilization was present without concomitant improvement in the dermatitis. The overall incidence of slight to pronounced beneficial effect attributed to reserpine and chlorpromazine was placed at 60 per cent in this group of 274 patients. Untoward reactions such as headache, nausea, vertigo, drowsiness, nasal congestion and depression were so pronounced in many instances as to necessitate discontinuance of the drug.

It was apparent from these early clinical observations that evaluation of the efficacy of the tranquilizers could best be accomplished by using double blind controls. Pillsbury, Livingood, and others aptly stressed that clinical investigation without controls can be misleading and inaccurate. This is especially true when dealing with such subjective symptoms as emotional stress, anxiety, nervous tension and pruritus. In order to attempt clarification of this problem, a study of the effect of a reserpine tranquilizer in these symptoms was instituted using controls. Fifty-two hospitalized patients were given either 0.25 mg. of reserpine or a placebo four times daily and clinical response was observed by the dermatology staff. No person participating in the study knew whether a patient was receiving the drug or the placebo, although in some instances side reactions indicated active medication. Local therapy other than a bland ointment or starch baths was withheld.

The following conditions were studied: Atopic dermatitis, 22 patients; neurodermatitis, six patients; eczematoid dermatitis, 14 patients; psoriasis and lichen planus, five patients; chronic urticaria, five patients. Of the 30 patients treated with reserpine, 16 showed improvement of varying degree, while 14 were unimproved. Tranquilization was considered a symptom of improvement even though not accompanied by significant skin change, inasmuch as subjective complaints were less. Of the 22 placebo-treated patients, four improved and 18 showed no improvement.

It is realized that no conclusion can be drawn from so small a series, but the results are considered indicative. The ratio of benefited to nonbenefited patients receiving reserpine therapy approximates the previous clinical experience wherein response was varied, inconsistent and unpredictable. The incidence of unpleasant side reactions was sufficiently great to cause many patients to discontinue use of the drug.

For the foregoing reasons, a new tranquilizing agent meprobamate, a carbamate derivative marketed under the trade names of Miltown and Equanil and related to mephenesin or Tolserol, was subjected to clinical testing. Meprobamate possesses, in addition to muscle relaxing properties, a pronounced emotional and psychic tranquilizing effect. Its mode of action is by blocking interneuronal stimuli between cortex, thalamus and hypothalamus. Unpleasant side reactions, in the authors' experience, are infrequent and toxicity is low. Selling reported that one patient took 50 and another patient 100 400-mg. tablets in a 24-hour period without serious consequences.

Either Miltown or Equanil (400 mg. four times daily) was given to 164 patients with the various kinds of inflammatory diseases of the skin dealt with in the previous study of the effect of chlorpromazine and reserpine. A tranquilizing effect, as manifested by relaxation of nervous tension, diminution of anxiety and emotional stress and lessening of pruritus, was more consistently observed and was greater in degree than was obtained with reserpine therapy. Almost all patients troubled with insomnia volunteered their sleeping habits had considerably improved. Side reactions were minimal, principally drowsiness which usually diminished after three days of therapy. Two patients complained of nausea, but it abated without continuance of treatment. Selling reported urticaria and angioneurotic edema in three of 137 patients. No reactions of that kind were noted in the present study.

Clinical response of the dermatoses, while varied, was more consistent than in the patients who were given reserpine. Even in cases of severe dermatitis not responding significantly to tranquilization, the calming effect, nevertheless, was sufficient to make management easier. Agitation, which was not infrequently observed in patients given reserpine, was noted in but one instance in the study with meprobamate. Meprobamate was found to be particularly useful when steroid therapy was being discontinued. The results were sufficiently encouraging to indicate meprobamate may be the drug of choice in many cases in which tranquilization is desired.

THERAPEUTIC PROCESS IN ELECTROSHOCK AND THE NEWER DRUG THERAPIES

Leo Alexander, M.D.
Director, Neurobiologic Unit, Division of Psychiatric Research,
Boston State Hospital, Boston, Massachusetts

The nature of the therapeutic process in shock therapy is unknown. One fact, however, emerges with increasing clarity: the patient successfully treated with electroshock is no longer frightened into panic or paralyzed into depression by his own warning or tension anxiety.

Six years ago I first presented my observation that in certain patients depression, defined as a state of sadness with self-reproach and psychomotor inhibition, can be converted into anxiety, defined as a state of tension with fear and psychomotor excitation, by the use of shock and reversed back into depression again by the use of nonconvulsive electrostimulation in a controlled, predictable, and repeatable manner. This finding has promoted me to conceive of depression not as a defense against anxiety but as a state of overwhelming anxiety with hopelessness: anxiety from which the ego can see no hope of escape, or, anxiety that has resulted in an inhibitory state. However, in itself the shock therapy does not directly affect either the original quantity of the anxiety or the psychological issues that precipitated and perpetuated the original warning anxiety; but, when anxiety comes to the fore again, depending upon its original quantity, it does so because it has been released by the shock procedure, due to the lifting of the depression, which had exerted a reciprocal inhibitory effect over the original anxiety (fig. 1 and 2). The conflict-laden psychological issues as well as the primary warning anxiety they aroused must await relief by concurrent and follow-up psychotherapy, by management of the patient and his family, and by a variety of rehabilitative measures—in other words by a totality of psychiatric therapy in which the physical treatment merely represents an essential facilitating measure, especially if the physician has succeeded in avoiding certain undesirable side-effects that might potentially aggravate specific psychological issues. Shock therapy itself, therefore, does not relieve the primary traumatic neurosis that originally evoked the warning or tension anxiety (fig. 1), but it does interrupt the vicious cycle between the warning anxiety on the one hand and panic and depression on the other (fig 2), thus relieving the secondary traumatic state of the ego, i. e., the secondary traumatic neurosis induced by the warning anxiety itself.

How does shock therapy accomplish this result? The paralysis of the ego in the form of depression, resulting as it does from the impact of excessive quantities of excitation by warning anxiety (fig. 1), has all the earmarks of a paradoxical reaction in the Pavlovian sense, in that it appears to be a state of profound inhibition or paralysis induced by excessive excitation. Furthermore, we are justified in assuming that warning anxiety, which is largely unconscious and which can be precipitated or aggravated by an injection of epinephrine, is essentially a subcortical phenomenon. Panic and depression, on the other hand, pervade the conscious mind and cannot be precipitated or intensified by intravenously injected epinephrine and hence appear to be mediated and perceived chiefly within the cortex of the brain.

Electroshock diminishes cortical excitability, and it appears to be for this reason that the subcortical warning anxiety can then no longer overstimulate the

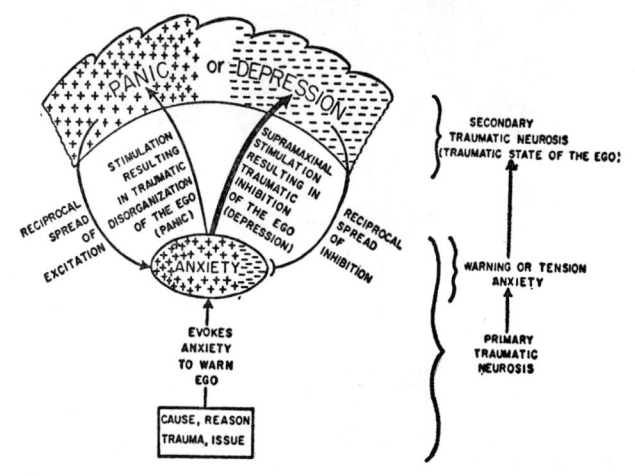

Fig. 1.—Relationship of trauma, anxiety, panic, and depression. + denotes excitation; — denotes inhibition.

cortical ego into panic or depression. The ego and its defenses appear strengthened after electroshock therapy, for the excitation threshold of the cortex has been raised (fig. 2). This dynamic alteration in the threshold gives the ego an opportunity to strengthen and regroup its defenses, a process that can be aided by psychotherapy, although it often takes place spontaneously after successful electroshock therapy.

Warning or tension anxiety, while no longer disruptive to the ego because of the latter's raised threshold to stimulation, can of course still be perceived at certain stages or intensities of treatment. This anxiety may come even more prominently to the fore (fig. 2) because its presence is no longer obscured through its secondary paralyzing effect upon the ego, which in turn had an inhibitory effect upon the anxiety due to spread of inhibition (fig. 1). This obviously explains the apparently reciprocal relationship between warning anxiety and depression that I pointed out earlier, based on the fact that I was able to convert and reconvert one into the other by specific physical measures.

The residuum of warning anxiety, conscious or unconscious, that the patient is likely to be left with after electroshock therapy has to be dealt with in one way or another. Often in his improved state the patient is able to look at the underlying issues that aroused the warning anxiety in a new light, much as we all are able to do with minor problems after a good night's sleep or when we find that something we had dreaded did not materialize. This resurvey in turn diminishes the anxiety engendered by the issue. A beneficent cycle has been set up. A similar result can be brought about by follow-up psychotherapy in

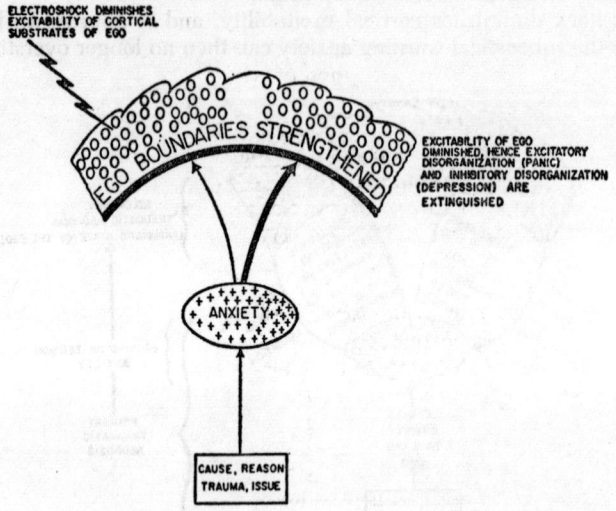

Fig. 2.—Effect of convulsive electroshock therapy. + denotes excitation; O denotes extinction.

patients who may not be able to attain this strengthening and maturing by themselves.

In particularly severe illnesses, massive shock therapy may be utilized to the point where not only excessive response to, but even awareness of, warning anxiety is suppressed temporarily. The disadvantage of this last method is that the warning anxiety is merely suppressed and during the convalescent phase is likely to erupt again disturbingly and precipitate relapse. I prefer release and ventilation of the warning anxiety by the added use of nonconvulsive-stimulation treatment, which enables the therapist to deal simultaneously with it and the underlying issues, thus paving the way for subsequent psychotherapy of the primary traumatic conflict.

Tranquilizing Drugs

The action of the new tranquilizing drugs, chlorpromazine and reserpine, is fundamentally different from that of shock therapy, in that these drugs appear to suppress the primary, epinephrine-precipitable, subcortical warning or tension anxiety while exerting only an indirect influence on the secondary cortical manifestations—the traumatic state of the ego—in inverse proportion to the degree to which important ego functions have been disrupted in the direction of paralysis or inhibition by the anxiety. For this reason tranquilizing medication, especially with chlorpromazine, is most effective in manic states. This may be due to the fact that the manic state is a condition most directly power-driven in the direction of excitation by epinephrine-precipitable tension anxiety, as I pointed out elsewhere, and in which important ego functions are least weakened. Conversely, for the same reason, and in remarkable accord with the fact that inhibitory cortical processes are more readily extinguishable than excitatory ones, manic psychoses are least readily relieved by electroshock therapy, which is an extinction type of treatment, unless the treatment is carried to the point of obliterating even the mere perception of warning or tension anxiety. Another reason for the superb clinical results of chlorpromazine therapy in manic patients is that manic psychoses tend to be of naturally short duration. Hence, if the manifestations of the psychosis can be suppressed for the natural duration of the manic episode, the patient can continue to live a rather normal life and may even be able to keep on working without experiencing either the social disadvantages of morbidity or the undesirable supression of cortical functioning produced by electroshock.

Depression is at the other end of the scale of effectiveness of the new tranquilizing drugs. Chlorpromazine and reserpine not only are entirely ineffective in most cases of depression but are actually contraindicated because they may aggravate the condition. The reason for their ineffectiveness is obviously the fact that, in depression, paralysis of the ego is most profound, the ego being in an inhibitory state already. Inhibition of ego functions is not only not relieved but is actually aggravated by these drugs, because not only has this inhibition of ego functions become independent of continued overstimulation of the ego by the warning anxiety that originally paralyzed the ego into depression but, by a process of negative induction leading to spread of inhibition, the inhibited state of the ego has extended to include the original warning anxiety as well (fig. 1). This fact explains the reciprocal relationship of anxiety and depression in contradistinction to the simple vicious-cycle type of relationship that exists between warning anxiety and panic (fig. 1). Thus it comes about that further suppression of the original warning anxiety by means of drugs will actually deepen the existing depression (fig. 3), or it may even precipitate depression. Conversely, enhancing the warning anxiety by injection of epinephrine, for instance, may relieve depression temporarily.

Depression is indeed the most significant mental and emotional complication arising from the use of these tranquilizing drugs. If administration of chlorpromazine, for instance, is continued too long after control of a manic psychosis (as occurred with three patients in my own experience, in whom this drug was administered over periods ranging from four to seven months in an attempt to tone down mild residual hypomanic states) or if reserpine is given to depression-prone individuals for relief of hypertension, these drugs may precipitate depression, which, however, can be promptly terminated by withdrawal of the drug. Gastrointestinal symptoms of withdrawal of chlorpromazine can be avoided by administration of Donnatal (a combination of hyoscyamine sulfate, atropine sulfate, hyoscine hydrobromide, and phenobarbital), which is then rapidly withdrawn.

The new tranquilizing drugs are less consistently effective in catatonic and excited schizoaffective states than they are in manic states. In catatonic and hallucinatory paranoid states I have found reserpine relatively more effective than chlorpromazine. In most other anxiety and panic states and in related regressive neurotic and psychotic syndromes, I have found the use of chlorpromazine and reserpine generally unsatisfactory from the long-range point of view, with a few remarkable exceptions in which patients responded very well. All

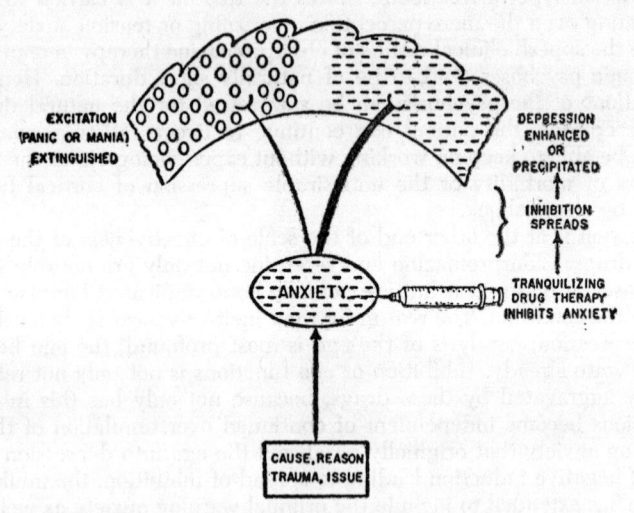

Fig. 3.—Effect of tranquilizing drug therapy. — denotes inhibition; O denotes extinction.

those who did respond well were marked by agitation and overactivity, and these are the patients who seem most amenable to chlorpromazine therapy. Reserpine, on the other hand, was useful in some patients in phobic states. All these patients, however, had one thing in common with manic patients: while the ego boundaries had been breached by panic anxiety, any secondary paralysis of important ego functions was absent or relatively slight, the clinical picture being dominated by excitation. As might then be expected, none of the obsessive-compulsive patients was benefited at all, not even temporarily.

The great variety in the response of patients with neurotic and borderline states to tranquilizing drugs may be in part explained by the fact that one of the more important effects of these drugs is that they enhance suggestibility. West has shown that the use of these drugs increases the ease with which these patients can be hypnotized or otherwise influenced by suggestion. This highlights the fact that additional therapeutic actions and/or attitudes of the physician may play a decisive role.

Chlorpromazine is useful in relieving states of excitation in the psychoses arising from chronic alcoholism and in states of pathological alcoholic intoxication as well as in cases of drug addiction for relieving nervous-system excitation released by withdrawal of narcotics. Both chlorpromazine and reserpine are useful in senile psychoses. In a patient with presenile sclerosis (Alzheimer's disease) with marked agitation, overactivity, and increased stream of talk, a remarkable degree of social improvement was brought about by administration of chlorpromazine. Chlorpromazine and reserpine have also been found helpful in the control of chronically disturbed patients in mental hospitals. In the majority of these patients, this method of control merely suppresses symptoms without bringing about actual recovery; however, physicians who have used large doses of reserpine in such hospital populations of persons with apparently chronic, incurable schizophrenia have consistently reported a social recovery rate of 20%, so that many such patients are able to return home after many years of hospitalization.

Other New Drugs

A number of additional new drugs have become available that differ from the tranquilizing drugs in varying degrees. I should like to divide these into three groups: (1) relaxant drugs, (2) ataraxic (deconfusing) drugs, and (3) antiphobic drugs. The action of relaxant medication, such as that exemplified by the new drug meprobamate (Miltown), is similar to that of the tranquilizing drugs, except that its inhibitory effect is less profound. This is an advantage in the psychoneuroses, in which marked reduction of drive such as that brought about by tranquilizing drugs is often anxiety provoking and thus tends to counteract the desired effect of the medication. Because of its less profound inhibitory action, meprobamate also does not tend to precipitate or aggravate depression, but for the same reason it is also much less effective in the treatment of psychotic states of excitement.

Ataraxic (deconfusing) action has been described as the characteristic effect of Frenquel [a-(4-piperidyl) benzhydrol hydrochloride]. In contrast to the tranquilizing drugs, Frenquel does not depress the activity of the hypothalamus either clinically or in the electroencephalogram; it counteracts the effects of lysergic acid diethylamide (LSD-25) and of mescaline without inducing sedation and restores the resting activity in the electroencephalogram after its disruption in the form of enduring arousal by lysergic acid diethylamide or mescaline.

Antiphobic medication, as with Benactyzine (2-diethylaminoethyl benzilate hydrochloride), is fundamentally different from tranquilizing medication in that it selectively abolishes "neurotic" inhibitory avoidance responses engendered by stress without inhibiting the orienting response and conditional reflex responses. Consistent with the conceptual scheme presented in this paper, this drug has proved itself in the hands of others as well as myself to be a mild antidepressant in clinical states of depression in human beings, of both manic-depressive and involutional-type. Further studies of these and related compounds promise to shed further light upon the neurophysiological and biochemical aspects of emotional and mental disorders and to aid in their treatment.

Summary

Electroshock therapy relieves the secondary traumatic state of the ego (panic and/or depression) by reducing the excitability of the nervous system, especially the cortex. Unconscious (subcortical, epinephrine-precipitable) warning anxiety can then no longer overstimulate the cortical ego and thus frighten it into panic or paralyze it into depression, as it did formerly along the lines of Pavlov's paradoxical reaction. The ego and its defenses appear strengthened after electroshock therapy, because its excitation threshold has been raised. The new tranquilizing drugs (chlorpromazine and reserpine) relieve the primary, unconscious, subcortical, epinephrine-precipitable warning and tension anxiety that impels states of excitation. They are thus capable of relieving states of agitation and overactivity, especially manic psychoses and organic-toxic states, in which secondary inhibitory or disorganizing effects upon the ego are slight or readily reversible. The action of certain newer groups of drugs, which may be classified as relaxants (such as meprobamate [Miltown]), ataraxic (deconfusing) (such as Frenquel [a-(4-piperidyl) benzhydrol hydrochloride]) and antiphobic such as Benactyzine (2-diethylaminoethyl benzilate hydrochloride), is different from that of the tranquilizing drugs. They require further study of their psychophysiology and clinical indications.

TREATMENT OF DEPRESSION WITH MERATRAN AND ELECTROSHOCK

Henry E. Andren, M.D.

Depressive illnesses, affecting individuals in nearly every age group, have become a therapeutic problem of ever-increasing magnitude to the psychiatrist and general physician. Whether the increase which has been noted stems from better recognition of these conditions or is due to a growing incidence in the number of such cases, is difficult to say. The fact remains that large numbers of individuals with varying degrees of depression are presenting themselves to physicians and improved forms of therapy are sorely needed.

While all forms of depression usually respond fairly quickly to electroshock therapy, a certain percentage of individuals are fearful of this procedure for various reasons, and an additional small group of patients are not suitable candidates for this type of therapy due to their poor physical condition. Particularly in milder forms of depression electroshock therapy may be regarded as relatively rigorous treatment. When effective, drugs with mood-lifting qualities are frequently satisfactory. A new drug of this type, Meratran, has been investigated recently by the author in a relatively small number of patients with reactive depressions.

The chemical structure of Meratran is quite different from that of older drugs which are known to stimulate the central nervous system, and pharmacologic studies which have been reported indicate that clinical differences may be expected to result. The absence of effect upon heart rate, blood pressure, and appetite is of considerable significance and the freedom from post-medication depression reported by Brown and Werner, if confirmed in human subjects, would be another major advantage not possessed by many central nervous system stimulants now available.

The original report on the clinical use of Meratran has been followed by a number of others. All of these investigators have achieved very favorable responses in mildly depressed patients whose condition was not complicated by a substantial overlay of anxiety. A convenient test procedure to determine suitable candidates for oral Meratran therapy has been described previously by the author. This consists of a single intravenous injection of 2.0 mg. (2.0 cc.) Meratran. Transient but obvious improvement occurs some time during the following sixty minutes in those patients who later respond well to oral Meratran.

My own series has consisted of a total of 44 depressed patients classified in Table I. Definite symptomatic improvement occurred in about half the patients. The degree of improvement depended largely upon the severity of the depression. The relatively more favorable response in reactive depression reported by other investigators was confirmed.

The doses of Meratran used in the patients varied from 1.0 mg. to 2.0 mg. t.i.d., and, in general, were well tolerated. Three patients, however, while receiving therapy, developed a macular rash which disappeared fairly promptly when the drug was stopped. One patient complained that the drug caused her face to become flushed. Two patients developed nausea while taking the drug and its administration had to be discontinued. Six other patients complained of a tense feeling while receiving Meratran. Of these, two were being treated for reactive depression, one for obsessive-compulsive neurosis, one for involutional depression, and two for psychotic depression.

Many of the cases which failed to respond to treatment with Meratran were subsequently given electroshock therapy and, as we expected, a satisfactory

TABLE I

	Significant Improvement	Moderate Improvement	Slight Improvement	No Change
Reactive Depression	3	3	5	3
Endogenous Depression	0	2	1	0
Psychotic Depression	0	1	2	10
Involutional Depression	0	1	1	5
Depression with Anxiety	0	0	1	3
Neurosis, Obsessive-Compulsive	0	0	0	2
Depression associated with arteriosclerosis	0	0	1	0
Totals	3	7	11	23

improvement occurred. It was noted, however, that these patients seemed to respond to electroshock therapy somewhat better than could be anticipated.

Since Meratran had been beneficial in many of the depressed patients who received it as the sole form of therapy, I continued to administer it to patients about to receive electroshock. The procedure was to inject 1.0 cc. intramuscularly one-half hour prior to the electrical treatments and on the days which intervened between them.

It is my impression that the confusion and amnesia which ordinarily follow electroshock therapy occurred far less frequently and to a much lesser degree. The suicidal drive which is on occasion increased after the first few electrical treatments seemed to be dampened in the few psychotically depressed patients in whom it had been observed on previous occasions. Similarly, the accentuation of the depression which occurs in about 10 per cent of the patients in this same group receiving electroshock therapy was notably absent when Meratran was administered one-half hour prior to shock therapy and on the days between electroshock treatments. Elevation of the mood, as a matter of fact, seemed to occur earlier than usual, and recovery appeared to proceed at a more uniform and consistent rate.

Since patients treated with electroshock therapy tend to become depressed on occasion after a course of treatment has been completed, maintenance electroshock is commonly required. In a small number of patients, the administration of Meratran, intramuscularly, at these critical periods has greatly diminished the need for such interim therapy.

These observations concerning the combined use of Meratran and electroshock therapy are, of course, preliminary in nature and additional studies are now being conducted.

Summary

1. A new central stimulant, Meratran, has been studied in a series of patients with depression. The oral dose is 1.0 mg. to 2.0 mg. t.i.d. and the single parenteral dose, 2.0 mg. given intravenously or intramuscularly.

2. A satisfactory therapeutic response was obtained in patients with reactive depressions, while less frequently favorable results were obtained in the endogenous, psychotic, and involutional types.

3. In patients who require electroshock therapy, the adjunctive use of Meratran appears to hasten the recovery and diminish the frequency of maintenance electrical treatments.

CHLORPROMAZINE AND RESERPINE AS ADJUNCTS IN ELECTROSHOCK TREATMENT

Merritt W. Foster, Jr., M.D., and R. Finley Gayle III, M.D.

It is the purpose of this paper to give a brief review of our clinical experience in the combination of electroshock treatment with these two drugs over the past 18 months. Furthermore, it is our purpose to discuss the conclusions, which we have drawn from these cases and to present our feeling as to the usefulness of these drugs at the present time in our particular type of practice. Our experience has been limited to patients treated in the fifty-bed psychiatric unit in a general hospital. This setting imposes certain limitations in the treatment of psychiatric patients, particularly in terms of duration of hospital stay so that the limited bed space may be used more effectively in serving the hospital community. All of the cases presented will be those in which the patients suffered an acute psychiatric illness and who we felt would benefit from relatively short-term hospitalization with intensive treatment. The cases reported are those in which (prior to the advent of these two drugs), the patients would have been treated with electroshock treatment alone. Diagnostically, they fall into the involutional psychotic reactions, psychotic depressive reactions, chronic brain syndromes with marked affective disturbances, and certain selected schizophrenics. We have chosen to disregard in this communication certain other types of disease which ordinarily would not be considered for electroshock treatment. These include alcoholism, psychoneurosis, organic psychoses without marked affective disturbances, and transient behavioral disorders. Our findings in these latter cases agree with those generally reported, namely, that when given alone, chlorpromazine particularly and reserpine occasionally, are helpful as part of our treatment armamentarium.

Use of Drugs Alone

Early in the summer of 1954 both reserpine and chlorpromazine were receiving enthusiastic reports by investigators in this country for their efficacy in controlling disturbed behavior in psychotic patients. Joining in this enthusiasm, we began by using reserpine alone in an attempt to control increased psychomotor activity in acutely disturbed patients. In the midst of our early use of this drug we felt that, when given by itself, it was not always effective in making patients more tractable and amenable. In some cases reduction in motor activity did occur, but upon cessation or withdrawal of the drug the disturbed behavior again presented itself. We also noticed that reserpine principally affected the pattern of behavior and showed little effect on actual thought content. Unwanted side effects which occurred were an increase in depression in some patients, and certain aspects of physiological intolerance in others necessitating withdrawal of the drug.

The early patients to whom reserpine was given, however, showed very dramatic behavioral responses leading to easier and safer management in the hospital. The first patient given reserpine was a young disturbed schizophrenic girl who had received both electroshock and insulin coma with no appreciable reduction in her overactivity both in the motor realm and in cerebration. Prior to the use of reserpine she was denudative, completely untidy in her person, was fed and nourished with extreme difficulty, and rested at very infrequent and short-lived intervals. When the physical therapies described were discontinued and the patient was given reserpine, she immediately became tractable, interested in her surroundings, fed herself, and slept at night. In a short time she was able to care for her youngest child whose advent had precipitated much of her psychotic behavior. There followed three other patients whose courses were essentially the same, with dramatic but temporary improvement on reserpine alone. Subsequent patients, however, did not show this type of response and those who did respond initially were beginning to relapse and require further hospital treatment. Because of this tendency to relapse it was felt that perhaps the most useful role of reserpine would be to assist in maintaining initial gains made by electroshock treatment alone. We then began using the combination of these two therapies with longer-lasting symptomatic improvement and resultant ease in management of disturbed patients. Our enthusiasm was short-lived, however, when it was noticed that an occasional patient would show an adverse physical reaction to electroshock treatment when combined with reserpine. This was in the nature of prolonged apnea, cyanosis and cardiac irregularity and occurred even though minimal amounts of electric current were used. This reaction led to a fatality in one case. Suffice it to say that this experience dictated a definite contraindication to the simultaneous combination of these two procedures.

Knowing that reserpine required several days of administration before reaching its maximum effective level, we assumed that withdrawal of the drug would require a similar period for reduction. It would, therefore, be necessary to wait several days after discontinuing the administration of reserpine before electroshock could be instituted. Our results indicated that this waiting period should last at least seven days.

Considering the necessity for this latent period between the two types of treatment, and considering the relapses which were beginning to show up in those treated earlier with this combination of electroshock and reserpine, we began focusing our interest on the useful possibilities of chlorpromazine. We felt it inadvisable to combine electroshock and chlorpromazine therapy at the outset due to the similarity in action of this drug and reserpine. We began, as with reserpine, using chlorpromazine alone in a series of patients since others were reporting favorable results with this method. Increasing the dosage to tolerance, we noted a similar type of response to this drug. Those patients who were initially symptomatically improved, relapsed with gradual withdrawal or lowering of the dose. This was true in several cases in spite of the fact that the dosage was carried as high as 1,200 mg. per day for periods of one to three weeks. When electroshock therapy was added, however, we were quite gratified by the effectiveness of combining these methods of treatment consecutively. We evolved the procedure of using electroshock therapy initially in acutely disturbed patients until there was definite evidence of symptomatic improvement. At this point electroshock treatment was discontinued and chlorpromazine was added to the regimen. The drug was given in doses of 100 mg. per day by mouth, augmented by 50 mg. doses by injection. Following the second or third day, the oral dosage was increased as needed and the intramuscular dosage was omitted. It was during this post-electroshock period that more intense efforts were made to deal with the patient's problems on a psychotherapeutic basis. At the time of discharge the dosage of chlorpromazine was usually reduced to the starting point of 100 mg. per day by mouth. The patient could be maintained at home on this amount and followed with psychotherapy as an outpatient. We have found that this drug facilitates an earlier psychotherapeutic endeavor with the patient and is helpful in managing the period of confusion which is not uncommon following electroshock treatment.

Drugs Combined with Electroshock Therapy

Our results in the use of these two drugs with electroshock therapy include 126 patients treated during the past 18 months. A rough diagnostic breakdown (Table 1) reveals that 63 patients were classified in the involutional psychotic group, 39 patients were diagnosed as having some type of schizophrenic reaction, 7 had a manic-depressive psychosis, 8 were classified as having psychotic depressive reactions, and 9 patients fell in the chronic brain syndrome group. It will be noted in surveying the totals in the two drug groups that there is an overlap of 19 case reports. These 19 failed to respond to a combination of electroshock and one of the drugs and were subsequently treated with a combination of electroshock treatment and the other drug. Therefore, they are in common to both the reserpine and chlorpromazine series.

In surveying the patients who were given a combination of electroshock treatment and reserpine (Table 2), we found a total of 88. Of these 46 achieved a social recovery, were able to leave the hospital and have not required further hospitalization since. Therefore, 42 of those treated with this combination were initial failures. We have arbitrarily decided for the purpose of this report to use the need for further hospitalization as our criterion of social recovery or failure. Of the 42 initial failures, 14 subsequently responded to the addition of further treatment with electroshock treatment alone, chlorpromazine alone, or a combination of the two. This indicates that of the initial 88 patients 28 ultimately failed to recover.

Our second group of patients (Table 3) namely those receiving a combination of electroshock treatment and chlorpromazine numbered 57. Among these 57, 49 achieved an immediate social recovery. Of the 8 remaining, 4 subsequently obtained a social recovery when given a further course of electroshock therapy, with one of them receiving reserpine in addition. The other 4 failed to recover.

TABLE 1
Diagnostic Grouping of Treated Patients

Involutional psychotic reaction	63
Schizophrenic reaction	39
Manic-depressive reaction	7
Psychotic depressive reaction	8
Chronic brain syndrome	9
Total number patients	126

TABLE 2
Electroshock and Reserpine Treatment

Recovered initially	46
Recovered with additional treatment	14
Failed to recover	28
Total patients treated	88

TABLE 3
Electroshock and Thorazine Treatment

Recovered initially	49
Recovered with additional treatment	4
Failed to recover	4
Total patients treated	57

Conclusions

1. In those disorders formerly treated with electroshock alone, we have found that a combination of chlorpromazine and/or reserpine with electroshock treatment is more effective than the use of either the drugs or electroshock alone.

2. Of these combinations, electroshock treatment followed by chlorpromazine proved more effective than electroshock treatment followed by reserpine. In the former group receiving chlorpromazine roughly 14 out of 15 recovered, whereas in the latter group receiving reserpine only 2 out of 3 recovered. Furthermore 10 of the 42 initial failures with the combination of electroshock and reserpine subsequently recovered when chlorpromazine and/or electroshock treatment were added to the initial regimen. Conversely, only one of those who failed to recover initially with electroshock and chlorpromazine was able to leave the hospital with the addition of further electroshock treatment and reserpine.

3. It was our clinical impression based on our facility in working with these patients that chlorpromazine was the more effective adjunct to electroshock treatment.

4. We would emphasize that the final evaluation of the concepts which we have presented must wait on larger series of cases, a more prolonged follow-up period, and more detailed and convincing explanation of the modus operandi of both these drugs and electroshock treatment.

Discussion

Dr. Jackson A. Smith, Omaha, Nebr. There seems to be an increasing agreement that chlorpromazine and reserpine, alone or in combination, have a definite place in the management of the disturbed patient in the state mental hospital. There have been too few reports of the effectiveness of these drugs in the treatment of the patients routinely seen in the private practice of psychiatry.

Dr. Foster's and Dr. Gayle's paper emphasizes the need to evaluate possible hazards resulting from combining these drugs with electric shock treatments. The tendency to presume an alarming hypotension or a depression of the vital functions may not exist because the patient does not expire, is not recommended as a criterion. Rather an extended series with a routine check of the control and post-treatment, blood pressures, pulse, and the rapidity with which respiration is resumed would be desirable for a valid evaluation. Previous reports have indicated that in some instances a very marked hypotension does exist. The combining of reserpine or chlorpromazine with a short acting barbiturate, and finally with a "blocking agent" before giving routine electroshock presumes these drugs in no way potentiate each other nor increase the hazards of the procedure.

Dr. Frank J. Ayd, Jr., Baltimore, Md. Chlorpromazine and reserpine are not always a satisfactory substitute for other somatic methods of psychiatric treatment, especially electroconvulsive therapy. As Drs. Foster and Gayle have pointed out electroconvulsive therapy is preferable to these drugs as a treatment for certain illnesses, particularly the endogenous depressions. However, in certain circumstances, a combination of these drugs with electroconvulsive therapy may be superior to either alone.

Drs. Foster and Gayle have observed that combined reserpine and electroconvulsive therapy may be hazardous. This method of treatment has caused adverse respiratory and cardiac reactions which may be fatal. Their fatality is one of several which have been reported in this country. Nevertheless, it is difficult to concur in their opinion that electroconvulsive therapy should not be administered to patients receiving reserpine. Thousands of patients have been safely treated with combined reserpine and electroconvulsive therapy. In my experience the incidence of alarming cyanosis, prolonged apnea, or cardiac irregularities in patients receiving combined reserpine-electroconvulsive therapy is quite low. These reactions occur most often in patients receiving relatively large doses of reserpine or when the convulsive treatment is administered within three hours after the last dose of reserpine. It is important, however, for the psychiatrist who employs this method of treatment to be aware of this potentiality and to be cautious in the administration of combined treatment.

Combined chlorpromazine and electroconvulsive therapy is also not entirely safe. Prolonged hypotensive reactions and fatalities have occurred in patients who received this combined treatment. Whether the fatality can be attributed to the combination of chlorpromazine and electroconvulsive therapy is debatable. In my opinion it is improbable that chlorpromazine played a role in the patient's demise.

The possibility of a prolonged hypotensive reaction in patients receiving chlorpromazine and electroconvulsive therapy should not be overlooked, and adequate preparation for counteracting it should be available. Norepinephrine, rather than epinephrine, is recommended to restore the blood pressure in such cases of hypotension since pharmacologically it has been demonstrated that chlorpromazine nullifies or inhibits the hypertensive effect of epinephrine.

Adverse reactions to combined chlorpromazine-electroconvulsive therapy are rare. As with reserpine, these are most apt to occur when the convulsive treatment is administered within three hours after the last dose of chlorpromazine. For this reason it is prudent to defer electroconvulsive treatment for at least three hours after the last dose of chlorpromazine or reserpine. By observing this rule I have not encountered any adverse reactions to combined chlorpromazine-electroconvulsive therapy, even in patients receiving as high as 1,000 mg. chlropromazine daily.

On the basis of my experience with over a thousand combined chlorpromazine and electroconvulsive treatments, I have found this technic advantageous for the following reasons:

(1) Chlorpromazine is effective in eliminating or controlling post-shock anxiety and excitement.

(2) Chlorpromazine reduces the number of electroconvulsive treatments required in hypomanic and manic reactions, catatonic excitement, and agitated depressions, thereby lessening post-treatment confusion and memory impairment and leaving the patient more accessible to psychotherapy.

(3) The physiologic action of chlorpromazine makes this drug ideal for combination with electroconvulsive therapy. As a sympathetic depressant it counteracts the excessive sympathetic stimulation that so often accompanies electroconvulsive therapy.

Essentially the same may be said with respect to combined reserpine-eletroconvulsive therapy.

There is no doubt that chlorpromazine and reserpine can be safely combined with electroconvulsive therapy, and that such a combination is therapeutically advantageous in certain situations. This method of treatment should be preferred to the technic of using electroconvulsive therapy followed by these drugs.

As a general principle it is unwise to administer reserpine to depressed patients who have improved following electroconvulsive therapy. In such patients reserpine may cause a relapse necessitating further electroconvulsive therapy. The reason for this clinically established fact is unknown at present. This particular propensity of reserpine to cause depressions, especially in cyclothymic individuals, demands further research on the part of all of us.

It is very difficult to assess the therapeutic results reported by Drs. Foster and Gayle since they have not indicated the number of electroconvulsive treatments or the dosage and duration of chlorpromazine or reserpine therapy. Schizophrenic patients, in particular, apparently require large doses of these drugs for prolonged periods even after electroconvulsive therapy is discontinued. It may well be that some of the therapeutic failures listed by Drs. Foster and Gayle could be attributed to insufficient dosage or premature termination of treatment.

Dr. Pete C. Palasota, Kingsport, Tenn. I have had some of these same experiences that Dr. Foster is speaking of, in my short stay at Kingsport. I had begun to feel something like Dr. Ayd, that I could use both of these drugs, until I had an unfortunate experience with the reserpine in one patient. After having two internists check this particular patient and follow her course very closely, we were able to determine that this person had probably had some coronary insufficiency. I am wondering if the hypotensive effect was what we were seeing there.

The other thing I am wondering about is the various phases we go through in starting a patient on reserpine or the Rauwolfia compounds, knowing, for instance, that it takes 8 to 10 days to reach the maximum effect, or at least the dosage that is giving us the effect we want. If there has been any work along the line of determining at which stage in the use of the medication, or the best point at which to give the electroshock treatment, I would like to hear it discussed. Now, from the series you reported, can you enlighten me a little on that item?

Dr. L. M. Foltz, Louisville, Ky. In Louisville, the practicing psychiatrists operate more as a unit, and we treat about 50 to 60 patients a day, every day, and we use a pretty standard technic of electroshock therapy when the patient is on reserpine or Thorazine. Most of our patients, I would say, at the present time get a combination of electroshock treatment and Thorazine or reserpine, or maybe all three.

We have not even had a glimmer of a problem in relation to any adverse effect of electroshock treatment combined with these drugs.

We have a pretty standard procedure in treating patients and have had no deaths with electroshock treatment. We have had no problems at all for at least six years. Patients do not receive any medication, that is any of the drugs, reserpine or Thorazine, for about six hours prior to treatment. Every patient receives atropine gr. 1/50 within an hour before treatment, and we use Pentothal or Surital on every patient. We use the relaxing drugs, Anectine and Quelicin in all the patients. These are given prior to treatment. When we give the electroconvulsive therapy, every patient has an airway inserted, and immediately after the current is discontinued every patient receives oxygen, by the positive pressure technic. With that technic we have not had any apnea, nor any difficulty—not even a shade of a problem in any patient receiving electroshock combined with Thorazine and Serpasil.

Dr. Foster (Closing). I appreciate the discussion and was expecting a certain amount of this reaction.

As to the cause of death in the patient about which you asked, this patient did not breathe and we could get no evidence of circulation following treatment. The postmortem examination was done by the state medical examiner, but he could find nothing anatomically to explain the death of the patient. There were no other drugs complicating the case. The patient was 45 years of age.

It has been suggested that reserpine can cause coronary insufficiency even without electroshock, so that may have been a factor.

I would agree with Dr. Ayd about the use of norepinephrine. We have utilized this drug when we have found hypotension with either drug.

As to the hazards of Thorazine and electroshock, in combination: in addition to our feeling about the similarity between this drug, and reserpine, there have been two cases reported in one of the other hospitals in Virginia. I did not feel justified in reporting it in the paper, but I mention it in passing in the discussion, my reason being that a variation in standard technics was used, and I do not know about the controls. When there are too many variables results may be inconclusive. In addition, I have a communication from Dr. Dale Console, who is the chief of research for one of the pharmaceutical houses, describing two similar deaths.

The question of whether dosage or premature drug termination accounted for our failures is valid. This would lengthen our discussion quite a bit. I would say ordinarily in using chlorpromazine following electroshock, we rarely go higher than 600 mg. a day by mouth and maintain that in the hospital for a week or ten days prior to discharge, before reducing the amount. This would seem sufficient in view of the fact that only four of our series required further hospitalization. Again, I might emphasize the relatively short follow-up period.

Finally, we do not check the blood pressure routinely unless there are objective symptoms.

DRUG THERAPY IN THE EMOTIONALLY DISTURBED AGED

Sol Levy, M.D.

Improvements in medical care and general living conditions have definitely lengthened the average span of human life. Each year a greater percentage of the population reaches advanced age and statistics indicate that this trend will continue. Consequently, there are constantly increasing numbers of persons subject to degenerative changes, especially in the central nervous system. Therefore, there has been an ever increasing demand for admission of aged patients to private and public, general and mental institutions. At the present time, more than one-third of all persons admitted for the first time to public mental hospitals in the United States are over 65 years of age. Magnitude of the problem posed by this group of persons needs no further emphasis but its significance is widened when one considers that for each person whose condition requires care in a general or mental hospital or even in a nursing home, there must be several others who can be cared for at home and who are not admitted to such institutions. Thus, as physicians we have increasing numbers of aged patients to deal with, and the problems they present are rather complex.

Because many of them are extremely difficult to handle, management of aged patients, in the past, has been viewed with extreme pessimism. However, we cannot close our eyes to this problem, hence more and more interest and attention have been given to the problems of the aging and the aged, both physical and emotional. New methods and ways are continually being searched for and being found to help in dealing with the aged.

We have learned, for instance, that to age is to change. The aging and the aged are different persons than they were in youth. Nutrition, anatomy, physiology and emotional equilibrium are peculiar to this age period and quite different from other periods of life. It also has been found that the group of the aging and aged presents a field in which disease can be prevented and health built. For instance, many of the milder forms of emotional and mental disorders, which are characteristic of the aging process, can be prevented, and with not much more than proper education.

Much of the stress of later life, which seems responsible for the onset of mild emotional and mental disorders, can be predicted and prevented. It is just a matter of preparing the adult for the coming senescence and telling him what to expect. This should include giving him new interests and values to make him feel useful within his own limitations. Attempt should be made to produce greater sense of security, of belonging, and of worth.

These factors are extremely important for the entire group of the aging and aged. There are many in this group who, in spite of these efforts, will present emotional and mental problems which must be taken care of by the physician in office or institutional practice.

We know that it is not uncommon for emotional or even major mental disorders to occur first in old age. Symptoms are similar to those occurring in the younger age groups. Therapeutic measures utilized for the younger persons can also be applied to this group. Overt psychotic reactions, if they should occur in the aged, should be treated as such. All newer therapeutic methods, as for instance convulsant therapies, should be utilized fully.

For milder forms of emotional and mental disorders treatment should be the same as in younger persons. Good results can be obtained. It is no longer true that because of advanced age, emotional and mental disorders are results of irreversible pathologic brain changes for which nothing can be done. Many so-called functional types of emotional and psychotic reactions develop late in life. Treatment can be given.

During recent years psychiatry has entered a new era, that of pharmacotherapy. With introduction of such drugs as chlorpromazine, the reserpines, Metrazol, Meratran, and Frenquel, to name just a few, great strides have been made in treatment of mental disorders. These drugs have been found to be extremely helpful, in conjunction with others, in treatment of emotionally and mentally ill aged patients. They may be given with as much safety as to the younger patient.

Chlorpromazine has been found to be extremely helpful in cases showing manic type of behavior characterized by agitation, hyperactivity and overproduction of speech and thought. It has the property of calming this type of patient, regardless of age. Many aged patients, because of their sense of insecurity and loss of self-worth and self-respect, become increasingly restless, agitated and irritable. It is in these cases that chlorpromazine has proven to be most successful. Before administering this drug to the aged, one must be familiar with possible complications, such as disturbance in liver function.

Reserpines can also be used with success in treating the aged. They are indicated where anxiety, tension and general nervousness, with or without psychosomatic manifestations, exist. Naturally, because of the hypotensive effect of these drugs, care should be taken in their administration. Indiscriminate use could lead, just as in the case of chlorpromazine, to tragic results. If properly used, they can be a major tool in rehabilitation of the aged.

Many of the aged become depressed because of their feeling of unworthiness, loss of self-respect and self-value. If depression is too severe, convulsant therapy, with or without prior administration of intravenous Coramine, is definitely indicated. In the milder forms of depression, which might be characterized by only autonomic symptoms, Meratran has been successful. Action of this drug is roughly similar to that of the amphetamines but appetite loss and cardio-vascular effects are not encountered. It does not interfere with nocturnal sleep. The drug is indicated, however, only if depression is not coupled with anxiety and tension. If this should occur, Meratran together with one of the reserpines should be given.

Frenquel, which is pharmacologically related to Meratran, has produced encouraging results in acute schizophrenia, regardless of age. It has also been found to be helpful in the periodic dissociation reactions which occur in senile patients with organic brain syndromes. In this group it has been able to relieve some of the noisy confusion and fears based on paranoid and hallucinatory experiences.

For many years a great deal of importance was attached to cerebral anoxia as the factor responsible for milder mental symptoms in the aged. These included confusion, emotional lability, errors in judgment, and inability to concentrate. Various therapies were introduced with the ultimate goal of correcting the presumed anoxia. One agent proven to be fairly successful is Metrazol, which has long been effective in respiratory and circulatory stimulation. Through its ability to stimulate the respiratory center in the aged, it was reasoned that it would improve pulmonary ventilation and, indirectly, the circulation. Thus it was expected to help overcome the anoxia frequently present in the aged. Numerous reports have appeared pointing to beneficial effect of Metrazol in treatment of the aged. This drug has proven to be especially helpful in care of institutionalized aged.

Several years ago I introduced the combination of Metrazol and nicotinic acid. It has been found to be of great value in treatment of aged patients. It is particularly useful in those with only mild memory defects, confusion and deterioration, in the absence of the more serious emotional and psychotic disturbances. It was found to be especially helpful in combating symptoms of abnormal behavior. These are the symptoms most objectionable to relatives of the aged.

Symptoms attributable to intellectual impairment are not combatted so successfully with this combination of drugs. This might be due to the fact that intellect and memory are first to suffer, while personality changes occur later. Thus, it may be assumed that intellectual deterioration depends upon more definite organic changes that may be irreversible. Symptoms of impaired behavior, to some extent, may still be reversible. Elixir of Metrazol and nicotinic acid has proven to be safe, practical and inexpensive. It may be used, without hesitation, on ambulatory patients of this group. Many of the aging and aged, therefore, with the help of this elixir or possibly other drugs of similar action, would not inevitably have to be committed to psychiatric institutions or placed in nursing homes. They could be permitted to live in the community with safety and without harm to others.

Thus, in conclusion from the foregoing, it can be seen that these drugs have proven to be of great value in certain cases of emotional and mental disorder in the aged. They have greatly enlarged our therapeutic arsenal for care of the aged. However, it should be cautioned that, although these drugs have proven to be of definite value, they are not wonder drugs in any sense. They should not be used to replace previously established successful treatment procedures. They are definitely valuable adjuncts, but over-enthusiasm and over-reliance may lead to tragic results. It should be mentioned that modern psychiatry—and this is especially true for geriatric psychiatry—deals with the individual and not with a label of illness pinned on this individual. Therefore, each case has to be considered on its own merits and specific treatment has to be prescribed for the individual case. This, in turn, should change our previously held pessimistic and even nihilistic attitude as far as treatment of emotional and mental conditions in the aged is concerned.

THE TREATMENT OF ANXIETY, AGITATION AND EXCITEMENT IN THE AGED
A Preliminary Report on Trilafon

Frank J. Ayd, Jr., M.D.

The pharmacologic management of the psychiatric disorders of geriatric patients challenges the therapeutic acumen of the physician. He must choose a drug which will produce a satisfactory remission as quickly as possible and with the least risk. For this reason the new tranquilizers represent an advance over the barbiturates, bromides, and chloral hydrate. However, these drugs are not the final answer to the troublesome emotional problems of senescence and the need for other new compounds exists.

Trilafon, or 1-(2-hydroxyethyl)-4-[3-(2-chlor-10-phenothiazl)-propyl]-piperazine, is a new tranquilizer which is rapidly active and therapeutically effective with a minimum of side-effects. It calms psychomotor excitement, agitation and anxiety but has little or no effect on an endogenous depression. Because of its potency and rapid absorption, small doses are usually therapeutic. This has the additional advantage that the physiologic and neurologic responses to Trilafon are minimal, thus avoiding side-effects which might complicate treatment.

These pharmacologic properties suggested that Trilafon could be useful for the treatment of elderly psychiatric patients. To determine the validity of this surmise, the drug was administered to 25 patients between the ages of 60 and 80. Diagnostically, these patients were classified: severe neurotic reactions 9, psychosis with cerebral arteriosclerosis 2, paranoid psychoses 5, schizophrenic reactions 3, and agitated depressions 6. However, they were selected for therapy primarily because anxiety, agitation or excitement was the predominant symptom of their illness.

TECHNIQUE OF THERAPY

In mildly and moderately disturbed patients the initial dosage of Trilafon was 4 mg. twice daily. If further tranquilization was needed the dosage was increased by increments of 4 mg. until the therapeutic level for the patient was reached. The most effective therapeutic dosage for this type of patient was found to be between 12 and 24 mg. daily. The drug was then gradually discontinued over a period of several months. In a few instances symptoms recurred as the dose was reduced, but disappeared on re-institution of Trilafon; these patients are now on maintenance therapy.

The treatment of acutely disturbed patients was initiated by administering Trilafon orally or intramuscularly. Most patients were given 8 mg. to 16 mg.

orally twice daily. When parenteral medication was employed, the dosage was 5 to 10 mg. every six or eight hours. This quickly induced a quiescent state characterized by somnolence or sleep. After three or four intramuscular injections, oral medication could be substituted. Thereafter, the dosage was adjusted for the patient and gradually reduced as improvement occurred.

Since Trilafon is not a powerful hypnotic, barbiturates were prescribed occasionally in addition, whenever insomnia was severe. Such combined therapy was found to be safe and practical, because Trilafon does not potentiate the action of barbiturates.

Therapeutic Results

To assay the benefits of Trilafon therapy the following criteria were employed: 1) marked improvement indicated complete remission from overt symptoms of a psychosis or neurosis, and 2) moderate improvement signified a sufficient degree of symptomatic relief to permit the patient to function satisfactorily. By these standards 19 of the 25 patients studied were improved (Table 1).

TABLE 1
Diagnostic Grouping and Therapeutic Results

Diagnosis	Marked	Moderate	None
Severe neurotic reactions	4	3	2
Psychosis/cerebral arteriosclerosis		1	1
Paranoid psychosis	3	2	
Schizophrenic reactions	1	1	1
Agitated depressions		4	2
Total	8	11	6

The symptomatic response varied with the severity of the condition treated. The more pronounced the emotional distress, the more striking was the effect of Trilafon. Consequently, the most dramatic improvement was observed in acutely ill patients in whom emotional turbulence and disturbed behavior were replaced by placidity. Comparable therapeutic results were observed in the neurotic and mildly disturbed psychotic patients, but in these individuals behavioral changes were less prominent.

Most of the improved patients experienced an onset of symptomatic relief within three to seven days after the beginning of Trilafon therapy. Initially, this consisted of subjective relief from anxiety. It was followed by behavioral changes proportionate to the affective changes. In the psychotic patients there was no apparent alteration in thinking, but delusions died out or were not verbalized for lack of emotional reinforcement. Neurotic patients reported that their obsessions or phobias were still present but no longer concerned them. The physical manifestations of disturbed autonomic function associated with anxiety were minimized or eradicated in the improved patients.

Trilafon was not an effective treatment for endogenous depressions. However, if the depression was accompanied by anxiety or agitation this drug relieved these symptoms. In such patients it was found that a combination of Trilafon and electroconvulsive therapy was safe and effective. The drug was also administered concomitantly with electroconvulsive therapy to prevent postconvulsive excitement and anxiety precipitated by the shock treatment.

Two patients in this group had nausea and vomiting associated with physical disorders. Trilafon absolished these symptoms almost immediately. In another clinical trial, which included patients with nausea and vomiting due to various causes such as pregnancy, Trilafon was found to be a potent antiemetic.

Illustrative Cases

Case 1: This man, aged 73, complained to the police that an attempt to murder him by poisonous gas had been made by his enemies. During the psychiatric examination he revealed that he was the victim of a conspiracy and that various attempts on his life had been made by unknown people who pumped gas into his room through the walls and tried to contaminate his food. With considerable anxiety and agitation he described being tortured by physical pains which his persecutors caused, and of being spied on and followed constantly.

The diagnosis was paranoid psychosis. The patient was given Trilafon, 4 mg. three times a day, increased to a maximum of 20 mg. daily. Within two weeks he no longer spontaneously mentioned his paranoid ideas. Three months later he was still taking Trilafon, 8 mg. daily, though there was no overt evidence of his psychosis. This man was staid, and when his former delusions were recalled to him he acknowledged that he still had the same ideas but commented that they caused him no concern.

Case-2: This 60-year-old woman's husband was informed by the FBI that she was pestering them with calls about communists. When examined she was very agitated and spoke of being persecuted. She revealed that she had procured a gun which she intended to use if necessary. She accused her children of attempting to poison her, and her husband of withholding money which was sent to her to help her wage her fight against enemies. She mentioned hearing voices and communicating with deceased acquaintances. She rejected the idea that she was ill, and considerable force was required to hospitalize her.

In the hospital, a diagnosis of schizophrenic reaction, paranoid type, was made. Trilafon therapy was started in a dosage of 4 mg. twice daily, with Nembutal, 3 grains at bedtime. Within a week the patient had improved considerably and was granted ground privileges. Some motor restlessness appeared after a month on Trilafon; this was abolished by an anti-Parkinsonism drug. Three months after admission she was discharged. She had recovered from her overt psychosis, but delusions could still be elicited on examination. For this reason, Trilafon was continued in a dosage of 8 mg. daily.

Case 3: This man, aged 80, was hospitalized for the treatment of an agitated depression with suicidal rumination. His physical condition was such that electroconvulsive treatment was contraindicated. He refused to eat, cried often, and paced the floor wringing his hands, and expressing delusions of unworthiness and despair; he slept poorly. He was given 10 mg. of Trilafon intramuscularly.

This erased the agitation and engendered somnolence. After three intramuscular injections of 10 mg. he slept for fourteen hours. Oral medication (8 mg. twice daily) was substituted, and this was gradually reduced to 4 mg. twice daily. After six weeks the patient was discharged to his home, improved. He is still depressed but no longer agitated, crying or preoccupied with suicidal thoughts. He sleeps fairly well, his appetite is improved, and he is gaining weight.

Case 4: A 68-year-old woman was treated on an ambulatory basis because of an exacerbation of a chronic anxiety reaction. She complained of persistent apprehension, numerous phobias, attacks of cardiac palpitation associated with dizziness and shortness of breath, episodic gastro-intestinal discomfort and diarrhea, difficulty in falling asleep, and nightmares. Trilafon was prescribed in a dosage of 4 mg. three times daily. This produced partial improvement and the dose was increased gradually to 24 mg. daily. Within four months this patient was symptom-free and Trilafon was gradually discontinued.

Case 5: A 75-year-old woman with a terminal carcinoma and cerebral arteriosclerosis was hospitalized on the medical service because of dehydration due to vomiting. She became extremely agitated and uncooperative. This impeded her medical treatment and transfer to the psychiatric service became necessary. Trilafon was administered on a schedule of 4 mg. intramuscularly every six hours for four doses. The patient became tranquil and cooperative, and her nausea and vomiting ceased. Until her death two months later, oral Trilafon in a dosage of 4 mg. four times a day controlled this patient's psychotic behavior, eradicated the nausea and vomiting, and obviated the need for more than a modicum of narcotics for pain.

SIDE EFFECTS

Trilafon may cause the following side-effects: weakness and fatigue, aching arms and legs, dryness of the mouth, miosis, constipation, and increased dreams. These usually occur in the early weeks of treatment when the larger doses are required. They are transient, even with continued medication, and do not require the addition of other drugs to counteract them. Trilafon may also cause motor restlessness, tremulousness and Parkinsonian manifestations. These extrapyramidal symptoms are related to the dose, and seldom occur in patients taking less than 30 mg. daily. A reduction of the dose, or administration of anti-Parkinsonism drugs will abolish them, so that it is unnecessary to interrupt Trilafon treatment when neurologic symptoms appear.

COMMENT

With advancing age, drug sensitivity and intolerance increase. Barbiturates, for example, may induce stimulation instead of sedation and the ensuing anxiety or restlessness may lead to the injudicious prescribing of more barbiturates. Idiosyncratic reactions to chlorpromazine and promazine, such as sudden hypotension with syncope, dermatitis, jaundice and granulocytopenia, occur most often in geriatric patients. Meprobamate-induced dermatitis and anaphylactic reactions also are most likely to occur in the older patients.

Although any drug may cause unusual reactions, especially in geriatric patients, no case of sensitivity or intolerance to Trilafon has been observed in elderly patients thus far. Nevertheless, since this compound is a phenothiazine derivative and because of the propensity of geriatric patients to be drug-sensitive, physicians must be alert for adverse reactions to Trilafon and institute counteracting measures immediately.

Summary and Conclusions

This paper describes Trilafon, a new tranquilizer, and its use in the treatment of the psychiatric disorders of geriatric patients. The technique of therapy, dosage, therapeutic results, and side-effects are discussed. Trilafon is a valuable drug for the symptomatic treatment of any psychiatric illness in which anxiety is paramount. This drug is especially suitable for geriatric patients, since it has not caused hypotensive reactions, dermatitis, hepatitis or granulocytopenia. It is a welcome addition to pharmaceutical agents for treating emotional and mental aberrations on an ambulatory basis.

IMPROVING SENILE BEHAVIOR WITH RESERPINE AND RITALIN

John T. Ferguson, M. D., and William H. Funderburk, Ph.D.

The advances made in medicine during the past few decades have been nothing short of miraculous. Man is healthier, and he lives better; he also lives longer. Consequently, we have produced a new and ever-increasing problem—the sociomedical complications created by these extra years. Today several million persons are involved; the number will be astronomical in the future unless prevention and control are found. An analysis of the situation reveals that abnormal behavior manifestations are predominant in those elderly individuals requiring special care, hospitalization, or institutionalization. Medical prevention and control of these abnormalities in the elderly by those closest to them, general practitioners, should be the starting point of attack.

In an effort to establish a therapeutic regimen for this type of patient that would assist in management at home, thus decreasing the need of institutionalization and the heartaches associated with it, this project was started. Our objective was to evaluate the effectiveness of reserpine (Serpasil), a tranquilizing drug, and Ritalin (methyl phenylpiperidylacetate), a psychoanaleptic drug, in controlling, ameliorating, or eliminating the abnormal behavior manifestations seen in elderly hospitalized patients. This report covers our observations after approximately 11 months of the oral administration of the drugs to 215 patients over 60 years of age who were management problems due to one or more manifestations of abnormal behavior.

Selection of Patients and Preliminary Evaluations

Although our original investigation of the geriatric population at Traverse City State Hospital revealed no correlation between the chronological age of the patients and the degree of senescence present, the arbitrary age of 60 was chosen as our base age. The 15 female halls and cottages, often called "backwards," which cover the complete range from seclusion to open as well as an infirmary, were chosen for the project because they represent a cross section of the usual state hospital geriatric population as well as a cross section of those geriatric patients who present the problems in behavior management in private practice. In our hospital these wards contain about one-third of the patients over 60 years of age, so that over two-thirds of our geriatric population acted as controls. Those patients from each of the 15 wards who were over 60 years of age, were known to have some behavior abnormality, or were management problems were chosen as participants, regardless of the diagnosis or pathological complications. The project, therefore, included patients with the types of behavior—overactive, underactive, and mixed—that were the basis for our use of the tranquilizing drug reserpine and/or the psychoanaleptic drug Ritalin.

Our preliminary studies revealed no correlation between aging, disease, or behavior, and there were no changes common to the group, although the largest portion of the 215 had some degree of deteriorated senile or arteriosclerotic change, with the subsequent mental symptoms and behavioral patterns associated with these changes. The number of abnormal nonprotein nitrogen values, cephalin flocculation tests, blood sugar levels, and urinalyses was compatible with a geriatric group of this size. There were no abnormalities of the total blood picture, including the number or relative proportion of the white blood cells that could be associated with the advanced ages of the group.

From the cardiac standpoint, due to our use of a drug that has some influence on the blood pressure, it is worthwhile to note that 81 of the 215 patients had cardiac abnormalities ranging from mild arteriosclerotic changes to marked electrocardiographic changes. The blood pressures of the 215 patients varied from 90/60 to 280/180 mm. Hg. The pulse rates varied from 36 per minute in two patients with heart block to 120 in several others. Forty-two of the 215 were receiving therapy with some digitalis preparation.

The ages of the 215 patients ranged from 60 to 84 years, with the average of the group being 66 plus. The length of time each patient had been in the hospital varied from one year to more than 53 years, with the average time spent in the hospital being 18 years.

Dosage Plan

The project was limited to oral medication. We used the standard 0.1 and 1.0 mg. reserpine tablets and the standard 0.2 mg. per teaspoonful elixir of reserpine. For the Ritalin we used the 10 and 20 mg. scored tablets. No special schedules were set up for the project; the drugs were given at the regular time used by each ward for dispensing medicine. This allowed a three-time-a-day schedule. One hundred one of the 215 patients received their medicine 30 minutes to one hour before meals, and 83 of the 215 received their medicine 30 minutes to one hour after meals. The remaining 31 of the 215 tended to resist the medicine, so their tablets were crushed and put in their food or beverage at mealtime.

Our first doses were based on an evaluation of the individual patient's behavior. This was accomplished by using an 11-category check system, which covered the following points of behavior: (1) personal appearance, (2) personal care, (3) motor activity, (4) aggressiveness, (5) eating habits, (6) toilet habits, (7) night behavior, (8) socialization, (9) supervision needed, (10) cooperation in routine, and (11) rehabilitation. Those patients showing predominance of overactivity in these categories were started on therapy with reserpine. Those showing a predominance of negative characteristics were started on therapy with Ritalin. Those showing a mixed type of behavior were started on therapy with reserpine and Ritalin at the same time. At the start, 62 of the 215 were given Ritalin alone. One hundred thirty-one of the 215 were given reserpine alone, and the remaining 22 of the 215 were given reserpine and Ritalin at the same time. From previous investigation of the two drugs we felt that a lower dosage schedule would be better for this group of patients. The starting dose for those receiving Ritalin alone was 10 mg. three times a day and for those receiving reserpine alone 0.25 mg. three times a day; those receiving both were given 0.2 mg. of reserpine and 10 mg. of Ritalin three times a day.

For the first 30 days the patients were checked each day and a minimal increase or decrease of each dose (0.1 mg. of reserpine or 5 mg. of Ritalin three times a day) was made every 24 to 48 hours as individually needed. By this method clinical behavior changes were gradual and controllable. We found that approximately 10% of the underactive group required more Ritalin than the 10 mg. three times a day used at the start. However, when 20 mg. of Ritalin three times a day did not produce a clinical response within two weeks, we reevaluated the patients and usually found their underactive clinical pattern was secondary to much internal anxiety and tension. By using reserpine to relieve this phase of behavior, we were then able to adjust the Ritalin for an improved over-all clinical behavior pattern.

In the overactive group we found approximately 15% who required more reserpine to control their aggressiveness and motor activity than the 0.25 mg. three times a day used at the start. By adding 0.1 to 0.2 mg. of reserpine three times a day every 24-48 hours on an individual basis, we were able to produce clinical change. In some patients this extra reserpine produced drowsiness, stuffy nose, red eyes, increased salivation, or diarrhea. However, the addition of 5 mg. of Ritalin three times a day, then, after 24 to 48 hours, the gradual reduction of the dosage of reserpine to a maintenance level eliminated these side-reactions.

After a period varying from three days to three weeks it was felt that 57 of the 62 patients receiving Ritalin alone and 116 of the 131 patients receiving reserpine alone would do better if given both drugs. Consequently, in each case the second drug was added at the rate of 0.1 mg. of reserpine three times a day to the patients receiving Ritalin and 5 mg. of Ritalin three times a day to the patients receiving reserpine as individually needed each 48 hours. As the clinical behavior pattern of each patient shifted toward normal, we found she needed less reserpine and/or Ritalin. Therefore, in an effort to establish a maintenance dose level for the patients, after they showed clinical improvement, we changed the reserpine dose 0.1 mg. three times a day and/or the Ritalin dose 5 mg. three times a day every 48 hours, based upon each patient's individual improvement toward normal and the amount of overactivity or underactivity present. We have by this method been able, after periods varying from four to eight months, to discontinue use of the drugs completely in 67 of the 215 patients without a return of the original abnormal behavior.

In order to maintain the optimal improvement in the behavior of the remaining 148 of the 215, it has been necessary to continue use of the drugs, although all of them have had use of their medicaments discontinued one or more times during the 11 months of the project. At the time of writing, 136 of the 148 are receiving 0.1 to 0.2 mg. of reserpine and 5 to 10 mg. of

Ritalin three times a day, while 8 of the 148 are receiving 0.5 to 1.0 mg. of reserpine and 5 mg. of Ritalin three times a day and 4 of the 148 are receiving 0.2 mg. of reserpine and 20 mg. of Ritalin three times a day.

Whenever it was necessary to adjust the medicines, we found that the clinical observations were most satisfactory, and, although behavior charts were made and laboratory work carried on in conjunction with the project, these were not found to be necessary. We were quite pleased with these findings, inasmuch as this allows for the use of these drugs by the general practitioner when he is unable to do routine follow-up laboratory procedures. To illustrate the type of patient in the project and to give examples of our method of administering the reserpine and/or Ritalin, three cases are presented.

Report of Cases

CASE 1.—This patient is a 76-year-old female who was admitted in 1910. She was a talkative, wandering, disoriented, and confused woman who resisted help but was unable to help herself. She required extra nursing care, as she was a feeding problem; she was untidy and soiled most of the time. She spent most of her time in the "specialing" room for her own protection. She was started on therapy with 0.25 mg. of reserpine three times a day. Within five days she was much quieter and more friendly. Her appetite picked up, and she went to the toilet with help. Within 15 days she was sleeping in the daytime, so 5 mg. of Ritalin three times a day was added. She became more alert and stopped sleeping within three days, but her motor activity was slow. Dosage of reserpine was then reduced to 0.2 mg. She continued slowly to awaken to reality, showed a decrease in confusion, and started participating in off-ward activities during the next month. After three months the dosage of reserpine was reduced to 0.1 mg. three times a day. Her condition was without change for two weeks, then she started becoming overactive. Dosage of reserpine was then increased to 0.2 mg. three times a day, where it has remained. She has continued to improve slowly on therapy with the 0.2 mg. of reserpine and 5 mg. of Ritalin three times a day for six months. However, her age and fragility have limited her activities to the sedentary type. She has ground parole and could go home or to a nursing home.

CASE 2.—This patient is a 67-year-old mentally retarded female who was admitted in 1929. She was noisy at times and had "jerkiness" of arm and feet at times. She never bothered others or caused trouble on the ward. She is partially blind and feels her way to the dining room and toilet. She made her own bed, but otherwise spent the remainder of the time away from others in a side-room. Our aim was to eliminate the noise and excess movements while still trying to decrease her underactivity. She was started on therapy with 0.2 mg. of reserpine and 10 mg. of Ritalin three times a day. After three days she was noisier, so dosage of reserpine was increased to 0.3 mg. three times a day and dosage of Ritalin reduced to 5 mg. three times a day. Within a week her noise had subsided, so the dosage of Ritalin was raised to 10 mg. three times a day. She gradually became more friendly and started a friendship with another patient. This second patient helped her to the dining room and to entertainment. The patient seemed to be slightly underactive after another month, so the dosage of reserpine was reduced to 0.2 mg. three times a day. After four months therapy was reduced until she was without any for better than a month. However, her old pattern started to reappear, and she lost much of her mental alertness. Therapy with 0.1 mg. of reserpine and 5 mg. of Ritalin three times a day was restarted. Within four days she was back to her optimal improvement. She has remained on therapy with this dose since then. She has ground parole, which she uses with the help of her friend. She could go home or to a nursing home, but the change, due to her poor eyesight, might be too much for her to surmount.

Case 3.—This 65-year-old female was admitted in 1922. She never talked unless prodded and was slow in movements. She needed help for all routine procedures, was a very finicky eater, and never moved by herself except to toilet. She was started on therapy with 10 mg. of Ritalin three times a day. There was no change after five days, so the dosage of Ritalin was raised to 15 mg. three times a day. There was no change at the end of four days on this regimen, so the dosage of Ritalin was raised to 20 mg. three times a day. After the third 20-mg. dose she was seen to get in line for dinner without having to be helped. She gradually started entering ward routine for the next two weeks and then started talking. However, it was felt she was showing a trend toward overactivity, so 0.1 mg. of reserpine was added to her regimen. This produced no change, so three days later the dosage of reserpine was raised to 0.2 mg. three times a day. After three days she was quieter in her activity but was talking too much. The dosage of Ritalin was reduced to 15 mg. three times a day and then after three days to 10 mg. three times a day. With this dose she has improved considerably. She participates in ward activities, enjoys television, goes to church and the movies, and went to the hospital picnic this year for the first time in 31 years. She has ground parole but will not leave the ward unless there is a group accompanied by a nurse. Her personal appearance is improved, as she likes to go to the Swap Shop (our volunteers' clothing and knick-knack shop) and pick our beads and other accessories. Her eating is normal, and she has gained weight.

Results in Relation to Behavior

At the start all 215 participants were chosen because they had some abnormal behavior manifestation. At the time of writing 171 of the 215 show a reduction in their original abnormal behavior while 44 of the 215 remain essentially the same. Changes within the control group during this period are negligible. As our investigation progressed we found our records were giving us an evaluation of the drugs in relation to the specific behavior covered by each category of our records. Consequently, we are reporting our observations (fig. 1 and 2) for each category in the hope that this new approach will help in establishing more specific indications for the use of reserpine and/or Ritalin in the management of the elderly patient.

Personal Appearance.—In the category personal appearance, 97 of the 215 patients were careless or were unable to take care of their manner or mode of dress. At the time of writing 81, or 83.5%, of the 97 show improvement. The most noticeable change is in the patients' ability to take an interest in what they wear and how they wear it; they also show increased interest in such things as jewelry, permanent waves, and dentures.

Personal Care.—In the category personal care, 134 of the 215 were either resistive to or were unable to handle washing, bathing, and other personal

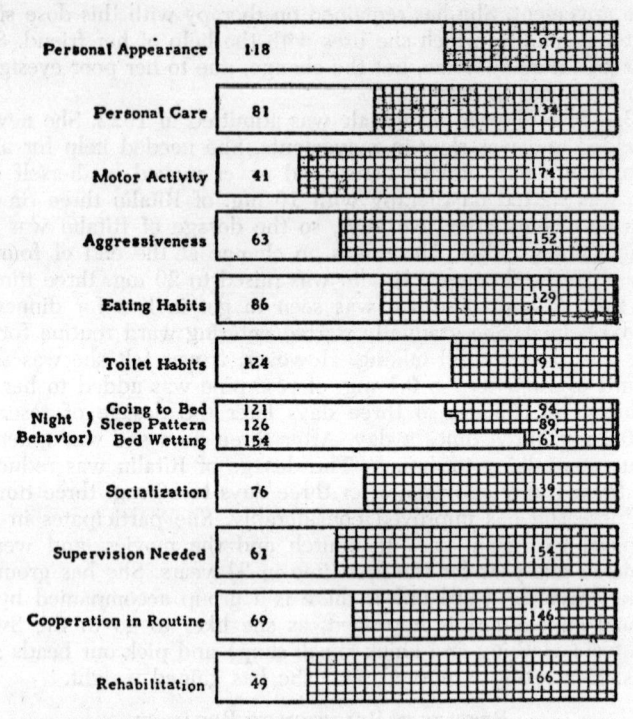

Personal Appearance	118	97
Personal Care	81	134
Motor Activity	41	174
Aggressiveness	63	152
Eating Habits	86	129
Toilet Habits	124	91
Night Behavior) Going to Bed	121	94
Sleep Pattern	126	89
Bed Wetting	154	61
Socialization	76	139
Supervision Needed	61	154
Cooperation in Routine	69	146
Rehabilitation	49	166

Fig. 1.—Behavioral patterns in 215 mentally ill aged patients before Ritalin-reserpine therapy. White areas, normal or adequate behavior; checked areas, abnormal behavior pattern.

hygiene. Now 110, or 82.1%, of the 134 show improvement. This is manifested by more personal cleanliness without help or supervision, although in most cases the total improvement is the result of retraining by the attendant-nurses of the wards.

Motor Activity.—In the category motor activity, 174 of the 215 had some abnormal overactive or underactive manifestation, such as pacing the floor, picking at themselves or others, exploring, remaining in bed, or sitting motionless unless prodded. Now 121, or 69.5%, of the 174 have improved. This is most noticeable by the decrease in movement on the wards and the decrease in patients remaining in bed or lying on the floor. There is a marked trend toward normal motor activity in both the underactive and the overactive group.

Aggressiveness.—In the category aggressiveness, 152 of the 215 were either overaggressive to themselves or others or were underaggressive and withdrawn from others at all times. Now 109, or 71.7%, of the 152 show a marked improvement toward reality. There is less fighting and destruction and fewer accidents, along with fewer patients hiding. This appears to be the secondary result of decreased confusion and as a result has increased the patients' ability to understand what is happening about them.

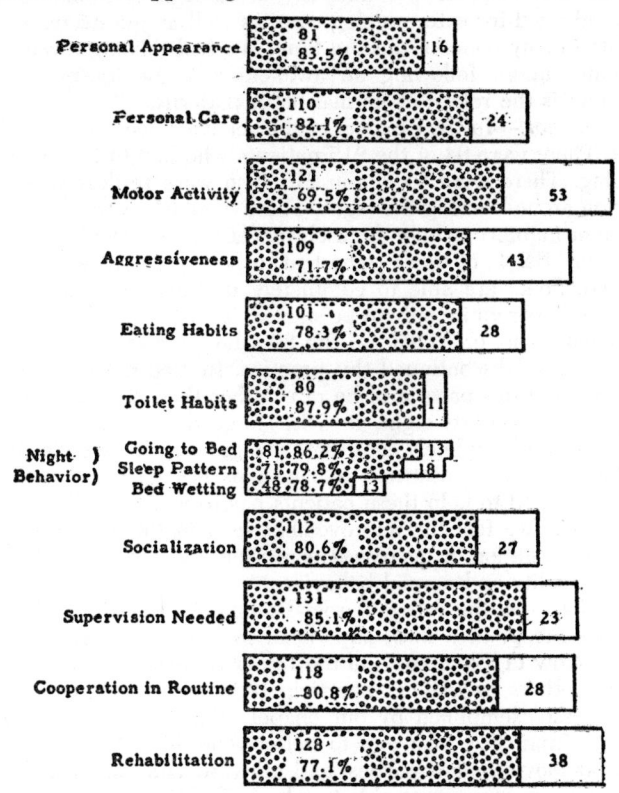

Fig. 2.—Behavioral changes after Ritalin-reserpine therapy in group showing abnormal behavior pattern (fig. 1). Dotted areas, improved with Ritalin-reserpine therapy; %, percentage of improvement with combination; white areas, unchanged.

Eating Habits.—In the category eating habits, there were 129 of the 215 who were unable to or did not eat properly in relation to messiness, greediness, need to be fed, or proper balanced caloric intake. Now 101, or 78.3%, of the 129 show marked improvement in eating habits. There is a marked decrease in those needing to be spoon-fed and in the finicky eaters. It appears that there has been an awakening toward old manners and better balance in that which is eaten. One hundred thirty-one of the 215 have gained weight during the project. Consequently, the over-all health of the group has improved. The decrease in nursing time is quite noticeable in this category.

Toilet Habits.—In the category toilet habits, 91 of the 215 were occasionally untidy, needed toilet supervision, or had no comprehension of the toilet at all during their waking hours. Now 80, or 87.9%, of the 91 are improved. At the start there were 27 who soiled regardless of the help given them. At the time of writing 23 have stopped spontaneously, while 2 are responding to training. The decreased need for extra nursing care, as well as the decrease in laundry, has eliminated many hours of nursing time. We feel this improvement is a secondary manifestation, following an awakening to reality produced by the medicines, and is the return of normal habit patterns.

Night Behavior.—In the category night behavior, we divided behavior into three parts. There were 94 of the 215 patients who had to be helped to bed or resisted going. There were 89 of the 215 who were restless sleepers or were up wandering around during the night. There were 61 of the 215 who because of confusion or inability to help themselves wet the bed regularly or occasionally. Now 81, or 86.2%, of the 94 who had to be supervised when going to bed are improved. Some are able to completely undress and take care of themselves, while others require only to be started. There are no longer any resistive patients. Seventy-one, or 79.8%, of the 89 who were restless sleepers or were up wandering have discontinued this practice. In fact, the night nursing notes of the wards show this pattern to be rare rather than regular as it was before starting the project. Forty-eight, or 78.7%, of the 61 who wet the bed at night have stopped completely, and there is a gradual decrease in the regularity of the remaining group. Mattress replacement has been cut over 75%, and nursing time needed to help these patients has been drastically reduced. From our observations, we feel the improvement seen in this category is again the secondary manifestation of decreased confusion and the awakening of the patients toward reality and normal behavior.

Socialization.—In the category socialization, 139 of the 215 were unable to participate except in a most superficial manner or resisted any efforts at socialization. Now 112, or 80.6%, of the 139 are able to enter into more sociable relations with others, as well as to participate in supervised reaction and activities. This is best exemplified by our chapel attendance within the group: It has increased from 35 a year ago to better than 110 at the time of writing. Attendance at movies, ward parties, and off-ward entertainment has increased over 300%. This year we were able to take 167 of the group to picinics, which necessitates a 14-mile bus ride, while last year only 42 were able to go. Improvement in this category, both subjectively and objectively, has led to much more enjoyment in living for the group.

Supervision Needed.—In the category supervision needed, there were 154 of the 215 who needed supervision or help in order to complete their daily tasks. Now 131, or 85.1%, of the 154 have improved to the degree that 102 of the 131 have ground privileges and come and go on the campus as they choose. This did not happen spontaneously, as many who were able to go out refused to do so until helped and reassured by our attendant nurses. In this category, we also find less supervision needed in all facets of daily living. The members of the group make more decisions for themselves, so that in all phases of activity the nursing time and care has been reduced and we have been able to spend these hours in constructive rehabilitation. This freedom from need of supervision has also allowed the patients to pursue their own personal pleasure outlets.

Cooperation in Routine.—In the category cooperation in routine, 146 of the 215 were either uncooperative or were unable to cooperate due to confusion or inability to understand directions. Now 118, or 80.8%, of the 146 show improvement. The improvement here parallels that in the category supervision needed, in that the rehabilitative efforts of the personnel have increased the final results as the patients awakened toward reality and lost some of their confusion.

Rehabilitation.—In the category rehabilitation, 166 of the 215 either resisted or were unable to participate in any form of rehabilitation. Now 128, or 77.1%, of the 166 show improvement in their ability to help in daily housekeeping tasks, to help in the dining room, and to go to occupational therapy. There is new interest in knitting and allied crafts to the degree that we have expanded our on-ward activities threefold. There is a new interest in music, and several of the patients now use our pianos regularly, whereas they were unable to enter into any of this activity previous to starting the project.

COMMENT

Improvement was seen at all age levels within the group so that age, per se, is no contraindication to the use of either reserpine and/or Ritalin. The length of time the patient has been ill is not a contraindication to treatment, as many of our patients in the 30 to 40 year bracket of time in the hospital have shown good improvement. None of the patients presenting abnormal physical findings at the start of the project are worse because of having participated. As a result of this, we feel that the usual physical abnormalities associated with elderly patients are no contraindication to the use of the drugs.

Throughout the period of investigation, we found no contraindication to giving the reserpine and/or the Ritalin to any of the 81 patients with cardiac disease. There was a slight gradual decrease of blood pressure in the majority of the hypertensive group receiving reserpine alone, although the hypotensive patients receiving reserpine alone showed no gross changes. The group receiving Ritalin alone and the group receiving Ritalin and reserpine combined showed no blood pressure changes of consequence. None of the patients showed any significant changes beyond normal. At the start, 72 of the 215 patients had some degree of senile tremor. At the time of writing, 61 of the 72 show improvement, manifested by a marked decrease in the rate and degree of the tremors.

During the progress of the project we conducted two withdrawal tests for verification of drug activity. In one, we substituted reserpine placebos for the reserpine in 50 patients, only to find an increase in activity within a few days. In the other, we substituted Ritalin placebos for the Ritalin in 47 patients and found most of them had reverted to their negative pattern within a matter of a few days. In each case, upon restarting therapy with the medicines we found that the patients were back to their improved level within 48 to 72 hours. No evidence of habituation was seen.

We witnessed a slight accumulative type of action with both drugs when they were used alone. This, however, was overcome by a reduction of the dose or the addition of the second drug. Consequently, we do not believe this is a true accumulation but a manifestation of change within the patient and an indication of the need for less medicine. It also leads us to believe that, when this is seen in a patient, it is an indication that the patient is establishing a balance to the degree that the drugs may be eliminated. The same is true of the so-called side-reactions reported for reserpine, inasmuch as we feel these are a manifestation of faulty balance due to improper dosage. It is rather difficult to confirm our beliefs at this time; however, with further investigation of the drugs and the physiological and biochemical actions of the brain, we feel that new light will be shed on the processes involved in mental illnesses.

There is a belief that too much therapeutic intervention in elderly patients is harmful, as it upsets the delicate balance nature has provided. This led us to be more cautious and more observant with this group; however, we believe that the chemotherapeutic management of elderly patients with reserpine and/or Ritalin should be further investigated, as many of the manifestations associated with senescence have been ameliorated or reversed during this project. We are led to believe that most of the improvement we have seen is a secondary manifestation, the primary action being a lessening of confusion and an increase in orientation, or, less specifically, a mental awakening toward reality. We were unable to pin-point this change anatomically, so we are led to believe that we are dealing with internal chemical reactions that in turn give us the manifested changes.

Our work with this group did not allow for psychotherapeutic procedures, but we feel that the complex nature of the illnesses manifested by the patients is such that one approach to the problem is not sufficient. With use of the medicines we saw a marked mental awakening of the patients to the degree that they were better able to participate; however, unless a patient was helped into new situations the improvement was minimal. This means, then, that the treatment of the elderly mentally ill patient is not chemotherapeutic alone but is a team effort in which the adjunct therapies must be used to their fullest to obtain the desired results.

Conclusions

From our work with 215 women over 60 years of age at Traverse City State Hospital, we feel that the oral administration of Ritalin (methyl phenylpiperidil-acetate) and/or reserpine (Serpasil) has a definite place in the therapeutic procedures of those treating elderly patients, as these drugs have opened an entirely new and most promising approach to the problem. Further investigation of this new chemotherapeutic approach to better management of elderly patients is recommended.

HYDROXYZINE: A NEW THERAPEUTIC AGENT FOR SENILE ANXIETY STATES

Mervin Shalowitz, M.D.

Stritch School of Medicine, Loyola University, Chicago, Illinois, and Department of Medicine, Edgewater Hospital, Chicago, Illinois

An oral preparation, Atarax, with the generic name hydroxyzine hydrochloride, has been used by various clinical investigators both here and abroad for treatment of psychoneurotic-like symptoms. The consensus appears to be that this agent has a definite calming effect on nervous and agitated subjects with symptoms such as fatigue states produced by an inability to relax, often encountered in industry; anxiety before college examinations and before important speeches; premenstrual tension; menopausal disturbances; and other situations where emotional stress is prominent.

In the later years of life, some patients may develop psychosomatic complaints caused by changes in living conditions, the loss of spouse, and economic changes following retirement. The symptoms then cause fears which produce further anxiety and symptoms, resulting in a vicious cycle of worry and incapacitation.

Psychoneurotic-like symptoms are often found in hypertensive states, such as generalized arteriosclerosis. Keys states that physical and emotional stress have some effect on the cholesterol metabolism in man. The appearance of micromolecules of low specific gravity and containing cholesterol have been reported in the blood serum of more than 90 per cent of patients with arteriosclerosis of the coronary arteries.

CHEMISTRY AND PHARMACOLOGY

Atarax is a p-chlorobenzhydryl piperazine derivative, chemically designated as 1-(p-cholorbenzhydryl)-4-[2-(2-hydroxyethoxy) ethyl] diethylenediamine (figure I). The hydrochloride of this compound is a crystalline solid readily soluble in water and rapidly absorbed from the gastrointestinal tract.

Administration of an oral toxic dose of hydroxyzine hydrochloride to mice produced only depression, while rats responded with depression, tremor, and ataxia. Rats given hydroxyzine hydrochloride became quiet within a short time and their movements became slower and steadier, but when threatened from the outside, they got up and ran with their customary agility and alertness.

Four groups of monkeys, with two animals in each group, were given hydroxyzine hydrochloride in oral doses of 25, 50, 100, and 200 mg. per kilogram of body weight. An additional group of four monkeys received oral doses of

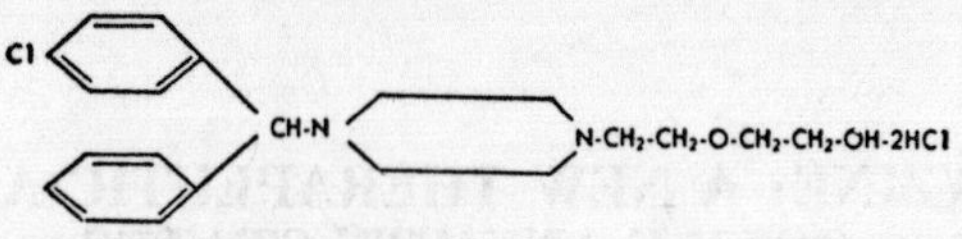

FIG. 1. *Structural formula of hydroxyzine hydrochloride.*

400 mg. per kilogram of body weight. No effect on the behavior of the animals was noted after oral administration of 25 to 400 mg. of hydroxyzine hydrochloride per kilogram of body weight.

Farah observed that the preparation produced more calmness and peace of mind in overemotional patients with anguish and anxiety symptoms than any drug used previously. Settel found that 73 per cent of 30 patients experienced relief of tension, felt more relaxed, and had better control of their tempers.

CLINICAL STUDY

Our study series consisted of 54 patients ranging in age from 65 to 90. Some of the patients had generalized or cerebral arteriosclerosis, alone or combined with other conditions, such as arteriosclerotic heart disease and essential or renal hypertension. Some had duodenal ulcers and diabetes mellitus. Placebos were given to 5 patients for the control of therapeutic results. Two of the control patients were later institutionalized for cerebral arteriosclerosis with senile dementia, manifested in severe agitation, loss of affect, and erratic behavior. Atarax, in the form of 10- and 25-mg. sugar-coated tablets, was administered in doses of 3 to 4 tablets daily after meals, during a period of one to five months.

RESULTS

Most of the patients assimilated the tablets rapidly. According to clinical and laboratory studies, hydroxyzine hydrochloride probably acts on the subcortical area of the brain. A calming effect was noted after three to four days and persistent effect after six to seven days. No increases in the calming effect was observed after seven days of therapy.

In an evaluation of the results, 41, or 76 per cent of the 54 patients treated, showed pronounced improvement; 10, or 18.5 per cent, showed good improvement; and 3, or 5.5 per cent, showed no improvement (see table 1). No evidence of toxicity has been observed to date. Complete liver function tests and blood studies were made on all patients after two months of therapy (tables 2, 3, and 4). In a period of forty-five minutes there was bromsulphalein retention range from 2 to 14 per cent; hemograms showed a range of 12.5 to 17.2 gm.; red cell blood count ranged from 4,010,000 to 6.600,000; and white cell blood count ranged from 5,400 to 14,000 with normal differentials. As can be seen, there were no significant abnormalities.

Hydroxyzine therapy showed no adverse effects on cerebral and generalized arteriosclerosis; cerebral arteriosclerosis; or on generalized arteriosclerosis combined with rheumatoid arthritis, carcinoma of the right antrum, or carcinoma of the breast (postoperative). Arterial hypertension of essential and renal origin, duodenal ulcers, and diabetes mellitus remained unchanged. The white blood

TABLE 1
CROSS SECTION OF RESULTS AFTER TWO MONTHS OF ATARAX THERAPY

Patient	Age	Sex	Dosage	Diagnosis (see key*)	Calming effect
E.E.	73	F	10 mg. q.i.d.	GA	Pronounced
M.W.	76	F	10 mg. q.i.d.	GA	Good
E.A.	75	F	25 mg. q.i.d.	CA	Pronounced
M.L.	68	M	25 mg. q.i.d.	CA	Good
M.H.	69	F	10 mg. q.i.d.	CA	Pronounced
N.B.	72	M	10 mg. q.i.d.	CA & AH	Pronounced
J.B.	76	M	25 mg. q.i.d.	CA & GA	Pronounced
A.W.	78	F	25 mg. q.i.d.	CA & GA	Good
N.M.	80	F	10 mg. q.i.d.	CA & GA	Pronounced
M.N.	76	M	25 mg. q.i.d.	CA & GA	Good
A.S.	68	F	25 mg. q.i.d.	CA & TP & CB	Pronounced
R.A.	71	M	10 mg. q.i.d.	GA & CRA	Pronounced
L.R.	78	F	10 mg. q.i.d.	GA & DM	Pronounced
O.A.	69	M	10 mg. q.i.d.	GA & RA & AH	Good
B.O.	65	F	10 mg. t.i.d.	GA & DU	Pronounced
J.R.	67	M	10 mg. q.i.d.	GA	None
G.O.	78	F	25 mg. q.i.d.	CA & GA	None
E.A.	74	F	Placebo	CA	None
A.W.	78	F	Placebo	CA & OMV	None

*Key to diagnosis:
GA—generalized arteriosclerosis
CA—cerebral arteriosclerosis
TP—taboparesis
CB—carcinoma of the breast
CRA—carcinoma, right antrum
DM—diabetes mellitus
RA—rheumatoid arthritis
DU—duodenal ulcer
AH—arterial hypertension
OMV—occlusion of major vessel

TABLE 2
RESULTS OF LIVER FUNCTION TESTS AFTER TWO MONTHS OF ATARAX THERAPY

Patient	Sex	Bilirubin (1-45 min.)	Thymol turbidity	Bromsulphalein (% retention)
V.G.	M	0.15	0.5	6.0	10
J.M.	M	0.6	1.0	4.0	2
A.R.	F	0.3	0.5	8.5	3
B.M.	F	0.6	0.8	7.5	14
A.P.	F	0.4	0.6	4.5	12
E.E.	F	0.15	0.3	8.0	3
M.H.	F	0.2	0.4	3.0	8
M.W.	F	0.3	0.5	2.5	6
R.A.	M	0.25	0.6	11.0	7
N.B.	M	0.15	0.3	6.0	9
O.A.	M	0.2	0.3	10.0	7
L.R.	F	0.65	1.0	9.0	6
N.M.	F	0.3	0.5	7.0	8

TABLE 3
BLOOD COUNTS AFTER TWO MONTHS OF ATARAX AND PLACEBO ADMINISTRATION

Patient	Sex	Hemo-globin gm.	R.B.C.	W.B.C.	Poly-nuclears	Lympho-cytes	Mono-cytes	Eosino-phils	Baso-phils	Young lymph-ocytes
Atarax:										
V.G.	M	14.5	4,340,000	12,000	60	37	2	1		
J.M.	M	14.9	4,650,000	12,100	75	24	1			
A.R.	F	15.3	4,590,000	9,300	75	24	1			
B.M.	F	14.9	6,200,000	14,000	80	16	4			
A.P.	F	12.5	4,010,000	8,600	64	33	1	2		
E.F.	F	15.7	5,010,000	9,200	64	34	1	1		
M.H.	F	15.3	4,660,000	8,000	64	30	6			
M.W.	F	16.2	5,160,000	8,200	55	44		1		
R.A.	M	17.2	5,220,000	11,200	64	30	6			
N.B.	M	16.6	6,600,000	8,200	72	20	6		2	
O.A.	M	14.9	4,360,000	9,000	57	38	3	Bands 2		
L.R.	F	14.5	4,500,000	6,200	43	51	5			1
N.M.	F	13.7	4,010,000	5,400	66	32	2			
Placebo:										
E.A.	F	10	3,500,000	8,000	65	30	3	2		
A.S.	F	14	4,930,000	4,300	64	32	4			
M.L.	M	13.5	4,250,000	4,750	64	31	2	3		
J.B.	M	13.5	4,570,000	9,200	58	33	4	2		3
A.W.	F	12.5	4,370,000	9,700	68	26	3	3		

cell count made after two months of hydroxyzine therapy showed no evidence of agranulocytosis (table 3).

Complete electroencephalographic tracings were made of 3 additional patients, before and one week after therapy with hydroxyzine, 1 mg. four times a day and 10 mg. preceding the second electroencephalogram. Two patients, C.W., an 85-year-old woman, and J.L., an 88-year-old man, had normal tracings before and after therapy with no changes. The third patient, S.R., a 75-year-old woman, had an abnormally slow electroencephalogram with no focus before hydroxyzine and no change after therapy. It is well known that many sedatives, particularly barbiturates, will alter the normal electroencephalogram. Usually fast activity is increased, but no evidence of this or other changes were found in the patients examined.

When placebos were substituted in some of the patients, a recurrence of symptoms was noted. Administration of Atarax was thought to be especially indicated for cerebral arteriosclerosis, in which use of the common depressants may cause bromide and barbiturate intoxication. It was found that patients with occlusion of a major cerebral vessel did not respond to treatment. Patients who were in an agitated or a somewhat depressed state—conditions which may result after multiple little strokes—responded best to hydroxyzine therapy. All patients treated, except those who responded poorly, reported that they did not feel as fidgety after therapy, and were able to sleep better. In this group, no drowsiness, dryness of mouth, or nasal stuffiness was reported. In most patients, the administration of 10 mg. of Atarax three or four times a day appeared to be

TABLE 4
LIVER FUNCTION TESTS AFTER PLACEBO ADMINISTRATION

Patient	Sex	Direct Bilirubins (mg. %)	Indirect Bilirubins (mg. %)	Total (mg. %)	Thymol in units (Normal = 0 to 5 units)	Bromsulphalein 5 mg./kg./body wt. (Normal = 0 – 5% in 45 min.)
E.A.	F	0.15	0.15	0.3	10.5	15% in 45 min.
A.S.	F	0.4	0.2	0.6	2.5	5% in 45 min.
M.L.	M	0.2	0.2	0.4	1.0	11% in 45 min.
J.B.	M	0.3	0.3	0.6	2.0	3% in 45 min.
A.W.	F	0.15	0.1	0.25	1.0	19% in 45 min.

sufficient to induce a calming effect. Doses of 25 mg. three or four times a day were not superior in action.

DISCUSSION

In 5 patients, hydroxyzine hydrochloride, 10 to 25 mg. three times daily, was substituted for chlorpromazine hydrochloride, 25 to 50 mg. three times daily with good or even superior calming effect. It was further noted that, in hypertensive patients, the therapeutic effect of Rauwolfia serpentina in 50 mg. doses given two to four times daily was potentiated by hydroxyzine therapy.

CHLORPROMAZINE (THORAZINE) TREATMENT OF DISTURBED EPILEPTIC PATIENTS

Vincent I. Bonafede, M.D.
Clinical Director of Craig Colony, Department of Mental Hygiene,
State of New York

This report covers the treatment of 78 epileptic patients at Craig Colony for a period varying from 30 to 60 days. All of the patients were female, and the group under treatment for the longest period represented the worst, most actively disturbed patients in an institution of 2,300 patients. The patients were selected in consultation with the ward physician, ward supervisor, and other ward personnel, and the method of selection was simply, "Name your 50 most troublesome patients." All of these patients lived in a closed service and were allowed to continue their daily activities as before. Later, additional cases were added. All were kept under close observation, and laboratory studies were undertaken when indicated by clinical judgment.

Behavior difficulties were characterized by episodic disturbed states and chronic disturbed states, involving hyperactivity, aggression, hostility, assaultiveness, noisiness, resistiveness, temper outbursts, furor states, and destructiveness. Many frequently required large doses of sedation or some form of restraint or seclusion. The majority had shown varying degrees of deterioration. With the exception of 3 patients, all were mentally defective, with 12 in the idiot group, 22 in the imbecile group, 25 in the moron group, and 16 borderline.

Mental Status		Age Groups,Yr.	
Idiot	12	12-15	7
Imbecile	22	16-20	10
Moron	25	21-29	21
Borderline	16	30-39	19
Normal	3	40-49	12
		50-59	7
		60+	2

Some of the patients were frankly psychotic. Twenty-eight of these patients were inaccessible by reason of mutism, mental defectiveness, and/or deterioration. Fifty-one were classified under idiopathic epilepsy and 27 under symptomatic epilepsy.

The ages of the patients varied from 12 to 61 years. Twelve patients had been afflicted with epilepsy for periods of 4 to 9 years; the others had suffered epilepsy for periods varying from 10 to 52 years, with an average of over 26 years. Five patients have been in the institution less than 6 months; 25, from

Idiopathic	51
Symptomatic	27
Agenesis and birth injuries	9
Meningoencephalitis	9
Metabolic defects	2
Postnatal trauma	6
Endocrinopathy	1

1 to 9 years, and 48, from 10 to 29 years, with an average institutionalization of approximately 17 years.

Administration and Dosage

Chlorpromazine was administered orally to all patients except six, who received it parenterally when they refused oral medication during acute excitement states. It was never necessary to give more than two successive parenteral injections, as the excitement states were fully controlled and the patients willing to take oral therapy. Parenteral chlorpromazine was given in 100 mg. doses, with 50 mg. given intramuscularly in each buttock. However, to control any possible discomfort, 1 cc. of 2% procaine was added to each 50 mg., the drug injected rapidly, and the area of injection massaged. No special precautions were taken to compel the patient to lie down.

The oral dose varied initially from 200 to 300 mg., with almost two-thirds of the patients receiving 300 mg. daily. These doses were maintained, decreased, or increased as clinical judgment indicated. All except one received a barbiturate singly or in combination with other anticonvulsants.

The 78 patients under therapy were separated into three equal groups. The first group had no reduction of phenobarbital, and their average daily intake was 4½ grains (0.28 gm.). In the second group, each patient's phenobarbital dose was reduced one-third, and 12 patients had an additional reduction of barbital sodium, varying from 2½ to 10 grains (0.15 to 0.6 gm.), average 6.7 grains (0.4 gm.). The intake of phenobarbital in this group averaged 2.92 grains (0.175 gm.). In the third group, phenobarbital was reduced 50% and 17 patients had a further reduction of barbital sodium of 2½ to 20 grains (0.15 to 1.2 gm.), average 8.9 grains (0.534 gm.). The daily phenobarbital intake averaged 1.81 grains (0.108 gm.).

Purpose of Research

Three questions were of paramount interest in this study:
1. Was chlorpromazine of any value in controlling episodic and chronically disturbed epileptics?
2. What effect would it have on convulsions?
3. Was there any intensification of barbiturates, and to what degree?

In evaluating the use of chlorpromazine in epilepsy, it is well to emphasize, at this time, three facts that are axiomatic with epileptics. First, they are subject to varying periods of remissions from seizures; second, they are subject to exacerbations of seizures, and, finally, they run the hazard of status epilepticus and/or serial seizures whenever there is an abrupt reduction or withdrawal of any anticonvulsant. Many of these patients had their epilepsy fairly well controlled, but since their psychomotor disturbances, excitements, and furor states constituted a problem of serious magnitude, the hope and promise of a new therapy to ameliorate these states was worth any risk that could be potentially involved. However, the risk was minimized by close supervision on closed wards.

RESULTS

Acute Excitement States

The parenteral injection of 100 mg. of chlorpromazine was rapid and highly effective in the acute excitement states, quieting and relaxing the noisy, hyperactive, resistive patients within 30 to 45 minutes. While this series of six patients is small, chlorpromazine proved to be a very effective therapeutic agent and is far superior to scopolamine, apomorphine, and the various barbiturates previously used in treatment.

Chronic Disturbed States

The behavioral response in the chronic disturbed states was also exceedingly gratifying. The patients exhibited considerably less irritability, hostility, aggression, and assaultiveness. Noise subsided appreciably. They became quieter, more relaxed, and more cooperative, and those whose deterioration or mental defect was not pronounced became interested and participated in ward activities. Anxiety and tension states were reduced—patients volunteered statements such as, "I lost my temper," "I can control my temper better," or "I don't feel as nervous as I did." There were fewer outbursts of temper, and, when present, the outbursts were less intense and of shorter duration than those previously shown. Restraint and seclusion were minimal. There was less destruction to clothing, linen, and windowpanes. The administration of parenteral and oral sedation was markedly reduced. Appetites increased in the majority, with 56 patients showing a weight gain of 1 to 21 lb.; 23 gained 1 to 5 lb.; 17 gained 6 to 10 lb.; 10 gained 10 to 14 lb.; 4 gained 15 to 19 lb., and 2 gained 21 lb. Thirteen lost 1 to 5 lb.; 3 lost 6½ lb., and 6 had no change in weight.

The behavioral response was markedly improved in 32, or 41%; moderately improved in 20, or 25.6%; slightly improved in 13, or 16.7%, and unimproved in 13, or 16.7%. The results were essentially identical in all groups in the total number of patients responding favorably to chlorpromazine.

The behavioral response in relation to reduction in phenobarbital intake was as follows:

Behavior	No Reduction	33.3% Reduction	50% Reduction
Markedly improved	8	10	14
Moderately improved	9	8	3
Slightly improved	3	5	4
Unimproved	6	3	5

Significant improvement was evident in all age groups.

A few illustrations of patients markedly improved follow.

A. M., a 13-year-old girl of normal mentality (I. Q. 103), had been an epileptic with uncinate fits since 5 ½ years of age. She has been in the institution over two years. Epilepsy was minimal (two grand mal and two petit mal seizures since admission), but her behavior was a major problem because of

Ages	Totals	Markedly Improved	Moderately Improved	Slightly Improved	Unimproved
12-15	7	4	2	..	1
16-20	10	2	3	2	3
21-29	21	9	4	1	7
30-39	19	12	3	3	1
40-49	12	4	4	4	..
50-59	7	1	4	2	..
60-61	2	..	..	1	1
Totals	78	32	20	13	13

hyperactivity, aggressiveness, irritability, and extreme emotional instability, with almost daily explosive temper outbursts. Stuttering was prominent, but worse during excitements. Restraint and seclusion was no novel experience, and she was classified to a closed service. Chlorpromazine was begun at 300 mg. and currently is maintained at 150 mg. daily. Phenobarbital was reduced 50%. Improvement has been dramatic from the first day. She has become quiet, cooperative, and productive. There has been no explosive outburst. Full ground privileges have been restored. This patient's release from the institution at this time is precluded by reason of her status as a deportable alien.

C. S., a 31-year-old patient, an uncommunicative idiot, has been an epileptic for 28 years and has lived at the institution for the past 25 years. Her epilepsy has been well controlled in recent years, but she has been chronically disturbed for many, many years, her behavior being characterized by guttural noises day and night. Heavy sedation was prescribed frequently, with little or no effort. She quieted almost immediately with chlorpromazine, has required no further sedation, and is maintaining her improvement on a daily maintenance dose of 50 mg.

R. B., a 24-year-old epileptic of moron intelligence, has lived at the institution for the past 15 years. Epilepsy has been present since birth and quite severe until the past year. Periodically, she has had severe temper outbursts, has been noisy, hyperactive, and aggressive, particularly at the time of her menses, and has required frequent sedation and restraint. These episodes had become so intense in frequency and duration that she had to be kept on a closed service. Except for a minor momentary outburst of anger with a provocative patient, there has been no rage reaction either at her menses or at any other time.

M. D., a 30-year-old imbecile, has been an epileptic for 27 years and has resided in the institution for 24 years. Her epilepsy has been well controlled, only one grand mal and two petit mal attacks having been observed since January, 1950. She has been chronically disturbed for many years, her behavior being characterized by yelling in a deep, hoarse, masculine voice, obscenity, aggression, resistiveness, hyperactivity, and destructiveness. Under treatment she has made excellent progress and has become quiet, pleasant, cooperative, and productive in ward activities, and her voice has lost its hoarseness and masculine quality.

Effect on Seizures and Intensification of Barbiturates

Patients in the first group, the majority of whom were under treatment for 30 days, received an average of 4½ grains of phenobarbital daily. Only two patients (S. J. and S. S.) could possibly be considered as having shown an increase in seizures; for example, S. J. had four grand mal seizures within 30 days after treatment, whereas no seizure had been observed during the previous 14 months. S. S. had a grand mal seizure on the 22d day after treatment, whereas none had been observed during the previous 15 months. Five patients had no seizures for 30 days, while four other patients had no seizures for 60 days. However, one of the patients without seizures did develop a coma, and this will be mentioned later.

The second group, which had a 33.3% reduction in barbiturates, has been under observation for 60 days. In this group, 4 patients had no seizures, 11 had no apparent change in seizure frequency, and 11 patients showed an appreciable alteration of their previous seizure frequency. Of the last group, four (M. B., R. M. G., S. H., M. A. R.) had a marked increase in seizure frequency for varying periods up to 12 days; four (R. B., M. D., C. K., M. R.) had a moderate increase, and three (S. K., B. L., F. S.) had a questionable increase. Seizure control was completely reestablished in six (M. B., M. A. R., M. R., R. B., M. D., S. K.) upon restoring the previous phenobarbital dosage.

The third group, with a 50% reduction in barbiturates, was also under observation for 60 days. Four patients had no seizures; seven patients had no change in seizure frequency; six patients had a questionable increase (A. M., E. R., C. S., M. I. D., S. S., M. McG.); four (E. N., Y. G., A. McG., M. S.), a moderate increase, and five (G. B., C. C., L. M. D., M. McQ., E. B.), a marked increase.

	No Reduction	Reduced 33⅓%	Reduced 50%	Total
No seizures	9	4	4	17
No change	15	11	7	33
Questionable increase	2	3	6	11
Moderate increase	..	4	4	8
Marked increase	..	4	5	9

The results for these three groups show that 17 patients developed no seizures and 33 had no essential alteration of previous seizure frequency, whereas 11 patients showed a questionable increase, and 17 patients a moderate to marked increase, in their seizure frequencies. It is highly significant that 26 of the 28 patients who showed any questionable or appreciable increase in their seizure frequencies were in the groups in which barbiturates were reduced one-third or one-half, thus strongly indicating that the seizure increase was due essentially and specifically to the reduction of phenobarbital rather than to any action of chlorpromazine.

For example, M. A. R. had 40 grand mal and 4 petit mal seizures in 1954 and none in 1955 before treatment, but during the first eight days after chlorpromazine was started and barbiturates reduced she had 27 grand mal seizures. Since restoration of phenobarbital no seizure has occurred. M. B., a patient who had an inadvertent reduction of diphenylhydantoin (Dilantin), in addition to the barbiturate, developed seizures daily for 13 consecutive days, totaling 37 grand mal and 5 petit mal, whereas she had 38 grand mal and 10 petit mal seizures in 1954 and none the three weeks prior to chlorpromazine. Seizures were abruptly controlled with restoration of the previous dose of phenobarbital and diphenylhydantoin. Where seizures became aggravated, seizure control in most instances was easily reestablished by returning to the prechlorpromazine level of phenobarbital except in one patient (G. B.), who died. On the other hand, a few patients stabilized themselves after demonstrating a seizure increase for seven days without recourse to additional phenobarbital.

In the single death, it is, at best, difficult to evaluate the role of chlorpromazine, but here the drug is suspect of precipitating serial seizures or status epilepticus. However, it again should be emphasized that a similar picture can and does frequently occur in epileptics not under treatment with chlorpromazine. The death (G. B.) occurred in a 29-year-old mute of idiot mentality who had been an epileptic since 4 months of age and who had spent the last 17½ years of her life within the institution. She had been chronically disturbed for many years, was resistive, aggressive, noisy, and destructive, and frequently required heavy doses of sedation and/or frequent restraint or seclusion. Her seizures had been very well controlled for the previous four years, only three grand mal and three petit mal attacks having been observed since January, 1951. From 1937 to 1951 she averaged 24 grand mal seizures annually and had never exceeded more than 2 grand mal seizures in any one day. The barbiturate medication prior to treatment consisted of 4½ grains of phenobarbital and 10 grains of barbitalsodium daily. This was reduced to 2¼ grains of phenobarbital daily. The chlorpromazine dosage started at 200 mg. and reached a maximal dose of 600 mg. The patient had been under therapy for 41 days when the first grand mal seizure occurred. This, incidentally, was 48 hours after the maximal dose had been reached. This was followed by two grand mal attacks on the 42d day, a single grand mal seizure on the 43d day and eight grand mal seizures on the 44th day. On the 44th day the drug was discontinued, with the beginning of serial seizures. Fifty-two grand mal seizures developed within the next 31 hours, and the patient died of pulmonary edema on the 46th day of treatment.

Intensification or potentiation of barbiturate is again a difficult question to evaluate, but if marked drowsiness and incoordination can be used as a qualitative gauge, then only 5 of the 78 patients were so affected and 1 of these became comatose. This occurred in a 21-year-old mute patient (M. A.) of idiot mentality who was placed under treatment because of hyperactivity, destructiveness, self-mutilation, and noisiness. She had been an epileptic since birth and had lived within the institution for 16½ years, averaging one grand mal seizure annually for the five previous years. The daily dose of phenobarbital was 4½ grains when she was placed on chlorpromazine therapy. The dosage began at 100 mg. daily and was gradually increased to 400 mg. She had been under treatment for 47 consecutive days and had experienced no seizures. One week after her maximal dose she became deeply comatose, with a weak and slow pulse, slow and shallow respiration, and initial blood pressure of 82/68.

She remained in coma for two days before reacting. No seizures had occurred during chlorpromazine therapy. In this single coma and in the four other cases of severe drowsiness, chlorpromazine undoubtedly was a contributory factor, but an element of doubt is raised as to whether these side-reactions are due to an intensification of the barbiturate or to an individual idiosyncrasy or intolerance of the patient for chlorpromazine or to a combination of the two.

COMPLICATIONS

A slight to moderate fever developed in 11 patients and was usually present between the 7th and the 10th day. Fever was invariably associated with constipation and subsided within 3 to 24 hours after adequate elimination. The ward personnel reported that patients under chlorpromazine therapy were more constipated and required more cathartics and enemas than before. Five patients (M. I. D., M. G., H. F., F. S., L. D.) developed a macular or maculopapular rash, which was irregularly distributed except in a single case, in which it was generalized and symmetrical. One patient (L. D.) developed an intermittent fever and rash and finally had to be dropped from therapy. Coarse tremors of the upper extremities were present in five patients; drooling, in four, and ringing of the ears, in two. Two patients (C. S. and B. L.) developed jaundice and clay-colored stools, and both conditions cleared up within six days after discontinuing the drug. Eosinophilia (13% and 22%) was noted in two cases. The previously reported coma and death complete the list of complications. The coma and death and the jaundice in one case occurred in patients receiving daily doses of 400 to 600 mg.

SUMMARY AND CONCLUSIONS

The period of observation is admittedly quite short and the series small, but the results so far observed among the most disturbed epileptics in the institution indicate the following conclusions:

1. Chlorpromazine (Thorazine) has been highly effective and dramatic in controlling behavior disturbances.
2. The drug can be safely administered with fairly large doses of phenobarbital with minimal risk.
3. Doses of 300 mg. or less are less likely to be involved in complications.
4. A maintenance dose may be necessary to retain control of both episodic and chronic disturbed states.
5. Chlorpromazine does not appreciably reduce the frequency of seizures when maintenance therapy of phenobarbital or diphenylhydantoin (Dilantin) is reduced.

MERATRAN WITH RESERPINE
Adjunctive Use in the Treatment of Parkinson's Disease

John C. Button, B.Sc., D. O.

The evaluation of drugs in the treatment of Parkinson's disease is extremely difficult. The illness is chronic, progressive, and incurable with present technics, although symptomatic improvement does occur, often in a dramatic way, when proper therapy is employed. Pharmacotherapy has been directed largely toward the control of the two major symptoms, tremor and muscle rigidity. Many synthetic drugs—antihistamines, antispasmodics, sedatives, central nervous system stimulants, and muscle relaxants—have been used successfully in various combinations, and as substitutes for one another, in the symptomatic treatment of the patient. They do, however, have in common the production of disturbing side-effects which limit their usefulness. Moreover, except for the central nervous system stimulants they do not influence the depression characteristic of advanced cases. In Parkinson's disease, as in other chronic disabling diseases, a deep-rooted and lasting depression of spirit is the reaction of the patient to the disabilities caused by his illness.

Certain of the antihistamines exert a tremendously beneficial effect upon the unique and uncontrollable trembling and the muscular rigidity because of their sedative and relaxing properties, yet they often make the patient extremely drowsy and apathetic. Likewise, the antispasmodic drugs quiet the tremor and lessen the rigidity in varying degrees, but with few exceptions their effectiveness is likely to lessen with continued use. Sedatives prescribed to combat the restlessness in these patients whose muscles are cramped and painful should be excluded. The addition of one of the usual central nervous system stimulants is effective in counteracting drug-induced drowsiness and in elevating the mood, but here again, concomitant side-reactions such as pressor responses and hyperglycemia, restrict their use over long periods.

The use of various combinations of these drugs, depending upon the predominating symptom, and the changing of these combinations at regular intervals have minimized drug tolerance and have enabled the patient to achieve a maximum degree of comfort. All too frequently, however, the severe tremor is refractory to treatment with the standard medications, and the pessimistic mental outlook is not altered.

Knowledge of the tranquilizing and gently sedative effects of reserpine, a chemically pure single alkaloid derived from Rauwolfia, and of the freedom from side-effects of a new antidepressant, Meratran, pipradrol, (a-[2-piperidyl] benzhydrol hydrochloride) suggested the use of these two drugs, adjunctively, in an attempt to control or modify the tremor and depression of Parkinson's disease.

Material and Methods

The present study concerns the use of a combination of Meratran and reserpine in the treatment of 22 cases: 8 of these were of the idiopathic type, 5 arteriosclerotic, and 9 postencephalitic. The ages of the patients ranged from 44 to 85 years, with an average age of 55.5 years; 13 of the patients were males and 9 were females. The duration of the disease varied from 3 to 20 years. The predominant symptoms in descending order of frequency were tremor, disability, rigidity, disturbance of locomotion, loss of initiative, contractures, tension, muscle cramps, and lethargy.

Early in the course of the study, separate tablets of Meratran and reserpine were employed. The dosage varied from 1 mg. to 3 mg. of Meratran and 0.25 to 0.75 mg. of reserpine (Serpasil) daily. In two cases 4 mg. of Rauwiloid at bedtime was used in place of Serpasil. Later a compound tablet designated as Meratran with Reserpine was substituted. Each of the compound tablets contained 1 mg. of Meratran and 0.25 mg. of reserpine. The effective dosage of Meratran with Reserpine was 1 to 3 tablets daily, except in one instance in which 4 tablets were administered. In all cases, the usual antiparkinsonism therapy was continued.

Results and Discussion

Definite improvement occurred in all twenty-two patients.

Tremor and feelings of tension which previously had been refractory to treatment with the antiparkinsonism drugs alone were modified, and indeed, the effectiveness of the initial therapy seemed to be enhanced. It has long been known that in such patients the regular rhythmic trembling which occurs in Parkinson's disease when the limbs are at rest tends to disappear during sleep. Reserpine, by its central tranquilizing effect, produced a state of relaxation and quietude which was conducive to more restful sleep and resultant amelioration of the involuntary trembling and quivering.

Perhaps even more impressive was the transformation which occurred in mental or emotional outlook. Depression is encountered in many of these disabled Parkinsonian patients; it is a natural reaction to their inability to carry on their usual pursuits. The future to them is dark, gloomy, and hopeless. They dread the prospect of another day. They feel listless and useless, and often they become suicidal. Meratran, to which these reactive depressions respond so dramatically, proved to be the ideal antidepressant drug because of its wide margin of safety. It has been demonstrated, both experimentally and clinically, that Meratran has little or no effect upon blood pressure, pulse, or respiration. Meratran can be used with safety even in older patients.

The virtual freedom from effects upon the appetite, normal sleep pattern, and cardiovascular system makes possible the use of Meratran in patients in whom other central stimulants might be contraindicated. It is significant that in this small series of patients diabetes was present in three and cardiovascular disease in three. There was no increase in blood sugar in the diabetic patients, and there was no pressor response in those with cardiovascular disease.

It is of interest to relate briefly a few of the more dramatic responses to Meratran and reserpine, which might categorize their action adjunctively in Parkinson's disease facilitating rehabilitation.

Case Reports

Case 1. A white male, 54 years of age, was badly disabled from idiopathic Parkinsonism; his mental depression was severe. He had lost his job as an engineer, and his sole activity consisted of taking a few steps around the house. In October, 1954, when he had been out of work for 5 years, he began receiving, in addition to antiparkinsonism medication, Serpasil, 0.25 mg., and Meratran, 1.0 mg., three times a day. More recently he has been taking Meratran with Reserpine, 1 tablet three times a day. In February, 1955, he started on a new job, giving estimates on engineering work. He is able to travel alone from New York City to Orange, N. J.

Case 2. A white female, 45 years old, who had formerly been active as a horseback rider, had idiopathic Parkinsonism of 10 years' duration. Physically, she could hardly drag herself around, and she was extremely depressed. In October, 1954, Meratran and reserpine, administered as separate tablets, were added to her treatment. Her general condition is now much better, and she is able to go out and visit friends. Her mood has improved to the stage where she talks of wanting to ride again.

Case 3. A white male, 52 years of age, had postencephalitic Parkinsonism of 5 years' duration. He was ready to close up his business because of his disability, and he threatened suicide. On March 1, 1954, Meratran, 1 mg., and reserpine, 0.25 mg., twice a day, were added to his routine medication. After a month of treatment, his symptoms cleared and he was able to return to work. A recent checkup revealed little evidence of disability except for a slight tremor. He is doing a full day's work at present, and he is being continued on the same schedule of treatment.

Case 4. A white female, 46 years old, a former schoolteacher, became completely disabled because of postencephalitic Parkinsonism of 20 years' duration. She was unable to walk; in fact, she was bedridden. Because of contractures she could not open her hands. Her mental outlook was very bad. She improved on antiparkinsonism therapy to a stage where she could walk unaided. The contractures were relaxed under anesthesia, and she was able to use her hands. Tremor and depression persisted, however, until Meratran with Reserpine was added to her routine medication. The tremor was modified and a definite change occurred in her mental outlook. Whereas previously she had no interest in anything, she is now taking a course in short story writing.

Summary and Conclusions

1. The use of Meratran and reserpine, adjunctively, in the treatment of twenty-two patients with Parkinson's disease has been discussed. The neurologic manifestations usually respond to various combinations of antiparkinsonism drugs, but tremor that is refractory to such therapy is modified and the deep-rooted depressions are relieved by the addition of Meratran and reserpine to

the standard medication.

2. Because of its freedom from pressor reactions and from an effect upon blood sugar, Meratran and reserpine can be given safely to Parkinsonian patients who suffer also from diabetes or cardiovascular disease.

3. Four cases have been summarized which demonstrate that Meratran and reserpine aid in the social and economic rehabilitation of patients with Parkinson's disease.

COMBINATION RESERPINE-METHYLPHENIDYLACETATE IN EPILEPTICS WITH PSYCHOSIS

G. Donald Niswander, M.D., and Earl K. Holt, M.D.

The Arthur P. Noyes Institute for Neuropsychiatric Research, New Hampshire State Hospital, Concord, New Hampshire

For the past three years reserpine has been widely used in the treatment of mental illness. Barsa and Kline have reported their experience with reserpine in the treatment of psychotic patients with convulsive disorders. These investigators found reserpine "not as effective in psychotic patients with convulsive disorders as in psychotics without convulsive seizures . . . in the former, the maximum effect to be expected is usually one of sedation." Previously, they had found that patients with convulsive disorders did not respond well to reserpine medication. Ferguson has reported the effective use of a new analeptic drug, methylphenidylacetate, in off-setting reserpine induced depression. He has also found that the combination of reserpine and methylphenidylacetate is a useful chemotherapeutic medication for improving the behavior patterns of 225 chronic hospitalized mental patients.

From the report of these investigators, it was felt that it would be worth while to evaluate the use of combination reserpine-methylphenidylacetate medication in psychotic patients with convulsive disorders. This paper reports the results of the first sixteen weeks of a study in which this drug combination was administered to a group of 26 hospitalized epileptic patients.

METHOD OF STUDY

The 26 patients were all women with epilepsy who were cared for on one of the chronic wards in the hospital. The age of the patients ranged from 16 to 64 years, with a median age of 40.5 years. The duration of hospitalization extended from 4 months to 30 years, with a median duration of 9.7 years.

Table I summarizes the diagnostic categories of the 26 patients.

TABLE I—Diagnostic Categories

Diagnosis	No. of Patients
Chronic Brain Syndrome Associated with Convulsive Disorder (Idiopathic)	16
Schizophrenic Reaction, with Associated Convulsive Disorder	6
Mental Deficiency with Associated Convulsive Disorder	3
Chronic Brain Syndrome due to Infection, Post-Encephalitis, with Convulsive Disorder	1

Observations: Those relating to ward behavior were recorded by psychiatric nurses in charge of the ward on which the patients resided. Symptoms of hyperactivity, over-talkativeness, assaultiveness, destructiveness, agitation and tension, were rated daily before and during the study. A simple rating scale for observations was as follows:

> 3 Severe (maximum rating)
> 2 Moderate
> 1 Mild
> 0 Absent (minimum rating)

This method of observing and rating ward behavior had been previously used by the authors in evaluating the effects of reserpine in mental illness. Convulsive seizures were recorded during the study, and compared with the number of seizures each patient had experienced during the preceding six months.

Medications: At the outset, each patient was placed on reserpine, 4 milligrams daily, in a single dosage. In addition, each patient was given methylphenidylacetate, 30 milligrams, twice daily. One, two and four milligram reserpine tablets, and ten and twenty milligram methylphenidylacetate tablets were used as medications.

TABLE II—Anti-Convulsants

Drug	No. of Patients
Diphenylhydantoin Sodium	23
Phenobarbital Sodium	18
Methyl-phenyl-ethyl hydantoin	1
Primidone	1
Trimethadione	1
Combination: Diphenylhydantoin Sodium Phenobarbital Sodium	14
Combination: Diphenylhydantoin Sodium Phenobarbital Sodium Trimethadione	1

Withdrawal of Anti-convulsants: All 26 patients were receiving some type of anti-convulsant medication when the project started. The following table depicts those medications.

The withdrawal of these anti-convulsants was initiated during the first week of the study, and the following schedule for discontinuing these drugs was carried out.

Diphenylhydantoin sodium was withdrawn first; this drug was reduced in dosages of 90 milligrams every five days. The procedure was accomplished by first withdrawing 90 milligrams of the drug from the group who were receiving the drug more than once daily, until all patients were receiving 90 milligrams daily. This last daily dosage was withdrawn from the entire group on the same day.

The same procedure was then used in withdrawing phenobarbital sodium, except when the group of patients was receiving 90 milligrams a day, the dosage was reduced to 45 milligrams a day for one week, and then was discontinued completely. This method was an attempt to alleviate the possibility of seizures associated with withdrawal symptoms in a drug which has a tendency to cause physiologic habituation.

The patient receiving primidone had the medication reduced 250 milligrams every 5 days until the medication was discontinued.

The patient receiving methyl-phenyl-ethyl-hydantoin had the medication reduced 100 milligrams every 5 days until the medication was discontinued.

The patient receiving trimethadione had the medication reduced 300 milligrams every 5 days until the medication was discontinued.

If there had been no change in the patients' ward behavior after having received the initial reserpine dosage, this medication was increased at weekly intervals. During the first one and one-half weeks of the study, 14 patients had the reserpine dosage increased to 5 or 8 milligrams daily. It was not necessary to change the reserpine medication in the other 12 patients. The methylphenidylacetate dosage remained constant throughout the study.

Results

The following summarizes the results observed in the symptom categories during the study.

Ward Behavior: The personality characteristics of all 26 patients changed remarkably during the study. The following summarizes the improvement of the symptomatology observed by the rating scale:

Hyperactivity: Twelve patients were rated as being hyperactive before receiving the drug. In 2 patients this was severe; in 4 moderate; in 2 mild, and in 4 others this symptom varied from absent to severe. While receiving the drug hyperactivity subsided in all but 2 patients. For the most part it was absent in those two patients, but occasionally rated moderate to severe.

Overtalkativeness: Twelve patients were rated as being over-talkative before receiving the drug. In 5 patients this was severe; in 4 moderate, and in 3 others this symptom varied from absent to severe. While receiving the drugs all patients improved. In 4 patients this symptom was absent for the most part, but at other times present, rating mild to severe.

Assaultiveness: Three patients were occasionally mildly assaultive before receiving the drugs. While on the drugs this behavior was not present.

Destructiveness: Three patients were rated as being destructive before receiving the drugs. In one patient this was severe; in another mild or moderate and in the third occasionally mildly present. On the drugs destructiveness was absent.

Tension and Agitation: Twelve patients were rated as being tense and agitated before receiving the drugs. In one these symptoms were severe; in 4 moderate; in 3 mild, and in 4 absent to severe. Tension and agitation subsided completely in all but one patient while receiving the drugs. In this patient it was almost always absent, but occasionally mildly recognized.

The patient's individual personality changes were even more dramatic. Whereas many of the patients were irritable, cantankerous, impulsive, demanding and hostile before receiving reserpine, they all became more pleasant and cooperative on the drug. Consequently, interpersonal relationships between patient-patient and patient-ward personnel were greatly improved. The bettered personalities made the patients more accessible toward occupational therapy activities and recreation.

Convulsive Seizures: At the end of the first 16 weeks of the study these 26 epileptic patients had become classified into three distinct groups.

Group I: This group included 4 patients who began experiencing a marked increase in the incidence of convulsive seizures after the first week of the study. As the study progressed the incidence of seizures increased. However, the program as outlined here was carried out until the end of the seventh week. At this time these four patients were markedly confused, extremely lethargic and bed-ridden. The clinical picture appeared serious. Reserpine and methylphenidylacetate were discontinued and the patients were returned to anti-convulsant medications. The response was dramatic and for the next four weeks none of these 4 patients had a convulsive seizure. At that time 3 of the patients began having occasional periodic convulsive seizures, and this has been better controlled by readjusting the anti-convulsant medications. The other patient in this group did not have the convulsive seizures which were characteristic of her clinical picture before the study started.

Group II: This group included 11 patients. As the anti-convulsant medications were withdrawn a slight increase was noted in the incidence of convulsive seizures in a few of these patients. At the eighth week 6 of these patients were having more seizures than previously. However, the clinical picture was in no way as alarming as those patients in Group I. The reserpine dosage for the patients in Group II was between 4 and 8 milligrams of the drug daily. At the eighth week this reserpine dosage was halved for each patient. For the next two weeks the incidence of seizures reverted to the previous normal picture. During the tenth week of the study 3 of the patients began having more frequent convulsive seizures, but no anti-convulsant medication was added to their treatment program. Therefore, these 11 patients in Group II have been carried on reserpine and methylphenidylacetate medications only, and except in a few instances, there was no increase in the number of convulsive seizures.

Group III: This group included 11 patients. All these 11 patients showed an increase in the number of convulsive seizures during the first six weeks of the study. At the eighth week the reserpine medication was halved. Previously they had been receiving from 4 to 8 milligrams of reserpine daily. For the following two weeks the incidence of seizures dropped markedly, but the frequency of seizures was much greater than before the study started, and greater as compared with the patients in Group II. Therefore, in addition to receiving reserpine and methylphenidylacetate these patients were gradually replaced on the anti-convulsant medications, which they were receiving before the study started. When the anticonvulsants were added the convulsive seizures reverted to the frequency rate at the early part of the investigation.

COMMENT

The patients were divided into three groups classified as to the clinical response while receiving combined reserpine-methylphenidylacetate medications. After anti-convulsants were withdrawn the patients in Group I did not tolerate the reserpine-methylphenidylacetate medication and their clinical picture reverted to its previous state and they were put back on anti-convulsants.

The patients in Group II were carried on a medical program using only reserpine and methylphenidylacetate as medication, without the addition of anti-convulsants, and those in Group III were on a combination of reserpine and methylphenidylacetate plus anti-convulsants. In Group II there was a marked decrease in seizures when the reserpine dosage was reduced fifty per cent. This likewise occurred with those patients in Group III before anti-convulsants were added. This fact would seem to verify the observations of Barsa and Kline, that smaller doses of reserpine are better tolerated by psychotic patients with convulsive disorders. These authors also observed in their study that the incidence of convulsive seizures decreased markedly when the dosage of reserpine medication was reduced from large doses, 5 to 10 milligrams a day, to 2 to 3 milligrams of reserpine daily.

All three groups experienced an increase in the frequency of seizures during the anticonvulsant withdrawal period. This was more evident in Group I and III. The increase in seizures in some patients undoubtedly was due to the withdrawal of these medications. However, in evaluating the entire 26 patients, there was no significance between the seizure frequency and the previous medications, which were gradually discontinued. After anti-convulsants were prescribed again for the patients in Group III the incidence of seizures lessened but was still much greater as compared with Group II.

Throughout this sixteen week period, the side effects of lethargy, transient diarrhea, etc., which is frequently encountered when reserpine is used alone, in small or large doses, did not occur in these patients, except those in Group I. Neither did Parkinson-like symptoms appear. This has been attributed to the methylphenidylacetate which apparently tends to offset the undesired side effects of reserpine in most patients.

It has been impossible to determine a significance between diagnosis and response to the reserpine-methylphenidylacetate combination in this group of epileptic patients. The patients who were classified into Group I were considered moderately deteriorated epileptic individuals, although similar patients are found in Groups II and III.

The authors are continuing this study to compare the data collected during this initial sixteen week period with other observations as they become available in the future. This group of 26 will likely be permanent hospital residents and in addition, other patients will be included as they are admitted to the epileptic ward. In the continuation of the program a comparison will be made between the patients in Groups II and III. Anti-convulsant medication will be manipulated between the groups, and an evaluation will be made when placebos are substituted for reserpine and methylphenidylacetate. As new patients come into the study the opportunity will be afforded to compare the experience gained during the first sixteen weeks with other treatment programs using reserpine and methylphenidylacetate for epilepsy, with or without anti-convulsant medications.

The authors feel that the combination of reserpine and methlphenidylacetate is valuable in the treatment of the chronic hospitalized epileptic patient. The personality improvements alone bring about a quieter, more pleasant and cooperative group of patients. Some epileptic patients can be carried on these drugs in combination without anti-convulsants as part of their treatment program. Others need anticonvulsants for seizure control when receiving reserpine and methylphenidylacetate and a few patients cannot tolerate the latter drugs.

It is suspected that the use of reserpine in combination with methylphenidylacetate for the treatment of epilepsy has to be extremely individualized; it would seem that it is necessary to evaluate how each patient is going to respond to such a treatment program, with or without anti-convulsants, before abandoning the drug combination even when results seem intolerable.

Summary

The results of a sixteen weeks study with a group of 26 hospitalized epileptic patients are reported. Reserpine and methylphenidylacetate in combination, have been used with or without anti-convulsant medication.

A remarkable improvement occurs in patients who are either hyperactive, over-talkative, assaultive, destructive, or tense and agitated. The individual personality changes make the patients more accessible for activities, recreation, and other interpersonal socialization.

Four patients did not tolerate the reserpine-methylphenidylacetate routine. Eleven patients needed anti-convulsants with the new drug combination. Eleven other patients got along as well on the combination, without anti-convulsants, as they had previous to receiving reserpine and methylphenidylacetate.

Acknowledgments: The authors wish to express their appreciation to Bohdan T. Nedilsky, M.D., Barbara F. French, R.N., and Audrey C. Raspiller, R.N., who assisted in the collection of the data in the study; and to George M. Haslerud, Ph.D., Professor of Psychology, University of New Hampshire, and Research Consultant to the New Hampshire State Hospital, who assisted with the preparation of the manuscript.

USE OF MEPROBAMATE (MILTOWN) IN CONVULSIVE AND RELATED DISORDERS

Meyer A. Perlstein, M.D.
Northwestern University Medical School, Chicago, Illinois

Clinical reports to date on the new drug meprobamate (Miltown) have dealt almost exclusively with its action in psychiatric patients suffering from anxiety and tension states. Reports on both the chemistry and pharmacology of the drug, however, suggested the possibility that meprobamate might also have value in the treatment of epilepsy and cerebral palsy.

PHARMACOLOGY

The parent compound of meprobamate is mephenesin, a muscle relaxant that also exhibits marked anticonvulsant action in animals but not in patients with clinical epilepsy. In the search for compounds more potent as anticonvulsants than mephenesin, it was found that 2-substituted-1, 3-propanediols, though possessing a weaker muscle-relaxant action, are much more powerful anticonvulsants than mephenesin. Unfortunately, all these compounds have an exceedingly short duration of action. The most promising compound of this series, 2, 2-diethyl-1,3-propanediol (DEP or Prenderol) was found to be of value in treatment of petit mal when used in conjunction with retarders. The rapid inactivation of these compounds is due to oxidation of the free hydroxyl groups. Esterification of the hydroxyl group with various acids prolonged the duration of action. The dicarbamate derivatives of the 2,2-disubstituted 1,3-propanediol showed the greatest promise, and of these meprobamate, which is 2-methyl-2-*n*-propyl-1,3-propanediol dicarbamate, was best.

Pharmacologically, meprobamate produces muscle relaxation without significantly affecting the autonomic functions such as heartbeat and respiration. In animals the drug is a potent anticonvulsant. As little as 30 mg. per kilogram of body weight (about one-thirtieth the lethal dose) will prevent death in convulsions from pentylenetetrazole (Metrazol). In this respect, meprobamate is about eight times more effective than mephenesin. Meprobamate is also an excellent antagonist to strychnine convulsions. As little as 134 mg. per kilogram of body weight (about one-sixth the lethal dose) will prevent death from a lethal dose of strychnine. In addition, meprobamate is about three times as effective as mephenesin and eight times as effective as trimethadione (Tridione) in preventing electroshock seizures in animals.

An unusual and interesting property of meprobamate is its ability to exercise a taming or tranquilizing effect on animals. This may be related to the effect of the drug on diencephalic areas. It has been shown that the electric potentials picked up from the thalamus are markedly increased in amplitude and decreased in frequency after administration of the drug. The toxicity of meprobamate is remarkably low. In animals, as well as in humans, it is about one-fifth as toxic as barbiturates. Two occasions of attempted suicide were reported in which 50 to 100 400-mg. tablets taken in one dose resulted in complete recovery without special treatment. One of my own patients, a 20-year-old girl, took 25 tablets in an unsuccessful suicide attempt.

Present Study

Patient Sample.—Patients for the study came from private practice, from the children's neurology service of the Cook County Hospital, and from the St. John's Home and Hospital for Crippled Children. The sample consisted of 130 patients, 60 with seizures and 70 with other neurological conditions; 21 of these patients had multiple ailments, so that a total of 151 conditions (76 epileptic and 75 nonepileptic) were available for study (table 1). Nearly all the epileptics in this group had refractory conditions, and administration of many other medicaments had previously been tried without success. This was also true of the 29 patients with behavior problems, all of whom were severely disturbed and 7 of whom were psychotic. The disturbances in behavior were of functional and/or organic origin and included tantrums, autistic and negativistic behavior, and various infantile regressions. Of the patients with cerebral palsy, 26 were athetoid and 18 spastic, and all had severe involvement with marked muscular tension. There were six adults in the study. The rest were children from 6 months to 16 years of age, with an average age of approximately 8 years.

Dosage.—The dosage was regulated to give the maximum therapeutic result without producing drowsiness or other side-reactions. Doses of from 100 to 800 mg. were generally given two to four times a day. In a few instances dosages of 1,600 mg. four times a day were tolerated without any side-effects. For children the dose was naturally smaller than for adults, but not proportionate to their weight. As a rule, the initial dosage was 200 mg. or less three times a day, and it was generally increased until clinical benefit or drowsiness resulted. Adults appeared to be less susceptible to drowsiness with use of higher doses than children. When meprobamate was effective, clinical changes generally began to show within 15 to 30 minutes, reaching a maximum in one to two hours and tapering off at the end of four to six hours. The drug was supplied in 400-mg. scored tablets. Because of the bitter taste of the crushed tablets, some problem arose with children too young to swallow pills. In these cases disguises of various kinds were used, such as cola drinks, sweet-and-sour flavors such as sweetened lemon juice or raspberry syrup, or thick, cold vehicles such as applesauce or ice cream. The most effective disguise was a base of cinnamon and sugar.

Method.—Treatment was in all cases intensive. Patients were seen as frequently as necessary and feasible, most of them once a week, and a few even as often as once a day. The drug was given both alone and in combination with other drugs. In patients with cerebral palsy, meprobamate, like other drugs, was used as an adjuvant to therapy.

In evaluating the results of treatment, the following rating scale and criteria were used: (1) marked benefit: in epileptics, spells reduced in number and severity by over 75%; in nonepileptics, symptoms completely or almost completely controlled; (2) moderate benefit: in epileptics, spells reduced in number and severity by 50 to 75%; in nonepileptics, symptoms controlled to a significant degree; (3) no benefit: seizures reduced in number by less than 50%; nonepileptic symptoms not controlled or controlled to an insignificant or doubtful degree; and (4) aggravated: spells and nonepileptic symptoms worse after administration of the drug than before.

The principle was followed that in order to be considered effective a drug's therapeutic effect must precede its toxic effect. Meprobamate was accordingly classified as ineffective (no benefit) in those cases in which patients became sleepy before therapeutic results were achieved. All patients who were helped by meprobamate were subsequently given placebos. These were also supplied by the manufacturers of meprobamate and were labeled "Piltown." Only those patients were considered helped who showed improvement after administration of meprobamate only. Those patients who also showed improvement after administration of the placebo were rated as unimproved (no benefit).

Results

Results of the study in 130 patients are summarized in tables 1 and 2. Table 1 shows that when epileptic and nonepileptic conditions were considered to-

TABLE 1.—*Effect of Treatment with Meprobamate of 151 Convulsive and Related Disorders**

	Total Diag- noses	Marked (over 75%) No.	Marked %	Moderate (50-75%) No.	Moderate %	Total No.	Total %	None (under 50%) No.	None %	Aggra vated No.	Aggra vated %
Total Series	151	22	15	24	16	46	31	95	63	10	6
Total epileptic	76	15	20	12	16	27	36	40	52	9	12
Grand mal	19	1	5	2	11	3	16	10	52	6	32
Petit mal	33	13	40	7	20	20	60	13	40	..	..
Other seizures	24	1	4	3	12	4	16	17	72	3	12
Myoclonic	10	1	.	2	.	3	.	7	.	.	.
Focal and cortical (Jacksonian)	8	..	..	..	..	..	..	6	..	2	..
Psychomotor	2	..	..	1	..	1	..	1	..	..	..
Vegetative	4	..	..	.	..	.	..	3	..	1	..
Total nonepileptic	75	7	10	12	16	19	26	55	73	1	1
Cerebral palsy	44	3	7	7	16	10	23	33	75	1	2
Athetoid	26	3	12	5	19	8	31	18	69	..	..
Spastic	18	..	..	2	11	2	11	15	83	1	6
Emotional and behavior	29	2	7	5	17	7	24	22	76	..	..
Psychotic	7	1	15	1	15	2	30	5	70	..	..
Nonpsychotic	22	1	5	4	18	5	23	17	77	..	..
Other	2	2	..	..	..	..	..	2	..	..	..

* The patient sample consisted of 130 patients, 21 with multiple conditions, making a total of 151 conditions treated.

gether, 31% were found to be alleviated and 6% aggravated by meprobamate. The epileptic patients showed greater benefit (36%) than the nonepileptics (26%); they also showed a higher percentage of deleterious responses (12%

TABLE 2.—*Results of Treatment with Meprobamate of Epilepsy of Idiopathic and Organic Origin*

	Total Diagnoses	Benefit						No Benefit			
		Marked (over 75%)		Moderate (50-75%)		Total		None (under 50%)		Aggravated	
		No.	%	No.	%	No.	%	No.	%	No.	%
Total epileptic	76	15	20	12	16	27	36	40	52	9	12
Idiopathic	24	10	42	6	25	16	67	5	21	3	12
Petit mal	18	10	55	5	28	15	83	3	17	..	..
Grand mal	5	..	..	..	..	..	..	2	..	3	..
Psychomotor	1	..	..	1	..	1	..	..	..	..	..
Organic	52	5	10	6	12	11	22	35	67	6	11
Petit mal	15	3	20	2	13	5	33	10	67	..	..
Grand mal	14	1	7	2	14	3	21	8	57	3	22
Other	23	1	4	2	9	3	13	17	74	3	13

of epileptic as against 1% of nonepileptic patients made worse). The results acquire clearer meaning when epileptic and nonepileptic conditions are considered separately.

Epileptic Conditions.—Analysis of the epileptic conditions by types of seizures (table 1) shows definite selective beneficial action of the drug on petit mal seizures. Whereas only 3 out of 19 patients with grand mal seizures (16%) were benefited by meprobamate, with the conditions of twice that number being aggravated, 20 out of 33 patients with petit mal seizures (60%) were benefited, with none becoming worse. The epileptic group also included 10 patients with myoclonic spasms of infancy (often called "lightning grand mal" and characterized by hypsarrhythmia [mountainous arrhythmia] in the electroencephalogram), 8 with focal and cortical (jacksonian) seizures, 2 with psychomotor seizures, and 4 with vegetative seizures (the latter characterized by abdominal cramps, sweating, or other visceral manifestations and often associated with 14 and 6 per second positive spikes in the electroencephalogram). Among these groups the patients with myoclonic seizures were the only ones to show appreciable benefit, 3 out of 10 being improved, with none made worse.

When seizures are analyzed according to etiology (table 2) the specificity of meprobamate appears even more striking. Of the patients with idiopathic seizures (combining all types), 67% were benefited, whereas only 22% of those with spells due to organic brain disease were benefited. Best results were achieved in patients with idiopathic petit mal, where 83% were helped and none made worse. Worst results were found in the five patients with idiopathic grand mal, where none was helped and three were made worse. In the group whose conditions were of organic origin, likewise, patients with petit mal derived greater benefit (5 out of 15 improved, with none made worse) than those with grand mal seizures (3 out of 14 helped and 3 made worse). To summarize, then, meprobamate proved most effective in the treatment of idiopathic petit mal (83% of cases) and somewhat effective in treatment of petit mal due to organic brain disease (33% of cases). It was less effective in patients with grand mal associated with organic brain disease (21%) and least effective in idiopathic grand mal (none of 5 cases). In fact, 32% of the patients with grand mal and none of those with petit mal were made worse by meprobamate.

Two possible explanations suggest themselves for these results. The first arises from the differences in the electroencephalographic records of patients with idiopathic and organic petit mal. The patient with idiopathic petit mal exhibits the typical 3 per second spike and wave record. In patients with organic petit mal, on the other hand, the record is more like that seen in the grand mal type, with spikes, petit mal variants, and focal abnormalities in rhythm, rate, and amplitude. This may account in part for the fact that patients with organic petit mal responded less favorably to treatment with meprobamate than did those with idiopathic petit mal. The second possibility is that the emotional reaction that often triggers spells may be blunted by meprobamate and that this tranquilizing action may be the basis of at least a part of its benefit in many patients with epilepsy. If this is so, then the drug may be expected to have a greater effect on patients with idiopathic than on those with organic petit mal, since the former group is on the average older and brighter than the group with organic brain disease and therefore perhaps more sensitive to emotional trigger situations in the environment.

Nonepileptic Conditions.—Meprobamate was of moderate benefit in 7 of 44 patients with cerebral palsy and of marked benefit in 3 (table 1). The athetoid patients, with extrapyramidal involvement, were helped most (8 out of 26), while the spastic patients (pyramidal tract involvement) were infrequently helped (2 out of 18). It is not likely that the selective benefits in athetoid patients as compared to spastic patients are due to any normalizing effect of meprobamate on the electrical activity of the brain, since the frequency of normal electroencephalograms in athetoid patients is two to three times that in spastic patients. It is possible that the selective effect of the drug in athetoid patients may be partially explained by its tranquilizing influence, since athetosis is characterized by marked aggravation of symptoms under emotional stress. The best effect from meprobamate occurred in a tense young athetoid woman whose involuntary movements and muscular tensions were extremely affected by emotional turbulence.

Of the 29 patients presenting serious behavior problems (including 7 psychotics) here treated, only 7 showed benefit that could be attributed to meprobamate. It should perhaps be mentioned that many more of these patients appeared to be helped at the beginning of the study. However, when the adopted criteria were applied—namely, that the patient must be helped more by meprobamate than by a placebo and that the effect must precede any onset of drowsiness—the number of patients benefited was reduced to that indicated in table 1. The two patients listed in the "other" nonepileptic column were both adult females in the 40's, one with severe tension headache, the other with acute rheumatoid myositis (fibrositis). Meprobamate dramatically relieved both conditions promptly and completely.

Side-Effects.—With the exception of drowsiness in some patients, no side-effects of any kind were noted during or subsequent to treatment with meprobamate. The tendency to sleep that was observed in some patients appeared to be a result of the drug's tranquilizing action rather than of a true soporific effect. Patients would often take one or two naps during the day but could easily be awakened. The ataxia in the twilight stage between the waking and sleeping state often seen in patients to whom the usual sedative drugs have been given was less noticeable or absent after administration of meprobamate. Blood, skin, liver, or urinary changes were not encountered.

COMMENT

It is generally recognized that epilepsy due to organic brain damage is more resistant to all forms of therapy than the idiopathic forms of epilepsy. It is not surprising, therefore, that meprobamate, like most other antiepileptic drugs, is less effective in the prevention of seizures due to organic brain disease. On the other hand, petit mal is less susceptible to control by drugs than grand mal, and it is in the treatment of idiopathic petit mal that meprobamate proved most useful. A new drug for the treatment of petit mal invites comparison with trimethadione (Tridione), which up to the present has shown greatest specificity for this condition. The improvement with meprobamate is generally not so complete, nor its effect so precipitous, as with trimethadione. With the latter drug the remission of spells may be complete and immediate, whereas with meprobamate remission is more typically of the order of 90 to 95%, with improvement being effected more gradually over several weeks of treatment. On the other hand, in treatment with trimethadione, where control is incomplete, residual spells may be more severe and of longer duration than the original spells and very resistant to therapy. No patient treated with meprobamate responded with such severe residual attacks; on the contrary, residual spells after administration of meprobamate are likely to be less severe than the original spells.

An unusual characteristic of trimethadione is that it often normalizes the electroencephalographic findings immediately and concurrently with clinical control of seizures. This does not generally occur when barbiturates or the other commonly used antiepileptics effect clinical control of seizures, nor does it happen after treatment with meprobamate. With meprobamate, as with other antiepileptic drugs, clinical improvement may antecede or exist without normalization of the electroencephalographic findings. Improvement and often normalization of the electroencephalographic picture, however, usually does occur after several weeks or months of control under therapy.

The great advantage that meprobamate has over trimethadione is its apparent complete freedom from toxic effect. With the exception of the drowsiness experienced by some patients, no toxic reactions of any kind were observed. The patient was either asleep or awake, but was rarely ataxic or "drunk." Blood dyscrasias, skin rashes, or gastrointestinal disturbances were not encountered. In my judgment, it is often more desirable to reduce a child's spells to a residual minimum without toxic reactions than it is to eliminate them completely at the cost of possible toxic effects or ataxia. The patient may be better off leading a normal life between occasional spells than living seizure-free in a perpetual fog of drug-induced confusion and hangover. This is especially true in children with petit mal, in whom spontaneous improvement in clinical and electroencephalographic findings occurs with the passage of time.

Another advantage of meprobamate is that it may often exert a tranquilizing effect in addition to its anticonvulsant and muscle-relaxant activity. As is well known, one of the factors determining both the frequency of spells in the epileptic and the severity of muscular tension and athetosis in the cerebral palsied is the emotional state of the patient. Meprobamate, possibly by diminishing the anxieties and tensions that beset these patients, may often remove the mechanism that triggers the seizure. Meprobamate showed no tendency to produce habituation. Doses did not have to be increased to sustain the therapeutic effect; neither did sudden withdrawal precipitate status epilepticus.

In evaluating any new antiepileptic drug, the general comment should perhaps be made that drugs that control petit mal are likely to aggravate grand mal and vice versa. This sometimes happens when meprobamate is used, as it does with many other drugs that help petit mal, notably trimethadione (Tridione), paramethadione (Paradione), and Prenderol. It should also perhaps be mentioned that relapses may occur with any medicament even after control has been achieved; and conversely, that control effected by any medicament may continue even after that medicament has been discontinued. Meprobamate behaves in these respects no differently from other medicaments. Unlike Prenderol, meprobamate had no beneficial synergistic action when given with trimethadione or paramethadione.

It is of particular interest to speculate about the mode of action of meprobamate. Present evidence suggests that petit mal is due to a focal disturbance in one or more midline subcortical structures located between the thalamus and brain stem. It appears likely that the patients who derived particular benefit from treatment with meprobamate are those with a lesion in that region of the thalamus that is specifically affected by the drug. This may also explain some of the beneficial effects in patients with athetosis and in those with behavior disturbances. It is also of interest to note that both trimethadione and Prenderol, which are effective in petit mal seizures, are also frequently beneficial in patients with athetosis and in some with behavior disturbances.

Conclusions

Meprobamate (Miltown) appears to be of greatest benefit in the control of petit mal, particularly of the idiopathic variety. It may also have some benefit in treatment of the tense forms of cerebral palsy, some behavior disturbances, and tension headaches and rheumatoid myositis (fibrositis). It occasionally aggravates grand mal, especially the idiopathic type. It is less effective than trimethadione (Tridione) in controlling petit mal but is at least as effective as paramethadione (Paradione) and Prenderol (2, 2-diethyl-1,3-propanediol) and is superior to other drugs that counteract petit mal. Its advantage over trimethadione and paramethadione lies in its relatively innocuous nature; its advantage over Prenderol lies in the fact that it has a sustained period of reaction and need not be used with retarding agents.

RESERPINE (SERPASIL) IN THE MANAGEMENT OF THE MENTALLY ILL AND MENTALLY RETARDED

Robert H. Noce, M.D., David B. Williams, M.D., and Walter Rapaport, M.D.

The last quarter century has seen many forward strides in the management of patients with mental disease. During this period modes of therapy have been available that are far superior to the old-time method of whirling patients on wheels or ducking them into cold water. Sedation produced by various chemical compounds marked one step, and this was followed by the development of insulin shock, pentylenetetrazol (Metrazol), electroconvulsive therapy, nikethamide (Coramine) combined with electroshock, hydrotherapy, rehabilitation, and many others. None of these measures has proved completely satisfactory, for in each there are inherent disadvantages and, often, danger. "Hangovers" follow heavy sedation, and the physician is wary of possible brain damage following insulin therapy or of fractures concurrent with convulsive treatment. While the use of curariform compounds will decrease practically to nil the incidence of fractures, one then may have to deal with a new side-effect, namely, respiratory embarrassment. Therefore, psychiatrists have long been seeking a safe method or an agent that can help the mentally ill toward normalcy.

For centuries the Indian plant Rauwolfia serpentina has been used in the treatment of mental patients as well as those who suffer from insomnia, snake bite, anxiety states, and various other conditions. Hakim, the Indian psychiatrist, claimed a recovery rate of 51% in 146 mentally ill patients using various Rauwolfia preparations and recovery in 80% when Rauwolfia was combined with electroconvulsive therapy. Results such as these naturally arouse both interest and skepticism as well as a desire to investigate the agent responsible. Recently, it has been demonstrated that reserpine, a chemically pure derivative of Rauwolfia serpentina, is the chief active alkaloid in the plant and one that can be used safely and effectively both by mouth and by injection. Since this compound apparently exerts its hypotensive and sedative effects through action on the hypothalamus, the seat of emotional behavior, a rational basis for trial in the mentally ill is evident. Because our results in the first seven months of treatment with reserpine are so dramatic, we are presenting our preliminary findings to stimulate others to study reserpine in all types of mentally ill and mentally retarded patients.

USE WITH MENTALLY ILL

Selection of Patients.—Our first nine patients, all schizophrenics, began to receive medication Oct. 15, 1953. In January, 1954, four additional patients were given reserpine, and, during February, seven more psychotic patients were added to the study. The general response of our original group of patients after four and a half months of treatment led us to expand our study as rapidly as possible. At the time of this report we have 68 female and 6 male mentally ill patients taking reserpine by mouth or injection or both. For this investigation we have selected only those mentally ill patients who had the worst prognosis as far as recovery was concerned. They were the so-called back-ward patients who had been regarded as hopeless. A great majority had been mentally ill for a long period of time and had been entirely refractory to other methods of treatment. Some had shown temporary response to shock only to regress on discontinuation of the treatment. Three or four of this group had received over 100 electroshock treatments each. In fact, all of the first nine patients were selected from our maximum security wards.

Prior to this study these wards presented the usual picture of wards of this type, namely, 10 to 12 patients in seclusion, some also in camisole or other types of restraint. In addition, heavy sedation and electroconvulsive therapy, as well as hydrotherapy and wet packs, were necessary and being utilized daily. Owing to the raucous, hyperactive, combative, sarcastic, resistive, uncooperative patients, the ward was in a continual turmoil. Necessary daily tasks, such as feeding, dressing, and bathing the patients, were arduous and had a depressing effect on the personnel assigned to these wards. Large numbers of physically strong technicians were needed to supervise and care for such patients, many of whom had to be spoon fed because they were too uncooperative to go to the dining room. They kept other patients awake at night because of their noisy behavior, and some continually ran up and down the hallway. Although frequently attempted, the administration of electroconvulsive therapy was difficult because of the resistance of these patients to treatment and their intense fear reactions.

Dosage and Side-Effects.—When we began treatment we had no idea what dose of reserpine would be required to calm these violently disturbed patients; therefore, we had to "feel" our way along to determine an effective, yet safe, dose. Arbitrarily we started patients on 0.5 mg. of reserpine twice a day for one week and then increased the dose to 0.5 mg. three or four times a day during succeeding weeks. More recently, since obtaining a supply of the injectable form of the drug, we have initiated therapy with intravenous doses of 1 to 10 mg., starting reserpine by mouth 0.5 mg. four times a day. Frequently, it is necessary to repeat the injection each day or every other day during the first week of therapy, presumably until such time as effective blood or tissue levels of reserpine are attained. Now that a vehicle is available that permits intramuscular or subcutaneous use of reserpine, we believe that there will be much less need for use of the intravenous route. In our experience to date, no reactions have occurred at the site of intramuscular or subcutaneous injection. No alarming reaction has occurred even after intravenous or intramuscular injections of 10 mg. In all of the intravenous injections the full dose has been given at one time, i. e., no infusions of reserpine have been given. Currently we are administering reserpine in doses up to 0.2 mg. per kilogram of body weight when therapy is first started, and on that same day beginning oral medication of 0.5 mg. four times a day or 1 mg. twice a day.

We have encountered little difficulty from side-effects. When 5 mg. or more of reserpine is injected intravenously one usually sees almost immediate flushing of the face and extremities, and often the patient will shiver. Some complain mildly of vertigo or weakness, but none have been forced to remain in bed. Many of these patients have had blood pressures of 80/50 mm. Hg and have not complained of vertigo. They are fully ambulatory, and not one has fainted or fallen. Many of these patients are now on work detail in the dining rooms or laundry. One 38-year-old woman experienced five epileptic episodes while taking 2 to 2.5 mg. of reserpine daily. With reduction of reserpine intake to 1 mg. daily and the addition of diphenylhydantoin (Dilantin) sodium and desiccated thyroid to her regimen no further episodes occurred; she is now in a remission. Although this woman had not previously shown any epileptic tendencies, she had received more than 100 electroshocks. We do not know whether reserpine had any relation to her seizures, but we shall watch our patients closely for such developments in the future.

Results.—Since the advent of therapy with reserpine by the oral and parenteral routes, changes in the patients' attitudes and behavior have been noted. The patients do not manifest a fear reaction to the alkaloid and gladly express a preference for this drug over electroconvulsive therapy. Patients have undergone a metamorphosis from raging, combative, unsociable persons to cooperative, friendly, cheerful, sociable, relatively quiet persons who are amenable to psychotherapy and rehabilitative measures. Most patients have shown favorable weight gains, and they have further expressed a desire to be assigned to work details. Hyperactive patients have become quiet, sedate, and cooperative in their behavior. Noisy patients have become quiet, while withdrawn and depressed patients have become alert and cheerful in their demeanor. At present on the wards where patients are receiving reserpine, seclusion, restraint of all types, sedation, and electroconvulsive therapy have been almost eliminated. It seems incredible that a drug can replace electroconvulsive therapy in this manner, but apparently such a drug has been found, and we expect it to revolutionize and facilitate modern psychiatric treatment.

Not only the patients have benefited but the ward technicians have adopted hopeful, optimistic attitudes, which are required for any positive and effective approach to therapy. They are overjoyed at the prospect of being converted from custodians to rehabilitation therapists. They are constantly requesting reserpine for all types of disturbed patients and would be alarmed if such therapy were discontinued, because they know that their duties would again entail restraining combative patients.

It is still too early to say what the ultimate classification of all these patients will be, for it appears that the longer a patient takes reserpine the better the chance for response. Every one of the first 20 patients improved to some degree, and 12 have shown marked improvement. Twenty are no longer psychotic, and eight persons have been discharged from the hospital. We hope and expect that the rest of our patients will show similar improvement as they continue to receive the drug. In psychiatry it is difficult to assess improvement by objective means. Prior to the availability of reserpine, "special incident reports" were filed at the rate of two to four per day from one maximum security ward. During six weeks after we began reserpine treatment only one report came from this same ward. One patient who was in the habit of striking someone at least once daily struck another patient only once in six weeks.

Comment.—While many patients show marked depression of blood pressure and pulse rate, many others show no change whatsoever. We have seen no correlation between effect on blood pressure and pulse and the calming effect. Patients whose pressure is reduced by one-half become no more tranquil than those whose blood pressure is unaffected. In reference to the effects of reserpine it is believed that some remarkable assistance to the homeostatic mechanism had been induced. Disturbed, confused, disoriented patients become rational, oriented, pleasant, and more interested in their surroundings and other persons. They become more considerate of the feelings of others and are more responsive to their environment. We cannot simply describe the effects of reserpine by confining them to the tranquilizing action of the drug. In addition, we believe that a reorganization of the personality is taking place in an amazing, rapid, satisfactory manner. This belief is borne out by the favorable reorganization shown in some of the electroencephalograms after therapy with this alkaloid. We believe that in 75% of mentally ill patients reserpine will substitute for and excel electroconvulsive therapy, both in acute states and for maintenance. To date it has proved far superior to shock therapy for the maintenance of disturbed patients in a sociable manner. The undesirable "organicity" that results from numerous electroshock treatments is not noticed with reserpine.

The drug provides a far more rational approach to the treatment of the chronically and acutely disturbed patient than any other method we have used to date. It is still too early to state with certainty whether reserpine therapy must be continued indefinitely. We withdrew medication from four patients for two months. Two maintained their improvement, and two started to regress. Therapy was resumed and both improved again.

Use with Mentally Retarded

Selection of Patients.—For our study of the use of reserpine in mentally retarded patients we selected on Feb. 5, 1954, 13 female patients whose intelligence quotients varied from 2 to 34. In age the patients ranged from 20 to 55 years, although most were in their 20's. The patients selected had the worst prognosis insofar as treatment, management, and possible recovery were concerned. As a group they were noisy, untidy, intractable, unable or unwilling to take care of bodily functions, and resistive both to ward personnel and to rehabilitation training.

Dosage and Side-Effects.—These 13 women were placed on a regimen of 1 mg. of reserpine by mouth daily after control blood pressure readings were obtained. Two additional patients, one man and one woman, were added to the series during March. No side-effects have been observed in any of the group.

Results.—After three months of treatment we feel that reserpine is of value to mentally retarded patients. Two have made remarkable improvement in their behavioral patterns. One 25-year-old woman with an I.Q. of 20 formerly had refused to dress or feed herself or to take any interest in her surroundings. She is now amenable to rehabilitation training, and at the same time she is dressing herself, feeding herself, acting in a friendly manner, and smiling frequently. Although she still does not talk, she appears to be more mentally alert and responsive to her environment and behaves in general as if she understands requests from the ward personnel. She sits at the table and eats acceptably. She is more sociable and gives the impression that she is grateful for her improvement. Another mentally retarded patient, a 42-year-old with an I.Q. of 34, formerly sat on the ward in a semicatatonic stupor, refusing to do anything for herself. Now she is more alert, not stuporous, regularly feeds and dresses herself, and has undergone a metamorphosis from a vegetable to a person who, though limited in her capabilities, is far more responsive to her environment.

A third patient, a 23-year-old man who had shown marked improvement, was a chronic "head beater" who required restraint 24 hours a day. His face, ears, and scalp were constantly bruised and cut from banging his head against the wall or from kneeing or punching himself. Reserpine, both parenterally and orally, has converted him into a different-looking person. Even without restraints he no longer tries to harm himself. His depression is partially relieved, and he now mingles occasionally with other patients on the ward.

The effect of reserpine on this group has not been confined to the patients alone. The morale of the ward employees has improved considerably, and they have assumed a positive, optimistic approach to the further training and treatment of these mentally retarded patients. While the other subjects have not responded like the three mentioned above, the afternoon and night shifts of psychiatric technicians report the patients to be much quieter and less hyperactive in their behavior. As a result, the ward is quieter at night and all the patients are more content.

Comment.—From this short term study on the most intractable retarded patients at Modesto State Hospital, we think it reasonable to predict that mentally retarded patients in the higher I.Q. ranges will respond to a correspondingly greater extent in their socialization programs. Since reserpine has not produced a single side-effect in this group of 15 patients over a three month period, even at the doses employed, we believe that a further study of its use with this type of neuropsychiatric patients should be widely expanded.

Summary

Seventy-four mentally ill and 15 mentally retarded patients received reserpine (Serpasil) for periods ranging up to seven months. All of these patients were given reserpine by mouth in an average daily dosage of 2 mg.; many had parenteral injections also. From our experience to date, we believe that about 80% of psychiatric patients show improvement that is attributable to the alkaloid. Depressed patients become alert and sociable, while the hyperactive, noisy, **assaultive group becomes tranquil. The use of restraints, seclusion, and electro-**

convulsive therapy has decreased by at least 80% since this study began. Remissions have been produced in 20 patients, and 8 have been discharged. In the near future, leave of absence for all patients in remission is contemplated. As reserpine is used for longer periods of time, we expect remissions to occur in a higher percentage of patients. The response of four of the mentally retarded patients has been so encouraging that we are expanding our study in that area. Even though the dosage of reserpine has been high, side-effects have been infrequent and minor. We do not suggest that reserpine is a panacea in the treatment of the mentally ill and mentally retarded; however, the response of these patients has been so promising that we urge other investigators to evaluate the drug in all types of mental disease.

SOME CONSIDERATIONS ON THE USE OF CHLORPROMAZINE IN A CHILD PSYCHIATRY CLINIC

Herbert Freed, M D., F.A.P.A., and Charles A. Peifer, Jr.

The use of chlorpromazine in psychiatry has been largely restricted to adults. The major deterrent to the exhibition of this drug in the behavioral manifestations of children would seem to be the incidence of disturbing side effects. This appears to be an important argument against the usage of this drug when it has been traditional in the field of child psychiatry to rely only on psychotherapy and environment manipulation. We have not observed disturbing side effects except drowsiness to date.

We have been interested in the combining of drug administration with psychotherapy in the child psyhiatry clinic for more than four years. In May, 1955 we reported our observations on the effect of the prolonged administration of chlorpromazine in 25 hyperkinetic emotionally disturbed children observed for periods up to 16 months. This was, to our knowledge, the first controlled study reported with an extended period of observation. We have since extended our observations and in addition accumulated some unpublished data from other observers in the field of child psychiatry that should prove interesting.

Our observations in adults as well as the further reports of the diminution of attendant abnormal or excessive movements spurred us on to treat the hyperkinetic emotionally disturbed child. In our first 25 cases observed from 4 to 16 months, improvement in varying degrees was noted in 21 (84 per cent) and was marked in 70 per cent. Diminution in hyperactivity was the outstanding response, while assaultiveness was reduced considerably. The psychologic testing program as well as the clinical evaluation by the therapist and teachers suggested that the learning process was facilitated with definite improvement in the willingness to learn. Finally, trends toward increased emotional control were evidenced although the basic personality structure remained fundamentally unchanged. In the above group the team approach of establishing therapeutic relationships with both the child and the parents was not utilizable since 80 per cent of these children were either illegitimate or came from broken homes, and a parental figure was not available for cooperation. On the other hand, a smaller group of patients of similar background had responded satisfactorily to activity group therapy. Because of a lack of therapists available for individual therapy, it was decided to extend the use of chlorpromazine therapy to the larger category of the primary behavior disorders of children as well as selected cases in every diagnostic group treated in our clinic.

There are now 30 boys and girls in the group of hyperkinetic emotionally disturbed children. In all categories 70 children are receiving the drug. The therapeutic indications varied from temper tantrums and frequent nightmares through disturbances in reading to the need for an immediate palliative procedure when psychotherapy was not initially available.

It is difficult to evaluate adequately the behavioral responses of children to any form of drug therapy because of the underlying influence of the associated interpersonal relationship. We discussed this aspect in the reported series where the children acted as their own controls, and 20 per cent showed a positive response to placebo medication. The remainder of the cases to be reported now did not.

We now, however, feel that we probably underestimated the psychic value of placebo therapy with children. A communication from Adamson (Austin, Texas, Community Guidance Center) highlights this. In his double-blind study of 40 mentally defective children with severe behavior problems, 8 (80 per cent) of the first 10 children who were given the placebo showed improvement, a figure that dropped to 40 per cent when the first six weeks of observation were finished. Incidentally, 9 (90 per cent) of the 10 children receiving chlorpromazine showed improvement. Krush noted the following sequence: 50 institutionalized children were given chlorpromazine and told it was "a means of helping you to get along better." During the first day, as the children were able to compare observations, they got the idea that these were actually vitamins to pep them up and a large number became much more active whether on placebo or on drug. On the second and third day word got around that they were getting a sleeping medicine, and a large number of the children spent much of these two days asleep or dozing, again unrelated to whether they received placebo or drug.

The general impression that relationship therapy in any form is effective with children would seem to be supported by these observations. The flexibility of the growing organism to adapt to various forms of treatment and changes in the environment both internal and external is certainly suggested. One can, therefore, appreciate the reliance of most child therapists on psychotherapy alone.

Nevertheless, there is a specific effect of chlorpromazine that can be observed in children. The report of Gatski was followed by an exhibit at the American Medical Association convention in Atlantic City in June 1955, where Flaherty and Gatski described the 45 children who were the most difficult conduct problems and who resisted "psychotherapy guidance and milieu therapy. When given various barbiturates they were still inaccessible to the therapist." After being treated with chlorpromazine for one week or longer, "39 of the 45 children improved . . . and continued to improve as they continued the drug. Having become amenable to supervision they were no longer resistant to psychotherapy . . ."

The above patients were hospitalized cases and for the most part not comparable to the other series reported thus far. Kinross-Wright listed a series of 19 cases of behavior disorders in children who were ambulatory. Seventy-nine per cent responded favorably. He commented on the favorable responses seen in cases with brain damage that manifested hyperactivity and in 1 boy with multiple tics.

At this time we have observed the therapeutic response in 70 children ranging in age from 3 to 15 years. All of them have been outpatients. Our criterion for the use of chlorpromazine was not based on diagnostic categories. It was essentially the formulation that hostility or tension was underlying the complaints for which the parents brought the children to the clinic. Five of the children admitted to significantly disturbing fears, but as yet we have not been able to study the clear-cut effect in a child with a marked phobia.

The observation that was readily made by all observers was that hostility was diminished consistently in those children who had taken medication regularly for at least two weeks. Free-floating anxiety is not commonly complained of by children and therefore could not be studied adequately. However, it was noted by us that children did not routinely drop their fears of the dark, of ghosts, etc.

It was our impression that the primitive type of psychomotor response that Cannon labeled the fight-flight response was presumably influenced. The treated children now seemed more willing to encounter and to tolerate new situations. The possible neurophysiologic basis for this has been described.

Krush has noted that a few schizophrenic children have become more regressed after medication. We do not doubt that a small number of children, particularly institutionalized cases, may show some evidences of withdrawal after treatment. We have not seen this degree of response in our cases. Two children we followed were described as worse in that they became more hostile. It was our feeling that we did not get adequate child-parent cooperation in these cases. So we would like to commit ourselves to the conservative observation that at least 3 out of 4 children were benefited to some degree while very few, if any, were made worse.

At this point one may ask, what are the contraindications? Thus far, we cannot list any that are clear-cut. The possibility exists that apathy and withdrawal may be accentuated, as Krush observed. We can speak only from the experiences with psychotic withdrawn adults, where we found the responses to be unpredictable and in many cases favorable. It is likely that further observation is necessary to determine contraindications as well as the most satisfactory technique for the termination of prolonged courses of medication in these children.

A comment that should be considered more than passing concerns our experience with 2 children with hitherto uncontrolled epilepsy who were controlled with chlorpromazine combined with anticonvulsives.

The usual effective oral dosage in our series was found to be 25 mg. three times a day. The proper dose was determined clinically by the therapeutic response and the observation that the child's activities were not interrupted by drowsiness rather than by body weight. The maximum dosage was 300 mg./day. Flaherty informed us that he used a wider range of dosage—60 mg. to 1000 mg. daily—in his series of intitutionalized severely disturbed boys. The patient who was given 250 mg. four times a day developed some manifestations of Parkinsonism that disappeared with dose reduction. Adamson reports an average dosage of 300 mg./day with the range being 100 to 400 mg. Significant posologic modifications may evolve if combinations of chlorpromazine and reserpine or chlorpromazine and dexedrine now under trial prove more effective. The advantage of a single daily dose, especially for the school child, is obvious.

Do our experiences with children suggest new perspectives in psychiatry? We think so. There are the confirmed observations that overactivity in the spectrum ranging from restlessness through marked assaultiveness can readily be controlled. At the same time there is some evidence both from psychologic tests and from the reports of teachers and counselors that the child resumes the learning process. Such implications should encourage us in our work with both children and adults, for Freud as well as Dollard and Miller and others has stressed that psychotherapy must include re-education as well as resumption of the learning process.

Finally, we offer a speculation arising from the absence of a finding in children that is relatively common in adults. A number of observers have reported on the frequency of the complications of Parkinsonism in chlorpromazine therapy in adults. The incidence ranges from 4.8 to 7 per cent in adults, while there is as yet no report on the incidence in children. This may simply be due to the fact that relatively few children have been treated in comparison with adults. But there is another consideration in the development of Parkinsonism in children. The preliminary experiments were made by nature. We have known for the last 30 years that there is usually a difference in the postencephalitic sequelae of epidemic encephalitis in children, particularly between the ages of 3 and 10. They manifest destructiveness and impulsive behavior rather than Parkinsonism. Our observation and inquiries suggest thus far that chlorpromazine administration does not produce the complication of Parkinsonism with the expected frequency noted in adults. This would take into account the reported relationship to the size of the dose. Should we assume that the child, in contrast to the adult, does not develop Parkinsonism in response to noxious stimuli for biologic reasons, perhaps because the degree of adaptability of the young nervous system is different? We may find it easier to answer this when we have accumulated more data from the use of reserpine (which seems to be more "Parkinsongenic") as well as chlorpromazine in children.

Buerger and Mayer Gross have theorized that ruminative thinking in postencephalitic Parkinsonism was the response to the release of motor impulses that were turned into thoughts instead of being directly discharged. We have been impressed with the diminution in motor activity without the apparent development of ruminative thinking either clinically or in the test material in our subjects. Thus far in our studies of adults who developed Parkinsonism we have not seen the expected increase in the incidence of obsessive thinking of the above theory were substantiated.

The idea has been put forth that the encephalitic process in children interferes with the development of superego manifestations in children. Allowing for possible differences in brain areas influenced in epidemic encephalitis and those in the chlorpromazine effect, should we anticipate any distinctive superego effect in the long-term administration of the drug to the young child?

Do the child and the adult who develop a drug-induced Parkinsonism have a psychic vulnerability exposed by the drug effect? Stengel felt that such individuals were dealing with destructive impulses by freezing the movements through Parkinsonism. We are pursuing further investigations, thus attempting to answer these questions. If some are answered, perhaps chlorpromazine will have opened new perspectives in dynamic psychophysiology while fulfilling the hopes of pharmacodynamics.

CHLORPROMAZINE FOR THE CONTROL OF PSYCHOMOTOR EXCITEMENT IN THE MENTALLY DEFICIENT

Judith H. Rettig, M.D.
Columbus State School, Columbus, Ohio

The findings of Lehmann and Hanrahan who studied chlorpromazine in 71 hospitalized psychiatric patients, revealed that this drug is of unique value in the symptomatic control of almost any kind of severe excitement. They were particularly impressed with the favorable results in manic depressive patients, all of whom had been continuously manic or hypomanic for more than a year and had previously failed to respond to standard therapeutic procedures or had had only brief remissions. The study of Sheatz brought out that patients with irreversible brain damage who were extremely overactive were successfully quieted with relatively small doses of chlorpromazine. Moreover, Elkes and Elkes from a trial of the drug in patients from the disturbed wards of the Winson Green Hospital, Birmingham, England, reported that their patients had become quiet, responsive and less destructive.

Since our review of the literature indicated that there was little or no published information on the use of chlorpromazine in mentally deficient patients, we undertook this evaluation to assess its usefulness in controlling psychomotor excitement in such patients.

Material and Methods

For the study, 27 mentally-deficient patients—5 males and 22 females—whose chronological age ranged from 14 to 64 years, were selected from the population of Columbus State School. The clinical characteristics of these patients are summarized in table 1. All were highly disturbed, hyperactive, and violent. They were destructive to their surroundings and clothing, screaming and uncontrollable. Some had to be restrained almost continually; others had to be secluded for long periods of time. Temper tantrums were frequent, often accompanied by self-injury, threats of suicide, assaultiveness against the staff and other patients. Several patients actively experienced hallucinations and delusions and were disoriented as to identity, time, and space. The problems of soiling were great. Duration of custodial care ranged from 7 months to 19 years, with an average of 5 years.

Intelligence quotients determined by commonly used tests, including the Stanford-Binet and Wechsler-Bellevue, indicated that of the 24 mentally-deficient patients tested, 12 were judged to be high-grade (I.Q. 70-51), 6 middle

TABLE 1.—CLINICAL DATA OF 27 PATIENTS: STUDY OF EFFECT OF CHLORPROMAZINE THERAPY

Patient	Age	Sex	I.Q.	Diagnosis	Length of Institution-alisation	Behavior before Chlorpromazine	Behavior after Chlorpromazine Treatment	Results in Terms of Manageability
J. B.	15	F	71	Familial c̄ behav. react.	7 mo.	Destructive, screaming incessantly	Quiet and cooperative	Excellent
M. L. R.	16	F	17*	Idiopathic c̄ psych. react.	20 mo.	Restive, unruly	Sleeps well, manageable	Fair
M. G. T.	32	F	27*	Familial c̄ psych. react., c̄ convul.	18 mo.	Surly, untidy	Better disposition, grooming	Good
M. O'G.	33	F	11	Familial c̄ psych. react.	4½ mo.	Hyperactive; in restraint	Some restraint still necessary	Fair
L. H.	20	F	63	Familial c̄ psych. react.	16 mo.	Manic, hyperactive	Severe depression	Poor
E. A. W.	17	F	30	Idiopathic, severe	4½ yr.	Violent, screaming	Less tense	Fair
T. C.	46	F	62	Idiopathic c̄ psych. react.	15 yr.	Hyperactive, destructive, irritable, with temper tantrums	Quiet, more occupied, relaxed	Excellent
I. K.	41	F	61	Idiopathic c̄ psych. react.	7 yr.	Disoriented, violent	Quiet, cooperative, less psychotic	Good
G. S.	29	F	44	Brain injury c̄ neurotic react.	12 yr.	Sullen, self-injurious	Pleasant, and cooperative	Excellent
M. W.	16	F	14	Idiopathic c̄ catatonic react.	22 mo.	Hyperactive, mute, unmanageable	Communicative, happy, and cheerful	Good
E. C.	30	F	59	Familial c̄ schizophrenic react.	19 yr.	Too unruly for ward	Calmed, no seclusion needed	Excellent
J. E.	19	F	54	CBS c̄ intracranial infection	10 yr.	Fighting, secluded from others	Quiet; no need for seclusion	Excellent
D. A. L.	19	F	40	Familial c̄ psych. react.	3 yr.	Manic, unruly	Quiet, manageable	Excellent
P. C.	19	F	48	Familial c̄ behavioral react.	2½ yr.	Violent, in seclusion	Manageable, relaxed	Excellent
J. L. McN.	14	F	23	CBS c̄ intracranial infection	4 yr.	Babbling, tense	Speech coherent, quiet	Fair
E. G.	64	F	33	Iodiopathic c̄ behavioral react.	21 mo.	Soiler, truculent	Tidy, helpful, good; slight depression	Good
J. E.	15	F	†	Psychotic disorder c̄ hebephrenic react.	3 yr.	Self-abusive, assaultive	Quiet and cooperative. On "trial" visit home	Excellent
D. S	15	F	38	Idiopathic c̄ behavioral react.	4 yr.	Temper tantrums with destructiveness	Tantrums less frequent, quiet, manageable	Good
T. A. J.	16	F	65	Idiopathic c̄ psych. react.	4 yr.	Anti-social; frequent tantrums	Manageable and cooperative; temper tantrums much less frequent	Good
M. A. W.	23	F	62	CBS c̄ psych. react.	10 yr.	Aggressive, moody	Manageable and cooperative	Good
G. S.	31	F	64	Familial c̄ behavioral react.	11 yr.	Trouble-maker, aggressive	No change	None
A. U.	33	F	57	Familial c̄ behavioral react.	2½ yr.	Suicidal	Quiet, less introspective	Good
W. B.	17	M	73	CBS (birth trauma) c̄ behavioral react.	2 yr.	Combative, obscene, and sadistic	Quiet and a bit more manageable; at times friendly and cheerful	Good
D. R. McK.	14	M	20	CBS (constitutional influence) c̄ congenital plegias and behavioral react.	3 yr.	Disoriented, mute; restraints needed on occasions	Quiet; restraints not necessary	Good
R. A. McC.	16	M	5	CBS (birth trauma) c̄ behavioral react.	3 yr.	Facial grimaces, hyperactive, destructive	No change	None
R. L. T.	23	M	10	CBS c̄ behavioral react.	4 yr.	Agitated, spastic flexion of left forearm and hand	No change	Poor
N. S.	17	M	40	CBS (birth trauma) c̄ behavioral react.	7 yr.	Alternately hyperactive and depressed	Quiet and cooperative	Good

* Social quotient. † Resisted testing.

grade (I.Q. 50-31), and 6 low-grade (I.Q. 30 or under). Of the remaining three patients, two were tested using the Vineland Social Maturity Scale and showed social quotients of 17 and 27, respectively. One patient could not be tested because of her hyperactivity.

All of the patients selected for this study failed to benefit from previous treatment which included barbiturates, electroshock therapy, occupational therapy, and psychotherapy. They remained manageable only with extreme difficulty—a burden to themselves as well as to those who cared for them.

When chlorpromazine therapy was started, all other medication was discontinued. Initially, 25 mg. to 50 mg. were given intramuscularly, augmented by 25 mg. to 50 mg. orally, as needed to maintain the patient calm. Once under control, they were switched to oral medication in doses of 25 mg. to 50 mg., usually four times daily.

The dose for each patient was tailored to give optimal results, increased or decreased, so as to establish a level of behavior in which control was possible without resorting to barbiturates, restraints, or seclusion.

All patients but one have received chlorpromazine for more than 6 months. The exception is a patient who reacted with severe depression necessitating withdrawal of the drug.

RESULTS

Table 1 summarizes our results with chlorpromazine in managing disturbed mentally-deficient patients. The efficacy of the drug was judged on the basis of the following criteria: (a) degree of cooperation; (b) absence or presence of destructiveness; (c) habit training; (d) disposition; (e) sleeping habits. Persistence at a given task and initiative were taken into account when differentiating between "excellent" and "good" results.

An *excellent* result was characterized by complete cooperation of the patient with the staff and with fellow patients, a cheerful disposition, absence of soiling and destructiveness, normalization of sleeping habits, and little need for supervision because of a certain amount of initiative and persistence at a given task. The result was judged *good* when there was a clear-cut improvement in the physical management of the patient, that is, the disappearance of destructiveness, soiling, and generally, of hyperactive behavior. Patients in whom results were judged to be *fair* became tidy and manageable for lengthy periods of time although occasionally there were relapses to overactive and destructive behavior —with the need for restraining them. *Poor* results were judged when only transient, non-recurring betterment in manageability or, in one case, adverse side-effects occurred necessitating discontinuance of therapy. When there was no perceptible change in the clinical picture of the patient, the results were graded *none*.

Using these criteria, results in this series of 27 patients were judged as *excellent* in 8 patients, *good* in 11, *fair* in 4, *poor* in 2, and *none* in 2. The failures occurred mostly in those patients who had suffered severe brain injury and in whom large areas of the brain were actually destroyed.

The changes which our units have undergone since the introduction of chlorpromazine into the regimen are marked. Generally speaking, most hyperactive patients who had been extreme conduct problems became quiet, manageable and cooperative. At night almost all slept well. As temper tantrums occurred with much less frequency, the need for isolation and restraint was virtually eliminated.

With the patients calm and more receptive to their social environment, more efficient training and rehabilitation are possible, or, at least, more efficient custodial care can be carried out for those with extensive brain damage. Some of the institutional personnel released from the time-consuming duty of disciplining and restraining overactive patients may be employed more profitably in recreation, in the training of patients, and in ways more profitable emotionally to themselves. On the whole, this and the savings resulting from less destruction make for a better balanced institutional economy.

Case Histories

The following case histories illustrate some of the typical results obtained with chlorpromazine:

Case 1: J. B., a 15-year-old girl, was admitted on May 24, 1954, because of severe disorderly behavior in the community. She was found to be a borderline mental defective, familial, with behavioral reaction. Her I. Q. measured by the Wechler I test was 71. In the various cottages where she lived, the patient was labeled by the nursing attendants as "uncontrollable" and "unmanageable." Her frequent temper tantrums provoked altercations with the other girls and, in general, upset the unit and its routine. She was constantly in motion, jumping through windows, walking the floor at night, playing hide-and-seek, and so on. The other girls expressed thorough dislike for her, and even the attendants, who were inured to such behavior, hesitated to tangle with her unless aided by other personnel.

On October 18, 1954, she was placed on chlorpromazine therapy and reacted with an almost remarkable improvement of behavior. She became quiet, easily managed, cooperative, and attentive to other patients, particularly those who were physically handicapped. She showed interest in her surroundings and in the school in which she was placed. Today she is progressing well with her school work. Moreover, her matron describes her as a constructive helper in her cottage, the attendants comment on her cooperativeness, and her companions find that she has become more sociable and they in turn have become friendly to her. At present she is being maintained on 50 mg. orally, t.i.d. and has sustained her improvement.

Case 2: G. S., now a 29-year-old woman, suffered a fractured skull in an automobile accident when she was 14. Shortly afterward her behavior changed markedly in that she became unruly, high-tempered, nervous, wandered about the house, and was unable to sleep. She grew progressively worse, until, three years later, it became necessary to confine her to an institution. Her condition was diagnosed as chronic brain syndrome associated with trauma, brain trauma through gross force, with neurotic reaction and mental deficiency.

Since her admission she has had a long history of bizarre behavior, self-inflicted injuries, temper tantrums, sullenness, and antagonistic behavior toward attendants and other patients in her cottage. At times she would refuse to eat; in cold weather she would run outside scantily clothed and there parade flauntingly or lie on the ground. Barbiturates had very little effect on her behavior.

This patient was first given chlorpromazine on October 20, 1954. She responded to the drug immediately and improved remarkably. At present she is a cottage worker and doing a better than average job of helping physically handicapped patients. She has shown considerable initiative in performing numerous errands with little or no direction, in helping the cottage physicians with the preparation of patients for injections, and so on. She is pleasant, cooperative, capable, and has become a useful member of the institutional society. Her present maintenance dose of chlorpromazine is 50 mg., orally, t.i.d.

Case 3: T. C., a woman now 46 years old, was first admitted to a mental institution 15 years ago when she became acutely disturbed, violent, and destructive. Psychological testing revealed mental deficiency with psychotic reaction. Although the patient was known to have been mentally-deficient since birth, she had managed to get along fairly well in the community, working about the house and creating no particular problems. When her mother died, however, her behavior changed for the worse, and 4 years later she had to be committed to a state hospital. She was later transferred to Columbus State School where she has remained since 1942 except for one year's stay at a sanatorium, when she was found to have active tuberculosis. Because of temper tantrums and destructiveness she had to be secluded often. Even when not secluded her periods of hyperactivity and extreme irritability were frequent; she avidly sought the attention and sympathy of the attendants and, with equal vigor, fought frequently with other patients.

In January, 1954, the patient began to express bizarre ideation, depersonalization, and seemed to be hallucinating both auditorily and visually. Between February 17 and March 24, 1954, she received 26 electroshock treatments resulting in improvement; that is, she no longer had bizarre ideas although her destructive behavior persisted. Sedatives produced only slight behavioral improvement. Chlorpromazine therapy was therefore instituted on October 20, 1954, and resulted in rapid behavioral improvement. The patient could be easily managed and was helpful around the ward. She no longer required seclusion at any time for her manifestations of hyperactivity or irritability. Consequently, the patient was permitted to go home for a trial visit—*the first time in 15 years*. It proved highly successful, and the patient's family reported that she was a model of good behavior during her stay at home. She was returned to the hospital, greatly delighted about her progress, and apparently quite content with the thought that she would be permitted future visits at home.

SIDE EFFECTS

Drowsiness, which proved to be the principal side effect, was considered more helpful than disadvantageous in these hard-to-manage patients. Usually it was transient and subsided after the first few days of therapy.

Other side effects were rare: Two patients complained of anorexia; one, of vomiting. The case of severe depression following chlorpromazine therapy has already been mentioned. Another patient became slightly depressed, but her over-all response was good. She became tidy, helpful on the wards, and friendly in contrast to her former slovenly, irascible, and churlish behavior.

SUMMARY AND CONCLUSIONS

Twenty-seven highly disturbed, mentally-deficient patients were treated with chlorpromazine (25-50 mg., four times daily) for a period of 6 months. Results were judged excellent in 8, good in 11, fair in 4. Four patients did not respond to the drug. Results were best in those patients whose disturbance was primarily emotional in nature, that is, the greater the actual brain damage, the less the effectiveness of the drug. Generally speaking, chlorpromazine was highly useful in bringing about better manageability of overactive and destructive patients.

The impact of the drug on the attendants personally and administratively was equally important. Relieving them of time-consuming duties, chiefly custodial and disciplinary, permitted them to spend more time in therapy and has consequently raised their morale considerably. With less destructiveness and through better manageability, maintenance costs should be reduced.

Side effects were minimal and consisted principally of transient drowsiness, which was considered an asset with these overactive patients. Two patients complained of anorexia; one, of vomiting. In one patient it was necessary to discontinue the therapy because she became depressed.

The author wishes to thank Myra Chatters, M.D., and Willa Caldwell, M.D., without whose help this study could not have been done.

POTENTIATION OF HYPNOTICS AND ANALGESICS
Clinical Experience with Chlorpromazine

Robert Wallis, M.D.

As a result of experimental work conducted by Courvoisier et al., a new compound was discovered which possesses diverse pharmacologic properties, generalized as marked ganglioplegic and sympathicolytic activity. Among these properties is its ability to intensify and prolong the action of drugs such as hypnotics, anesthetics, and narcotics. This new compound, known as chlorpromazine, is 10-(v-dimethylaminopropyl)-2-chlorophenothiazine. Although structurally related to Phenergan and Diparcol, chlorpromazine exhibits relatively weak antihistaminic and anticholinergic activity. Developed in France by Rhone-Poulenc-Specia Laboratories, chlorpromazine, in addition to its drug-potentiating action, blocks apomorphine-induced vomiting and alters conditioned reflex responses in animals. Friend and Cummins recently reported on the clinical usefulness of this compound in controlling drug-induced and disease-induced nausea and vomiting. In psychiatric work Delay et al. and Sigwald and Bouttier have found chlorpromazine effective in managing psychomotor excitement seen in states of anxiety, confusion, mania, obsessions, and phobias. Moreover, Lehmann and Hanrahan, using higher than usual dosage levels, observed improvement of various degrees in treating schizophrenics.

Use of chlorpromazine to potentiate other drugs in surgery and in anesthesia has been demonstrated by the French investigators, Laborit et al. and Forster et al. They observed that patients who received the drug with hypnotics preoperatively later required less hypnotic and anesthetic and that use of narcotics postoperatively also could be reduced. These results prompted me to investigate the usefulness of chlorpromazine in potentiating drugs used in the treatment of conditions commonly seen in everyday office practice.

This report, then, relates my experience with chlorpromazine to potentiate the action and prolong the duration of action of other drugs in three groups of 39 nonsurgical patients: patients unable to sleep in spite of their taking Seconal, Nembutal, or Tuinal before bedtime; patients with acute and chronic pains unrelieved to any appreciable extent by usual analgesic therapies, and anxious and tense patients with psychosomatic complaints.

Results

Seventeen patients whose complaints of insomnia were not amenable to sedatives in usual doses were benefited immeasurably when chlorpromazine, 25 to 50 mg. orally, was given with sedatives. A portion of the group in whom

Seconal, Nembutal, and Tuinal (1½ grains) had previously proved ineffective obtained singularly good results when these drugs were supplemented with chlorpromazine. Patient response to phenobarbital, ½ grain, or to chloral hydrate, 15 grains, given with chlorpromazine was equally satisfactory; in some cases as little as ¼ grain of phenobarbital was adequate. These combinations generally permitted the patients to sleep at least eight to ten hours. On awakening patients felt refreshed and experienced none of the hangover effects that so often follow taking soporifics. We have had practically no failures, regardless of whether the cause of insomnia stemmed from physical or emotional origin. Although chlorpromazine and Phenergan (12.5 to 25 mg.) proved effective for inducing sleep, patients given this combination reported being somewhat drowsy and uncoordinated the following morning.

In using chlorpromazine with sedatives to re-establish normal sleeping patterns, it appears undesirable for patients drinking alcohol or for inebriated patients to take the drug. We observed that not only is the depressing effect of alcohol increased, but that the postalcoholic state is aggravated as well. Chlorpromazine has, however, been successfully used for controlling nausea and vomiting resulting from Antabuse-alcohol reactions.

In a series of nine patients with pain of diverse origin, including cancer, severe neuralgias, sciatica, and neuritis of the brachial plexus, chlorpromazine was added to determine whether it would augment the action of various analgesics. Although providing only symptomatic relief, there is no doubt that the combined administration of chlorpromazine and 1-dromoran, morphine, Demerol, codeine, or salicylates increases the efficiency of these analgesics.

As an example, a patient with cancer of the prostate and bone metastases had been maintained fairly free from pain on estrogen therapy following orchiectomy. Within two years, however, the liver became involved, and the patient now required Demerol or morphine to relieve his pain. When Demerol or morphine was given with chlorpromazine, he could be kept comfortable with doses of 100 mg. or 1/3 grain, respectively. Another terminal cancer patient was completely free from pain when given 1-dromoran (1 cc. every six hours) and Tuinal (3 grains) in combination with chorpromazine, 25 mg. orally three times daily. Aside from the resultant potentiated and sustained drug action noted, it was observed that the concurrent use of these drugs seemed to induce a state of emotional indifference, which replaced the justified fear of death.

In the vast majority of patients requiring relief from pain, the analgesic-chlorpromazine combination proved very effective. It was unsuccessful, however, in providing adequate analgesia in migraine, premenstrual pelvic pain, and radicular sciatica complicated with sacroiliac dislocation.

In view of the fact that chlorpromazine slightly depresses blood pressure, it might not be amiss to speculate on its usefulness in hypertension when given in combination with hypotensive agents. An eighty-one-year-old hypertensive woman (260/140 mm. Hg) whose trigeminal neuralgia could no longer be managed by alcohol nerve block, began taking codeine, ½ grain, and chlorpromazine, 25 mg. orally, three times daily. Her pain was relieved, and she later learned that an imminent attack of neuralgia could be obtunded, if not obviated, by taking chlorpromazine, 25 mg. orally, with aspirin 10 grains—*without codeine.* After two months on this medication intermittently, her blood pressure became stabilized at 190/120, even though her diet and normal activities remained unchanged.

On the basis of 13 patients' subjective reports and my clinical impressions, chlorpromazine appears to be quite useful in the treatment of psychosomatic complaints resulting from anxiety and tension states. Twenty-five milligrams, given before each of three meals, together with specific therapy, such as phenobarbital, Trasentine, Belladenal, and Phenaphen, undoubtedly made these drugs effective when they had previously been ineffective. If the drugs had previously been effective, adding chlorpromazine augmented their activity, thus permitting their dosage to be reduced. When given singly in the treatment of psychosomatic conditions, chlorpromazine appeared to produce only slight to moderate effects in contrast to its remarkable effects when given in combination. In only two cases, anxiety reactions previously treated for many years by psychoanalysis, could a real improvement be attributed to chlorpromazine without adjuvant therapeutic measures.

Chlorpromazine was, in general, well tolerated. Since it depresses blood pressure slightly, patients with postural hypotension or low blood pressure were given the drug only at bedtime to prevent dizziness or fainting. Except for patients treated to re-establish sleep patterns, chlorpromazine had to be given continually, for symptoms returned when it was withdrawn. However, the minimum dose which is active for a certain person remains active at the same level when given over a period of months.

Comment

Clinicians have long sought a drug that by depressing hypothalamic centers of the sympathetic nervous system would inhibit cenesthesia. That chlorpromazine is such a drug seems obvious from its diverse pharmacodynamic effects. If not, how can it simultaneously alter the *reaction* to pain, relax skeletal muscle, reduce body temperature, slow metabolism, inhibit psychomotor agitation, and facilitate sleep? These physiologic effects focus its action in those subthalamic vegetative nuclei of the diencephalon which Harvey Cushing, with great foresight, said were the essential spring of instinctive, vegetative emotional life that mankind has tried to cover with a cortex of inhibitions. Previously, only by lobotomy or limited topectomy were we able to modify the neural circuit between the cortex and—what J. F. Fulton and J. Delay have called—the "affective brain." Now, with chlorpromazine, it appears possible to interrupt pharmacologically synaptic transfer between the cortex and diencephalon by less drastic means. Moreover, it is this sympatholytic action of chlorpromazine on hypothalamic centers that alters reaction to pain and thus enhances the effectiveness of analgesics given with chlorpromazine.

Observations of the reactions following the injection of chlorpromazine erroneously into the cerebrospinal fluid of a human have contributed further evidence that the potentiating effect of this drug is predominantly centrally acting. Briefly, these observations, reported by Dr. J. Schneider, of Rhone-Poulenc-Specia Laboratories, at the Therapie Kongress in Karlsruhe, August 30, 1953, are as follows:

A few minutes after 1 cc. of chlorpromazine solution (25 mg.) was injected by error into the cerebrospinal fluid, the muscles in the patient's legs became flaccid. Thirty minutes later the patient became very sleepy, and a paraplegic state involving the pelvis and the lumbar region ensued. Paralysis and sphincteric relaxation persisted approximately three hours; however, the patient was able to stand without assistance five hours later. He slept well that night, and on the following day paralysis subsided and sphincteric control returned. The patient completely recovered within forty-eight hours. Examination of the cerebrospinal fluid at this time revealed data essentially within normal limits. The fact that at no time did the patient experience pain indicated that the drug is relatively nonirritating, producing only a diffuse neuroplegia ascending toward the diencephalic centers and resulting in sleep.

All this enables us to have a clearer insight into the deeper mechanism of shock (in the initial alarm sympathetic phase) and to understand better the transition between hibernation and sleep, between physiologic sleep and anesthetic sleep, between subcortical pain and cortical homologation.

Summary

Clinical experience with a new phenothiazine derivative, chlorpromazine, indicates that this drug potentiates or augments the action of hypnotics, narcotics and analgesics. Patients whose difficulty in sleeping had been inadequately solved by barbiturates and other soporifics were benefited when chlorpromazine was added to their medication. Similarly, the compound proved effective in augmenting the action of narcotics, thus permitting lower doses of narcotics to be used in relieving pain of terminal cancer. Patients with psychosomatic complaints reported a better response when specific therapy was supplemented with chlorpromazine.

Part Four

SIDE EFFECTS

COMPLICATIONS AND CONCOMITANTS

Otis R. Farley, M.D.
Chief of Medical Service, St. Elizabeths Hospital, Washington, D. C.

I shall discuss the clinical and laboratory data of those patients admitted to the Medical and Surgical Division during the past 13 months with significant concomitants or complications incident to treatment with Serpasil or chlorpromazine. I will also very briefly discuss certain highlights of our use of these drugs in patients within the Medical and Surgical Division of the Tuberculosis Service. Incident to the presentation I shall try to point out certain observations and impressions we have developed that seem to be of value as guides to better and safer use of the two drugs.

One or the other or both drugs have been administered during the past 13 months to a total of almost 2,000 patients. The dosage in most cases has been continued over a period of 60 days or more in each patient treated. In general, Serpasil has been given in divided doses 2 times daily and chlorpromazine in doses 3 times daily. The individual doses of Serpasil have varied from fractions of 1 mg. per day to 12 or more mg. daily in a few cases. The dosages of chlorpromazine have varied from 75 mg. per day in some medical patients to 1,200 mg. or more per day in some psychiatric patients.

Based on available experience in the use of Serpasil in the treatment of hypertension, Serpasil was administered to no patient known to have malignant hypertension with azotemia, nor was it given to any patient known to have an active peptic ulcer or other potential bleeding lesion of the gastrointestinal tract.

It should be stated that the physicians throughout the Hospital have, for the most part, a tremendous respect for both of these drugs because of their extreme potency. Almost without exception they have been highly suspicious of potential complications from the use of either of the drugs. Because of this respect and low threshold of suspicion, most of the patients with significant complications were referred to the Medical and Surgical Division for observation and treatment.

For convenience' sake, I will discuss first the data in regard to the Serpasil-treated cases; second, the chlorpromazine-treated cases, and then briefly the experience of the Medical and Surgical Service staff in the use of the drugs within the Medical and Surgical Division and the Tuberculosis Service. In conclusion, I will point out what appear to be pertinent observations and impressions to be derived from our experience with the 2 drugs.

Among the Serpasil-treated patients, 3 aged women were admitted to the

Medical and Surgical Division in varying degrees of acute weakness, inertia, apathy and hypotension. In each of these patients the symptom complex was of sudden onset and responded promptly to symptomatic and supportive treatment.

Two patients were admitted to the Service with urticarial dermatitis of insidious onset during Serpasil therapy. One of these showed a positive intradermal reaction to the drug and the other was not tested. Both patients cleared up rather promptly on cessation of the therapy. Three patients were admitted to the Service with generalized edema of severe degree. Two of these reactions occurred in association with congestive heart failure and 1 occurred in a patient with far advanced myxedema.

One patient was admitted for observation because of a massive lower gastrointestinal tract hemorrhage. The hemorrhage was not recurrent, and after extensive study we were unable to find the site of the bleeding. One patient was admitted in profound shock and failed to respond to supportive measures.

One young man died suddenly on the Psychiatric Service after a few days of Serpasil therapy and is included in this group for the sake of completeness.

Among the patients described above there were 4 deaths. All of these patients were carefully examined at autopsy. The patient with myxedema and generalized edema was found at autopsy to have a generalized severe septicemia and a phlegmonous cellulitis of the soft tissues of the mouth and neck.

The patient with the profound shock was found to have a massive perforation and bleeding of a duodenal ulcer. One of the patients was found to have severe congestive heart failure which failed to respond to digitalis and diuretics and supportive measures. The myocardium showed generalized brown atrophy.

The patient who died suddenly on the Psychiatric Service was found to have generalized congestive phenomena of all the viscera, including the kidneys.

Careful consideration of the deaths in this group leads us to believe that the sudden death occurring in the young man was probably not related to Serpasil therapy except in so far as Serpasil masked the recognizable signs of impending renal failure in a hyperactive, confused young psychotic.

The case of the myxedema patient with the terminal septicemia was complicated by the fact that she had had a similar exacerbation of edema previously on the initiation of Thorazine therapy. It is well recognized in medical circles that myxedema patients respond in bizarre and sometimes hazardous fashion to many drugs, including narcotics, barbiturates and sometimes even salicylates, and we think the death in this case could be attributed to Serpasil only in so far as it constitutes a bizarre reaction to a drug, and in so far as the seriousness of her illness was masked in some measure by the ataractic effect of Serpasil.

We think it quite likely that the bleeding and perforation of a duodenal ulcer which proved fatal can be justly attributed to Serpasil therapy. Unfortunately, we were unable to elicit any history from this patient or her family that gave a clue to the presence of a duodenal ulcer prior to the institution of therapy.

The death of the patient in congestive heart failure while he was simultaneously receiving Serpasil in some measure supports our suspicion that Serpasil complicates edema states due to other causes.

In reviewing the second group of patients, namely, those with symptoms incident to Thorazine therapy, we find a wider range of complications which included the following. Eleven patients were admitted with jaundice. Each of these showed elevation of the alkaline phosphatase, elevation of serum bilirubin both in the direct and indirect fractions, and little or no clues to hepatocellular damage.

Because of the atypical nature of the jaundice in 1 case, an exploratory celiotomy was accomplished early in the course of her disease, at which time the liver and biliary tract were found to be within normal limits on gross inspection; and the liver biopsy showed nondescript changes including some bile stasis in the canaliculi. She developed intercurrent paratyphoid enteritis. This patient is at the moment profoundly cachectic and has required colostomy for idiopathic low bowel obstruction; it is our impression that she suffers intrahepatic biliary obstruction, probably due to causes other than chlorpromazine therapy, but in the last analysis the diagnosis is as yet unknown and she must be considered a potential complication of chlorpromazine therapy.

Four patients were admitted with hypothermia, hypotension and depression of consciousness of a variable degree. Ten patients were admitted with dermatitis of moderate to severe character. In 6 of these patients the dermatitis was clearly of a photosensitive nature. In all patients considerable edema of skin area involved also was noted. Four patients were admitted with fever alone.

Six patients were admitted with variable degrees of leukopenia or agranulocytosis or developed the symptom-complex while in the Medical and Surgical Division. One of these latter cases is included only for the sake of completeness since the patient also had advanced carcinomatosis with bone marrow depression, and had a significant degree of agranulocytosis due to her carcinomatosis and the phosphoramid therapy being given for her malignant disease prior to the institution of chlorpromazine therapy. A second patient in this group developed the agranulocytic reaction while simultaneously receiving both propylthiouracil and chlorpromazine and showed a prompt remission on discontinuance of both drugs. We think it likely that both of these patients developed their agranulocytosis, at least in part, due to causes other than chlorpromazine therapy. Of the remaining 3 patients, 1 died shortly after admission and before the effects of supportive and substitution therapy could be brought to bear. The others recovered after a reasonably short interval of supportive therapy with cortisone, ACTH and antibiotics.

We have had occasion to use reserpine or chlorpromazine in 36 psychiatric patients who also had pulmonary tuberculosis, many of whom were simultaneously receiving streptomycin, PAS and/or isoniazid. The indications for the use of the drug and the results of the use of the drug in these patients are approximately those described by Dr. Waldrop and Dr. Riesenman in their series of patients. In one of these patients we noted the appearance of fever and sore throat and a leukopenia with a fall in the total white blood cell count to 3,350 but with no significant disproportion in the cell constituents of the total count. In this patient the fever, the leukopenia, and the sore throat remitted when the dose of the drug was cut in approximately half, and it was not necessary for that reason to discontinue the drug.

We carried 1 grossly psychotic patient through a full-term pregnancy and to remission of psychosis and delivered a viable, healthy infant in spite of otherwise intractable hyperemesis gravidarum, and in spite of a known history of postoperative hypoparathyroidism. It is worthy of note that both the mother and the child are out of the hospital at the moment and apparently doing very well.

Within the Medical and Surgical Service we have had occasion to use the ataractic drugs for control of anxiety, agitation, hostility and overactivity, particularly in those patients in whom those symptoms interfered with nutrition and with about the same results that have been described by Dr. Riesenman and Dr. Waldrop.

We have used chlorpromazine in conventional doses for the treatment of radiation sickness and nausea and vomiting due to other causes, including the nausea and vomiting of uremia. In 1 case we used the drug for control of anxiety and pain in a hopeless terminal patient with carcinomatosis. This patient has been referred to elsewhere under the discussion of chlorpromazine treatment in patients and represents 1 of our fatalities.

Based on clinical, laboratory and/or autopsy data in the cases studied, we believe the following observations to be pertinent:

1. Lesions of the gastrointestinal tract are prone to bleed under the stimulus of Serpasil therapy and should be considered relative or absolute contraindications to the use of the drug until or unless further evidence is accumulated that speaks to the contrary.

2. We believe that Serpasil acts in some way to aggravate or exacerbate the derangement of salt and water metabolism or excretion in patients predisposed to edema for other reasons and that the drug should be given with caution to patients with hypothyroidism or myxedema and those with edema states due to congestive heart failure, renal failure or cirrhosis.

3. The sedative and ataractic effect of Serpasil may appear abruptly and in profound degree in patients with organic brain disease, including those with arteriosclerosis and traumatic brain disease, but this complication is readily reversible when recognized and does not constitute a contraindication to the use of the drug.

4. Both drugs modify the subjective response of patients to a point where they tend to mask the symptoms of intercurrent medical and surgical illness, and in some cases they complicate the diagnosis of other diseases to a significant degree. In our experience the single most striking effect in all patients receiving adequate doses of Serpasil is the marked slowing of the heart that goes along with such therapy. This slowing of the heart persists in the presence of congestive heart failure in some cases and in some cases of shock, and profoundly alters the conventional signs of disturbance of intracranial pressure.

5. Both drugs produce in adequately treated patients a reaction pattern that in some ways mimics the witzelsucht seen in lobotomized patients so that they are prone to develop a rather detached attitude toward pain, bleeding or otherwise alarming symptoms.

6. In chlorpromazine-treated patients there is a high incidence of eosinophilia early in the course of treatment which may go as high as 50 per cent of

the total count. Leukocytosis is common and may go as high as 15,000 or more, and there is often an elevation of the serum gamma globulin to levels of 10 to 40 per cent increase over normal. The serum bilirubin is commonly elevated to levels above the normal renal threshold for serum bilirubin without the spilling of the pigment in the urine and without clinical jaundice. It is our impression that the blood cell and serum phenomena occur as concomitants of chlorpromazine therapy and offer no clues to impending complications or their severity. The jaundice remits in all cases when the drug is withdrawn.

7. We believe all the complications of chlorpromazine are reversible if detected in time and if the drug is discontinued.

8. We wonder at the absence of dermatologic manifestations of reserpine or chlorpromazine therapy in the colored male, whereas we have seen it in colored females and both sexes among the white.

9. It is our impression that Parkinsonism in all of its manifestations and gynecomastia and lactation among young females is most common among the colored race, but that these manifestations are completely reversible on discontinuing the drug and probably on reducing the dose of the drug.

10. Fever occurs rarely among patients receiving chlorpromazine, and when it does occur must be considered a warning of impending complications, some of which are of potential severe import. In our experience fever occurred before jaundice in most of the cases in which the record is complete. Each of the patients with agranulocytosis had both pharyngitis or angina and fever for variable intervals before the agranulocytosis was actually discovered.

11. We believe there are no reliable criteria at the clinical or laboratory level for rejecting patients as poor medical risks for either drug except, as mentioned elsewhere, that gastrointestinal tract lesions or edema states make Serpasil therapy hazardous. At least one of us believe that the presence of liver disease makes chlorpromazine more hazardous.

12. In the Medical and Surgical Service we use chlorpromazine as the ataractic of choice because of its much more rapid onset of action.

13. We believe that chlorpromazine should be given in small doses and with care in patients with extensive malignant disease, particularly when nitrogen mustard, phosphoramids or X-ray therapy are being given.

14. We feel that these extremely potent chemotherapeutic agents represent a distinct advance in the approach to the treatment of the psychiatric patient, but that each drug, and particularly chlorpromazine, exerts widespread effect on many organs, tissues and functions. We believe the acute toxic side-reactions to be readily reversible in each case if detected early enough. We are sure that further experience will teach us more about optimum and maximum safe doses and the physiologic and pathologic effects of both drugs.

INEFFECTIVENESS OF CHLORPROMAZINE AND RAUWOLFIA SERPENTINA PREPARATIONS IN THE TREATMENT OF DEPRESSION

Lawrence H. Gahagan, M.D., Ph.D.

It has been our observation and contention for more than a year that almost every depressed patient whom we have examined or treated had received somewhere along the line an ineffective course of chlorpromazine or a Rauwolfia preparation [1] or a combination of these drugs. Such treatments were, of course, given with high expectancy of success.

But it seems to me that only a short experience with these drugs is required to find out that neither are, as a rule, effective in the treatment of depression. Since there exists a highly effective, well known and reasonably safe method of treatment of depression—early and adequate electrotherapy—the question comes to mind: why has electrotherapy been more or less abandoned or at least subordinated to drug therapy? This is the inevitable conclusion one draws from reading the glowing reports which emanate from the state hospitals. It is, of course, unquestioned that it is much simpler to give a patient a pill than to administer an electrical treatment, but this does not settle the question. The question bears only on the relative effectiveness of two competing methods of treatment; in this paper we refer to the treatment of depression only.

It is generally recognized that electrotherapy, even when done under careful conditions, carries a small but significant risk of serious injury or death. It must also be recognized that neither chlorpromazine nor reserpine is innocuous. There are also scattered reports of death, which has been associated with their use. It is my contention, as mentioned, that neither chlorpromazine nor reserpine is usually a satisfactory treatment of depression; in fact, either of these drugs may induce or aggravate depression. This latter statement is particularly relevant in the case of reserpine.

Since the experience of any private practitioner of psychiatry is necessarily limited in numbers and may, therefore, be atypical, it seemed to me that it would be useful to compare my experience with that of other physicians, who are observing the effects of these new drugs. So, largely through correspondence, we obtained the opinions of 25 other physicians—21 psychiatrists and 4 internists—who ranged alphabetically as well as geographically in the United

---

[1] In the interest of simplicity, Rauwolfia serpentina preparations will be referred to as reserpine, which is actually one of the component alkaloids of the whole root. Reserpine is, on a weight basis, 1,000 times as effective as the whole root; otherwise, there is no significant difference.

States from Leo Alexander at Boston to Eugene Ziskind at Los Angeles. The others are: R. W. P. Achor (Rochester, Minn.), Frank J. Ayd, Jr. (Baltimore), Herman C. B. Denber (New York), John Donnelly (Hartford), John Dunne (Dublin, Ireland), Joseph Epstein (New York), Howard D. Fabing (Cincinnati), Hamilton Ford (Galveston), R. Finley Gayle, Jr. (Richmond), Jacques S. Gottlieb (Detroit), Paul H. Hoch (Albany), David J. Impastato (New York), Lothar B. Kalinowsky (New York), Vernon Kinross-Wright (Houston), Louis M. Lipton (New York), Harry R. Lipton (Atlanta), Walter S. Maclay (London, England), Robert B. McGraw (New York), Milton Mendlowitz (New York), Benjamin Pollack (Rochester, N. Y.), Henry A. Schroeder (St. Louis), Leon J. Warshaw (New York), and Joseph Wortis (Brooklyn). Our thanks are due to these physicians for their prompt and unambiguous replies. Several have published significant reports on these new drugs; all are known for their interest in the clinical applications of neuropharmacology.

The consensus so obtained was in good agreement with our contention, but there were several noteworthy exceptions and qualifications; these will first be cited. Ford writes: "We have had some success [with chlorpromazine] in true depressions...I would say it worked only in those patients who had been chronically anxious for a long time and finally became depressed or there was a great deal of agitation."

Kinross-Wright writes: "...in a number of cases of depression, particularly the agitated involutional variety, but also in the simple retarded type, excellent responses have been achieved with chlorpromazine alone. It is necessary to give intensive dosage and to persevere with a full course of chlorpromazine treatment, despite the fact that initially the patient seems to grow more depressed. Why only a relatively small percentage of depressed patients respond satisfactorily, I do not know."

McGraw writes: "Chlorpromazine is good in depressions if there is agitation and reserpine is sometimes good if there is anxiety."

Pollack writes: "There are, however, a number of patients who do well under chlorpromazine alone, and these are depressions which are accompanied by a great deal of anxiety, restlessness, and projections and introjections."

Joseph Wortis writes: "I have seen a few cases of depression (usually agitated depression) which were helped by reserpine."

These excerpts are the only ones which favor in any way the use of either reserpine or chlorpromazine in the treatment of depression. These statements can be fairly summarized, I believe, by saying that the successful use of these drugs in the treatment of depression is quite limited, and whenever these drugs are so beneficial, the effect is mostly upon certain accompaniments of depression, particularly agitation or anxiety or both.

We shall now turn to the excerpts, in which there are expressions of dissatisfaction with the use of these drugs in the treatment of depression. Because of limitations, we are not permitted to report all the relevant statements; we have selected a fair sample so as to hear from both the psychiatrists and internists.

Achor writes: "I am personally convinced that all Rauwolfia preparations have the same propensity for increasing the vulnerability of patients to depressive episodes."

Donnelly writes: "It is my feeling that in agitated depressions, [chlorpromazine and reserpine] are useful in controlling the anxiety and agitation but seem to have little effect on the depression itself. It appears to me that the depression may seem to become deeper but it is my impression that this is due to the removal of anxiety...It is also my impression that initially the use of electroshock therapy decreased considerably in hospitals, public and private, but I have also gathered recently that the use of electroshock therapy is again increasing...In depressions chlorpromazine is of use as an adjuvant and as yet it has not been proven that it can replace electroshock therapy...I have seen manic episodes converted into depressions (through the use of these drugs) but have not seen the reverse."

Dunne writes: "I have not found [chlorpromazine] to be of any use in the treatment of depressive states. In fact, I have observed that the depression has become very much increased following the use of chlorpromazine. I have had the unfortunate experience of two cases with mild depressive states who, following the administration of chlorpromazine, committed suicide and I am quite convinced that it was the drug which was responsible for increasing the depression to such an extent...I have also found that [reserpine] produces a severe depression in a number of cases where depression had not existed before, and the drug had to be withdrawn on this account. Furthermore, a number of cases of depression did not clear up following the withdrawal of reserpine and E.C.T. had to be administered. E.C.T. was successful in all cases in clearing up the depression."

Epstein writes: "[Reserpine] is distinctly contraindicated in depressions and, in fact, there is a distinct danger, not only of causing a depressed patient to become more depressed, but in actually making him suicidal."

Gayle writes: "Reserpine and chlorpromazine are not effective in depressions, and...reserpine often makes them worse."

Gottlieb writes: "[Chlorpromazine and reserpine] gave little, if any, benefit to patients with depression and, in fact, somtimes made them worse, so that they were discontinued...It has been some time since I have used these drugs or suggested their use for patients with depressions."

Hoch writes: "[Chlorpromazine and reserpine] are no help in patients who are suffering from depressions."

Kalinowsky writes: "I agree with you on the uselessness [of chlorpromazine and reserpine] in the treatment of depressions, and I have the same experience you have that most patients who are sent to me for ECT in a depression and who had been taking these drugs for varying lengths of time, had no benefit from them...It has also been more and more recognized that reserpine, used in hypertension, can produce depressions in patients who never had such conditions before."

Kinross-Wright writes: "Reserpine should not be given to patients who are, or have been, depressed. In many cases, it is a powerful depressant agent."

Mendlowitz writes: "I have within the last month seen four cases of reserpine depression and I believe that the warning signals appear several months before the depression sets in. It may last as long as two or three months after cessation of depression."

Schroeder writes: "The interesting thing to me is that [reserpine], used so widely for psychosis and psychoneurosis, will actually produce the disease."

Warshaw writes: "This danger of depression makes me reluctant to use this drug [reserpine] except in cases where the conventional sedatives have failed...I believe that those patients who complain of persistent and troublesome nightmares under reserpine therapy will go into depression if the drug is continued...Many patients with depression present themselves with symptoms of nervous tension, anxiety and agitation. It is difficult to separate this group from those who present similar symptoms without the underlying depression."

Joseph Wortis writes: "I have also seen several cases of depression caused by reserpine which was administered for hypertension."

Ziskind writes: "Some patients have gone on to suicide in addition to others who have been prolonged in their period of illness, because these drugs [chlorpromazine or reserpine or both] have been given in place of electrotherapy."

Space does not allow us to enlarge on these remarks or to cite the statements, which are equally pertinent, from the other physicians with whom we discussed this problem, but may I assure you that their opinions are similar to the above.

In concluding this presentation, I should like to take this opportunity to speculate briefly upon the reason why the failure of these drugs, reserpine and chlorpromazine, to relieve depression is regarded so lightly. I believe that this situation is largely due to the fact that the main reports about these drugs emanate from the state hospitals and similar institutions. In general, the results and conclusions derived from studies of state hospital patients are at best only marginally applicable in the care of private psychiatric patients. This is due primarily to the fact that the kinds of patients, state hospital as compared with private patients, are so unlike. In the state hospitals, the main varieties of illness are chronic schizophrenia, senile psychosis and the related psychosis with cerebral arteriosclerosis. In private practice we are dealing mostly with anxiety, depression, character disorders, the gamut of psychosomatic complaints, and alcohol and other drug dependencies.

Since the advent of electrotherapy, depression is primarily a disease treated in private practice. As a result, the state hospital psychiatrist, in speaking of a disturbed patient, rarely has in mind a depressed patient; he is apt to be thinking of a chronic, deteriorated schizophrenic or an elderly patient with an organic psychosis. The commonness of the problem of depression in private psychiatric practice, as opposed to the rarity of schizophrenia, is well described by Fabing: "In all the talk about schizophrenia which is going around, the other great functional psychosis has been lost in the shuffle. This shouldn't be. Although schizophrenia is a far more chronic disease, and although it fills more long-term hospital beds, melancholia is a more common disorder. My associates and I, who meet all comers, and who can best be described as general practitioners of disorders of the nervous system...find that we encounter at least four or five new cases of melancholia to every one of schizophrenia in our consulting rooms."

This dissimilarity between state hospital and private psychiatric practice is the crux of the problem. Another facet of this problem is the difference in therapeutic aim between the two types of practice; this can, perhaps, best be explained by posing two questions. In private practice, the basic question is: How does the patient feel? In the state hospital, this question is: How does the patient behave?

Summary

Chlorpromazine and reserpine are, as a rule, ineffective in the treatment of depression. From the standpoint of psychiatry, these drugs are essentially anti-excitants: for this reason their usefulness is greater in state hospitals and related institutions, where there are large numbers of disturbed schizophrenic patients and those suffering from organic psychoses.

Chlorpromazine may be occasionally useful in controlling the excitement which accompanies certain cases of depression without, however, favorably affecting the depression itself. Reserpine may precipitate or aggravate depression. It should not be used in the presence of a depression or probably whenever there is a history of depression. Signs of early or impending depression, such as nightmares and other sleep disturbances, should be heeded in the patient who is receiving reserpine.

"All new drugs are overrated before they find their proper place as therapeutic weapons."

DISCUSSION OF DR. GAHAGAN'S PAPER

Edwin J. de Beer, Ph.D.
Associate Research Director of The Wellcome Research Laboratories,
Tuckahoe, N. Y.

Dr. Gahagan's interesting and pertinent paper raises several fundamental points. If the treatment of depressed patients with chlorpromazine (or the Rauwolfia derivatives) can be used interchangeably with electroshock treatment, it seems reasonable to expect that the two therapeutic processes would produce similar physiological and pharmacological reactions. This is not the case, however, for as Dr. Gahagan has pointed out, electroshock treatment produces the effects of a general autonomic discharge, all the way from such typical signs of sympathetic stimulation as pilomotor action to the characteristic slowing of the heart which accompanies parasympathetic discharge. Chlorpromazine, on the other hand, is a strong adrenolytic drug which antagonizes the sympathetic system and blocks many effects of the parasympathetic as well.

These two treatments then are diametrically opposite in mechanism. Electroshock is fundamentally stimulating and chlorpromazine is fundamentally depressing; one wonders about the use of this drug in treating the already depressed patient.

The central depressant effect of this drug has been observed in laboratory animals. It is especially evident in cats. If the doses are large enough chlorpromazine will produce a state of narcosis.

Smaller doses of chlorpromazine, however, can cause definite changes in the behavior patterns of cats. This is especially noticeable in the hostile animals. After single doses of the drug the behavior pattern will shift so that the antagonistic animal will become friendly or docile, even purring on occasion. This drug effect is not to be interpreted as stimulation or excitement for the excitement pattern is quite different and the cats show no tendency to display signs of stimulation.

Dr. Gahagan is to be congratulated for his very timely observations on the proper fields of use of electroshock therapy and of drugs such as chlorpromazine.

COMPLICATIONS OF CHLORPROMAZINE THERAPY

Irvin M. Cohen, M.D.
Associate Professor of Neurology and Psychiatry, University of Texas Medical Branch, Galveston, Texas

Critical evaluation of a drug requires that untoward effects as well as therapeutic efficiency be considered. Although the ultimate position of chlorpromazine in therapeutics is yet to be determined, there is ample evidence attesting to its usefulness in the management and treatment of a variety of psychiatric disorders. In comparison, our present knowledge of its toxicity is meager.

This paper describes the complications encountered in a large series of chlorpromazine-treated patients. The term "complications" here includes all effects of chlorpromazine which from the standpoint of the clinician are considered therapeutically undesirable, regardless of the degree of severity. They range from minor symptoms of limited clinical significance to major reactions of alarming proportions.

This report has been derived primarily from clinical observations, but final conclusions regarding the toxicity of chlorpromazine will be possible only when the physico-chemical mechanisms involved in the production of its adverse effects have been defined.

Material and Methods

This study covers 14 months' experience with a series of 1,400 cases, including both inpatients and outpatients, all of whom were being treated for psychiatric and neurologic illnesses. Dosages ranged from a minimum of 40 mg. per day to a maximum of 2,500 mg. per day, given as Thorazine (S.K.F.). The shortest duration of administration was 5 days, and the longest 6½ months. Although other therapeutic methods were often used in conjunction with chlorpromazine, the observations described are those we regard as peculiar to the drug.

In critically evaluating these data the following points should be considered. Observations were made by many physicians and nurses. As might be expected in a large series and with multiple observers, complete and reliable information was not obtained in each case. Also, in the early months of the study effects which were subsequently recognized as resulting from chlorpromazine were not faithfully recorded. Accurate computation of the incidence of each complication throughout the 14 months is impossible in view of these variables. With the exception of certain complications to which particular attention was directed, percentages of incidence have been derived from statistical analyses of random samples, are therefore approximate and are qualified as such.

RESULTS

The inconstant behavior of chlorpromazine and the intricate interrelationships of its adverse effects complicate presentation of the data in a clinically useful form. Our limited understanding of the site and mode of action precludes organization of the results on the basis of specific etiologies or loci or origin. Efforts to establish reliable correlations with such factors as dosage level, duration of administration, age, and sex, have been disappointing. Though many complications do occur with greatest frequency at certain dosage levels and phases of administration, consistent relationships which allow for prediction were not found. In the last analysis we must confine ourselves to simple description, discussing the adverse responses on the basis of the individual disordered organ systems.

Central Nervous System.—Effects on the central nervous system were common and among the most troublesome of the complications.

Disturbances of wakefulness were the most frequent and ranged from insomnia to hypersomnolence. Drowsiness occurred at one time or another in 85%. Except when sedation was desired, it constituted a most adverse effect. Single intramuscular doses of 25-100 mg. usually induced drowsiness and sleep lasting from 2 to 6 hours. Orally administered chlorpromazine caused drowsiness at all dosage levels but most often when total daily dosage was 75 mg. or higher; hypersomnolence usually began when the oral dosage exceeded 200 mg. daily. Despite apparent depth of sleep patients could be awakened easily, became alert with little or no disturbance in perception, and quickly returned to sleep when left alone. There was no interference with nocturnal sleep even though diurnal sleep might have been as much as 10 hours. In patients with considerable sleep difficulty, reassurance was often required because of their fear that nighttime sleep would be diminished. If dosage was maintained at a single level, drowsiness and hypersomnolence could be expected to disappear within 7 to 10 days. Mild degrees of drowsiness were counteracted by amphetamine or other central stimulating compounds. However, in some patients receiving very high dosages of chlorpromazine, drowsiness was not only persistent but intractible.

Approximately 0.5% of patients developed insomnia. It is difficult to determine whether this is a specific effect produced by chlorpromazine or is secondary to anxiety induced by other side-reactions. It was confined to neurotic patients in whom somatic preoccupation had been characteristic. Whether primary or secondary, the resulting insomnia was itself anxiety-producing and aggravated existing sleep disturbances. The effect that higher doses might have had was not ascertained since the drug was quickly discontinued in such cases.

Vivid dreams occurred intermittently in the early phases of treatment in approximately 5% of patients, and were independent of dosage level. Although the dreams were almost like motion pictures in clarity, the anxiety connected with them was inappropriately small. On the other hand, there was diminution in dreaming concomitant with the establishment of a state of tranquility.

Apathy, lack of initiative, and loss of interest in surroundings was commonly seen in patients receiving intramuscular doses exclusively and when the oral dosage exceeded 600-800 mg. per day. Affective disturbances of this quality seemed to be most prominent in previously agitated psychotic patients. Blurring of vision occurred, usually when dosage was high.

Disturbances in thermoregulation were among the earliest described effects of chlorpromazine. Although much has been written about hypothermia, it was neither a prominent nor consistent finding in this study. Reduction of temperature occasionally occurred during the first week of administration, particularly when doses were high, but it was never greater than 1.6°. Of more significance to the clinician was the occurrence of fever. Elevations of temperature usually to 102°-103°, but as high as 105°, without evidence of infection or leukocytosis frequently occurred in any phase of treatment. The pattern was variable but most commonly appeared as an evening spike for 1 or 2 days. Two patients who had received comparatively low doses for 1 week had fever and chills nightly for 3 and 6 days respectively. The drug was discontinued and on reinstitution the symptoms recurred.

Delirium occurred in 3 patients. Two were chronic alcoholics who had recovered from delirium tremens during the preceding week. In both cases the original picture of the delirium tremens was reproduced. The third case was a 9-year-old organically-driven child who had a history of allergy and who had frequently reacted to infection with delirium in the past. In all cases the delirium subsided within 24 hours after immediate withdrawal of chlorpromazine.

Parkinsonism with rigidity as the dominant feature developed in 4% of patients. It occurred only when dosage was high, the average being 800 mg. daily, usually after 2 weeks of administration. It was preceded in many cases by tremor of the fingers and diminished mimetic expression; there followed the insidious development of a typical Parkinson picture, including stooped posture, masklike facies, loss of associated movements, rigidity, and tremor. Rigidity was more prominent than tremor, and sialorrhea and seborrhea were common. Following withdrawal of the drug the syndrome resolved without apparent residue within 5 to 14 days. However, in one patient it persisted until his death from uremia some 4 months later. Ayd has described spontaneous resolution in one patient in whom the drug was not discontinued.

Transient episodes of tonic spasms of various muscle groups were observed in 2 patients, both of whom were being treated for psychiatric illnesses. In both cases opisthotonos, torticollis, and muscular twitchings were observed, and in one there were torsion movements of the trunk. The resemblance of the latter case to dystonia musculorum deformans suggests that Parkinsonism may not be the only basal ganglia syndrome induced by chlorpromazzine.

A number of patients developed dysphagia and dysarthria several hours after initial subjective complaints of "thick tongue," difficulty in talking, lisping, and a feeling that the tongue world would fall backwards. Objective swelling of the tongue occurred in only one case in which a skin eruption followed shortly on exposure to sunlight.

Cardiovascular System.—The most frequently encountered undesirable effects in this sphere were consequences of chlorpromazine-induced hypotension. Peripheral vascular effects were also noted.

Reduction of recumbent blood pressure occurred in over one-half the patients regardless of dosage or route of administration. Some decrease was a constant finding after intramusclar administration, readings usually dropping within 30 to 40 minutes, an average of 30-50 mm. systolic and 20-30 mm. diastolic, associated with a compensatory tachycardia of 20-40 per minute. The decrease was most pronounced if elevated blood pressure had been noted prior to injection. The most serious consequence of this precipitous fall in blood pressure was acute circulatory insufficiency. However, it was rare and occurred in only 2 cases.

A middle-aged normotensive female showed signs of vascular collapse 3 hours after a single intramuscular injection; the condition persisted for 6 hours and resolved after a short period of confusion.

A shock-like picture lasting 1 hour occurred suddenly in an 81-year-old normotensive arteriosclerotic male who had been receiving oral dosages of 100 mg. daily for 4 days.

Rea, Shea and Fazekas have noted shock and death due to subsequent renal insufficiency. Although Stevenson and Sjoerdsma found that following intramuscular administration of chlorpromazine there was no significant change in recumbent blood pressure and that hypotension was directly correlated with changes in posture, we found that the blood pressure was reduced even in the recumbent position but was maximal during postural change and on standing. They also found that the blood pressure drop was maximal in 3 to 4 hours, in contrast to our findings that it was maximal within 2 hours after injection with return to preinjection levels usually within 4 to 6 hours.

Recumbent blood pressure was also decreased to some extent during oral administration but in this situation its orthostatic quality was more evident. It usually became apparent sometime within the first 3 days of administration and generally lasted from 5 to 7 days. Approximately 50% of patients complained of "dizziness" on assuming erect posture, concomitant clouding of vision, and momentary imbalance. Despite often associated tachycardia, palpitation was a rare complaint. Syncopal attacks were also rare. They occurred in any age group but mainly in patients above 60. Not all patients developing hypotension suffered its effects; conversely, many who complained of orthostatic effects did not show significant blood pressure variations on postural change.

Some patients showing minimal signs of cerebral arteriosclerosis began to manifest increasing memory defect and difficulty in retention and recall while taking chlorpromazine. In some cerebral arteriosclerotic patients more severe degrees of clouding of consciousness were observed. This was regarded as being due to cerebral vascular hypotension, and frequently required discontinuation of the drug.

Ankle edema was observed in a few middle-aged and elderly patients. None showed evidence of cardiac decompensation.

Facial pallor was often seen in patients immediately following parenteral injection and when oral doses were high. We found it judicious to warn relatives that such an appearance would not be unexpected, and that this did not indicate that the patient's condition was deteriorating.

When strict control of the patient is not possible, particularly when he is in the elderly age group, gradual increase of dosage may minimize changes in blood pressure and its associated undesirable effects. When signs of cerebral arteriosclerosis are present intramusclar injection or initially high oral doses are unwise except when unusual indication exists.

Gastro-Intestinal Tract Manifestations.—With the single exception of jaundice, the undesirable effects referable to the gastrointestinal tract were minor reactions which almost never required discontinuation of the drug.

"Heartburn" localized either in the upper portions of the esophagus or at the level of the cardia was an occasional complaint following oral ingestion of chlorpromazine. Nausea was also seen in a few cases, but rarely was there associated vomiting.

Unusual increase in appetite, beyond what might be expected from relief of anxiety, was noted in over 40% of patients. This was generally related to high dosage and ordinarily appeared in the second to fourth weeks of administration.

Constipation occurred in over one-third of patients, usually when dosage exceeded 100 mg. daily. Patients on very high dosages required almost constant laxation.

Jaundice was the most serious complication. In this series there were 11 cases, an incidence of 0.9%. No criteria for its prediction could be established, except that there was a significantly high incidence of histories of previous allergic reactions. Its occurrence was unrelated to dosage or route of administration, age, sex, or psychiatric diagnosis. In the majority of cases icterus appeared 2½ to 3 weeks after chlorpromazine had been instituted. The shortest time was one week, the longest 1 month. Five of these patients had also developed dermatitis, one of whom had also begun to show early signs of Parkinsonism. Premonitory symptoms of the jaundice were generally very mild; the patients, though experiencing general malaise, were in no great distress. In several instances if icterus had not appeared the complication might have escaped detection, for often the complaints were at first attributed to the psychiatric condition. In the usual case there was a sudden elevation of temperature, followed by persistent or intermittent nausea, vague abdominal pain, and occasionally vomiting. Icterus usually followed in from 2 to 5 days, although in one patient there was a 2-week lag and in another no prodromal symptoms. The succeeding clinical course in most cases was comparatively uneventful, disturbing symptoms disappearing within several days, icterus clearing within 2 to 3 weeks. However, in one patient clinical and laboratory signs persisted for over one month. Treatment was supportive, consisting mainly of withdrawal of the drug, intravenous glucose when indicated, therapeutic vitamin regime, and high-carbohydrate-high-protein-low-fat diet. Laboratory findings were characteristic of obstructive jaundice, with hyperbilirubinemia, elevated serum alkaline phosphatase, and bilirubinuria, and no evidence of interference with cellular function. Chlorpromazine was later reinstituted in one patient who had previously developed both dermatitis and jaundice while receiving a maximum daily dosage of 1,000 mg. Neither complication recurred and clinical laboratory findings remained normal.

Clinical and laboratory studies of liver function in patients not developing jaundice showed no interference with hepatic function. We conclude that chlorpromazine-induced jaundice is a consequence of individual drug idiosyncracy and that under ordinary circumstances chlorpromazine is not hepatotoxic. However, it is probable that patients with histories of prior drug reaction should be given chlorpromazine cautiously and with adequate warnings of the possible complications that could ensue.

Dermatological Manifestations.—These were the most common of the major undesirable reactions to chlorpromazine. There is good presumptive evidence that they result from allergic sensitization. However, certain features are unusual, and further investigation by dermatologists is needed to clarify the mechanisms. Incidence was generally unrelated to dosage level. In the majority of cases an incubation period of 2 weeks preceded the outbreak of clinical manifestations. Histories of past allergic reactions to other chemicals were more frequent in this category than in any other.

Localized or generalized pruritis was the most common dermatological reaction. Most frequently affected were the extremities. Itching was often so intense as to require discontinuation of the drug, especially when excoriations were produced by scratching. Antihistaminic drugs afforded only partial relief.

Chlorpromazine appears to have photosensitizing properties. Controlled studies have demonstrated that increased reactivity of the skin to ultraviolet radiation may follow oral or parenteral intake. Sunlight was an impressive factor clinically in the precipitation and intensification of certain dermatological reactions, which were most apparent during the summer months. Intense erythema on exposure to sunlight and predisposition to sunburn occurred in several patients. Sunlight was also capable of inducing transient pruritis and dermatitis, aggravating existing cases, and was the apparent precipitating factor in some severe skin eruptions.

Dermatitis occurred in 8% of our cases. Though occasionally preceded by a prodrome of intense itching, it usually appeared suddenly about 2 weeks after treatment was started and was unrelated to dosage level. In some cases only 1 week had elapsed, in rare cases 1 month. Three forms were observed: the most common a localized or generalized maculopapular eruption. Sites of predilection were the face, neck, upper chest, upper extremities, or thighs. Vesicles were seen in some cases and in one case bulla formed. Erythema multiforme, in one case with hemorrhagic features, and generalized or localized urticaria were also observed. Such skin reactions disappeared spontaneously 3-5 days after discontinuation of the drug, even though the original appearance was florid or even alarming. In later phases of this study, we observed that the skin eruptions sometimes disappear even though medication was continued. This feature of chlorpromazine-induced dermatitis is unique and deserves further investigation.

Contact dermatitis occurred in 2 employees who handled syringes which had contained chlorpromazine.

Edema of the face and hands usually occurred in association with other skin manifestations but was frequently an independent finding. Angioneurotic edema of the lips was precipitated by sunlight in 3 cases.

An acute allergic reaction occurred after a single intramuscular injection of chlorpromazine in 1 patient who had sporadically taken 25 mg. orally for 6 weeks. Findings included swelling and itching at the site of injection, generalized pruritic papular rash, angioneurotic edema of the lips, orthostatic hypotensive effects, and generalized weakness. The condition reached maximum intensity 14 hours after injection and resolved in 3 days, with persistent arthralgia for 2 weeks thereafter.

Respiratory System.—Nasal congestion was very common (48%). It was not accompanied by rhinorrhea and usually responded to instillation of vasoconstrictor drugs. If not previously warned, some patients assumed they had "colds" and sought medical attention. Dryness of the mouth and throat occurred in approximately 76% of patients but was rarely a volunteered complaint. Both of these reactions disappeared within 2 weeks when dosage was low, but were more persistent when it was high.

A typical asthmatic attack occurred 1 hour after the first injection of chlorpromazine in one patient without previous asthmatic history.

Musculoskeletal System.—Muscular weakness was second only to drowsiness as the most common subjective complaint. It occurred at any dosage level but was intensified by increasing dosage. Ordinarily it disappeared within 14 days, but did not necessarily resolve when dosage exceeded 1,000 mg. daily. In some cases weakness did not become apparent until the patient exerted himself. Several complained of incoordination, and in extreme cases ataxia was observed.

Tremor, of either tension or action type, was observed in some patients on high dosage. Occasionally it preceded the development of Parkinsonism.

Arthralgia, either associated with dermatological reactions or as an independent finding, was not infrequent and probably represents an allergic manifestation.

Endocrine System.—Increased sexual urge was noted in 0.5% of cases, principally in female patients. Possibly this is related to relief of anxiety or other psychogenic causes. In contrast, the most common change in males was in the direction of decrease. Whether this was a specific effect of chlorpromazine or a reflection of apathy could not be determined as in each instance the dosage was very high.

Swelling of the breasts, occasionally accompanied by secretion of a thin colostrum-like fluid, was noted in a few female patients. The swelling was diffuse, and was not associated with tenderness or cyst formation. All such patients were between the ages of 20 and 40 and were receiving unusually high dosages.

Urinary System.—Effects on the urinary system ranged from oliguria to polyuria, most frequently the latter. Deep orange coloration of the urine without evidence of the presence of bilirubin occurred when dosage was high.

Hemopoietic System.—In recent months several reports have been published describing agranulocytosis due to chlorpromazine. The cases of Boleman and Prokopowycz terminated fatally. Goldman has reported 3 cases, successfully treated with antibiotics and corticotropin.

Leucopenia as low as 4,200 leucocytes per cubic millimeter was occasionally observed in patients who were receiving high dosages of chlorpromazine, but such reductions were transitory and of no apparent clinical significance. Transient leucocytosis and eosinophilia, often unexplainable, were more common.

Ayd, who has collected several cases of agranulocytosis, finds no correlation with dosage or duration of administration. He warns that the early symptoms are vague and difficult to evaluate, and that a blood count should be done if symptoms of excessive fatigue and anorexia appear.

Indirect Effects.—Patients in any age group who received combined ECT and chlorpromazine appeared to develop confusional effects earlier than when ECT was given alone. There is some indication that convulsive threshold during insulin coma is lowered in patients simultaneously receiving chlorpromazine therapy. Further studies regarding the influence of chlorpromazine on the shock therapies are in progress.

An indirect effect on the respiratory tract was the development of pneumonia in elderly patients. This may be regarded as a preventable complication, in all probability the result of pulmonary hypostasis occurring during hypersomnolence.

Discussion and Summary

The undesirable effects of chlorpromazine which occur most frequently seem to be reflections of direct or indirect action on various levels of the nervous system, particularly the reticular formation, hypothalamus, and autonomic nervous system. Although most effects of this type are objectionable, certain of them, e.g., drowsiness, are at times useful in therapy. A second group of complications appear to be the result of allergic sensitization even though they do not entirely fulfill the criteria of allergic reactions. The frequency of this type of response suggests that chlorpromazine possesses greater sensitizing properties than do most drugs commonly used in psychiatry. A third category of complications are of such curious quality that they cannot be understood on the basis of the limited data now available, e.g., vivid dreams. A fourth group are indirect expressions of the effect of chlorpromazine and are not wholly assignable to the drug, e.g., hypostatic pneumonia in hypersomnolent aged patients.

From a clinical standpoint the undesirable effects of chlorpromazine are divisible on the basis of severity into minor and major complications. Most are minor and of clinical significance only insofar as they may induce varying degrees of subjective distress. Major reactions, which occur in a much smaller percentage of patients, are relatively severe and occasionally of alarming proportions.

Most minor complications take place in the first 2 weeks of treatment, and are predominantly central depressant, sympatholytic, parasympatholytic, and myatonic effects. Such effects are generally self-limiting, tending to be maximal during the first 7-10 days of administration with progressive diminution thereafter even though medication is continued. Minor complications which occur later suggest interference with the metabolic and endocrinological aspects of hypothalamic function, and are more likely to be persistent. The most commonly encountered minor complications are nasal congestion, dryness of the mouth, drowsiness, weakness, and dizziness.

The majority of major complications occur in the second 2 weeks of treatment, and consist mainly of disorganization of extrapyramidal motor regulation and allergic-type reactions. Those which occur earlier are usually of vascular origin. There are no reliable standards by which a serious reaction may be predicted, although a previous allergic history is of suggestive value. Fortunately even the most alarming complications resolve rapidly and apparently without residual when chlorpromazine is withdrawn and in some instances even though medication is maintained. Major complications of chlorpromazine included acute circulatory insufficiency, sensorium changes due to cerebral vascular hypotension, delirium, symptomatic Parkinsonism, obstructive jaundice, dermatitis, acute severe allergic reactions, and exaggeration of confusional effects during electroconvulsive therapy. Agranulocytosis has recently been reported but was not encountered in this series.

Dosage level is of limited significance, individual sensitivity being the prime factor. With the exception of those reactions suggesting allergic sensitization, oral dosages of 50-75 mg. daily ordinarily produce few undesirable effects, although equivalent amounts administered parenterally commonly do. When oral dosage exceeds 200 mg. per day one or several harmless, but sometimes annoying, symptoms occur in approximately 60% of patients. Parkinsonism occurs only when dosage is high.

The final impression gained from this survey is that although the complications of chlorpromazine therapy are multiple, they are infrequently of major severity and do not outweigh the therapeutic advantages. It should be noted, however, that chlorpromazine is not without hazard, and its administration should be accompanied by a knowledge of the risks involved.

Conclusions

1. Chlorpromazine has many undesirable effects, most of which are transient and of relatively minor clinical significance.

2. Complications of greater severity occur in a significant number of cases but generally resolve rapidly and without residuals.

3. Four categories of complications are distinguishable: direct or indirect action on various levels of the nervous system, allergic-type reactions, responses of indefinite origin, and indirect effects of drug action.

4. Despite its numerous undesirable effects chlorpromazine is clinically a relatively safe drug.

COMPLICATIONS DURING RESERPINE THERAPY

C. H. Cahn, M.D.

This is a brief report on one out of 50 patients who have received reserpine therapy at the Verdun Protestant Hospital, Montreal.

The patient is a 67-year-old white female of English origin. She was admitted in 1935 with the diagnosis of involutional paranoid state, the chief symptoms being delusions of persecution with auditory and olfactory hallucinations and an attitude of marked hostility. During the 20 years of her hospitalization her mental condition changed very little; physically she was healthy except for marked obesity and slight dependent edema intermittently since 1944. Average blood pressure was 140/90.

On January 4, 1955, reserpine therapy was started using 2.5 mg. (1 cc.) intramuscularly twice a day. This dose was continued until January 7, when it was doubled. The early side-effect of flushing of the face was somewhat more pronounced in this patient than usual, but was at first discounted as being in keeping with her plethoric appearance. On January 8 the patient began to feel weak and could not walk to supper; she was perspiring profusely, and her blood pressure was 90/60. Other patients on even higher doses had shown similar changes, so the nursing staff were not particularly alarmed. The next morning the patient was given her usual dose of reserpine, 5 mg. intramuscularly.

Later that day physical examination showed marked prostration, fast pulse, blood pressure 120/65, moderate pitting edema of the legs and gross edema of the face and neck. Reserpine therapy was discontinued.

On January 10, the patient was given 1.0 gm. (10 cc.) of calcium gluconate intravenously and the following day the edema seemed to be subsiding. The patient was out of bed and was reported to be pleasant and cooperative.

On January 12, however, the edema increased again, and the next day the patient looked very ill, felt quite weak, and stayed in bed. She became increasingly dyspneic and cyanosed. On January in spite of oxygen, nikethamide and penicillin she reached a low point in her illness, expressing the fear that she was going to die. Much mucus accumulated in her throat which had to be suctioned. Temperature was 102°, blood pressure 90/50, and there was massive generalized edema (but no albuminuria). Abdominal paracentesis was attempted but was unsuccessful.

The patient was next placed on antihistaminic therapy, and she was made more comfortable by being allowed to sit up in a chair rather than having to lie constantly in bed in the orthopneic position. The blood pressure rose to

140/80, dyspnea and cyanosis gradually subsided, and the edema began to decrease on January 20. Thereafter the patient gradually recovered physically but mentally reverted to her pretreatment condition.

In summary, on the fifth day of reserpine therapy this patient developed a severe reaction of the angio-neurotic edema type. She was dangerously ill for 8 days, but then made a physical though not mental recovery.

ADVERSE REACTIONS TO MEPROBAMATE

Henry T. Friedman, M.D., and Willard L. Marmelzat, M.D.

Meprobamate is a drug that has received extreme widespread acceptance by the medical profession of the United States as well as by the general public. Scarcely a day goes by without some laudatory mention of this wonderful new tranquilizing drug in the daily press, in national lay periodicals, and even through radio and television mediums. Particularly in the area in which we practice is this compound being used indiscriminately for a tremendous number of patients by a large number of physicians. The desire for a harmless pill that will almost magically return man into a bucolic, idyllic emotional state free from everyday stresses and strains is a deep-rooted one. There is extreme paucity of pharmacological and clinical reports on this compound. Likewise, to our knowledge, no clinical reports have been published of toxic, idiosyncratic, or allergic reactions. The drug has been on the clinical market for only approximately one year, and we feel that it is time to warn the medical profession of possible toxic and allergic reactions to this compound. The only clinical reports published to date are by Selling and Borrus.

PHARMACOLOGY

Meprobamate, or 2-methyl-2-n-propyl-1, 3-propanediol dicarbamate, was first synthesized by Ludwig and Piech in 1950. It is stable in both gastric and intestinal juices and is relatively insoluble in water. The original pharmacological and toxic actions were studied in animals by Berger, utilizing rats, mice, dogs, cats, rabbits, and monkeys. Meprobamate resembles mephenesin in producing reversible paralysis of the voluntary muscles without significantly affecting autonomic functions. It acts on the central nervous system and, in fact, inhibits internuncial circuits. It is antagonistic to strychnine and counteracts symptoms from released inhibitions during light anesthesia. It also augments anesthesia with barbiturates. There is little direct action on the muscles, no effect at myoneural junctions, and no blocking of conduction of peripheral nerves. Closely related to mephenesin, it has a much longer duration of action and is rapidly absorbed through the gastrointestinal tract. The latent period for action of the compound is as long as the duration of action once it is established. No nausea or emesis is produced in dogs, monkeys, or man. Approximately 10% is secreted unchanged and the remainder conjugated with glucuronic acid in the urine.

REPORT OF CASES

CASE 1.—A 55-year-old female was placed on meprobamate therapy, 400 mg. twice a day. After the patient had taken the second pill, severe diarrhea developed, with cramps, gas, and nine watery stools in 24 hours. Medication was discontinued at once, and 48 hours were permitted to elapse before the readministration of one 400-mg. tablet orally, which produced diarrhea within one hour.

CASE 2.—A 73-year-old male was given meprobamate, in a 400-mg. tablet, to relax him because of coronary artery disease and chronic cardiac decompensation. Four hours after initial ingestion of the tablet he had chills, and within six hours he had an eruption that was purpuric and maculopapular in type. The rash occurred pubically and about the pelvic gridle, anteriorly and posteriorly, and in both antecubital fossae. Itching was marked and extreme in character. Twelve hours after the patient's ingestion of the pill, the eruption began to clear. It took three days to entirely disappear. One week later the patient was given 200 mg. of the same compound, in four hours itching began, and after five hours the eruption began to appear. It was less severe but in the same locale and presented similar primary lesions. On March 20, 1956, one 400-mg. tablet was given orally experimentally, and four hours later the eruption began to appear. This was quite severe, as in the original outbreak. There seems to be no doubt of the cause-and-effect relationship of this drug and the appearance of the rash. This patient had never had a drug eruption before nor had any known allergic symptoms.

CASE 3.—A 33-year-old female, without prior history of allergic disease or sensitivity to drugs, received 400 mg. of meprobamate four times a day for 15 days. On the 16th day she developed a small group of violaceous maculas on the midback. Rapidly, within a period of two days, the eruption became generalized over the entire body in a symmetrical fashion, with maculas, papules, and small vesicles. All the lesions were purpuric in nature and showed a tendency toward coalescence. The mucous membranes were not involved. Medication was discontinued, and the patient was treated with corticotropin (ACTH), 80 units per day intramuscularly, plus colloidal baths and topical therapy. She recovered in one week. Later she was given one 400-mg. tablet of the same drug and developed a similar eruption on the back of the trunk. Biopsy and histopathological diagnosis of the initial site on the back gave the following findings: The epidermis exhibited alternating exaggeration and diminution of the granular layer with slight surface hyperkeratosis. The capillary tufts were dilated, with moderate thinning of the suprapapillary plates. The most general change was noted in the cutis and consisted of plasmocytic and lymphocytic periadnexal and pericapillary infiltration in a collarette arrangement. The patient's serologic tests for syphilis were negative.

CASE 4.—A 49-year-old female had no history of any drug sensitivity except for the development of a pruritic dermatosis involving the right breast, both axillas, the back, and the inguinal region two years previously, after the systemic administration of penicillin. She had no other history of allergic or atopic disease. She had been instructed to take 800 mg. of meprobamate at six-hour intervals for nervousness. After the first dose of 800 mg. she developed an acute eruption involving the right breast, both axillas, the back, and the entire inguinal area. Examination revealed an acute process, involving the skin of the right breast, back, axillas, inguinal folds, and vulvar areas. This consisted of an erythematous base, with a loosely adherent furfuraceous scale. Borders of the lesions were not clearly demarcated. Diascopic examination produced a complete blanching of the erythema. Mycologic cultures and scrapings revealed no pathogenic growth. Therapy consisted of medicated baths, compresses with dilute alibour water, topical administration of hydrocortisone cream, and antihistamines given parenterally. The patient's eruption disappeared within 72 hours. Five days later 400 mg. of the meprobamate orally produced the same eruption in the same area within three hours.

CASE 5.—A 51-year-old female took four 400-mg. tablets of meprobamate per day for one week prior to the onset of an eruption on her back. In a 48-hour period the eruption spread rapidly to involve her neck, both upper extremities, and the upper thighs. The pruritus was most intense. There was no history of any previous allergic or atopic diseases. She had been given one x-ray treatment and medication topically by another physician and was seen by us five days after the onset of the original lesion. Examination revealed the presence of a symmetrical eruption over the back, neck, thighs, and upper extremities, with the wrists being particularly involved. Eruption showed a faint red morbilliform pattern, with a tendency toward confluence in the large macular areas. The mucous membranes were not involved. The patient improved rapidly under treatment with colloidal baths; corticotropin, 60 units per day for five days; antihistamines orally and by intramuscular injection; and hydrocortisone cream topically. One week later the patient took one 400-mg. tablet of meprobamate, and pruritic, erythematous maculas recurred in the identical areas previously involved within approximately three hours after the ingestion of the medicament.

CASE 6.—A 45-year-old male took one 400-mg. tablet of meprobamate, and three hours later there was a marked erythema of the genitalia and the inner aspects of both thighs. Itching were severe, and the lesion was red and macular in type. The patient was placed on therapy with antihistamines orally, and the rash cleared up in approximately three days.

CASE 7.—A 32-year-old female was given 400 mg. of meprobamate every morning for two days without any therapeutic effect or ill-effects. The next day she took 800 mg. at 4 p.m. At 8 p.m. diplopia accompanied by nausea developed. This lasted until she fell asleep. The next day she was well. The patient has developed generalized dermatitis from penicillin. She has had hay fever, eczema, and bronchial asthma since early childhood.

In addition, there were three cases of paradoxical reaction to meprobamate of extreme excitement rather than tranquilization. After two tablets in each instance the meprobamate therapy was discontinued. One tablet subsequently produced excitement and nervousness within one hour after oral administration.

COMMENT

Although there were only sparse reports in the literature regarding this new drug and no samples were sent out to practicing physicians for trial, meprobamate, marketed by two related established drug companies under two different names, has been sold from coast to coast in great quantity. Almost a year was required for the production to equal the demand. From various physicians in our area, we found that many internists have seen several patients with drug eruptions from meprobamate. Some cases have been so severe that hospitalization and treatment with intravenously given corticotropin were required. In an occasional case the life of the patient was in actual danger. No one to date, however, has reported these cases in clinical literature. We have learned of cases with generalized urticaria, the localized fixed drug-type eruption, and the morbilliform toxic-type drug eruption. Basically, the lesions we have seen fall into four categories, namely, muscular paralysis, intestinal hyperactivity, dermatological reaction, and paradoxical reaction.

From the pharmacology of the compound, muscular paralysis with a large dose would appear to be a real possibility. For ocular palsy to occur from two tablets (800 mg.) seems impossible; yet it occurred in one patient. Intestinal hyperactivity from a muscle-relaxing compound that is said to have no autonomic nervous system effects seems rather paradoxical, as in case 1. On the other hand, paradoxical reactions, where sedation is expected and excitement is produced, have long tradition in regard to the barbiturates and other sedative compounds.

The skin lesions were interesting, in that the sites of predilection appeared to be the pelvic girdle area, the breast area, and the flexor surfaces of the arm. Less commonly involved were the trunk, anteriorly and posteriorly, and the legs. More remarkable was the fact that a patient who had never taken the compound before would develop the reaction within three to five hours after taking one tablet. Usually in drug eruptions the patient has had prior contact with the compound before developing dermatitis medicamentosa. In other words, prior sensitization is required before a reactive state is created, which on reexposure gives a clinical allergic response. A possible explanation of this phenomenon is that these patients have been exposd in the past to chemically related compounds such as mephenesin. No percentages of toxic reactions can be given, as we have no idea of the morbidity of adverse reactions in a large definitive series of patients on therapy with this compound. However, Selling reported on 187 patients without any adverse responses in 1955.

Summary

As a result of administering a new tranquilizer, meprobamate, we have seen three cases of paradoxical excitement, one case of intestinal hyperperistalsis with rice water stools, one case of palsy of the extraocular muscles with diplopia, and five cases of skin lesions, chiefly but not solely purpuric in nature, extremely pruritic, and with a predilection for the lesions to appear first in the pelvic girdle area, genitalia, and groin in both males and females. As yet no severe exfoliative dermatitis has been seen, though this appears to be a likely prospect. Initial exposure with one 400-mg. tablet of meprobamate may produce the skin lesions in less than four hours. Meprobamate has the potential of producing a number of diverse dermatological patterns that may be confused with other dermadromes. No mucous membrane lesions were seen.

INHERENT DANGERS IN USE OF TRANQUILIZING DRUGS IN ANXIETY STATES

Herman A. Dickel, M.D. and Henry H. Dixon, M.D.
Department of Psychiatry, University of Oregon Medical School,
Portland, Oregon

A few months ago, not many opinions had been expressed about any dangers of the tranquilizing drugs, that rapidly growing list of pharmacological agents used chiefly for their effect in reducing anxiety, nervousness, emotional distress, and many abnormal mental states. Now, many authors have begun to voice opinions. We join them, fully aware that our original purpose has lost its urgency, but we have a particular point to emphasize, nonetheless.

"THE AGE OF ANXIETY"

It has been common in the recording of mankind's history for certain names to be given to eras in an attempt to characterize them. A number of historians and commentators of this particular era would designate it as "the age of anxiety." Whether this designation is to be accepted, only future historians can say, but certainly it is a descriptive term that has a good deal of merit. An apparent abundance of tensions, fears, worries, and anxieties confronts mankind at this time. Moreover, mankind has suddenly become aware that these elements of tension exist in and are common to each race and geographical sector of the world. It might be proper to call this the age of anxiety because we have the tremendous means of communication to allow men to know of one another's problems and tensions or because there are so many obvious stresses and anxieties that affect not only the individuals of whom we psychiatrists write but almost every other individual. Again, this term might be considered apt because many of the pharmaceutical companies of the world have discovered remedies that relieve the syndrome of anxiety and because several branches of medicine have made this syndrome a focal point of their therapeutic procedures. Finally, it might be apropos to call this the age of anxiety because anxiety has become a frequently used device by which political philosophies exert their influence on the masses, encouraging a rule almost medieval in character.

From the standpoint of the physician in practice, there has been a marked increase in the matters pertaining to anxiety since the end of World War II, approximately 10 years ago. Chief among the interesting developments of this decade has been the appearance of the large number of pharmacological agents that can be utilized by the physician for the specific treatment of the increasing number of patients who come to him seeking relief from tension, anxiety, and related somatic and emotional disturbances.

The physician has always had an interest in anxiety and has tended to treat that anxiety, whether it be an isolated symptom, a syndrome peculiar to itself, or a measurable part of some other illness. His procedures in handling anxiety have varied from the tact and humanness with which he related himself to his patients to administration of the various pharmacological and medicinal agents that were available to him in his time, such as opium, alcohol, or barbiturates. From time to time the physician has treated anxiety by a combination of factors. A specialty has even grown up in our midst for the specific purpose of dealing with anxieties. Certainly we can say the use of procedures, drugs, and agencies is not new in the treatment of anxiety by the medical profession.

But there has been a noticeable change in the last 10 years in the manner in which this treatment of anxiety has proceeded. Anxiety has become a disease entity recognized not only by the medical profession but also by the lay public, who, as they grow aware of the entities for which medicine has a treatment, demand not only the known procedures for treatment but the research that will supply advanced procedures and agents. This public interest has stimulated the quest for the tranquilizing drugs. Because of the interest of the medical profession, pharmaceutical houses, research scientists, lay health agencies, and the general public, who are characteristically influenced by the advertising and agencies of communication in the United States, the last 10 years may indeed be the age of anxiety.

Anxiety affects, according to some health statistics, 25 million to 50 million people in the United States alone, and it is devastating in its most advanced form. For these reasons, and because anxiety can be treated easily by all physicians, it could appear at first glance that the use of these new drugs is more than justified in medical practice, and particularly in general practice, where the patient is first seen. The use of these drugs might be considered justified because they are relatively safe, according to the early literature; because they are relatively inexpensive as compared to previously known remedies, such as psychotherapy or hospital care; and because many people can be practically treated in a short time with little inconvenience.

At the Conference on Meprobamate, held in New York in October, a representative of one of the drug companies announced that so far in 1956 some 30 billion tablets of one particular tranquilizing drug had been sold to the American public. This statement, which seems to indicate better than any other we know the tremendous usage of the tranquilizing agents, is only partially indicative of the great use of these pharmacological agents. The drug companies indicate that there is sufficient sale of the tranquilizing agents for us to infer that there are few people at the present time who have not tried some of the tranquilizing substances that we as physicians prescribe. There is an increase in the number of detail men who ask us to listen to their information and not only bring to our offices tablets, capsules, and liquids designed to appeal to the convenience of the physician and his patients but also arrange to send us luxurious neck rests and pretty slippers. The treatment of anxiety and anxious patients is big business, even without doctors, and the pressure is on the doctor to make it more so.

Our interest in the tranquilizing drugs goes back to 1949, when, in a practice limited to patients with anxiety states, we sought an agent that could be used as a supplement in the rapid training of our patients in techniques of neuromuscular relaxation. At that time we used mephenesin to real advantage and stated in a publication that mephenesin was a tremendously useful drug in teaching tense, anxious people the techniques of relaxation, allowing the patient a more rapid course in any psychotherapeutic procedure.

Material of Study

Since 1949 we have seen approximately 8,200 patients in whom anxiety is the chief finding. Almost all these people have been referred for psychotherapeutic treatment by other physicians in the medical field. This has presented us an opportunity of studying the interest in tranquilizing drugs as treatment for anxiety, their wide use, and the complications resulting from their use.

We define patients with anxiety states as those individuals of essentially normal physical make-up, possessing rather definite advantage or superiority in intellectual capacity, who either are steadily working or are capable of working at any time, and who come to the physician complaining of tension, worry, anxiety combined with such physiological disturbances as rapid heart, cold perspiring hands and feet, cervical tension, elevated blood pressure, distress in breathing, or gastrointestinal variations, together with varying moods of anxiety, depressiveness, morbidness, and occasionally mild obsessive-compulsive tendencies.

These patients who suffer anxiety, then, do not include the so-called neurotics, who complain but are certainly not driving, proficient individuals who are working but are doing so with anxious distress. We are referring here to that large number of American people who perhaps might more aptly be called the "psychosomatic cases," since their anxiety is frequently seen in connection with ulcers or hypertensive, asthmatic, dermatological, or gastrointestinal disturbances. We include as "anxiety cases," then, all those people who are living fully but doing so with anxiety and its direct effect or the effects of the many physiological variations seen in the "psychosomatic entities."

Dangers of Tranquilizing Drugs

In our analysis of 8,200 cases of such people, referred by physicians for psychotherapeutic procedures, some 7,500 had had some amount of the tranquilizing drugs already. In this group we have found certain definite complications and dangers arising from widespread use of the drugs and have grouped these into four categories: physical danger to the patient, emotional, moral, and philosophical danger to the patient, danger to medicine and the physician, and danger to society.

Physical Danger to the Patient.—We would like to point out that, even though the tranquilizing drugs seem to be of no general harm, nonetheless they constitute a definite threat to the health and even the life of many patients. The literature at present is beginning to note that there are definite toxic reactions to many of the tranquilizing drugs. Many individuals who seemingly should be "tranquilized" by the drugs instead develop most unusual, untoward reactions. Anxious people become depressed enough to commit suicide; calm easy-going people become hypomanic or manic after the use of the drugs; and many other unpleasant and unfavorable responses occur that require additional and often intensive treatment and hospitalization. The number of such instances has totaled almost 400 in 8,200 cases. This is not a large percentage, but it certainly is large enough to cause us to reconsider the benefits of these drugs.

TABLE 1.—*Physical Dangers to Patients Treated with Tranquilizing Drugs*

	No. of Patients
Death (4)	
Altered response to electric therapy	1
Altered physiological function	1
Acute depression and successful suicide	2(?)
Alteration of life processes with physical change (324)	
Convulsive disorder (etiology unknown)	1
Complication to pregnancy (1 abortion, 1 nearly)	2
Addiction	1
Habituation	72
Liver disturbances (severe)	31
Skin disturbances (severe only)	25
Gastrointestinal upheavals (severe)	18
Blood dyscrasias (noted by others)	0
Allergic phenomena	96
Generalized toxic effects	78
Total	328

Table 1 shows the physical problems we found and the number of patients in whom they occurred, some overlapping, of course. The deaths may have been due to several factors, but they occurred nonetheless. The liver problems, the toxic reactions, the allergic phenomena, and the skin changes are now known and seen by many. We have seen no blood dyscrasias as others have, but we have seen many cases of habituation. The one patient in our group who became addicted to tranquilizing drugs had previously been addicted to narcotics. The convulsive reaction (definite in one case and questionable in another) and the complications of pregnancy may have to be explained as sensitivity or allergic reactions.

Emotional, Moral, and Philosophical Dangers to the Patient.—When we consider the use of these drugs on a wide basis, there is a great deal of danger to the patient from an emotional, moral, and philosophical point of view. People at present obviously are undergoing many emotional disturbances, and the use of these drugs at times seems to be justified to ease these disturbances. However, we have noticed an increasingly large number of people who have been referred to us for psychotherapeutic procedures after having been treated by their physicians over a period of months in somewhat the following manner: They were normal people who went to their physicians for advice and counsel about mildly distressing problems that had produced tensions, worry, and anxiety. The physicians, busy and perhaps too casual in their examinations and their evaluations of the patients involved, often prescribed a new tranquilizer and sent the patient off to return later. The patients returned to complain of unpleasant, unwanted responses, often emotional, to the drugs, and the physicians misinterpreted the reponses as meaning a more "deeply seated" illness was present. They so stated to the patients and precipitated serious reactions. We have noted (table 2) about 1,700 instances in which serious problems were

TABLE 2.—*Nonphysical Dangers to Patients Treated with Tranquilizing Drugs*

	No. of Patients
Well persons complaining of minor problems (1,700)	
Acute anxiety	1,100
Acute depression	600
Emotionally ill persons (827)	
Acute manic state	11
Acute depression with suicidal threats	80
Actual amoral behavior never previously noted	13
State of well-being causing very ill people to stop therapy	126
Morbid fear of addiction or habituation	296
Fear of drugs	301
Guilt over fantasy or over religious thoughts	No accurate count
Total	2,527

created in the cases of essentially normal people for a time due to misunderstanding on the part of physicians. The doctors, rather than the drugs, should perhaps be considered at fault. In the obviously emotionally ill persons, problems arise when the patient's treatment with tranquilizing drugs has been poorly watched and regulated (table 2).

Dangers to Medicine and the Physician.—Medicine and the physician have always stood behind the basic philosophy that, if everything done for the patient could do no good, it should do no harm. The goal of all medical treatments is to help the patient attain the highest possible performance from his basic equipment, or to return the patient to a state as nearly normal as possible. At first glance the use of drugs for relief of anxiety seems to fit the goal. But actually, does it?

History has always recorded the many attempts on the part of man to avoid and withdraw from pressures, tensions, and anxieties. Yet, as we will note later, pressures, tensions, apprehensions, and fears may actually be very necessary stimulants to the finest and highest attainments of man. In the past man and medicine have had to learn very healthy respect for some of the "drugs" such as alcohol, opiates, bromides, and barbiturates that would relieve distress and anxiety. Many physicians were harmed by these and in being harmed were a danger to the medical profession. In the same way, we have noted eight or nine cases in which physicians themselves overused the tranquilizing drugs and three others in which they suffered further emotional problems due to them.

Now the physician and medicine find themselves confronted by a restless public, a growing pharmaceutical industry, an able advertising profession, and many truly anxious patients. They all apply a tremendous pressure on the medical profession, individually and collectively, to find, to make available, and to prescribe a large number of inexpensive tranquilizing drugs. This is a threat, just as each major advance in medicine, surgery, anesthesia, or antibiotic therapy has posed serious threats to the physician. To each, medicine has responded so that dangers and complications are minimized. The tranquilizing agents may yet prove to be the most serious threat to the sound principles of medical practice.

In a sense physicians have always avoided really learning the nature of anxiety, of the neuroses, the psychoneuroses, and the psychoses. To most doctors these were conditions of a "nonorganic nature," giving the patients no real reason to be ill and to take the doctor's time. Such patients were, however, always consulting the physician. Then came the tranquilizing drugs. Here was something the literature said helped tension, nervousness, and emotional illness of all degrees of seriousness. Without thoughtfulness many physicians, it would seem, began to give the tranquilizing drugs to any or all of these patients, with utter disregard for diagnostic categories. This has resulted in serious danger to the physician, for now it will take a long time to reestablish the simple fact that "psychotherapy" is not the easy ability to write prescriptions for tranquilizing drugs, any more than the ability to write prescriptions for antibiotics is characteristic of an internist's ability. The real knowledge of psychiatric illnesses is advancing, but there could be a serious setback to these advances if there is not competent use of these newer drugs.

Dangers to Society.—The comments that we will make must not be interpreted as an attempt to find fault with any of the present philosophies of political groups. Rather we are trying to point out what to us is an unusually important effect on people, as noted by our observations in our patients. The point that we wish to make is essentially this: In the last 25 years we all have seen a philosophy develop that is focused on the need for us to have freedom from several things, including fear. This philosophy is obviously a useful one, especially when looked at from afar. But, if we study the natural history of mankind, we cannot help noting that tension, alertness, alarmedness, fear, worry, anxiety, and apprehension have been, are, and always will be important elements in the shaping of progress. A great many authorities in the past have told us this, are telling it to us now, and probably will go on saying it for many years. As a nation we Americans have been strong, and we envision continued strength because we have been able to rise to the occasion of defending ourselves in the presence of stress, tensions, and apprehension. But now it would appear a philosophy has crept in that intimates that fear and anxiety are evidence of illness and are to be avoided or necessitate therapy.

Whether this is a political philosophy, whether it has come from psychiatric schools of thought, or whether it is a misinterpretation of the times, we are unable to determine. But certainly we see a malignant tendency invading our thinking, forcing us to believe that no one should ever be afraid, no one should ever feel anxiety, no one should ever feel so moved about his position in life as to do something about it. Rather we are to be completely tranquil under all circumstances and let someone else "do the worrying," try to get ahead, or be successful.

Among the 8,200 people whom we have seen, a large number were having difficulty interpreting their own course within the structure of the above-named philosophy. They would read or be told that no one should get upset about anything, and yet they would go to the office and find the pressure from their bosses, their supervisors, or their boards of directors. Conflict, turmoil, and distress appear everywhere when our national philosophy approaches things in one manner and our individual philosophy approaches it in another. The use of the tranquilizing drugs obviously numbs many of these disturbances. Many individuals who are otherwise unable to handle the tensions of modern conflicts in philosophy can do so under the use of the tranquilizing drugs. But the majority of these people are doing so without being of real value to themselves and to the group in which they work. It is our honest estimate that probably 1,200 to 1,300 of the 8,200 people fell into this category. They felt obvious dissatisfaction with the use of tranquilizing drugs as a means of treatment or a way of handling their tension and anxiety, for it seriously impeded their contributions to their company or their value to their group. They could see no good coming from the idea of everyone feeling completely placid, unless it would be the greater acceptance of certain future political philosophies.

From all the instances of dangerous reactions to tranquilizing drugs cited, a total of some 4,100 instances in 8,200 cases, we sincerely hope no one draws the conclusion that we are about to place the blame for all the wrongs in medicine, our political situation, or the world on the tranquilizing drugs. Rather, we are simply and humbly trying to bring forth one very important point, that the modern pharmacological agents known as the tranquilizing drugs are not any more safe for patient and doctor than any other drug of any other time. We physicians must not, although the effect of the drugs is to tranquilize, be led to believe that the drugs have no dangers. They do, and the various ones as we see them have been noted above.

Prevention of Dangers

One might ask, then, if there are no procedures that can be followed, or certain safeguards that can be used, so that an absolute minimum of danger is experienced. The following points are something in the way of suggestions along this line, and we offer them, as others have, for whatever value they may have in stimulating others' suggestions.

It would be well for physicians dealing with patients with anxiety states to use the oft-repeated advice of our medical school faculties that there be no prescribing until a full evaluation of the patient is made and we know his personality and emotional responses and needs as well as his physical and laboratory status. Doctors should consider urging the acceptance of the tranquilizing drugs as being just as much in need of legal restriction as any others and demanding that the frequent giving of these drugs to patients by well-meaning and friendly druggists be curtailed. Research groups might be requested to give us special laboratory techniques to measure as accurately as possible the best dosage for each individual patient from time to time, as they have with bromides, sulfonamides, hormones, and antibiotics. Pharmaceutical companies and their willing and able publicity departments should be urged to initiate public education about these drugs in much the same manner as some state liquor control boards have done.

Physicians as a whole must bring up to date their knowledge of anxiety states and their ability to ascertain and diagnose them and then to handle and treat the many thousands of essentially normal people who are worried, anxious, and depressed. These patients want no pills from their doctor, but instead an honest attempt on the doctor's part to help them do the best they can, to help them learn some way of living with, and even enjoying, the tensions of modern living. Finally, the modern medical philosophy must continue to be that basically man is better off having to fare for himself—that being too well cared for, having too little fear from cradle to crypt is not healthy and that all drugs are still only a small and essential part of medical practice, certainly no cure-all for modern trouble, to be dispensed indiscriminately without sound medical advice.

Conclusions

In our perusal of some 8,200 cases of anxiety in persons referred to us by other physicians for psychotherapy, we have found some serious complications and dangers resulting from the use of tranquilizing drugs. The physical danger to normal people and the danger to the physician, to medicine itself, and finally to society as a whole can be minimized by certain actions on the part of physicians. Finally, we would like to stress that our cautious attitude is not directed toward the drugs alone, because they are valuable to a certain degree when used wisely. Our attitude is directed toward the physician, who must inform himself well if he is to use these tranquilizers or any drugs wisely. Never have any drugs caused quite the same effect as these available today. Their future, as well as our own, will depend on the immediate reorientation each physician makes in his own thinking about the indications for, and the limitations of, these drugs.

James G. Shanklin, M.D., and Gerhard B. Haugen, M.D., collaborated in the writing of this article.

EDEMA AND CONGESTIVE FAILURE RELATED TO ADMINISTRATION OF RAUWOLFIA SERPENTINA

George A. Perera, M.D.
Department of Medicine, Columbia University College of
Physicians and Surgeons, New York, N. Y.

Following the administration of alkaloids of Rauwolfia serpentina, the occasional occurrence of temporary sodium retention has been reported. In the course of further experience with these drugs in the treatment of hypertension, fluid retention has now been encountered in five instances, even to the point of extensive edema, pulmonary congestion, and venous pressure elevation. The four women and one man who developed fluid retention all had documented hypertensive vascular disease with no previous history of dyspnea, edema, or cardiac pain. Four had negative urinalyses and one a 1+ proteinuria immediately prior to the episode. Three had been given 0.25 mg. of reserpine (Serpasil) twice daily by mouth, and two had been given Rauwolfia serpentina (Raudixin), 100 mg. twice daily by mouth, all five being on an ambulatory outpatient basis and on a self-selected diet but without extra salt.

In all instances moderate pitting edema of the ankles appeared within a week of the start of therapy. Two subjects went on to develop marked edema of the lower extremities and basal pulmonary rales, and one of these complained of moderate exertional dyspnea and exhibited some periorbital swelling. Both the patients with the more severe degrees of fluid retention, observed after three weeks of continued medication, had gained more than 4 lb. (1.8 kg.) in weight, with the venous pressure in an antecubital vein recorded as 116 and 130 mm. of saline respectively; both had a 1+ proteinuria; and a white blood cell count and differential smear was within normal limits in one. In only one patient of the group of five was there any significant reduction in blood pressure or pulse rate in association with drug administration. None complained of cardiac pain, and none exhibited any irregularities of cardiac rhythm.

No improvement was noted until therapy with the drug was discontinued, each patient having received from three to four weeks of sustained treatment without change in diet or dosage. Within one subsequent week all manifestations of abnormal fluid retention had vanished, one patient spontaneously remarking of her increased urine output. The weight of the two subjects with more marked edema returned to pretreatment levels by the end of the week, and in one of these it was possible to check the venous pressure, which had fallen to 80 mm. of saline. During a period of observation of from one to three months after treatment, no patient developed any recurrent edema or cardiac symptoms. At a later date, one of the patients who had developed marked edema while receiving reserpine was given the same drug in the same dosage for one week; definite pitting edema of the ankles was again apparent, and once more it vanished when administration of reserpine was discontinued.

COMMENT

The association of fluid retention in five patients treated with crude or purified alkaloids of Rauwolfia serpentina seems more than happenstance and, although no balance studies were undertaken, may possibly be related to the occasional sodium retention previously reported. It is difficult to attribute the accumulation of edema to changes in diet. Against the possibility of a coincidental cardiac decompensation in these hypertensive subjects are the negative previous histories, the temporal relationship to drug administration, the rapid remission following cessation of therapy, and the subsequent course. The minimal urinary findings do not suggest a nephrotic episode.

The observation that alkaloids of Rauwolfia serpentina may occasionally produce fluid retention needs further confirmation, and the mechanism remains to be elucidated. In the meantime, this possibility should be kept in mind, particularly in patients who already have a lowered cardiac reserve.

SUMMARY

In five patients with hypertensive vascular disease, fluid retention occurred after the administration of crude or pure alkaloids of Rauwolfia serpentina. In two of these patients, the fluid retention was severe enough to cause congestive failure.

RECURRENT THORAZINE INDUCED AGRANULOCYTOSIS

Benjamin Pollack, M.D.

At least 50 cases of agranulocytosis occurring during treatment with chlorpromazine (Thorazine) have been reported. That this should occur from time to time is not surprising in view of the chemical structure of this drug. Most of the reported cases have occurred within 1 or 2 months after the beginning of treatment. With few exceptions the reported cases have consisted of female patients. The writer is aware of only 2 male cases, including one previously reported by the author.

Reports of agranulocytosis following treatment with chlorpromazine have been reported by Munch-Peterson (1954), Lomas (1954), Pollack (1955) 1 case among 500 patients, Tasker (1955), Boleman (1955), Prokopowycz (1955), and Shapiro (1955). Giacobini and Lassenius (1954) reported 1 case among 147 patients treated, Goldman (1955) 4 cases in the treatment of about 1,000 patients, Barsa and Kline (1955) 2 cases among 300 patients. Lomas, Boardman and Markowe (1955) refer to 7 further unpublished cases of agranulocytosis following treatment with chlorpromazine. Other reports have been made by Ayd, Adams, Corti, Hobson, Tillim and Stone. Yules reported a case of agranulocytosis occurring in a 78-year-old woman which did not recur on retreatment.

As far as I can ascertain, there have been no cases reported in the literature similar to the present one. In our series of over 2,000 chlorpromazine-treated patients, there have been only 2 cases of agranulocytosis.

T.H. an 82-year-old woman was admitted to the Strong Memorial Hospital on July 9, 1955. About 1 year previously she began to exhibit memory loss and disorientation, with restlessness and excitement. Two months previously she had been placed on Thorazine by her family doctor (exact dosage unknown). On July 6, she became delirious, stuporous, and developed a fever. She appeared acutely ill. There was marked ulceration of her throat, with erythema of the posterior portions of the palate, the uvula and the tonsillar fossae. A diagnosis of Thorazine-induced agranulocytosis was made on the basis of a blood count on admission which showed only 700 white cells (almost entirely lymphocytes). The following day the white count fell to 425 and counts on the next 2 days showed white blood counts of 550 and 700. A report of the bone marrow obtained from a sternal puncture on July 11 was reported as follows:

Peripheral blood showed evidence of marked leucocytopenia. Differential smear showed only lymphocytes with occasional reaction forms and no young forms. Erythrocytes are normocytic and the majority are normochromic, with slight anisocytosis, and slight polychromatophilia. Platelets are of normal morphology and normal in number.

The bone marrow was hypocellular and obviously was markedly dilated with peripheral blood. Megakaryocytes appear to be mature and in the lower limits of normal number. Erythroid series was markedly hypoplastic with a few late stages seen. A very rare basophilic and prenormoblast form is found. It is normoblastic. Myeloid series—a very rare young neutrophil form is found along the edge of the smear. A very rare blast form was seen on searching one smear. Differential on 50 cells: 80% lymph, 20% monos. Lymphocytes display much pleomorphism—many showing toxic characteristics. No immaturity was noted. A rare plasm cell is present. The smear is suggestive of hypoplasia of the myeloid elements.

The patient was treated with massive doses of penicillin and streptomycin, and parenteral fluids. She became afebrile after 4 days and the mouth lesions cleared. The white blood count increased and on July 14 was reported as 1,600. The white count on July 18 was reported as 7,500 and on the 20th as 9,700, on the 21st as 12,800, and on the 22nd as 14,000. The count gradually returned to a normal level. A blood marrow examination from another sternal puncture taken 10 days after the acute onset indicated "a remarkable degree of recovery of bone marrow function, especially in the myeloid series and suggests that the patient had some overshoot." The patient made an uneventful recovery from this acute illness. She was then given an oral test dose of Thorazine, 10 mg. on one day and 25 mg. on the next day, without any subsequent change in her blood picture. She was transferred to the Rochester State Hospital on August 18, 1955, because of the continuation of her disturbed behavior. At that time the physicians had no knowledge of her previous agranulocytosis. At this hospital she continued to be extremely noisy. On January 10, 1956, she was given 200 mg. of Thorazine by mouth and this was repeated daily for the next 11 days. At first the patient became quiet and cooperative, and the drug was finally discontinued because patient's behavior seemed improved. During this period of medication no change was noted in her physical state. As time went on she gradually became noisy again and on June 21, 1956, she was placed on 50 mg. of Thorazine twice daily. She became quieter but still had periods of excitement and marked confusion. On July 4, she complained of dizziness, staggered about and seemed very drowsy. Her temperature was 103° and she became increasingly drowsy and finally almost stuporous. She appeared dehydrated, throat was inflamed without, however, any petechiae, and moderate exudate. There were no other abnormal new physical findings. She was placed in high doses of antibiotics such as penicillin, streptomycin, and terramycin. Her initial white count was 1,200 with no granulated leucocytes and 97% lymphocytes and 3% large monocytes. Platelets were slightly decreased; Thorazine was discontinued. On July 6 white count was 2,000; on July 9 it was 1,200; on July 10, 1,400; on July 11, 1,200; on July 12, 1,100; on July 13, 1,200; on July 16, 3,100; on July 17, 3,400; on July 18, 3,900; on July 19, 4,400; on July 20, 5,700 and on July 25, 8,700. Following this the patient made an uneventful recovery to her previous state.

This case is of interest because it is probably the first report of recurrence of agranulocytosis in a patient under chlorpromazine medication. Yules reported a 78-year-old woman who had developed a similar agranulocytosis, who on retreatment with chlorpromazine failed to reproduce "a leukopenic reaction or frank agranulocytosis."

The mechanisms responsible for the production of agranulocytosis in certain patients are still not clear. Further study and further reports are necessary before the complex etiology of this rare complication of chlorpromazine therapy can be elaborated.

DRUG-INDUCED BLOOD DYSCRASIAS

Stuart L. Vaughan, M.D..
Buffalo General Hospital and the University of Buffalo School of Medicine, Buffalo, New York

The complete physician must, among other attributes, be a student, scientist, and healer. It is to the healer within us that the patient appeals for help. Without full appreciation of the studies involved or the scientific methods that must be used, he expects us to intercede in the pathologic physiology that has shown itself through unpleasant symptoms and to cause the body's function to be restored to normal balance. Our desire to help is as great as the patient's need, yet we realize that whenever we interfere with the complex internal environment of living cells, our capacity to do good is balanced by a proportional capacity to do harm.

Nowhere is this concept better exemplified than in chemotherapy which was invented by Paul Ehrlich and which has burgeoned into a huge industry. Ehrlich's famous "606" illustrates the long search for a drug that will produce a desirable effect without too much danger. As early as 1910, this drug was known to produce purpura and anemia. Twenty years later the concern over agranulocytosis related to the widespread use of aminopyrine led to Federal legislation designed to protect the public. No doubt this Federal Food, Drug and Cosmetic Act has prevented much harm, but the continued development of blood disorders in the wake of drug administration has proved that laws cannot do the whole job of prevention. This is where the student and scientist roles of the physician must assert themselves in seeing that unnecessary harm is not done to his patients.

Study of the sequence of events which accompanies the discovery and trial of a promising new drug has shown that it has a rather definite pattern:

Laboratory Promise—Limited Clinical Trial—Initial Encouraging Results—Banner Headlines in the Lay Press—Pharmaceutical Fanfare—Rumors of Trouble—Definite Reports of Dangerous Complications—Condemnation—Revaluation.

Most of us are not directly concerned in the laboratory studies and early clinical trials, although we must appraise the results of such investigations critically before using the medicine. We have the right and the duty to ask searching questions about the drug's discovery, its relationship to other drugs, its standardization, its use in human subjects, follow-up observations, undesirable side-effects, the investigators themselves, and the sources of their financial grants before seriously considering the use of a new drug on our patients. When encouraging reports are published in the newspapers and magazines, we begin to feel pressure from our colleagues, our patients, their relatives, and from the detail men. We wish to be modern and up to date and to give our patient the benefit of the very latest "wonder drug," and yet at this stage we lack information about potentially harmful effects.

If we assume the privileges of using the newest therapy, we must accept the responsibility for observing its results. It is from us, to a great extent, that the medical world learns the unusual complications of drugs. This requires accurate records, a baseline of control observation, use of the drug alone where possible, and accurate systematic records during the period of observation which must be extended for a long follow-up. The longer the follow-up observations, the more valuable they are. The late effects of thorium and radium required over fifteen years to evaluate, and these studies are still not complete. It is obvious that there will be no mutual benefit from the observations unless they are reported.

From the hematologic point of view we must look for changes in the blood cells. The changes may be quantitative, as shown by comparing the pretreatment blood counts with those taken during the course of treatment and during the follow-up phase. They may also be qualitative with a variety of evidence of cell damage, toxic phenomena, and altered morphology. Careful appraisal of such evidence can be of immense help both immediately and later on.

Final appraisal of a drug's value and its potentiality for harm is often difficult. It is easy to confuse coincidental improvement during drug administration with favorable pharmacologic effect, and it is equally easy to attribute to the drug unfavorable manifestations that may occur in the wake of the drug's use. The recent investigations on Chloromycetin illustrate the difficulties even when we have tremendous resources for collecting information.

In spite of the difficulties, there is abundant evidence that many types of blood disorders are related to drugs. Among the more significant of them are the following:

1. Those in which the drug affects only one blood cell type
   A. Anemia
   B. Leukopenia
   C. Thrombocytopenia
2. Those in which the drug affects various combinations of blood cell types
   A. Polycytopenia, e.g., anemia and leukopenia
   B. Pancytopenia (anemia, leukopenia, and thrombocytopenia)
3. Other conditions in which the drug produces blood abnormalities
   A. Infectious mononucleosis-like disease
   B. Systemic lupus erythematosus-like disease
   C. Leukemia?

Practically all of the blood cell types may be affected, sometimes selectively and sometimes more universally. Thus we may see anemia, leukopenia, thrombocytopenia, or various combinations including depletion of all of the marrow-produced cells at once in the form of pancytopenia or aplastic anemia. In addition, leukemia, infectious mononucleosis-like disease, and systemic lupus erythematosus have been ascribed to drugs.

NORMAL EQUILIBRIUM
Supply = Dissipation

DEPLETION

Normal Supply + Excessive Dissipation

Reduced Supply + Dissipation $\begin{cases} \text{Normal} \\ \text{Excessive} \\ \text{or even} \\ \text{Somewhat Reduced} \end{cases}$

FIG. 1. Depletion of circulating blood cells (anemia, leukopenia, or thrombocytopenia).

An understanding of the physiologic forces involved in maintaining supplies of red cells, white cells, and platelets at adequate and relatively constant levels is desirable in approaching the study of drug effects. Many details of knowledge are missing, but we may be in a position to fill in the gaps by recalling a few fairly well-established concepts. For instance, we may remember that the process of blood cell turnover is extremely dynamic. Blood cells are being destroyed or dissipated continuously, and new cells are being formed and released to replace those lost. Maintenance of a normal level involves a delicate

TABLE I.—EXAMPLES OF DRUGS WHICH MAY INDUCE BLOOD DISORDERS

Antimicrobial	Antineoplastic and anticellular
Arsenobenzols	Aminopterin
Chloramphenicol	Benzene
Para-aminosalicylic acid	6-Mercaptopurine
Quinine	Myleran
Quinacrine	Nitrogen mustards
Streptomycin	Phenylhydrazine
Sulfonamides	T.E.M.
Thiosemicarbazones	Urethane
Analgesics and antipyretics	Anticonvulsants
Acetanalid	Dilantin
Acetophenetidin	Mesantoin
Aminopyrine	Phenurone
Phenylbutazone	Tridione
Antihistamines	Antithyroid drugs
Antergan	Thiouracil
Dramamine	Tapazole
Pyribenzamine	Diuretics
Antiarrhythmics	Mercurials
Quinidine	Diamox
Procaine	
Miscellaneous	
Apresoline	Gold salts
Diethazine	Naphthaline
Dinitrophenol	Sedormid

TABLE II.—TYPES OF BLOOD DYSCRASIA PRODUCED BY VARIOUS DRUGS

Anemia	Granulocytopenia
Phenylhydrazine	Aminopyrine
Naphthaline	Thiouracil
Thrombocytopenia	Procaine amide
Sedormid	Antihistamines
Quinidine	Diamox
Pancytopenia	Thorazine
Mustards	Mercurial diuretics
Benzene	Mixed dyscrasias
Dinitrophenol	Quinine
Arsenobenzene	Urethane
Anticonvulsants	Aminopterin
Quinacrine	6-Mercaptopurine
Chloramphenicol	Myleran
Leukemia?	Sulfonamides
Radioactive drugs	Phenylbutazone
Thorium	Gold salts
Benzol	Infectious mononucleosis-like disease
	Para-amino salicylic acid
	Collagen disease
	Apresoline

equilibrium between supply and demand (Fig. 1). Depletion of any element means either a reduced supply or increased dissipation.

Dissipation of cells results from their destruction, from actual loss as in hemorrhage, or from removal from the circulation, at least temporarily, by sequestration. Reduced supply of cells may result from depletion of precursor cells, from failure of formative cells to divide or to differentiate and mature, or from failure of the mechanism by which the cells are released into the circulation.

Red cell destruction is the time-honored mechanism of depletion in the old standard forms of hemolytic disease. So-called maturation arrest (failure of cells to mature) was thought to be the mechanism in many other conditions such as agranulocytosis and pernicious anemia. The relative importance of these two processes has been the subject of debate for a long time, but recently there has been a noticeable shift in the weight of evidence to the side of destruction. Osgood, in discussing the subject, has intimated that maturation arrest is more illusion than fact. There are different explanations for the picture that simulates maturation arrest; Osgood favors the view that it is the result of a regenerative phase in which primitive cells previously depleted are returning to normal in a stepwise fashion, while Rohr emphasizes the view that it represents an equally stepwise destructive phase in which cells of greatest maturity are destroyed first with less mature cells destroyed in order. Moeschlin supported the latter concept. He felt that peripheral destruction involving increasingly immature elements might progress to a point where the picture would be that of "aplastic" anemia. He thought that this might explain the hemolytic anemias with aplastic marrows as described by Owren.

In any event the fundamental mechanisms of cell depletion and the methods by which drugs produce their damaging effects will become interesting to us. Again, we shall find that many questions must be left unanswered, but we can gain some insight into the processes of cell death and failure of normal cell proliferation as revealed by recent investigations.

There are different mechanisms in the events that lead to the death of cells or to disturbances of their proliferation, growth, or development. There may be profound alterations in vital chemical components, in enzyme functions, in chromosomes, etc. Some of these mechanisms are being studied intensively, as was true recently when the toxic actions of nitrogen mustard were examined. In this instance the mode of action seemed to be a direct chemical union between the drug and desoxyribose nucleic acid, thus interrupting mitosis and preventing cell proliferation.

Aminopterin and 6-mercaptopurine also interrupt orderly cell development by disturbing synthesis of nucleoprotein and purines. Presumably other drugs have characteristic methods of altering normal processes and interfere with blood formation.

The list of drugs capable of producing toxic changes in blood cells is now an extremely long one. Table I shows selected examples which are placed in a relatively few pharmacologic groups for convenience.

Earlier in this paper, mention was made of a selective tendency on the part of some drugs. Aminopyrine, for example, produced granulocytopenia almost exclusively. Other drugs such as benzene may have a selective effect on leukocytes in most cases, but if the dose is great enough and if other circumstances prevail, there may be pancytopenia and possibly even leukemia. In Table II are shown the significant blood disorders, under each of which is placed some of the drugs most likely to produce the disorder.

At this point it is only fair to state that the toxic actions of drugs are not all undesirable. In fact, such agents as nitrogen mustard, aminopterin, urethane, and myleran are used primarily because of their toxicity, which under proper circumstances is selective. The therapeutic results are most encouraging while the selective action is maintained, but all of these drugs may cause serious complications if the controlled selective action is superseded by an uncontrolled, nonselective toxic process.

Mention of this group of toxic drugs used therapeutically for their hemotoxic effects leads to an interesting observation. These drugs and a few others seem to act rather directly on vital cell processes in such a way that toxic manifestations are produced in all persons receiving a dosage in excess of their tolerance. In contrast we note another group of drugs, typified by aminopyrine and quinidine, which are capable of producing harmful effects in some persons but not in others, the harmful effects usually having little or no relationship to the dosage. For convenience we use the terms "poisonous" to characterize the first group and "idiosyncratic" to characterize the second (Table III). Evi-

TABLE III.—Examples of So-Called "Poisonous" and "Idiosyncratic" Drugs

Poisonous	Idiosyncratic
Mustards	Mesantoin
Urethane	Pyribenzamine
Aminopterin	Thiouracil
6-Mercaptopurine	Sulfonamide
Benzene	Gold salts
Myleran	Aminopyrine
Phenylhydrazine	Quinidine

dence suggests that the "idiosyncratic" drugs do not produce their toxic effects directly but that they do so quite indirectly through the mediation of some complex immunologic mechanism in which the affected person must be sensitized.

Some twenty years ago such workers as Kracke and Parker, Madison and Squier, and Dameshek and Colmes contributed important indirect evidence to indicate that many persons suffering from agranulocytosis had been sensitized to aminopyrine. It was not until 1949 that Ackroyd demonstrated the proof of this concept by producing clinical and laboratory manifestations of hemorrhagic disease in a person "sensitized" to Sedormid and by showing that such manifestations cannot be produced in a "nonsensitized" person.

From these experiments and others it has been concluded that administration of an "idiosyncratic" drug in certain subjects under circumstances that are not entirely clear will result in sensitization of body cells (absorption of protein upon the cells). Subsequent administration of the drug will result in a union of the drug with blood proteins in such a way that the sensitized cells become agglutinated or lysed. If this effect is relatively mild and of short duration, the damage may be reversible. If severe and prolonged, the process may go to an extreme as in "aplastic" anemia. It is only fair to mention that some workers in immunohematology feel that full acceptance of the validity of acquired sensitization as outlined should await further evidence.

Three mechanisms of drug hematoxic effects are as follows:
1. The "poisonous" effect is a rather direct one upon one or more cell types.
2. The "idiosyncratic" effect is an indirect one mediated through the development of immune bodies.
3. Constitutional or hereditary allergic susceptibility to drugs may explain some of the dyscrasias not accounted for otherwise.

Having learned that our chemotherapeutic agents can and do cause distur-

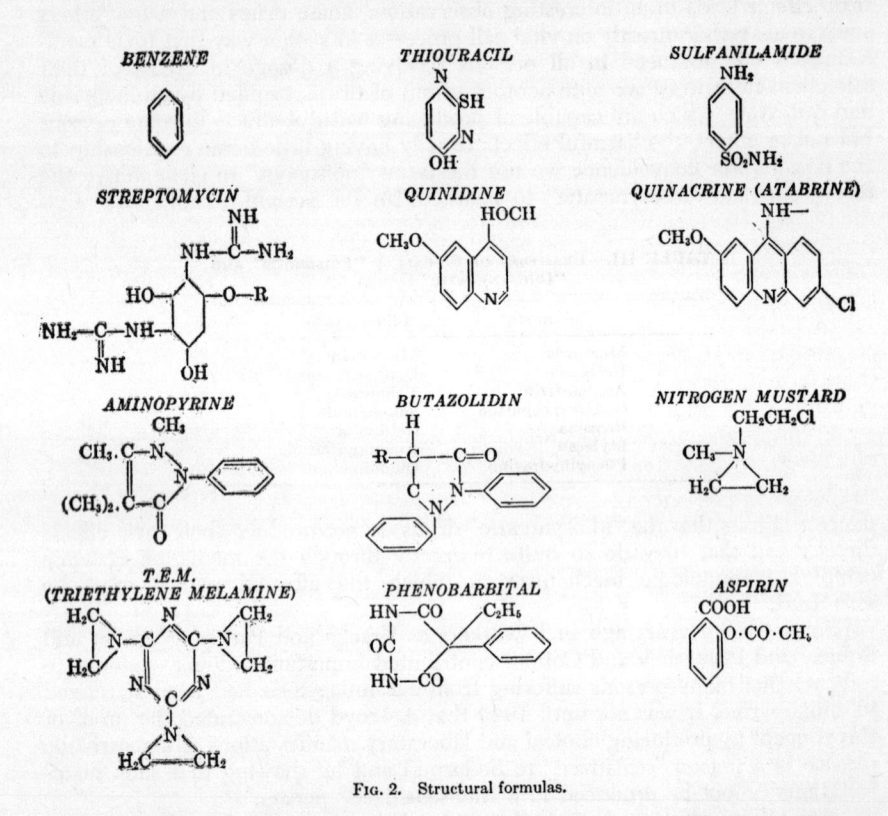

Fig. 2. Structural formulas.

TABLE IV.—PARTIAL CLASSIFICATION OF "IDIOSYNCRATIC" DRUGS ON THE BASIS OF RISK

High Risk	Low Risk
Arsenobenzenes	Sulfonamides
Mesantoin	Trimethadrine
Gold salts	Quinacrine
Aminopyrine	Procaine
Nitrophenol	Quinidine
Phenylbutazone	Streptomycin

TABLE V.—COMPARISON OF TOXICITY ON THE BASIS OF NUMBER OF NITROGEN GROUPS

Toxicity	Number of Nitrogen Groups
Greater	
T.E.M.	5
Mesantoin	3
Aminopterin	3
Lesser	
Nitrogen mustard	2
Tridione	2
Phenobarbital	1

bances of the blood of various types through a variety of mechanisms, we find that the problems are not quite exhausted. Why are some drugs toxic while others are not? Among the toxic drugs what determines the degree of toxicity? When a new drug is made available to us, is there a way to anticipate its dangerous effects? Finally, what are we to do if a drug-induced blood dyscrasia develops in one of our patients?

The benzene ring has been emphasized as an important hemotoxic factor ever since Selling produced marrow changes and corresponding anemia, leukopenia, and thrombocytopenia with benzene. Kracke concluded that N, NH, and NH$_2$ groups attached to the benzene ring were especially dangerous. He called this chemical arrangement the "benzamine linkage." Other workers have attempted to show the relationships between hemotoxicity and chemical structure (Fig. 2).

The degree of toxicity is probably determined by the interplay of several factors. One of these seems to be the number of nitrogen groups in the molecule. Among the "poisonous" drugs, triethylene melamine with five nitrogen groups is definitely more toxic than nitrogen mustard with three groups. Among the "idiosyncratic" drugs there seems to be a similar relationship. In Table IV an attempt is made to divide the drugs roughly into high risk and low risk types.

In Table V a comparison of the nitrogen groups with toxicity is made. It is clear that this is not the final answer since some drugs, such as streptomycin, show large nitrogen group counts but low degrees of toxicity. It has been suggested that the large molecule is less toxic than smaller ones.

From these considerations it seems reasonable to conclude that the formula of a given drug may suggest its potential toxicity, but this is not a completely reliable index.

We who have now assumed our responsibility of student, scientist, and healer in the field of chemotherapy as related to the hazards of blood complications are in a position to carry out our obligations regarding the administration or withholding of drugs in a rational manner. However, there is one final consideration which deals with the patient who develops a complication of one of the types we have discussed.

To stop the drug at once is logical and proper. If this is done early enough, the blood changes are apt to be quickly reversed, and no other measures may be necessary.

Antibiotics are to be used on the slightest provocation, especially in leukocyte disorders. Some people advocate their use prophylactically, and there is much to be said for this plan. On the other hand, there are advantages in delaying antibiotic administration until a reasonable attempt to establish bacteriologic diagnosis is made.

Steroid hormones are indicated early. Although we are not fully informed as to the precise mechanism of improvement, there is abundant evidence that these drugs help in a variety of ways.

Blood transfusions are given to maintain life and a good level of resistance. They are most useful in progressive anemias to elevate the hemoglobin to a level of compensation, especially during critical periods. There is no satisfactory evidence that recovery is ever hastened by transfusion.

Other agents, such as cobalt, chloride, iron, vitamin B_{12}, folic acid, etc., have not proved to be beneficial.

SUMMARY

One of the problems of the practicing physician in this era of rapid scientific progress is to recognize the potential harm in many of the wonderful chemotherapeutic agents available for our use. It is obvious that we owe it to our patients to use new drugs whenever the dangers of the disease outweigh the dangers of the drugs. In so doing we must know both the merits and the dangers of the drugs. With such knowledge we are in a position to assume a progressive attitude and avoid some of the pitfalls of being too radical.

The type of knowledge alluded to concerns such items as recognition of the pattern of drug promotion, the relationship of the practicing physician to the pattern, the experimental method as employed in use of a new drug, basic principles of blood production and blood cell depletion, the mechanism by which drugs may affect normal blood equilibrium, factors determining a drug's toxicity, and the risks involved in use of a drug. This same knowledge helps in devising a reasonable plan of treating the patient who may have been unfortunate enough to develop one of the hemotoxic manifestations.

HEMATEMESIS AND MELENA COMPLICATING TREATMENT WITH RAUWOLFIA ALKALOIDS

Leo E. Hollister, M.D.
Veterans Administration Hospital, Palo Alto, California

Alkaloids of Rauwolfia serpentina, especially reserpine, are being used widely in the treatment of hypertension and mental illness. In addition to their pharmacologic actions on the cardiovascular and central nervous systems, a variety of effects have been reported on the gastrointestinal system. Both gastric secretory and motor activity in dogs are augmented by reserpine. Increased volume and acidity of gastric secretions has also been found in man under the influence of reserpine. Hypermotility of the lower gastrointestinal tract is clinically evident in the occasional complaint of diarrhea in patients taking the drug. Emetic effects, suggesting hypermotility of the upper gastrointestinal tract, have been reported in animals and man. These actions on the gastrointestinal tract, produced in the main by the cholinergic-like action of the drug, suggest that duodenal ulcer might be activated. Such activation of ulcer in patients receiving reserpine has been reported.

Hematemesis and melena associated with the use of reserpine have been previously mentioned, but the circumstances were such that a direct causal relationship could not be established. Three of the cases to be presented occurred among over 600 patients treated for mental illness with large doses of various Rauwolfia preparations. The fourth case had been treated for hypertension with the drug. Although this complication must be rather rare, its potential seriousness merits consideration whenever these drugs are to be used in large doses or for prolonged periods of time.

REPORT OF CASES

CASE 1.—This 25-year-old man with a schizophrenic reaction was started on reserpine on April 24, 1955. In 1953, he had complained briefly about abdominal pain. A gastrointestinal series on Oct. 20, 1953, had been reported as negative. His general health was excellent.

A single oral dose of 12 mg. of reserpine was given by error on the first day of treatment. The patient soon developed severe vomiting and retching in addition to a marked cutaneous flush. These symptoms subsided in about 36 hours. A gastrointestinal series on April 27, 1955, indicated probable reflux esophagitis. On April 29, treatment was resumed with a daily parenteral dose of 5 mg. of reserpine followed soon by an oral dose of 3 mg. daily. He seemed to tolerate this program of treatment well. The daily oral dose of drug was increased to 6 mg. on June 11. On July 4, he returned to the hospital from a leave of absence complaining of abdominal distress. Soon after, he vomited a large amount of blood and passed a large bloody stool. His blood pressure quickly fell to 80/45, but his pulse rate did not exceed 100 despite the manifest clinical signs of shock. The erythrocyte count declined to 2.65 million, the hemoglobin to 8.5 gm. per 100 ml., and the packed cell volume to 26%. He received morphine, intravenous dextran solution, whole blood transfusions, and parenteral diphemanil methylsulfate (Prantal). Shock responded readily to treatment after 2000 ml. of whole blood and 2000 ml. of 6% dextran solution had been given. He was started soon on a Sippy regimen with methscopolamine (Pamine) bromide and phenobarbital given orally. A gastrointestinal series on July 11 again showed probable reflux esophagitis, with no evidence of ulceration.

Treatment with a daily dose of 400 mg. of chlorpromazine orally was started on July 29. On Sept. 22, while on both chlorpromazine and methscopolamine bromide, he developed a large fecal impaction. With some reduction in dosage of each drug, he has continued without further symptoms.

CASE 2.—This 64-year-old man with a chronic schizophrenic reaction was started on reserpine on Aug. 15, 1955. His previous health had been excellent. He received 5 mg. intramuscularly for seven days, with an oral dose of 3 mg. daily being started on Aug. 17.

On Aug. 20 he had several episodes of hematemesis, vomiting 200-300 ml. of blood each time. His blood pressure declined to 100/60, pulse rate was 80, and only mild clinical signs of shock were observed. The packed cell volume remained at 47%. He was treated with intravenous saline solution, parenteral diphemanil methylsulfate, and phenobarbital sodium. The following day he was started on a bland diet and methscopolamine bromide and phenobarbital were continued orally. No further bleeding occurred.

A gastrointestinal series on Aug. 24 showed evidence of a hiatus hernia without any ulceration, but with enlarged rugae. Reserpine was resumed on Aug. 30, at a daily dose of 1 mg., and has been continued without further adverse effects. An anticholinergic drug was continued along with the reserpine.

CASE 3.—This 62-year-old man with a chronic schizophrenic reaction was started on tranquilizing medication on Feb. 10, 1956. Except for his chronic psychosis, his general health was good. He had an episode of vomiting associated with a fecal impaction a few weeks before treatment was begun.

He was started on a preparation containing all the alkaloids of Rauwolfia serpentina with most of the reserpine removed, receiving 20 mg. three times daily by mouth. This preparation, similar to large doses of reserpine, produced a marked cutaneous flush and mucous membrane injection. He seemed to be doing well until Feb. 17, 1956, when he suddenly collapsed after having a massive hematemesis. Within a short time he passed a large amount of tarry stool and had several more hematemeses. His blood pressure became unobtainable, but the pulse rate never exceeded 100. Shock was treated with infusions of 6% dextran solution followed quickly by transfusions of whole blood. Mephentermine (Wyamine) sulfate, oxygen, phenobarbital (Luminal) sodium, and digoxin were also used. Despite the transfusion of blood under pressure through both femoral arteries, he remained in shock for 24 hours. Repeated hematemeses and massive melena occurred during this period. His blood pressure reached a borderline level on the second day, but promptly fell to shock levels with each new hematemesis or bloody stool during the next three days. Black liquid stools persisted for another five days, but no new hematemesis occurred. The erythrocyte count declined to 2.26 million, with a hemoglobin of 6 gm. per 100 ml. Blood urea nitrogen rose to 102 mg. per 100 ml. but quickly fell to normal when the bleeding ceased. Altogether, he received 10,000 ml. of whole blood before signs of hemorrhage stopped and his erythrocyte count was restored to normal.

As soon as feasible, he was started on a Sippy regimen with parenteral doses of an anticholinergic drug. A gastrointestinal series on March 1 was not satisfactory because of the presence of residual clots in the stomach. This examination was repeated on March 6, no abnormalities being found. His subsequent course has been satisfactory, without evidence of further bleeding.

CASE 4.—This 64-year-old man was admitted to the hospital on Feb. 18, 1956, because of hematemesis and melena. He had never had these symptoms before, though 25 years previously he had bled from hemorrhoids. For the past 11 months he had complained of intermittent epigastric pain, sometimes associated with vomiting. The day of admission he vomited dark liquid material, and soon after he passed a soft black stool.

He had been started on treatment for hypertension on April 4, 1955. Alseroxylon fraction of Rauwolfia serpentina was administered in daily doses of 8 mg. until July 8, 1955. At this time he was placed on a daily dose of reserpine, 0.6 mg., and hydralazine, 150 mg., which was continued until Jan. 19, 1956. On this date his medication was changed to a daily dose of reserpine, 0.5 mg., and protoveratrines A and B, 2.0 mg. He was taking this medication when he entered the hospital.

After admission (Feb. 18, 1956), he had one small hematemesis and a large soft black stool. Both specimens were strongly positive for blood. He complained of epigastric pain and tenderness, but no further evidence of bleeding was observed. His blood pressure was slightly elevated, his pulse within normal limits. Determination of the erythrocyte count was 4.72 million, the packed cell volume was 39%, and the hemoglobin, 11.5 gm. per 100 ml.

He was started on a progressive Sippy regimen, supplemented by methscopolamine bromide and phenobarbital. A gastrointestinal series on Feb. 24 showed an active duodenal ulcer. With continued treatment and discontinuation of the Rauwolfia medications, he showed symptomatic improvement. A gastrointestinal series on March 28 revealed a healed duodenal ulcer.

ADDITIONAL STUDIES ON RESERPINE AND BLOOD CLOTTING

The possibility that reserpine has some direct effect on blood clotting was raised by a report of failure of blood to clot and lengthening of the prothrombin time in patients on the drug, as well as inhibition of in vitro clotting by the addition of reserpine. To study such effects, we selected patients who had been on reserpine for two months or more and whose daily dose of the drug was 2 mg. or more.

Blood clotting and clot retraction were observed to be normal in 148 such patients. Determinations of prothrombin time were performed in 105 reserpine-treated patients and 32 control patients. The distribution of results was similar between the two groups, the lowest value for prothrombin activity in either group being 60%. The fall in prothrombin activity 48 hours after a single dose of 200 mg. of bishydroxycoumarin was compared in 21 reserpine-treated patients and 18 controls. The degrees of change were comparable between the groups and were not excessive. Capillary fragility tests were performed on 68 reserpine-treated patients. The test was negative in 56, equivocal in 10, and positive in two patients. Platelet counts in the 2 patients with positive tests and in 5 of the 10 patients with equivocal tests were normal. Bleeding and clotting times were normal in all 12 patients with equivocal or positive capillary fragility tests.

COMMENT

Each of the four patients experienced hematemesis and melena for the first time during treatment with reserpine or other alkaloids of Rauwolfia. The close time relationship between the onset of treatment and these symptoms in Cases 2 and 3 makes chance coincidence an unlikely explanation. The rather high dose of drugs used in the first three cases produced this complication early in the course of treatment, while the smaller doses of reserpine used in Case 4 did not evoke symptoms until later. The possibility of a preexisting duodenal ulcer in the latter case can not be excluded. Although reserpine was the alkaloid responsible for hematemesis and melena in three of these cases, the preparation containing all the alkaloids of Rauwolfia used in Case 3 produced a similar complication. Thus, other alkaloids of Rauwolfia besides reserpine may also produce this effect.

The most tempting explanation of these effects is to postulate the development of peptic ulceration aggravated by the drugs. However, clear-cut evidence of such ulceration occurred only in Case 4, and the possibility that such ulceration existed before treatment could not be excluded. Even without postulating the development of the usual type of peptic ulcer, the possibility remains that the combination of hypersecretion and hypermotility induced by these compounds could cause acute gastric erosions. If such erosions occurred in a mucosa which was the site of marked vasodilation, such as these drugs produce in the skin and visible mucous membranes, then massive hemorrhage might occur. Gastroscopic studies of the appearance of the stomach mucosa after use of these drugs would be most helpful in explaining such a possible mechanism.

A remote possibility exists that hematemesis and melena could be the result of some systemic disorder of blood clotting induced by these drugs. The absence of any other clinical evidence of bleeding in these patients makes such an explanation unlikely. Our own studies and others of which we are aware have failed to show any evident or consistent change in blood clotting of patients treated with large doses of reserpine for prolonged periods. The discovery that reserpine increases the excretion of a serotonin metabolite raises the possibility that some qualitative change in blood platelets might occur due to serotonin depletion. Here, too, one would expect that widespread systemic hemorrhage would be present. So far, the available evidence suggests that hematemesis and melena are due to local changes in the gastrointestinal mucosa rather than a disorder of blood coagulation.

The complication of hematemesis and melena during treatment with alkaloids of Rauwolfia serpentina is unusual enough to make this risk worth taking if the clinical indications for these drugs are strong enough. In patients with known ulcerative disease of the gastrointestinal tract or hemorrhagic diatheses, it would appear that these compounds are contraindicated unless closely covered by other treatment or laboratory control. Patients under treatment with large doses of these drugs for prolonged periods of time should be observed closely for any symptoms suggesting the development or activation of peptic ulcer.

Summary

Four cases of hematemesis and melena are reported which occurred during treatment with alkaloids of Rauwolfia serpentina. The lack of antecedent gastrointestinal hemorrhages and the close time relationship of these symptoms to the use of these drugs makes a causal relationship likely. Although reserpine may cause exacerbation of duodenal ulcer, frank ulceration was found by roentgenologic examination in only one of these patients. The hypermotility, hypersecretion, and vascular dilatation of the gastric mucosa produced by these drugs are thought to cause small gastric erosions which may bleed profusely. No evidence was found that these drugs cause a disorder of blood clotting. Gastrointestinal ulceration or hemorrhagic diathesis are contraindications to the use of these preparations unless the clinical indication is sufficiently great and close observation is possible.

Since submission of this paper for publication, the following report of a similar complication has also appeared: Dillon, D., and Swain, J. M.: Gastro-Intestinal Hemorrhage as a Complication of Reserpine Administration: Report of 2 Cases, *Am. J. Psychiat.* 113:462 (Nov.) 1956.

AGRANULOCYTOSIS WHILE RECEIVING COMBINED RESERPINE-CHLORPROMAZINE THERAPY

Joseph A. Barsa, M.D., and Nathan S. Kline, M.D.
Rockland State Hospital, Orangeburg, New York

It has been known previously that chlorpromazine potentiated the effects of hypnotics and sedatives. Because of this, we decided to investigate the effect of combining reserpine and chlorpromazine. At first only those cases which failed to respond to reserpine alone were given the combined medication. It was soon learned that chlorpromazine definitely potentiated the clinical effects of reserpine. Early results were so encouraging that a much larger group of patients was placed on this combined therapy. A report of the therapy has appeared elsewhere. The general dosage schedule used was as follows:

The patient was started on 3 mg. reserpine and 25 mg. chlorpromazine orally once a day. After about ten days the chlorpromazine was increased to 25 mg. twice a day. At the end of three to four weeks, if the patient was not showing satisfactory progress, the dose of chlorpromazine was increased to 50 mg. twice a day, reserpine remaining at 3 mg. daily. After another three to four weeks, if the patient's therapeutic progress was still unsatisfactory, 5 mg. reserpine intramuscularly was added to the oral regimen. This was continued for ten days. If the patient then showed signs of responding to therapy, intramuscular medication was gradually withdrawn, but the oral medication remained unchanged until the close of therapy. If, however, after ten days of intramuscular injections, the patient was not showing an adequate therapeutic response, the intramuscular dose was raised to 10 mg. and was continued until the response was adequate; then intramuscular injections were gradually withdrawn, leaving only the oral medication. A course of therapy lasted a minimum of three months.

If at the outset the patient was extremely disturbed, and an early quieting effect was necessary, the patient was started on 5 mg. reserpine intramuscularly, and 3 mg. reserpine and 25 mg. chlorpromazine orally once a day. After ten days the chlorpromazine was increased to twice a day, and, if the patient's progress was satisfactory, the intramuscular injections were gradually withdrawn. However, if progress was still not satisfactory, the injections were continued for another ten days. Then, if necessary, the intramuscular dose was raised to 10 mg. After improvement was sufficient to discontinue this initial course of intramuscular reserpine injections, the subsequent dosage regimen was the same as outlined in the preceding paragraph.

The purpose of this paper is to report two cases of agranulocytosis occurring while the patients were receiving combined reserpine-chlorpromazine therapy. These two cases were from a group of 303 female patients who had received the combined medication for three to seven months.

CASE REPORTS

M. S. is a 40 year old, married, white female. She has a diagnosis of Dementia Praecox, Paranoid type, and has been continuously hospitalized since 1942. At the time of her admission the patient was seclusive, withdrawn, preoccupied, delusional and hallucinated, with periods of abusive, assaultive and destructive behavior. Her general physical condition was satisfactory except for some evidence of malnutrition. Despite a course of twenty electroconvulsive treatments in 1947, the patient's mental state gradually deteriorated, and her disturbed periods became more frequent. She was uncooperative, resistive, destructive to her clothing, noisy, abusive and impulsively assaultive. She was started on reserpine therapy on August 13, 1954, receiving 5 mg. intramuscularly and 3 mg. orally once a day for the first ten days, and then receiving a daily maintenance dose of 3 mg. orally. She showed a moderate improvement, becoming clean, neat, cooperative, quiet, but remaining idle, seclusive, apathetic and hallucinated. In an effort to raise her level of improvement she was started on combined reserpine-chlorpromazine therapy on December 29. In addition to the oral dose of 3 mg. reserpine, she received 25 mg. chlorpromazine daily for the first twelve days. Then the chlorpromazine was increased to 25 mg. twice a day. Because she was not showing satisfactory improvement, the chlorpromazine dose was raised to 50 mg. twice a day on February 14. A few days later she complained of not feeling well physically, although there was no complaint referable to a specific organ. Physical examination at this time was negative. On February 24 she complained of a sore throat and suddenly spiked a temperature of 104°. On examination there was evidence of a moderate follicular tonsillitis. Blood count was as follows: hemoglobin 9 gms. per 100 cc., RBC 3,910,000 per cubic millimeter, WBC 2,000 per cubic millimeter; her differential showed 91% lymphocytes, 4% prolymphocytes, 5% segmented neutrophils. Reserpine and chlorpromazine therapy was immediately discontinued. On February 25 the WBC was 1,400 per cubic millimeter and the differential count revealed 100% lymphocytes. The platelets numbered 66,000 per cubic millimeter. Bone marrow examination showed islands of normoblasts, very few granulocyte precursors and an occasional increase in reticulo-endothelial cells. The patient was treated with procaine penicillin 300,000 units b.i.d., streptomycin 0.5 gm. b.i.d. and cortisone 100 mg. daily. On February 26 the patient's temperature was normal, and it remained so. However, it was not until March 4 that granulocytes reappeared in the peripheral blood. Blood count at that time was as follows: hemoglobin 11 gms. per 100 cc., RBC 3,530,000 per cubic millimeter, WBC 5,800 per cubic millimeter; differential 51% lymphocytes, 4% monocytes, 13% segmented neutrophils, 15% non-segmented neutrophils. In the next few days the patient developed a leucocytosis, and on March 8 her WBC was 24,800 with the following differential: 38% lymphocytes, 29% non-segmented neutrophils, 18% segmented neutrophils, 3% monocytes, 3% myelocytes, 9% metamyelocytes. Her blood count then began to return to normal gradually. On March 16 her WBC was 7,750 per cubic millimeter; her differential showed 37% segmented neutrophils, 58% lymphocytes, 2% monocytes, 3% basophils. On March 17 cortisone and antibiotic medication were discontinued. On April 22 her WBC was 8,000 per cubic millimeter with 63% segmented neutrophils, 1% non-segmented neutrophils, 35% lymphocytes and 1% eosinophils.

V. O. is a 40 year old, single, white female. She has a diagnosis of Psychosis with Mental Deficiency, and has been continuously hospitalized since 1943. At the time of her admission she was described as seclusive, childish, emotionally unstable, at times silly, at times apprehensive, and at other times extremely irritable, displaying temper tantrums in which she became self-abusive and assaultive. She expressed paranoid delusions and seemed to be reacting to auditory hallucinations. Her I.Q. was measured as 61. Through the years at the hospital her mental state deteriorated somewhat; she became completely idle, rather untidy, more withdrawn, and quite disconnected in her speech. On January 4, 1955, she was started on combined reserpine-chlorpromazine therapy. She received 3 mg. reserpine and 25 mg. chlorpromazine once a day for the first eight days. Then the chlorpromazine was increased to 25 mg. twice a day. She showed no improvement in her mental symptoms, and on February 14 the dose of chlorpromazine was raised to 50 mg. twice a day, the reserpine dose remaining at 3 mg. daily. On February 21 she complained of generalized aches and pains, a sore throat and diarrhea. Her temperature was 102°. On examination pharynx and tonsils were moderately infected, and the cervical lymph nodes were palpably enlarged and tender. Later that afternoon the temperature rose to 104.6°. The patient was given procaine penicillin 600,000 units daily, and aureomycin 250 mg. four times a day. The temperature fell to 100°, but spiked to 103° on the next afternoon. The following day it again dropped in the morning, and rose to 102.6° in the afternoon. On February 25 examination of the throat revealed the presence of a grayish pseudomembrane over both tonsils. A blood count at this time was as follows: hemoglobin 11 gms. per 100 cc., RBC 3,220,000 per cubic millimeter, WBC 900 per cubic millimeter; differential 2% prolymphocytes, 98% lymphocytes. Reserpine-chlorpromazine therapy was immediately discontinued, and the patient was placed on the following medication: procaine penicillin 300,000 units twice a day, streptomycin 0.5 gm. twice a day and cortisone 100 mg. daily. The next day the temperature was 99.6°, and her WBC was 1,100 per cubic millimeter with 3% prolymphocytes, 95% lymphocytes and 2% segmented neutrophils; platelets numbered 206,000 per cubic millimeter. Bone marrow examination revealed diminished erythroid elements, diminished granulopoiesis, and an occasional plasma cell. Subsequent blood count revealed the presence of more and more granulocytes. On March 4 her WBC was 7,950 per cubic millimeter with 54% lymphocytes, 2% monocytes, 8% metamyelocytes, 30% segmented neutrophils and 6% non-segmented neutrophils. In the next few days the patient developed a leucocytosis. On March 11 her WBC was 18,100 per cubic millimeter with 9% non-segmented neutrophils, 78% segmented neutrophils, 11% lymphocytes and 2% monocytes. The blood count gradually returned to normal, and on April 4 it was as follows: hemoglobin 12 gms. per

100 cc., RBC 3,830,000 per cubic millimeter, WBC 6,300 per cubic millimeter; differential 3% non-segmented neutrophils, 61% segmented neutrophils, 33% lymphocytes and 3% monocytes.

COMMENT

Reserpine has been used extensively, and, to our knowledge, there have been no reported cases of agranulocytosis due to the drug. However, there have been several instances of agranulocytosis in patients receiving chlorpromazine therapy. It can be assumed, therefore, that the agranulocytosis in our two cases was due to the chlorpromazine. Furthermore, the development of agranulocytosis does not seem to depend on the dosage of chlorpromazine, since we usesd relatively small doses of the drug.

We have reported these two cases of agranulocytosis not to discourage the use of combined reserpine-chlorpromazine therapy, but rather to call attention to a serious toxic effect so that it may be guarded against. We feel that this combined therapy is especially effective in psychotic states, and that it has certain advantages over reserpine when used alone. The chlorpromazine seems to have a definite potentiating effect on reserpine. Many cases that do not respond adequately to reserpine alone, do respond to the combined therapy. In the majority of instances it is possible to achieve satisfactory results without the use of intramuscular injections. Furthermore, the clinical course in combined therapy is less stormy and less distressing to the patient than with reserpine alone.

JAUNDICE CAUSED BY CHLORPROMAZINE (THORAZINE)

Lawrence R. Loftus, M.D., Kenneth A. Huizenga, M.D., Maurice H. Stauffer, M.D., Howard P. Rome, M.D., and James C. Cain, M.D..

Mayo Clinic and Mayo Foundation, Rochester, Minnesota

Chlorpromazine [10 - (y-dimethylaminopropyl)-2-chlorophenothiazine hydrochloride], better known in this country under the trade name of Thorazine, became available for general use by the American medical profession in May, 1954. It was first synthesized in France in 1951. In France it is known as Largactil; while it was being used experimentally in this country it was known as SKF 2601-A. It has been used in the symptomatic treatment of alcoholism, barbiturate intoxication and withdrawal symptoms, bronchial asthma, delirium tremens, emesis, epilepsy, hiccups, hypothermic anesthesia, hypertension, Meniere's disease, peripheral vascular disease, paralysis agitans (Parkinson's disease), pruritus, psychomotor tension incident to psychotic and psychoneurotic reaction types, and seasickness.

Among other side-effects of the drug jaundice has been described; however, only Moyer and his associates have described this type of jaundice in detail. They had one patient in a series of more than 500 patients treated with chlorpromazine. Winkleman performed a biopsy of the liver in one such case but was handicapped by the fact that underlying chronic disease of that organ obscured any acute changes referable to the agent. Recently we observed four patients in whom jaundice developed while they were receiving chlorpromazine as part of the symptomatic management of anxiety and psychomotor tension. Needle biopsy of the liver of one of these patients had been performed.

REPORT OF CASES

CASE 1.—A 48-year-old white man, manager of a grocery store, was admitted to the clinic on Sept. 5 1954, with jaundice of 16 days' duration. Previously he had been seen in July, 1954, when the diagnoses of mild essential hypertension and anxiety state were established, Rauwolfia serpentina had been prescribed; it had produced the undesirable symptom of drowsiness. Use of this agent had been stopped on the third day, and 25 mg. of chlorpromazine and 5 cc. of a sedative agent, such as elixir of aprobarbital (Alurate), were each given three times daily, starting July 20, 1954. The patient returned to his home and continued to receive regular doses of chlorpromazine and elixir of aprobarbital for 25 days. At that time the onset of a mild sore throat, chilly sensations, anorexia, and malaise were noted. There was no nausea, vomiting, or diarrhea. The temperature was not taken. Doses of chlorpromazine and aprobarbital were stopped at this time. The sore throat subsided by the next morning, but the other symptoms persisted. Two days later, on Aug 18, 1954, dark urine, clay-colored stools, and mild pruritus were noted. He visited his local physician on Aug. 20, 1954, at which time clinical jaundice was noted. The patient began to feel better and regained his appetite after two days in the hospital. The jaundice, however, did not abate. Tests of hepatic function did not suggest a diagnosis of infectious hepatitis. Biopsy of the liver was done on Sept. 1, 1954, and the results were reported as indicative of obstructive jaundice. Abdominal exploration was considered, but the patient decided to return to the clinic for further studies. On Sept. 2, 1954, the urine became lighter, and dark stools were noted for the first time in two weeks.

Physical examination at the clinic showed this patient to be apprehensive and moderately jaundiced but not acutely ill. Temperature was 98.4 F, and the blood pressure was 150 mm. Hg systolic and 100 mm. Hg distolic in both arms. There was a 1 by 1 cm. firm, nontender node in each axilla. The edge of the liver was palpable 2 cm. below the right costal margin with inspiration and was sharp and nontender. Results of the physical examination otherwise were normal.

The value for hemoglobin and the results of leukocyte counts, differential counts, urinalysis, and a roentgenogram of the thorax were normal. Serum bilirubin amounted to 5.2 mg. per 100 cc., with 4.0 mg. direct reacting and 1.2 mg. indirect. Alkaline phosphatase was 47 King-Armstrong units per 100 cc. of serum. Prothrombin time was 18 seconds (normal: 17 to 19 seconds). The value for cholesterol was 264 mg. per 100 cc. of plasma, and cholesterol esters amounted to 167 mg. per 100 cc. of plasma. The result of a thymol turbidity test was zero. A cephalin-cholesterol flocculation test gave a negative result at 48 hours. The value for blood urea was 32 mg. per 100 cc. Heterophil agglutination was 1:32. Roentgenograms showed a normal esophagus, stomach, and duodenum. A roentgenogram of the gallbladder was attempted on Sept. 10, when the value for bilirubin was 4.0 mg. per 100 cc. of serum, but the dye did not concentrate sufficiently to permit visualization. The procedure was repeated on Sept. 16, when the value for bilirubin was 2.4 mg. per 100 cc. of serum and was reported as indicating a "poorly functioning gallbladder." It was repeated again on Sept. 20, when the value for total bilirubin was 2.1 mg. per 100 cc. and was reported as indicating a "poorly functioning gallbladder with no evidence of stones."

A section of the liver obtained from the patient's local physician was studied, and it was reported as showing "bile stasis, particularly in relation to central vein areas. The picture is compatible with extrahepatic obstruction of the bile duct." The patient was put at rest in bed, and a high caloric diet was prescribed, with multivitamin capsules and vitamin K as supplements. He ate well and continued to feel well. The jaundice gradually cleared, and the patient was dismissed to return home on Sept. 21, 1954. At this time the value for total bilirubin was 2.1 mg. per 100 cc. of serum and for alkaline phosphatase, 32 King-Armstrong units per 100 cc. of serum.

CASE 2.—A 38-year-old single, white, woman schoolteacher was admitted on July 14, 1954, complaining of jaundice that had been present for a month. A course of chlorpromazine, 50 mg. daily, had been prescribed by her local physician on May 28, because of complaints of fleeting pains in the chest and chronic fatigue of 10 months' duration. Chlorpromazine had been taken for eight days, or until June 6. At that time, when a total of 0.4 gm. of the agent had been ingested, "flu-like" symptoms of chills, temperature as high as 103°F and malaise developed. The use of the drug was stopped, but the symptoms persisted for three days. At that time, anorexia was noted. It continued to a mild degree until the patient was seen here in consultation. On June 11, 1954, six days after the onset of symptoms, mild pruritus developed, and on the following day dark urine and light-colored stools were noted. On June 14, eight days after onset of the illness, jaundice was evident. The only other sign was slight tenderness in the right upper quadrant of the abdomen. Her local physician reported the van den Bergh reaction as direct; the total bilirubin content was 11.75 mg. per 100 cc. of serum. A low fat diet was prescribed, and the patient was advised to rest in bed. The jaundice did not remit, and the patient was referred to the Mayo Clinic.

Physical examination showed her to be a rather deeply jaundiced, moderately obese woman; otherwise, the results of the examination were essentially normal. Values for hemoglobin and results of an erythrocyte count, leukocyte count, differential count, urinalysis, and roentgenogram of the thorax were within a normal range. Serologic tests of the blood showed it to be normal. The concentration of serum bilirubin was 17.7 mg. per 100 cc.; in the direct test the value was 14.4 mg., and in the indirect, 3.4 mg. Cholesterol amounted to 260 mg. per 100 cc. of plasma. Cholesterol esters were recorded as 177 mg. per 100 cc. The prothrombin time was 20 seconds. Result of thymol turbidity test was expressed as 1 unit. Reaction of a cephalin-cholesterol flocculation test was negative at 48 hours. Alkaline phosphatase amounted to 35 King-Armstrong units, and total proteins, 6.4 gm. per 100 cc. of serum, 3.5 gm. of albumin, and 2.9 gm. of globulin. Gastrointestinal roentgenograms revealed a normal esophagus, stomach, and duodenum. No bile was obtained by duodenal intubation on July 19, but when intubation was repeated on July 22, yellow bile was obtained.

A regimen of rest in bed, high caloric diet, multivitamin capsules, vitamin K, and brewer's yeast was prescribed. On the 13th hospital day the patient felt well and the jaundice was less intense. The value for bilirubin had decreased to 8.5 mg. per 100 cc. of serum. The patient was dismissed from the hospital and advised to follow the same regimen until her jaundice completely disappeared. At that time it was suggested that she gradually resume her full duties. Three months after the onset of the jaundice, the value for serum bilirubin was normal, and a roentgenogram of the gallbladder showed it to be functioning normally.

CASE 3.—A 48-year-old white man admitted on July 13, 1954, complaining of jaundice of one day's duration. This patient had been seen at the clinic on five previous occasions, at which times the diagnoses of psychoneurosis and moderate essential hypertension had been made. He had been given 25 mg.

of a Rauwolfia derivative, reserpine (Serpasil), four times a day and 5 mg. of a hypotensive agent cryptenamine (Unitensen) acetate four times a day for about four months. On June 18, 1954, the patient had been given 25 mg. of chlorpromazine three times a day in an effort to palliate the symptoms. On July 11 dark urine and light-colored stools were noted. On July 12 he visited his local physician, who discovered scleral icterus and noted bile in the urine. No other symptoms were present. The next day chlorpromazine therapy was stopped, and the patient returned to the clinic.

Physical examination revealed the blood pressure to be 212 mm. Hg systolic and 108 mm. Hg diastolic. The scleras were icteric. On deep inspiration the liver was palpable 3 cm. below the right costal margin and was slightly tender. Otherwise, results of the physical examination were essentially normal. The value for hemoglobin and results of a leukocyte count, differential count, urinalysis and a roentgenogram of the thorax were within normal limits. The concentration of bilirubin was 3.5 mg. per 100 cc. of serum, with values of 2.5 mg. for the direct van den Bergh test and 1.0 mg. for the indirect test. Cholestervol amounted to 234 mg. per 100 cc. of plasma. The content of alkaline phosphatase was recorded as 119 King-Armstrong units. Prothrombin time was 21 seconds. Results of a thymol turbidity test were expressed as 2.5 units. Reaction of a cephalin-cholesterol flocculation test was negative at 48 hours.

The patient was put as rest in bed, a general diet was prescribed, and the use of all medicaments was stopped. He remained asymptomatic. By July 17, the scleral icterus had cleared. On July 21, the result of the direct test for bilirubin was negative, while the indirect test gave the value of 1.1 mg. of bilirubin per 100 cc. of serum, although the value for alkaline phosphatase was still 90 King-Armstrong units. On July 27 the content of bilirubin in the serum was normal, the value for alkaline phosphatase was reduced to 49 King-Armstrong units, and a sulfobromophthalein test showed no retention of dye at 60 minutes. The patient was dismissed from the hospital the next day.

CASE 4.—A 43-year-old housewife was admitted to the clinic on June 30, 1954, complaining of jaundice of eight days' duration. Chlorpromazine had been prescribed by her local physician on June 10, 1954, for chronic fatigue. Doses of 25 to 75 mg. of chlorpromazine had been taken daily for 10 days. On June 19 the patient awoke with malaise, chills, and a temperature as high as 100°F. The later persisted for two days and was followed by nausea, vomiting, dark urine, light-colored stools, and transient pruritus, at which time the physician noted clinical jaundice. During the next week the symptoms abated, but the jaundice persisted. It could not be established that the patient had been in contact with other victims of jaundice. Physical examination revealed moderate jaundice and tenderness in the right upper quadrant of the abdomen, but otherwise the patient's condition was normal.

The value for hemoglobin and results of an erythrocyte count, leucocyte count, differential peripheral blood-smear count, roentgenogram of the thorax, prothrombin time, thymol turbidity test, zinc sulfate turbidity, cephalin-cholesterol flocculation test, values for cholesterol and cholesterol esters, and heterophil antibody titer all were within normal limits. Clear, yellow bile was obtained on duodenal intubation. Bile was present in the urine. On July 1, 1954, the content of total serum bilirubin was 5.5 mg. per 100 cc., with the figure of 4.2 mg. from the direct test and that of 1.3 mg. from the indirect test. The value alkaline phosphatase was 27 King-Armstrong units. On July 9, a roentgenogram of the gallbladder revealed a normally functioning organ without stones. The jaundice had subsided clinically. In a letter written on Sept. 4, 1954, the patient's physician stated that she had remained asymptomatic.

Comment

The four cases presented in this paper appear to represent examples of jaundice caused by chlorpromazine. The medical department of the manufacturer of chlorpromazine states:

"Characteristically the patient in whom jaundice has been reported has been taking Thorazine without unusual side effects for a week or more, at which time an abrupt onset of temperature elevation may occur with mild grippe-like symptoms. This may be accompanied by mild abdominal distress and sometimes changes in bowel habits. Nausea and occasionally vomiting may occur even though Thorazine controlled these symptoms originally. Several days later jaundice becomes apparent, frequently accompanied by pruritus, dark urine, and clay colored stools. There may or may not be hepatic tenderness. During the period of jaundice the patient is seldom seriously ill. The jaundice lasts approximately three weeks with considerable variations of duration in individual cases. Biochemical tests of liver function are typical of those seen with obstructive jaundice. Histopathological examination of liver biopsy section reveals a characteristic picture of cholestasis in the biliary canaliculi with varying degrees of inflammatory infiltration. After clinical recovery, biochemical tests, including BSP and liver biopsies when done, have shown no evidence of residual hepatic damage."

In cases 1, 2, and 4 the onset and clinical course were suggestive of an acute viral hepatitis. This was particularly true of the patient who had chills and a temperature of up to 103 F. The laboratory features were those generally seen in obstructive jaundice, although occasionally similar findings are observed in viral hepatitis. The patient in case 3 was entirely asymptomatic, and the laboratory findings were similar to those in the other three cases. Therapy with chlorpromazine is the common factor in each instance, and it would seem unlikely that these four patients had atypical viral hepatitis. The biopsy findings in case 1 constitute partial evidence that the disease was not viral hepatitis. The incidence of jaundice occurring during treatment with chlorpromazine is difficult to determine. It has been noted in as many as 3 out of 71 patients treated in one series, and in as few as 1 among 506 patients treated in another series.

Two deaths have been reported during chlorpromazine therapy. Death occurred on the fourth day of treatment for delirium tremens in a seriously ill patient who had severe cirrhosis of the liver. It is not disclosed whether the patient was jaundiced, and no necropsy findings are given. It seems unlikely that this death was related to the chlorpromazine therapy. Boardman reported the death of an institutionalized psychotic patient receiving 500 mg. of chlorpromazine daily. Necropsy revealed mitral stenosis, chronic congestive failure, and "toxic hepatitis." At the time of death there were three instances of infectious hapatitis in the institution in patients on receiving chlorpromazine. Again, we are unable to determine if this death was related to the chlorpromazine. One author wrote that in about half of his patients treated with chlorpromazine there were slight changes in the results of cephalin-cholesterol flocculation tests and that 30% showed minor changes in the values for total serum protein and in the albumin-globulin ratio. Another author found the results of the sulfobromophthalein test "positive" in 10% of his patients treated. Most observers agree that they have found no evidence of abnormal results of these tests in their series.

Moyer used chlorpromazine in the treatment of several patients who had disease of the liver prior to receiving the drug. None of these showed any evidence of progressive hepatic dysfunction; however, some of these patients with preexisting disease of the liver exhibited increased responsiveness to chlorpromazine. Several authors have reinstituted chlorpromazine therapy after the icterus cleared in patients among whom jaundice had developed while they were taking chlorpromazine. In this limited number of cases, the chlorpromazine was tolerated without recurrence of jaundice.

In our experience with jaundice that occurs during treatment with chlorpromazine, results of the hepatic function tests are similar to those obtained among most patients with extrahepatic obstructive jaundice. There is elevation of the values for serum bilirubin and alkaline phosphatase. Bile is present in the urine. There do not appear to be significant abnormalities in the results of the cephalin-cholesterol flocculation procedure, the thymol turbidity test, or the zinic sulfate turbidity or values for serum proteins. This type of jaundice responds to a therapeutic regimen such as that prescribed in the treatment of viral hepatitis; that is, restricted activity, high caloric diet, and supplemental vitamins. Of course, the use of chlorpromazine, the presumed inciting factor, should be discontinued. There does not appear to be measurable evidence of hepatocellular damage during the course of treatment. The jaundice may persist from a few days to as long as several weeks. In case 2 the jaundice persisted for about three months. In all of these respects the jaundice that may occur as a result of treatment with chlorpromazine is similar to that that may occur incident to the administration of methyltestosterone. The microscopic picture seen from biopsy of the liver, with heavy concentrations of bile in the small canaliculi, appears alike in the two conditions.

The importance of jaundice caused by chlorpromazine lies neither in its incidence nor in the possibility of permanent hepatic damage. Rather, the importance resides in the nature of a warning: physicians who prescribe the use of chlorpromazine should be advised that jaundice may occur during this type of therapy and they should note that while the laboratory findings may be those usually associated with extrahepatic biliary obstruction, extreme caution should be exercised before surgical intervention is recommended.

Summary

In four patients in whom jaundice occurred during therapy with chlorpromazine [10-(y-dimethylaminopropyl)-2-chlorophenothiazine hydrochloride] biopsy of the liver was performed in one case. The typical picture and laboratory findings are similar to those of jaundice occurring from treatment with methyl testosterone. Thorough consideration should be given before surgical treatment is advised for a patient in whom jaundice develops during therapy with chlorpromazine.

Addendum

We have encountered 10 additional patients with jaundice occurring during the course of administration of chlorpromazine. The condition of these patients followed the same pattern outlined in this paper and will be the subject of a further report.

LIVER FUNCTION AND HEPATIC COMPLICATIONS IN PATIENTS RECEIVING CHLORPROMAZINE

Irvin M. Cohen, M.D., and John D. Archer, M.D.
Department of Neurology and Psychiatry and Pharmacology, University of Texas Medical Branch, Galveston, Texas

The use of chlorpromazine [Thorazine, 10-(y-dimethylaminopropyl)-2-chlorophenothiazine hydrochloride] is occasionally complicated by the development of jaundice. In our series of over 800 patients treated with this drug, 5 such cases have occurred. Results of laboratory studies in these instances have consistently indicated an obstructive process within the biliary system. The complication has proved to be benign, the ensuing clinical courses being characterized by rapid resolution of symptoms and uneventful recovery. Though this side-reaction occurred only rarely and was apparently confined to the bile passages, we believed that the possibility of damage to the liver cells demanded further investigation. Of particular concern to us was the question of whether patients receiving the drug over relatively long periods of time sustained subclinical liver damage. The presence of the phenothiazine nucleus in chlorpromazine further suggested the need for this determination, since phenothiazine itself, in sufficient high dosage, has been reported to produce liver disease.

The aim of the study, therefore, was to ascertain (1) whether chlorpromazine represented a highly specific hepatotoxin and, if so, the site of damage, or (2) whether liver involvement was simply a random effect that could be expected to occur in a certain number of patients hypersensitive to the drug. Though definitive conclusions must await further study, the results that follow represent impressions derived from a preliminary investigation of these questions.

MATERIAL

The study included a total of 89 patients, all of whom were being treated for psychiatric illnesses of various clinical types. In no case was there a history of liver disease, and physical examinations had revealed no findings of contributory significance. For purposes of this report the patients are divided into three groups. Group 1 consists of five cases in which clinically evident jaundice developed. Table 1 shows age and sex distribution, diagnosis, the presence or absence of allergic history, and other complications that developed during the course of therapy. Table 2 shows duration of administration of chlorpromazine prior to appearance of icterus; minimum, maximum, and average doses that had been given; and route of administration. Group 2 consists of 14 patients

TABLE 1.—*Descriptive Data on Patients Developing Jaundice During Chlorpromazine Therapy*

Case	Age, Yr.	Sex	Diagnosis	Allergic History	Associated Complications
1	21	F	Hysterical character	....	......
2	22	M	Situational reaction	Yes	Rash
3	30	M	Phobic neurosis	....	......
4	34	F	Chronic schizophrenia	Yes	Rash
5	43	M	Chronic schizophrenia	?	......

TABLE 2.—*Therapeutic Regimen in Patients Developing Jaundice During Chlorpromazine Therapy*

Case	Duration of Therapy,* Days	Dose per Day, Mg. Minimum	Maximum	Average	Route of Administration
1	8	200	300	210	Oral
2	17	100	200	123	Oral
3	21	150	200	160	Oral
4	22	150	1,000	660	Oral-I.M.
5	20	200	800	320	Oral-I.M.

* Prior to development of icterus.

who were subjected to an extensive battery of liver function studies prior to and during the administration of a generally constant dose of chlorpromazine for periods of time varying from two to six weeks. Group 3 consists of 70 cases in which less extensive liver function studies were done prior to and during treatment. Dosage and duration of administration varied widely in this group.

METHOD

Group 1.—Pretreatment liver function studies had been obtained in three of the five patients in whom jaundice subsequently developed; all had been reported as being normal. In one case the control study had revealed spotty but minimal evidence of hepatic disease. Chlorpromazine was then instituted at low dosage levels and increased progressively as the case warranted. Maximum daily dosage ranged from 100 to 1,000 mg. Use of the drug was immediately discontinued when jaundice became apparent, and serial laboratory tests were done frequently thereafter. These included quantitative van den Bergh determinations, serum alkaline phosphatase, blood cholesterol, urine bilirubin and urobilinogen, cephalin-cholesterol flocculation, thymol turbidity, total serum proteins with albumin-globulin ratio, prothrombin time, and sulfobromophthalein (Bromsulphalein) retention. All tests listed were not done in all patients.

Group 2.—In group 2, 14 patients were given chlorpromazine for varying periods that averaged more than one month. Ten received 25 mg. orally three times a day; four received doses that varied from 25 to 100 mg. given two to four times a day. To detect any possible early biliary obstruction or change in hepatocellular function, the patients were followed at regular intervals with tests of liver function. Typically, these tests consisted of (1) thymol turbidity determinations twice weekly, (2) 48-hour cephalin-cholesterol flocculation determinations twice weekly, (3) direct serum bilirubin determinations twice weekly, (4) urinary bilirubin and urobilinogen determinations three times weekly, and (5) a determination of sulfobromophthalein retention once before or near the beginning of chlorpromazine therapy and at least once after or near the end of therapy. Occasional exceptions to this procedure occurred, most of which were in the nature of laboratory or nursing errors, but these exceptions were taken into consideration in the evaluation of the results. Two pretreatment control studies were obtained in 10 of the 14 patients, one control study was obtained in one patient, and no pretreatment controls were done in the remaining three patients.

Group 3.—The third group, 70 patients, received chlorpromazine for varying periods of time and in varying dosage totals. The average duration was one month, with a range of one week to five months. Dosage ranged from 100 to 1,000 mg. daily. The usual procedure was to initiate therapy at a dose of 25 mg. four times a day, after which it was increased to therapeutically effective levels and then reduced. The average maximum reached was 800 mg. daily. Pretreatment controls were obtained in each case and consisted of tests for serum bilirubin, cephalin-cholesterol flocculation, and total serum proteins with albumin-globulin ratio. If there was suggestive evidence of any abnormality, further tests were done, which included sulfobromophthalein retention and thymol turbidity tests. Thereafter serum bilirubin determinations were done weekly on all patients. In the event of a rise in serum bilirubin level, more extensive tests followed.

Results

Jaundice.—The occurrence of jaundice was erratic, appearing sporadically in relatively widespread areas and at various times. An infectious factor was thought to be of little probability. There was no correlation among the factors of age, sex, and diagnosis. The total daily dose did not appear to be a significant factor. The route of administration was usually oral; two of the patients had received the drug intramuscularly during the early phases of treatment. One factor that may be of significance was noted in two of the five cases. In both there was a definite history of allergic skin reactions; both patients developed dermatitis and jaundice during the course of chlorpromazine therapy.

In the majority of cases icterus appeared approximately three weeks after chlorpromazine therapy had been instituted. With the exception of one patient in whom there was a generalized maculopapular eruption, no unusual sidereactions had previously occurred. Premonitory symptoms of the jaundice were generally very mild; the patients, though experiencing general malaise, were in no great distress. In several instances if icterus had not appeared the complication might have escaped detection, for often the complaints were at first attributed to the psychiatric condition. Symptoms usually consisted of persistent or intermittent nausea, vague abdominal pain, and occasionally vomiting. In three patients there was sudden elevation of temperature, which ranged from 100 to 102 F. One patient simultaneously developed a generalized urticaria. Generally these symptoms preceded the appearance of icterus by three to five days, although in one patient there was a two week lag and in another there were no prodromal signs.

The succeeding clinical course in each case was uneventful, disturbing symptoms disappearing within several days, icterus clearing within two to three weeks. Treatment was of a supportive nature, consisting mainly of withdrawal of the drug, intravenously administered glucose when indicated, therapeutic vitamin regimen, and high carbohydrate—high protein—low fat diet. Laboratory findings were characteristically those of obstructive jaundice, with hyperbilirubinemia, elevated serum alkaline phosphatase level and bilirubinuria. Cellular function did not appear to be impaired as determined by cephalin-cholesterol flocculation, thymol turbidity, and total serum proteins with albumin-globulin ratio. Unfortunately, in only one case was prothrombin time obtained; in this instance it was 100% of normal. Chlorpromazine therapy was later reinstituted in one patient who had previously developed both dermatitis and jaundice while taking a total daily dose of 1,000 mg. Neither complication recurred, and liver function tests remained normal.

Hepatotoxic Studies.—There was no evidence that hepatotoxic effects were occurring in the 84 patients studied for possible change in hepatocellular function. In the series of 14 patients who were closely followed by means of comprehensive batteries of liver function tests, there was no clinical or laboratory evidence of development of hepatic dysfunction. Bile excretion, as indicated by determinations of serum bilirubin, urinary bilirubin, and urinary urobilinogen, was not disturbed. Cellular function was likewise not impaired. Isolated increases in cephalin-cholesterol flocculation to abnormal levels (2+ to 3+) occurred during the course of treatment of four of the patients; however, the remainder of their tests were normal, and we were confident that they were experiencing no hepatocellular damage from therapy. Thymol turbidity units varied greatly, although variations generally remained within normal limits. The averages between the control studies and the studies during treatment were in most cases remarkably consistent. Only two patients ever showed thymol turbidity values greater than the normal 5 units. In one values ranged from 4 to 10 units. The mean before treatment had been 5.0; the mean during treatment was 6.2. In the other case a single elevation occurred 23 days after treatment had begun, but subsequent determinations were consistently within normal limits. In both these cases the possibility of liver involvement was discounted on the basis that all other tests remained normal. In the group of 70 patients in whom less extensive liver function studies were done, no changes of significance occurred. Serum bilirubin levels remained normal throughout the duration of therapy in all but three patients. Each of the latter showed a single elevation during the course of therapy, but more extensive batteries failed to corroborate this finding.

COMMENT

On the basis of results obtained in this study it would appear that under ordinary circumstances chlorpromazine does not interfere with normal liver function. There is furthermore no evidence that the drug is injurious to the liver cells, even on prolonged administration. This report has necessarily included only patients who were followed by serial tests of hepatic function. Not included are over 700 patients, some of whom have been taking the drug for as long as six months, who have manifested no clinical symptoms of liver involvement throughout the duration of therapy.

We are of the opinion that the development of jaundice is an expression of individual drug idiosyncrasy. We have been unable to correlate the appearance of this complication with any factors that we have considered. The process is apparently confined to the bile passages, the liver parenchyma being spared. Although our deductions are based solely on the results of biochemical tests, studies of liver biopsy material by others have revealed occlusion of the biliary canaliculi with stasis of bile and varying degrees of inflammatory cell infiltration but no parenchymatous change. Chlorpromazine therapy was reinstituted in one of our patients who had previously developed jaundice, without recurrence. This feature further suggests that rather than toxic specificity of the drug itself, an idiosyncratic, or perhaps allergic, factor exists. Another possible clew may lie in the finding that the only two patients in our series who developed both dermatitis and jaundice had shown allergic reactions to other chemicals in the past. We consider that chlorpromazine is not a specific hepatotoxin and that, in the absence of extenuating factors such as hypersensitivity, hepatocellular function and bile excretion will remain undisturbed.

Conclusions

Jaundice is an infrequent complication of chlorpromazine [10-(-3-dimethyl-aminopropyl)-2-cholrophenothiazine hydrochloride] therapy and is believed to be an expression of individual drug idiosyncrasy. The jaundice appears to be due to obstruction within the intrahepatic bile passages, hepatocellular function remaining unimpaired. Preliminary investigation suggests that under ordinary circumstances chlorpromazine is not hepatotoxic and can be administered over prolonged periods of time without undue risk.

FATAL ACUTE ASEPTIC NECROSIS OF THE LIVER ASSOCIATED WITH CHLORPROMAZINE

R. N. Elliott, M.D., A. H. Schrut, M.D., and J. J. Marra, M.D.

A 32-year-old white woman had been consecutively hospitalized in a state institution for 5½ years, her psychiatric diagnosis schizophrenic reaction, paranoid type; the clinical picture characterized by hostility, florid religious delusions, and combativeness. Two courses of EST in 1950 and 1951 resulted in only temporary improvement. The initial physical examination was normal and the patient had never had any significant physical illness. In recent years she had continually required the supervision of semidisturbed wards because of her unpredictable behavior.

On November 21, 1955, she was started on chlorpromazine. The dosage was increased rapidly following the intensive treatment method reported in the literature, with the exception that the dosage was increased every few days rather than daily in order to better observe the patient for improvement. Initially, on November 21, 1955, she received 50 mgm. t.i.d. intramuscularly. Thereafter, the drug was given by the oral route exclusively. By November 29, 1955, the dosage had been increased to 1,600 mgm. daily and was held at that level because of beginning improvement.

At about 7:00 a.m. on December 2, 1955, the patient was noted to have an erythema over the face, chest, and arms, and the drug was stopped. By 10:00 a.m. a diffuse, botchy, macular erythema had spread over the trunk and to the thighs. Small papules resembling urticarial wheals appeared superimposed on the macular erythema. The temperature was 102° rectally. No localized infection was found on examination. A CBC done on 12-2-55 showed: RBC 4,650,000, Hbg. 85%; WBC 10,300 with 76% PMN's and 4% eosinophils. Pyribenzamine was started. At 4:30 p.m. the same day, the rash was somewhat more extensive. No other change was noted in the patient's condition which appeared to be satisfactory. At 12:30 a.m. on December 3, 1955, she was found dead in bed.

Autopsy revealed hepatomegaly with an acute aseptic necrosis of the liver and acute hepatic insufficiency. The lobular architecture was almost completely lost. The central veins and radiating sinusoids were markedly engorged. Individual liver cells showed marked degenerative changes, and often appeared ghostlike in character. A large number of the cells showed fat infiltration. There were zones in which not a single liver cell was recognizable. There was a notable lack of exudate. The portal triads showed occasional collars of lymphocytes about the arterioles, but these were not extensive. Fibrosis and bile duct reduplication were not in evidence. The spleen was considerably enlarged and the sinusoids were congested, but showed no exudate. The significant remaining findings were limited to passive congestion of all visceral organs, pulmonary congestion and edema, and mild brain swelling.

A review of recent world literature revealed several cases of fatal agranulocytosis attributed to Thorazine but only one fatal case of toxic hepatitis. This latter case, reported by A. H. Boardman in England, had become jaundiced before death.

The authors feel the death reported here seems to be associated with chlorpromazine therapy. Whether the large dosage was a factor remains a problem for future study.

PSYCHOSIS AND ENHANCED ANXIETY PRODUCED BY RESERPINE AND CHLORPROMAZINE

G. J. Sarwer-Foner, B.A., M.D., and W. Ogle, B.A., M.D.
Department of Psychiatry, Queen Mary Veterans Hospital, Montreal and the Department of Psychiatry, McGill University, Faculty of Medicine.

We first referred to the production of psychosis by reserpine and chlorpromazine in our preliminary report on the use of reserpine in psychiatric patients. Freis, Doyle and other authors had previously mentioned mainly depressive reactions and an occasional anxiety reaction, as occurring in patients treated, on a long-term basis, with reserpine for essential hypertension. Recently, other authors have reported psychotic depressions occurring during treatment for essential hypertension with reserpine. These latter authors have emphasized these reactions, whereas earlier authors, with the exception of Freis, had not done so. We believe our work to be the first dealing specifically with psychiatric patients, and offering an explanation of the mechanisms involved in these reactions. To our knowledge, it is also the first to implicate chlorpromazine as well as reserpine.

In a study of the physiological and psychological effects of reserpine on affect, 55 carefully selected psychiatric patients were intensively studied over a one-year period (July 1954 to July 1955). The research design was novel. The data and conclusions of this study have been reported in detail elsewhere. Concomitantly chlorpromazine was used in 35 cases on a non-research basis, i.e. when indicated as an ordinary drug. Sixteen out of the above-mentioned groups are the subject of this paper, because they were characterized by the same general reaction types and by common psychodynamic elements. The present paper consists of a detailed report of these cases, a discussion of the factors involved, and a statement of how we believe this phenomenon is produced.

Dose: The average dose of reserpine in the 55 cases was 7 mg. daily orally or intramuscularly. The average duration of treatment was 26 days. For chlorpromazine the dose was 50-100 mg. three or four times a day orally or intramuscularly. Duration of treatment varied greatly in the 35 cases.

Intensive knowledge of the psychodynamics and interpersonal relations has enabled us to formulate opinions as to the psychological as well as the physiological factors involved in the psychic reactions.

Production of Psychosis or of Further Psychotic Disintegration with Reserpine. (B.P., P., R. = blood pressure, pulse and respiration.)

1. (Case 11). G.A., a 25-year-old man. Before receiving reserpine, he showed perplexity, indecision, ambivalence and ambitendency. He could not make up his mind as to proper course, was somewhat sad and unhappy, and had a bland expression. He was anxious, but masked all the above with a great need to move around, be tremendously active, and unrestrained in his motor activity, such as drinking, going out, cashing bad cheques or running up debts. His symptoms developed when he was removed from his paratrooper's job, involving frequent jumping, to one requiring very little actual duty or activity in a newly forming regiment. When frustrated in his outgoingness by being confined to the ward, he became increasingly tense and showed an inappropriate euphoria. He was given 2.5 mg. reserpine intramuscularly four times a day for two days, and 3 mg. orally four times a day for 11 days. Weight went from 210 to 218 lb. in seven days, stabilizing at 218 lb. There was no oedema. His appetite had been good, but the patient complained that he lost his "zest in eating" while on the drug. Blood pressure fell from 125/70 to 100/60 mm. Hg. Pulse rate fell from 80 to 60 (variation 80-50) respiration rate remained at 20. The patient felt that he was "worse." The results in respect of affect were considered poor. The patient was slowed down; his motor activity was markedly cut; he was tired, drowsy and irritable, and felt "held down." He could move his body, but tended to move it in one block, although he was able to do otherwise. He was unhappy, jittery and extremely anxious. He felt cut off from life, "unable to sleep, unable to stay awake." He felt he was "going queer", felt "cut off from outside things", and felt that his body was changing. Main observable changes were slowing down, inappropriate euphoria, panic at being chemically held, and a feeling of change and dissociation and of changes in body image and in his motor control. The natural course of the disease was changed for the worse; from an acting out person who mastered his anxiety through activity, he became an inhibited, unhappy frustrated man whose mental content became psychotic. The side-effect was nasal stuffiness. The patient was taken off the drug, and returned to his pre-drug state within a week. He was a very happy and relieved man at this, and remained with his acting out behaviour for the remaining month in hospital.

Comments: The drug removed his ability for vigorous motor activity at all levels. This rendered him more passive and he felt this as a lessening of his masculine prowess. He became paranoid.

2. (Case 16). S.O., aged 33, before receiving reserpine showed the beginnings of motor overactivity, flight of ideas, a tendency to dissociated thinking and a mild euphoria. He was aware that this was an abnormal state. On admission he was dependent, clinging, shaking hands, and speaking pleasantly to everyone. He was inclined to be passive in his interpersonal relations, and was open to verbal reassurance with good temporary effect. He had religious delusions and illusions, and grandiose ideas, and showed perplexity at his state, ambivalence, and ambitendency. His normal premorbid personality was marked by considerable drive in all activities and by social outgoingness. Physical findings were normal. Dosage: he received 5 mg. i.m. b.i.d.

stat, then 5 mg. i.m. t.i.d. for three days, then q.i.d. for two days. He received one extra 5 mg. i.m. dose on the last day. Weight went from 124 to 129 lb. in six days. No oedema. His appetite changed from poor to good. His B.P., pulse and respiration were 130/90, 112, 20 before receiving the drug and 130/90-90/60, 88-72 and 20 while on the drug. B.P. fluctuated with dose and averaged 100/70. Patient felt he was "not helped." The result on affect was considered poor. Patient became calm and drowsy and felt held down. He was able to battle with his delusions, grandiosity and disorientation. His flight of ideas stopped. His irritability and impulsivity remained. Thus, the initial effect was excellent, but only enough drug to calm him had been given, the aim being to permit him to be up and around. When an extra dose which cut his activity to a level that immobilized him was given, he became paranoic, fearful, agitated and suicidal. He feared a plot against him, he felt that things had changed. He couldn't move, he felt we were changing him, and he became afraid that he would have to kill himself. The natural course of the disease was unchanged. The patient moved head, trunk and upper limbs in one block when under the influence of the last dose. Because of his condition he was transferred to a closed hospital. Final diagnosis: schizophrenia, schizo-affective type.

Comment: This man had an early psychotic process which he was able to cope with as long as he had motor activity as a defence. His defensive mobility was chemically removed, and greater psychotic deterioration resulted.

3. (Case 45). J.R., aged 34, before reserpine treatment had marked anxiety. He was trembling, sweating, scratching, moderately sad and markedly irritable. There was dermatitis eczematoides, interdigital dermatitis, and now back pain without physical signs. Dose: 7 mg. daily p.o. for 21 days. He gained 5 lb. in 21 days. No oedema. Appetite remained fair. B.P., P. and R. before reserpine treatment 130/80, 90, 20; on drug, B. P. fell to 100/70 in a day, then fluctuated between 140/90 and 90/50, P. 90 to 68, R. 20 Patient felt he was "not helped." Results on affect were considered poor; the patient was slowed, lost his tremor, sweating, irritability and sleeplessness. He appeared less sad. The low back pain was unchanged, but he developed bowel symptoms which persisted, and marked projective thinking. Major observed changes were that he appeared slowed, tired, sleepy and drowsy. His ability to relate in the interpersonal field was reduced. The natural course of disease was changed for the worse; from obsessive compulsive state, with signs of anxiety and with somatization, to loss of anxiety but also loss of ability to function positively. He felt passive and frightened. He developed more somatic symptoms, and paranoid (projective) thinking. Side-effects were stuffiness in nose, nausea, and on one occasion hiccups. The patient was taken off the drug and given sub-coma insulin and supportive psychotherapy; he showed a little symptomatic improvement in 1½ months.

Comment: Here again the physiological effects of chemically "holding him down" were intensely threatening, and resulted in psychosis.

4. (Case 48). A.A., aged 38, complained of sleeplessness, headache, bowel complaints, and itching around the anus and genitals. Few overt signs of anxiety. He was thin, with dermatitis around anus, genitals and knees. Dose:

2 mg. daily for 15 days. He gained 3 lb. in 15 days. No oedema. Appetite changed from poor to fair. B.P. 140/80 before drug; on drug fluctuated from 140/80 to 100/50. P. fell from 90 to 60, R. remained at 16. Patient felt he was "helped." For one week patient slept better and was uncomplaining. He was quiet, was slowed, felt tired, and was socially more co-operative and outgoing. His activity was markedly cut down. His passivity during this week was accepted by his physician, and the patient felt better because of his acceptance by a strong masculine figure. After the week, the patient became afraid of his passive role in reference to the physician, and complained that he was being "held down" and didn't know why. In the space of two days he became suspicious of his physician, with marked paranoid distortions of all that happened in his environment. The natural course of the disease was changed for the worse in that, from the initial symptomatic improvement, the patient felt threatened by his chemically induced passivity and became overtly paranoid. The drug was stopped, his physician happened to go on vacation, and within two weeks the patient had returned to his pre-psychotic state. Psychotherapy continued, and the patient was discharged as improved after three months.

Comment: As the transference developed, he feared the passivity imposed on him by the drug since he distorted the physician's motives. He became psychotic.

5. (Case 50). M.J., aged 39, before reserpine was slow in his physical movements, gloomy, covertly hostile, sleepless, paced the floor, and showed considerable despondency. Neck movement was limited because of previous discectomy. Dose: 1 mg. p.o. for 10 days. He gained 2 lb. in 10 days. No oedema. Appetite remained fair. B.P. 130/90 went to 120/70, P. went from 100 to 70, R. remained at 16. Patient felt he was "made worse." Results on affect were considered poor. The patient became slowed, showed more psychomotor retardation and more despondency, and was gloomier. He had less ability for social contacts, and lost all ability for even subtle expression of overt hostility. He developed self-destructive nightmares, and became overtly suicidal. The major observable changes were that all symptoms of depression were increased except his pacing. The patient lay on his bed and appeared dejected. The natural course of disease was unchanged, in that depressive reaction became sufficiently severe to be considered a psychotic depression. The patient lost his small ability for outward expression, and his long-standing somatization through head ache, stiff neck, and arm pain increased. There were no side-effects. Patient returned to his pre-drug state within one week of discontinuation. He improved with about 1½ months of further psycho-therapy.

Comment: In this depressed patient, the drug removed the limited ability for psychomotor activity, and the patient felt even more helpless and inadequate. A deepening of the depression to psychotic levels followed.

6. (Case 51). M.A., aged 31, before reserpine showed anxiety, restlessness, fear, inappropriate affect, bodily delusions and auditory hallucinations. Physical findings were normal. Dose was 15 mg. i.m. daily for 8 days. Patient gained 9 lb. in 8 days. No oedema. Appetite changed from poor to good. B.P. went from 170/80 to 120/70 while on drug, P. from 100 to 72, R. remained at 16. Patient felt he was "helped." The results as to affect were considered

poor. The signs of anxiety, agitation and disorganized behaviour disappeared, and the patient became a quiet and resigned psychotic instead of one full of fight and turmoil and still battling with his illness. The major observable changes were that he became drowsy, lethargic, slowed down, and apparently resigned to his hallucinatory experiences. He was unable to use his previous psychotic mechanism of going through a ritual of active symbolic bodily movements to make his somatic delusions disappear. The natural course of the disease was unchanged, but an active, turbulent psychosis was changed into a quiet one. There were no side-effects. The patient was sent to another hospital where he received electroshock and insulin, but still had residual schizophrenic symptoms.

Comment: This psychotic patient was anxious and struggling with his illness. The drug removed the ability to mobilize energy into physical activity and he became a quiet, resigned psychotic.

Production of Psychosis or Further Psychotic Disintegration with Chlorpromazine

7. T.J., aged 33, before chlorpromazine showed signs of increased motor activity and speech, euphoria, flight of ideas, and a feeling that he alone was doing his job as it should be done. He had shown increasing evidence of the above for approximately one week, and had been sleepless, anxious and somewhat irritable for two or three weeks before that. He was given chlorpromazine 50 mg. i.m. q.i.d. for approximately 30 days. At the end of the second day, he was quiet, calm, and no longer overactive. He sat quietly by his bed, smiled at everyone who approached him, and when he felt "like doing something to keep busy" asked permission to wash the windows. In psychotherapeutic interviews, however, or if asked how he felt or what he thought, he stated that he could "see angels sitting in the tree tops outside the windows" and they were talking to him. He added that there was no longer a need for him to fight because all was now settled. He was waiting orders from God to join the Heavenly Father or to remain on earth awhile. He presented autistic thinking, delusions of grandeur and persecution, and ideas of reference. Thus, from an overactive person with hypomanic symptoms but no known hallucinations he was turned into a quietly hallucinated person with typical schizophrenic symptoms. He was treated over a four-month period with reality-testing psychotherapy, occupational therapy, and a therapeutic work programme. After three months he was free of delusions, hallucinations and ideas of reference. There was some residual autistic thinking.

Comment: In terms of time this was the first case in our hands to show an increased psychotic deterioration when activity, used as a major defence, was chemically removed (Sept. '54). A manic symptomatology covering a homosexual panic was changed to a quiet, but typical paranoid schizophrenia.

8. K.J.G., aged 22, before reserpine showed acting out and characterological defences (character neurosis) such as a surface affability, cheerfulness, and an apparent ease in his interpersonal relations. This latter was characterized by drive, energetic actions and much motility. Thus, he would drink beer "with the boys", boast, act "like a big shot", and spend a great deal of money to "prove" that he was a "big shot." On admission, he showed all of the above character-

istics, plus marked anxiety, fear that he was going insane, loss of appetite, pain in the right genito-femoral region, and, beneath his motor activity, a feeling of sadness and despondency. Because of his marked anxiety, he was given chlorpromazine 50 mg. i.m. t.i.d. for one day, then 50 mg. p.o. t.i.d. This resulted in a marked diminution of the patient's motor activity. He felt tired and weak, and complained of having "a dry mouth" and of being dizzy. He was unable to engage in his usual motor activities such as sports, and spent much time lying in bed. With this physical inactivity, he became more overtly sad, despondent, and irritable; at night time, he began to hear voices, which frightened him, although in the morning he was uncertain as to their reality. The drug was discontinued when the above phenomenon developed after six days. He became more active one day after the drug was discontinued, and within the next three days, with return of his motor outlet, much of the depressive element lessened, although he remained markedly anxious. He was transferred to another hospital because of ineligibility for treatment under D.V.A.

Comment: Here again removal of activity, which was a major defence and "demonstration of his masculinity", resulted in further psychic deterioration in a patient with a borderline state.

9. (Courtesy of Dr. C. Conway Smith—Montreal.) This 74-year-old man had had a previous manic episode 15 years ago, which had been treated by E.C.T. This latter had not interfered with his usual outgoingness, at the time.

In September 1955, he consulted a physician because of increased irritability, impulsiveness, and the beginnings of increased motor activity. Normally this patient was an extremely active, exacting, and aggressive business man whose sensorium and intellectual capacities were unimpaired, and who was considered to have an obsessive-compulsive personality with a tendency to marked mood swings. Because of increased symptoms his physician put him on an unknown dose of chlorpromazine. This dose was sufficient to markedly cut down his activity, and with the removal of this outlet the patient became increasingly disturbed. His irritability increased and the patient felt inwardly more excited, even though he was unable to express this at a motor level. The patient developed jaundice at this point, and an exploratory laparotomy was performed. Being thus further immobilized, he became even more excited and difficult to manage. A psychiatrist (Dr. C. C. Smith) was consulted at this point, and hospitalized the patient in a closed setting. Reserpine 1 mg. b.i.d. was substituted for the chlorpromazine. The patient became more mobile and physically active, since the dose of reserpine was insufficient to have the same chemically holding effect that the dose of chlorpromazine had had. As the patient became more physically active, his agitation and excitement diminished. He was given ground privileges shortly after arrival at the closed hospital, and improved markedly over a period of one to two months. Towards the end of his hospital stay, some peripheral oedema was noted and reserpine was discontinued. Dr. Smith felt that the use of reserpine in sufficiently low dosage to permit the patient recourse to activity as a defence helped him cope with his fear of being made helpless, and thereby less manly.

Comment: Here again, removal of the patient's long-established mode of reassuring himself as to his adequacy and manhood through activity produced further psychotic deterioration. Restoration of activity helped his recovery by offering an old and well-established pattern of expression.

Enhanced Anxiety Produced by Reserpine

10. (Case 9). S.J., aged 25, before reserpine showed marked anxiety, poor control over aggression, weakness in the knees and tremor of the hands and legs when angry. He often became panicky, and had a slow slurred speech. He had from his early childhood been awkward, and showed a marked inability to master muscular co-ordination. He had spontaneous hypoglycaemia with fugues. He hyperventilated when he was panicky, and at times had hypnagogic hallucinations. He was an asthenic, thin man, with a marked awkwardness which seemed to express his inability to master himself. Dose: 4 mg. orally daily for 8 days. The patient gained 5 lb. in 7 days. There was no oedema. His appetite remained good. His B. P., P. and R. went from 120/76, 72, and 20 before the drug to 120/70-90/68, 68 and 22 while on the drug. The patient felt he was "made worse." The results on affect were considered poor. The patient was made weak and dizzy, and his already intolerable awkwardness increased. He felt more helpless and passive, looked worse and felt worse. The major observable changes were weakness, tiredness, dizziness, increased awkwardness, and enforced passivity. The result on the natural course of the disease was unchanged, but the patient felt infinitely more anxious and less the master of himself. Side-effects were headache and nasal stuffiness. Investigation showed involvement of total body and psyche in the illness (i.e. autonomic nervous system, endocrine, psychic, muscular and E.E.G. findings). Reserpine was stopped and mild phenobarbital sedation substituted. Psychotherapy continued, and the patient felt considerable relief within three days (as the drug wore off). He improved under psychotherapy and was discharged 10 weeks later.

Comment: The drug increased his already intolerable awkwardness by removing his capacity for voluntary energetic movement. This made him feel less adequate, i.e., less manly, and increased his anxiety.

11. (Case 17). J.C.A., aged 39, before reserpine had somatic pains (low back pain, pain in right shoulder blade and right knee). He was unhappy and moderately despondent. He was irritable, hostile, and aggressive and insisted that the pain was organic in origin. Chronic prostatitis, an enlarged prostate and moderate essential hypertension (150/100 mm. Hg) were found on physical examination. Dose: 2 mg. orally for 5 days. His weight did not change and his appetite remained good. His B.P., P. and R. went from 150/100, 80, 20 to 100/70, 72, 20. The patient felt he was "made worse." The results as to affect were considered poor. The patient was made weak, dizzy and more passive. He reacted to this by increased anxiety and agitation. He felt useless, frightened, and weak, and his pains increased. The major observable changes were weakness, dizziness, agitation, and more passivity. The result on the natural course of the illness was unchanged. The patient remained an obsessive-compulsive with somatic symptoms and a marked dependency as manifested in his desire for a pension. Side-effects were diarrhoea for 24 hours and a stuffy nose. The drug was stopped, and he lost his fear of the effects of the drug in two to three days, and along with this the feelings of indecisiveness and frus-

tration. He continued on psychotherapy. His depression was significantly improved through working with his hostility. In the next two months his somatic complaints and his demands for pension persisted.

Comment: The physiological effects of the drug threatened this passive-dependent man by reducing his capacity to control his own body. He interpreted this as a "demasculinization" of himself and became markedly anxious, with increased somatic complaints.

12. (Case 28). C.J., aged 29, was weepy, unhappy, covertly hostile and manipulating in his interpersonal relations. He was effeminate in gesture and speech. He had headache and nausea, and seemed to be a very passive and dependent person. Physical findings were normal. Dose: He received 2.5 mg. i.m. the first day and responded with marked anxiety and more weeping, all directed at the nursing staff in an attempt to manipulate them into stopping the injections. On the second day he received 5 mg. i.m. and felt so terrible, with such marked panic at night, that the medication was cancelled. He stated that he could not stand the weak, helpless feeling the drug gave him, and that the thought of it made him sweat and shiver. The patient felt he was "made worse." The results as to affect were poor. His headache, sadness and anxiety were worse, and on the second evening he had a mild attack of panic. The major observable change was a marked increase in his anxiety to the level of panic. Nausea was the only side-effect, after withdrawal of reserpine. Psychotherapy plus the hospital milieu helped the patient. He left, improved, approximately one month later.

Comment: Here a passive dependent, somewhat effeminate man with considerable anxiety and a mild depressive reaction, panicked at the chemical effects of being made weaker and less active by the injections. He resorted to his characterological defence of manipulating the environment away from a "dangerous" situation.

13. (Case 37). Miss W.P., aged 21, before reserpine was intensely anxious, fearful, unhappy and impulsive. She was physically very active, and blinked her eyes continually. She had suicidal thoughts, and was very disturbed by her conscious awareness of being attracted to other women. Physical findings were normal. She received 5 mg. orally daily for 15 days. She gained 10 lb. in 15 days. There was no oedema and her appetite remained good. Her B.P., P. and R. went from 120/70, 68, 16 to 95/50, 72, 16 in 48 hours. B.P. stabilized at 110/60. She felt she was "made worse." The results as to affect were considered poor. The patient became "groggy", weak, dizzy and felt chemically held down. She was very frightened by this. She lay on the bed, slept continually except at meal time, and was very irritable and hostile. She began refusing the drug. The natural course of the illness was unchanged. There were no side-effects. The drug was discontinued, and she reverted to her pre-drug state with much relief. Psycho-therapy continued, and she improved to a limited degree in the next three months.

Comment: This girl had a marked attachment to the treating physician, and interpreted the drug as a seduction or assault by him. The physiological effects in making her weak, tired and relatively helpless were doubly threatening because they removed her ability for aggressive independent action as well.

14. (Case 53). C.M., aged 37, before reserpine was sleepless and moderately anxious with an obsessive-compulsive personality, and a right-sided spasmodic torticollis of 18 months' duration. He received 5 mg. i.m. daily for 10 days, then 3 mg. orally for 10 days. He gained 3 lb. in 20 days, his appetite went from fair to good and there was no oedema. B.P., P. and R. went from 124/84, 80 and 20 to 110/70, 72 and 20. The patient felt he was "not helped." The results on affect were considered poor. He was slowed, felt "lifeless, doped", "useless", had a sad facies, and looked dull and inert. He showed a marked diminution in his social activities. The natural course of the disease was unchanged. He became more depressed and anxious and discharged himself from the hospital.

Comment: The patient became more depressed and anxious, feeling threatened at being chemically held down. He considered this as an assault and a seduction, and ran away from it by discharging himself from the hospital.

Two other cases with reserpine will now be presented with the same psychodynamic and physiological constellations. Here however, in contradistinction to the other cases, circumstances were such that they were benefited by the drug.

15. (Case 26). C.J., aged 29, had been hospitalized for several months with some benefit. He went on a week-end pass and spent much of his time drinking beer with male friends. He panicked afterwards, and made a suicidal gesture by swallowing some barbiturates. He returned to the ward despondent, very anxious, and almost in panic. He was jittery, persiring, trembling, crying. He was given 2 mg. i.m. as night-time sedation, and he received the same dose nightly for seven days. The patient felt that he was "helped." Results as to affect were considered good. The patient was initially anxious and afraid of going to sleep. He remained awake most of the first two nights. When he was told that he was in a hospital, that his fear of what could happen to him was understood, but that nothing was going to happen to him here, he relaxed and calmed down, and at the end of the seventh day asked for further injections.

Comment: This patient had been in homosexual panic, i.e. he feared that an unconscious uncontrollable urge for some sort of homosexual contact would become conscious. He thus feared a drug that would render him more helpless. But in the "safe" reassuring atmosphere of the hospital, he relaxed and obtained unconscious but safe gratification of his need to be assaulted (i.e. injections) and felt better as a result. The safe hospital milieu and understanding physician made the difference between a good and bad therapeutic result in this case.

16. (Case 47). W.Y., aged 38, before reserpine was so angry at being jilted by a girl that he had been on a five-day binge and was shaking, sweating, pacing the floor, crying and expressing great fear of suicide or homicide. He was known to have a violent temper that was difficult to provoke, but once provoked he had in the past been known to give way to great physical violence. Physical findings included slight jaundice, a large tender liver and early bronchopneumonia. The diagnosis was acute depression with alcoholism, infectious hepatitis and bronchopneumonia. The patient received 40 mg. reserpine daily orally and i.m. for 20 days, and felt that he "was helped." The

results on affect were good. Anxiety and tremor were dispelled; the patient was inert and listless in bed and was therefore passive, and reassurable as to violence. On psychotherapy and medical treatment he moved towards aggression related to reality. He was slowed to the level of complete bed rest for one week, after which he was able to move, but moved like an automaton. The natural course of the disease was changed. The drug interrupted an acute psychotic episode by rendering impossible the threatened eruption of aggressive feelings and drives. Nassal stuffiness was the only side-effect. He returned to army duty mildly euphoric after reserpine was stopped.

Comment: Here the very passivity and helplessness, which in other circumstances this man would have probably feared as a feminizing thing, were welcomed and sought as protection against his aggressive impulses—with good therapeutic result.

Discussion

A series of patients have been presented in whom two drugs, quite useful in psychiatry and enjoying a current vogue, caused a psychotic process, further deterioration of a psychotic process, or enhanced anxiety. Both these agents have fairly standard physiological effects for a given dose. In psychiatry, these physiological effects are useful to relieve selected symptoms. The drugs are therefore not psychiatric "specific agents" but *symptomatic* drugs.

A standard physiological effect of both drugs is to chemically "hold down" the patient. It makes him feel tired, weak, and, in adequate dosage, incapable of mobilizing much energy into physical activity. There are other effects which are predominantly *psychological* and are the result of the way in which the physiological effects fit into the patient's way of handling and expressing his conflicts (i.e. defences). When a patient does badly, it is due to the way in which the physiological effect *psychologically* threatens him.

This report does not mean to imply that reserpine and chlorpromazine have no place in psychiatry. Rather, the good or bad effect depends on the last-mentioned consideration. In all the cases reported here, the desired physiological effect for which the drug had been given was reached. That is to say, the patient had been slowed, felt tired, was calmed, and had his activity cut, and it was precisely this physiological effect that was *psychologically* threatening to the patient.

1. *Fear of increased passivity.*—The chemical "holding down" action of these drugs removed activity as an outlet. A large group of patients with marked doubts about their masculinity, and with marked feminine identifications, express these in conflicts over their sexual, social, and intellectual potency. Many of these patients use activity in one or all of the above spheres as a means of reassuring themselves that they are adequate males. When this activity is used as a *major* defence, removing it chemically, by rendering them incapable of energetic action, is very threatening. These patients consider activity to mean masculinity and passivity to mean femininity. (Cases 1, 2, 3, 6 and 7 show this feature.)

Thus for the same intrapsychic conflict, a better integrated defence, i.e. one allowing better contact with reality (activity), was chemically removed. Under the threat of increased relative passivity (femininity) these patients reacted with more poorly integrated defences, because of the intolerable anxiety produced (see Dr. D. G. Wright's theory of schizophrenia). This results in either enhanced anxiety or further breaks with reality (i.e. psychosis).

2. *Fear of impaired body function or of body image changes.*—Another group showed essentially the same psychodynamic conflicts over psycho-sexual identifications as group 1 but expressed it clinically as fear of impaired body functioning or of body-image changes. This group interpreted the physiological effects of these drugs, and/or the multiple side-effects, as a lessening or impairment of body function. Again, as in group 1, and for the same psychological reasons, changes meant increased passivity (i.e. femininity). This lessened control over themselves caused increased anxiety, and if the latter proved intolerable, a "downward" rearrangement of the defences into psychosis. Patients with obsessive ruminations over bodily health often show increased anxiety when the multiple physiological effects and side-effects of these drugs increase somatic dysfunctioning.

3. *Increase in depression.*—The depressed patients became more depressed. The action of these drugs in further limiting the expression of hostility through psychomotor activity, or limiting ability for some interpersonal relations, increased the feeling of personal helplessness and unworthiness, and therefore unconscious aggression as well.

4. *Interpretation as assault or seduction.*—Several patients, including the only woman in this report, interpreted the physiological effects, in rendering them less active, weak, passive and less the master over themselves (i.e. more in the doctor's power), as an actual or threatened assault or seduction. This they interpreted as either homosexual or heterosexual. When this was too threatening, and therefore unwelcome, the psychiatric disability increased. It should be pointed out that safe unconscious gratification in the protective hospital milieu, of the same need to be seduced or assaulted can prove beneficial (cf. Case 15).

From the above, it becomes clear that the clinical nosological entity produced—e.g. paranoid reaction, enhanced anxiety, depression, or agitation—is not dependent on a specific action of the drug concerned, but is rather a result of the way in which the patient responds, with all his total assets, to the removal of one of his important defences, such as activity. Whether a depression or a paranoid psychosis is produced is the result of the interplay of many forces, the constellation of which has a high degree of individual variation for any particular person. This can only be evaluated by careful individual psychodynamic study.

We therefore believe that any variety of psychiatric condition is possible, depending on the interaction of the physiological effects of these drugs, the psychological effect of this on the very complex defences, and the reality situation. It is naive to attribute these effects to some possible vague specific action of these agents on the brainstem, since the physiological effects of these drugs are fairly constant for any one dose and were also present in patients who did well on these agents. As another example of this, Case 16 shows a good result, i.e. beneficial to the patient, from the physiological effects in holding this man down, because he feared eruption of his aggressive feelings. It is probable that the same man would have been threatened instead of supported in other circumstances than these, because of his fear of passivity.

SUMMARY

A study of 14 cases of psychotic reactions, further psychotic deterioration or enhanced anxiety, produced with reserpine and chlorpromazine, is presented. Two other examples of the same psychodynamic elements, with benefit, are presented in contrast. We believe this to be the first work to deal specifically with psychiatric cases and offer explanations for this phenomenon.

All these cases had common psychodynamic elements.

The physiological effects of the drugs were fairly constant for a given dosage and were present both in those patients who reacted badly and in those who did well on these agents.

It is felt that untoward reactions had nothing to do with the physiological effects *per se*, but rather with the way in which the physiological effects *psychologically* threatened the patient.

The psychological reaction produced was nonspecific as regards the drug but specific as regards interaction between the physiological effects and the particular psychic, interpersonal, and reality factors in the patient concerned. Thus any variety of psychiatric nosological entity is theoretically possible.

This paper presents some psychodynamic criteria from which clues as to the proper selection of cases have been deduced.

UNDESIRABLE EFFECTS AND CLINICAL TOXICITY OF CHLORPROMAZINE

Irvin M. Cohen, M.D.
University of Texas Medical Branch, Galveston, Texas

Although reporting of the therapeutic properties of chlorpromazine has been unusually extensive, there has been comparatively little systematic investigation of its toxicity in man. It is a remarkable fact that even though a bibliography of over 3000 papers has accumulated since its synthesis in 1950, its safety as a clinically useful drug is still debated. The consensus seems to be that although chlorpromazine possesses many undesirable side effects and occasionally produces serious complications, it is in general a safe drug that can be utilized without undue risk. It should be recognized that these conclusions have generally been based on clinical experience. On the other hand, the relatively few laboratory studies have produced no unanimous or unqualified conclusions.

Several factors indicate that an early answer to the problem should not be expected. The side effects and complications are multiple and extremely diverse in character and site of origin. They occur in widely disturbed and apparently dissociated organ systems, so that each may require individual investigation. Many of the reactions are unique, and do not fulfill the eitologic criteria previously established for reactions of similar clinical appearance. Some untoward effects occur infrequently and may escape recognition as being due to chlorpromazine, as was illustrated in the case of jaundice that was not recognized until 1954 even though chlorpromazine had been subjected to extensive clinical trial in Europe for nearly two years. Finally, our limited knowledge of neurophysiology and neurochemistry, inaccessibility of the brain, and ignorance of the biologic mechanisms that may be involved in the production of mental illness are basic factors that will preclude early understanding of many of the unusual responses that may be induced by this drug.

The side effects and complications of chlorpromazine are characterized by such a high degree of unpredictability that reliable correlations have been possible only within narrow limits. The following appear to be the most consistent: (1) the majority of the side effects occur during the first two weeks of administration; (2) most of the complications appear within the second two weeks; (3) side effects tend to be more intense during intramuscular administration and when oral dosages are high. With few exceptions, side effects resolve despite uninterrupted administration. This characteristic spontaneous resolution during treatment also applies to the dermatologic complications and may be true in the case of jaundice and Parkinsonism. An important feature of the complications is that they usually do not recur on subsequent administration.

Most of the undesirable effects of chlorpromazine may be attributed to action on various levels of the nervous system. Those that occur most frequently are central depressant, sympatholytic, parasympatholytic, and myatonic effects. Others suggest interference with the metabolic and endocrinologic aspects of hypothalamic function and disorganization of extrapyramidal motor regulation. Occurring less frequently are those complications believed to be due to allergic sensitivity. The validity of this concept is less disputed in relation to responses occurring in the skin and bronchi than it is when the liver and hemopoietic systems are involved. A third group of undesirable effects, including such diverse effects as excessive dreaming and depersonalization, defy explanation.

Central Nervous System Effects. The central side effects reflect more clearly than any others the possible loci of action of chlorpromazine. In general, those that occur earliest can be ascribed to a depression of the alerting function of the reticular activating system, while the later effects mostly indicate disturbed hypothalamic function and basal ganglionic release.

Drowsiness and hypersomnolence are the most common central side effects and, in fact, occur in a majority of patients receiving chlorpromazine. In rare instances, particularly in hypochondriacal or phobic patients, insomnia may be produced, but this is doubtfully a primary effect of the drug. Sedation is maximal during the first 7 to 10 days of treatment. The degree is based on dosage, route of administration, and individual sensitivity. Intramuscular injections of 50 to 100 mg. ordinarily induce sleep of from two to six hours. Oral dosages exceeding 75 mg./day may produce mild lethargy; when the dose exceeds 200 mg./day, most patients experience a nagging desire for sleep or actual hypersomnia. The patient can be awakened easily, and the perceptive and intellectual fogging so characteristic of barbiturates or other cortical depressants is minimal. If the patient cannot be aroused, other factors are present. While this potent sedative property is an effective instrument in the management of highly disturbed patients, it is troublesome and often distressing to the ambulatory patient. Fortunately it disappears rapidly, but may be protracted in those patients who must continue on very high dosage regimens.

Apathy, lack of initiative, and loss of interest in surroundings are a common response in patients receiving intramuscular doses exclusively and when the oral dosage is in the range of 600 to 800 mg. daily or higher. Affective disturbances of this quality seem to occur predominantly in previously agitated psychotic patients. Contrariwise, Hoch has observed restlessness and tension accompanied by feelings of depersonalization occurring after 7 to 10 days of treatment when the dose was but 100 to 200 mg. daily. Chlorpromazine also appears to be capable of worsening depressions and perhaps even of mobilizing incipient cases. Statistics supporting this observation are lacking, but in the author's experience the incidence is sufficiently impressive to contraindicate its use in this illness.

Errors in thermoregulation, endocrinologic and metabolic changes, and other untoward effects attributable to hypothalamic dysfunction may take place at any stage of treatment, but are generally seen during the later phases, particularly if dosage is high. In our experience, the most frequent disturbance in temperature control has been in the direction of fever, usually in the form of isolated spikes of from 101 to 103 F. Subnormal temperatures, never lower than 97 F., have been uncommon, contrary to numerous reports in the European literature describing the hypothermic capacity of chlorpromazine. Various manifestations of disorder water, fat, and carbohydrate metabolism have been reported. Courvoisier *et al.* found that chlorpromazine raised the blood sugar level in animals, and glycosuria has been observed clinically. However, we have been unable to detect any significant changes of this type. For purposes of this paper, aberrations in water and fat metabolism and endocrinologic function are described in other sections.

Other undesirable central effects are excessive dreaming, blurring of vision due to paresis of accommodation, and predisposition to convulsive seizures.

The signs and symptoms described above may be regarded as undesirable side effects, to be anticipated in a considerable percentage of patients. They are of clinical importance mainly because they are capable of causing subjective distress. In most cases they disappear rapidly despite continued administration, and the patient can be reassured to this extent. However, there are two central nervous system reactions that are of the proportions of complications and may require either reduction of dosage or interruption of therapy. They are the extrapyramidal syndromes and delirium.

Minor signs referable to the basal ganglia occur in approximately 20 per cent of patients receiving high dosages. These include sensations of restriction of movement, transient difficulties in swallowing and talking, and feelings of the tongue falling backward or that the head "wants to fly backward." Objectively there may be tremor of a static or tension type and moderate loss of associated movements. During the first two weeks of treatment many patients show a reduction in mimetic expression, which is almost masklike. Whether this is the result of apathy, a part of generalized reduction in muscular tone, a posterior hypothalamic effect similar to that which can be experimentally induced in animals by surgical lesions, or of extrapyramidal origin is disputed. These various signs and symptoms are in most cases isolated findings that do not progress. In approximately 4 to 5 per cent of patients, however, there develops a picture of Parkinsonism, most frequently of a post-encephalitic character. Rigidity is usually more marked than tremor, sialorrhea and seborrhea are common, and there are stooped posture, masklike facies, and loss of associated movements. The dosage in most of these cases is more than 500 to 600 mg./day. If it is reduced or the drug is withdrawn, the syndrome ordinarily resolves without apparent residue within two weeks. Various antiparkinsonism agents have been used effectively. Spontaneous resolution in patients in whom the drug was not discontinued has been described.

Tonic spasms of various muscle groups have occurred in 2 patients in a series of 1400 cases studied at the University of Texas Medical Branch Hospitals. Both patients exhibited torticollis, opisthotonos, and ticlike movements. In 1 there were also torsion spasms, reproducing the picture of dystonia musculorum deformans.

A 14 year old catatonic schizophrenic girl who had received intramuscular injections of 25 mg. of chlorpromazine for four days suddenly developed ticlike twitching of the face and arching of the back. The opisthotonic posture was intermittent and was accompanied by conjugate deviation of the head and eyes to one side. The syndrome disappeared within 18 hours after chlorpromazine was discontinued.

A 38 year old woman who had received four intramuscular injections of chlorpromazine but who had previously received high oral doses without incident suddenly developed hyperextension of the back, conjugate deviation of the head and eyes to the right, choreiform twitching of the fingers and right mouth angle, and torsion movements of the trunk to the right. Neurologic examination revealed hyperreflexia. Dismissed as being of hysterical origin, it recurred intermittently within the next hours. Later the patient became slightly cyanotic and complained of dysphagia, and a positive Chvostek's sign was elicited. Calcium level, however, was normal. Injections of phenobarbital and calcium gluconate terminated the episode. Subsequent investigation failed to show any organic neurologic disease.

A case similar to the latter has been photographically recorded by Ayd. In 1954, Labhardt described torticollis and torsion movements (*arc en cercle*) occurring in patients receiving chlorpromazine, but he regarded them as psychogenic complications of an hysterical nature.

Toxic states ranging from mild confusion to typical toxic delirium are rare complications of chlorpromazine therapy. Kinross-Wright has reported death in 1 patient during a toxic confusional state, with post-mortem findings of changes in the subthalamic body, globus pallidus, and hypothalamus. Confusion of this type must be differentiated from the exaggeration of existing sensorium defects that may occur in cerebral arteriosclerotic patients receiving chlorpromazine. In the latter case it is on an ischemic basis, and is due to cerebral vascular hypotension to which the aged patient is more susceptible.

Cardiovascular Effects. Interference with orthostatic control of blood pressure, transient arterial hypotension, and signs of peripheral vascular insufficiency are the principal untoward effects referable to the cardiovascular system. These manifestations reflect the potent sympatholytic and adrenolytic properties of this drug. As in the case of other blocking agents of this type, the action is on the peripheral vascular network rather than on the myocardium. A peripheral vasodilatation is produced; cardiac responses are compensatory. Tachycardia, for example, occurs very frequently, particularly in situations requiring rapid cardiovascular readjustments, such as change of position.

Temporary reduction in recumbent blood pressure may occur after either oral or parenteral administration of chlorpromazine. A transient arterial hypotension nearly always follows intramuscular injection, particularly when the dose is 50 mg. or higher. This finding is most prominent in elderly patients and those displaying functional hypertension during intense motor activity or in whom hypertension exists for other reasons. In these cases the drop may be precipitous and of such degree that shock would ordinarily be expected, the systolic pressure falling as much as 50 to 60 mm. and the diastolic 20 to 30 mm. However, measures to counteract shock are rarely required despite what appears to be an alarming picture. This margin of safety is probably based on chlorpromazine's capacity to reverse hypertension due to epinephrine while allowing minimal sympathetic activity to be maintained by norepinephrine. Cases of serious circulatory collapse, even in normotensive patients, and protracted tachycardia have occurred, and death has been reported, but successful termination is the rule. In the absence of complicating factors such as hypertension, the decrease in recumbent blood pressure is usually so small and short-lived as to be clinically insignificant, especially if oral administration is used exclusively. However, evidence of adrenergic blockade continues in the form of orthostatic hypotension for about the first 7 to 10 days of treatment. Approximately 50 per cent of patients receiving dosages greater than 150 mg./day experience dizziness on postural change and exertion, simultaneous visual blurring, momentary imbalance, and occasionally syncope. These effects are greatest in cerebral arteriosclerotics in whom there may also be intensification of sensorial clouding. In a few middle-aged and elderly patients, ankle edema without evidence of cardiac decompensation has occurred.

Facial pallor commonly occurs when parenteral and high oral doses are used, but usually does not persist for longer than the first week of treatment.

Gastrointestinal Effects. The most widely discussed complication of chlorpromazine therapy has been jaundice. The weight of evidence now available favors the concept that the process is a reversible reaction that confines itself to temporary occlusion of the biliary canaliculi and spares the parenchyma. However, the mechanism by which it is produced is a subject of great speculation. There is no convincing evidence that chlorpromazine is a specific hepatotoxin, capable of producing liver damage in the manner of, for example, yellow phosphorus. Patients who do not develop jaundice show no disturbance in bile excretion or cellular function. Prolonged administration or large dosages do not increase the incidence or induce laboratory signs of liver damage. We have been unable to confirm the observation of Moyer *et al.* that patients with preexisting liver pathology have an exaggerated clinical response to chlorpromazine, an observation that led to his conclusion that biotransformation of chlorpromazine may take place in the liver. Pelner and Waldman postulate that chlorpromazine may act as a biologic antagonist to choline. This theory is based, however, on the highly questionable assumption that chlorpromazine causes jaundice only in poorly nourished patients. Movitt *et al.* suggest that cholestasis may be secondary to hepatic cell injury preventing normal bile hydration.

Strong presumptive evidence exists that chlorpromazine-induced jaundice is an allergic reaction that occurs in sensitive patients. In support of this concept are: (1) the relative rarity despite widespread use; (2) experiments showing that chlorpromazine is not hepatotoxic; (3) occurrence on either small or large dosages after a relatively constant incubation period; (4) an unusual antigenic capacity as reflected in the frequent occurrence of other complications more closely resembling classic allergic reactions; (5) frequent histories of previous allergic reactions; and (6) a chemical structure commonly found in sensitizing drugs. Whether jaundice results from a previously existing sensitivity or develops when the patient becomes sensitized remains to be determined. The clinical course is unique and parallels that of the skin reactions: it rarely recurs on reinstitution of the drug and may even disappear without interruption of treatment.

The incidence is approximately 1.4 per cent. It is unrelated to dosage or route of administration. A review of fourteen reports in the literature reveals that of a total of 28 cases, 65 per cent were aged 40 or above, and 65 per cent were women. The clinical course is generally mild. Usually a fever occurs suddenly two or three weeks after the beginning of treatment, followed shortly by nausea or perhaps vomiting, vague abdominal pain, acholic stools, and the appearance of icterus within one to five days. Pruritus may be intense. Subjective distress is ordinarily minimal unless the patient is aroused by the physician's anxiety over the implications of liver involvement or laparotomy is performed. Symptoms disappear within a few days and icterus clears in from two to three weeks. Variations may occur. The incubation period may be shorter or longer than two or three weeks, but does not generally extend past one month. Treatment may be terminated and jaundice appear after a latent period. It may also remain subclinical, manifesting nothing but sudden fever and characteristic laboratory findings. Icterus may be persistent; the patient of Azima and Ogle was icteric for seven months. Laboratory findings are those characteristic of obstructive jaundice: hyperbilirubinemia, elevated serum alkaline phosphatase, bilirubinuria, and negative hepatocellular function tests. Biopsy studies almost routinely reveal bile thrombi in the canaliculi, varying degrees of inflammatory cell infiltration, and preservation of cell architecture. Following recovery, signs of liver damage are not discernible.

Other undesirable effects referable to the gastrointestinal tract occur frequently but are of small consequence. The most common is constipation, which usually occurs when the dosage exceeds 100 mg. daily. Unusual increases in appetite and excessive weight gain beyond that expected with relief of anxiety are often seen. This response begins during the second to fourth week of treatment and is probably a diencephalic effect. Anorexia, vomiting, and diarrhea may also occur. Pyrosis, localized substernally or in the epigastrium, may follow oral ingestion. The mechanism is difficult to understand, for chlorpromazine depresses hydrochloric acid secretion; local irritation is a doubtful explanation since the symptom tends to occur in the same patient but irregularly.

Dermatologic Effects. Of all the untoward effects of chlorpromazine classed as complications, dematoses are the most common. Like so many others, the character of these reactions strongly suggests an allergic mechanism. However, they do not fully satisfy the criteria of allergic reactions, for they rarely recur on subsequent administration. In fact, they possess the unique feature of usually disappearing while treatment continues. Until more precise understanding is reached, these skin responses must be regarded as allergic reactions of a peculiar sort. Incidence appears to be unrelated to dosage but can be correlated to some extent with duration of administration. They usually appear after two weeks of treatment, occasionally after only one but infrequently after four.

Four types of skin reactions may occur, either alone or in combination: (1) photosensitivity, (2) pruritus, (3) dermatitis, and (4) edema.

It has been demonstrated that chlorpromazine increases sensitivity of the skin to ultraviolet radiation. In a small percentage of patients, possibly because of individual hypersensitivity, this may become clinically apparent in the form of predisposition to sunburn, hypersensitivity to heat, dermographia, and precipitation of skin eruption and angioneurotic edema on exposure to sunlight. Pruritus, either localized or generalized, may be associated with photosensitization or may occur independently.

The figure of incidence of dermatitis varies widely from series to series, but is about 8 to 9 per cent. It is most frequent in the spring and summer, probably due to the photosensitization factor. Three forms can be recognized. The most common is an erythematous maculopapular rash, which often becomes vesicular or even bullous. Urticaria and erythema multiforme, occasionally hemorrhagic, are less common. Sites of predilection are the face, neck, upper chest, upper extremities, or thighs, but there may be generalized spread. Anti-histaminic drugs and topical antipruritic agents are of supportive value but provide only partial relief. Steroid hormones are almost never required. Even though the clinical appearance may be florid or even alarming, with rare exception the dermatitides resolve in from three to five days, whether or not treatment is stopped. If treatment is interrupted and later resumed, it rarely recurs. This is not true if dermatitis is due to contact allergy, which almost always recurs on repeated exposure. It also differs in clinical appearance, being of an eczematous type with edema, redness, vesicles, fissuration, and desquamation. Labhardt reports the case of a nurse who had blepharoconjunctivitis and palpebral edema each time she came in contact with chlorpromazine.

Edema of the face, lips, and hands usually occurs in association with other skin manifestations and tends to be more persistent than the dematitides.

Hematologic Effects. The changes in the blood picture that may occur during chlorpromazine therapy deserve special attention, for they indicate reactions that are the most likely to terminate fatally.

Several investigators have found that following initial injections of chlorpromazine, the peripheral leukocyte count is decreased for several hours. During the course of therapy, leukocytosis, eosinophilia, leukopenia, and neutropenia may be observed. More often than not such variations are insignificant except to signal close observation of the hemogram. Leukopenia and neutropenia, however, may herald the most fearful of all chlorpromazine complications, agranulocytosis. A review of seven cases in the literature discloses a strong correlation among the factors of age, sex, and duration of administration but none with dosage. All were females; excluding 1 patient aged 38, all were at least 57 years old, the average being 64.9 years. In every case a minimum of 41 days had elapsed after onset of administration. Three cases were preceded by jaundice and/or rash. The mechanism of this complication is not defined, but the factor of sensitivity must be seriously considered. There are no consistent prodromal symptoms of agranulocytosis. Renewed lassitude and weakness occurring four to six weeks after onset of treatment indicates a complete blood count, for prompt detection followed by antibiotics, corticotropin, and transfusions may prevent death.

Other blood elements do not appear to be similarly affected by chlorpromazine. Rizzo and Russo found that erythrocytes and hemoglobin decreased as did leukocytes after initial injections but that this was also transitory. Sedimentation rate is increased. There have been rare cases of anemia, and "bleeding tendencies" have been described, but in general, disturbances of this type are confined to the late stages of agranulocytosis.

Respiratory Effects. Nasal congestion without rhinorrhea, and dryness of the oral and pharyngeal mucous membranes, are two of the most common side effects. Only rarely do patients volunteer these complaints, usually assigning them to acute coryza. These effects usually subside within the first few weeks but may persist when large doses are used. Dyspnea has been observed in association with prolonged tachycardia. We have observed an asthmatic attack in a patient without previous asthmatic history. An indirect effect on the respiratory tract is the development of pneumonia in elderly patients. This may be regarded as a preventable complication, in all probability the result of pulmonary hypostasis occurring during hypersomnolence.

Musculoskeletal Effects. Facilitation of the lower motor neuron by the reticular activating system (via the reticulospinal tract) is depressed by chlorpromazine. The result is subjective musclar weakness, a complaint second only to drowsiness in frequency. It is also one of the earliest, usually resolving within two weeks but renewable by increasing dosage. Constant at first, it may later be apparent only during periods of muscular exertion. In extreme cases there may be ataxia and incoordination. Related effects have been discussed above in relation to Parkinsonism. Arthralgia, associated either with dermatologic reactions or as an independent finding, probably represents an allergic manifestation.

Urinary Effects. The disorders of urination that may occur are not believed to be primarily renal in origin. Moyer *et al.* found no evidence of acute renal toxicity or renal hemodynamic alterations either clinically or in laboratory experiments, although sodium and water excretion in animals increased slightly after parenteral administration. Patients receiving chlorpromazine drink excessive amounts of water because of mouth dryness, with resulting polyuria. Oliguria, which occurs much less frequently, is probably of neurogenic origin. Deep orange coloration of the urine that may be seen when dosage is high may be mistaken for bilirubinuria.

Endocrinologic Effects. Swelling of the breasts, frequently accompanied by secretion of fluid that has been found to be identical with mothers' milk, may occur in female patients receiving large doses of chlorpromazine. The swelling is diffuse and not associated with tenderness or cyst formation. In the author's series it occurred in women between ages 20 and 40 when doses were high. Increased sexual desire may occur, most commonly in females. In men the most common aberration is impotence. This discrepancy is not easily explained. Protracted amenorrhea is a rare complication. Bulimia and excessive weight gain have been described above in relation to the gastrointestinal system.

Precautions

Despite the multiplicity of side effects and complications, very few deaths have been reported. Certain precautions may minimize the occurrence of untoward reactions. When strict control is not possible, particularly when the patient is in the elderly age group, gradual increase of dosage may minimize changes in blood pressure and its associated symptoms. When signs of cerebral arteriosclerosis are present, intramuscular injections or initially high oral doses are unwise except when unusual indication exists. Since a significant number of patients who suffer complications have past histories of other allergic reactions, it should be prescribed in such cases with an awareness of the risks involved. It probably should not be given in cases of depression where retardation is prominent. Close observation of the blood picture is indicated if there is reduction of leukocyte count or if for no apparent reason the patients begin to complain of general malaise and weakness after these symptoms have originally cleared. The potentiation of barbiturates and narcotics by chlorpromazine appears to be overemphasized. There is no general agreement as to whether preexisting liver pathology is a contraindication to chlorpromazine therapy; in the author's experience it is not. Since chlorpromazine is being used so widely, it is becoming necessary to consider it in the differential diagnosis of every case of obstructive jaundice.

Comment

As has been noted, the most characteristic feature of the side effects and complications of chlorpromazine therapy is their unpredictability. There are few drugs in which the factor of individual response is as significant. This high degree of unpredictability plus certain other features, however, may have important implications, offering perhaps a clue to the physicochemical process mediating the action of chlorpromazine.

Current theories attempt to explain the action of chlorpromazine as an inhibitory effect on the reticular formation, hypothalamus, and other structures with which they are intricately interrelated. On a descriptive level this hypothesis accounts for most of the side effects and many of the complications, but the explanation is only partially satisfactory. A constant pharmacodynamic action presumably affects the same structures in all patients so as to regularly produce a more or less uniform set of "side effects" at relatively similar dosage levels. Clinically this does not occur during chlorpromazine therapy. On the contrary, there is no uniformity in occurrence, type, or degree of untoward effects. The hypothesis also does not answer the question as to why most side effects can be expected to disappear even though administration is uninterrupted. It also does not explain, for example, why the occasional patient develops Parkinsonism while receiving 800 mg./day while many others can tolerate many times that amount without any signs of basal ganglia involvement.

Certain parallels exist that seem to indicate that another factor must be present. It is well known that dermatitides due to chlorpromazine, which more than any others appear to be classical allergic reactions, disappear in the same way as the side effects, i.e., without the necessity of discontinuing therapy. Cases in the literature describe a similar course of events with jaundice and Parkinsonism. There is much to support the belief that jaundice and agranulocytosis are expressions of allergic sensitivity. It should also be noted that many of the extrapyramid syndromes due to chlorpromazine are of a postencephalitic character, and that toxic-confusional states can occur. Finally, just as acute allergic reactions may follow single doses of other drugs, dermatitis and jaundice have been produced by one dose of chlorpromazine. Parkinsonism has been produced within 24 hours after onset of administration.

The question therefore arises of whether the side effects of chlorpromazine occur through the production of some unusual type of transient, self-limiting, allergic-like process of which the "complications" are merely the extreme manifestation. To support this theory it must also be postulated that sensitivity of this sort is extremely common in human beings and that the classical criteria of allergic reactions, which demand reproduction on subsequent administration, are not met. This hypothesis is far from unassailable but deserves further investigation.

Conclusions

Chlorpromazine has many undesirable effects, most of which are transient and of relatively minor clinical significance. Complications of potentially serious degree occur in a significant number of cases but generally resolve rapidly and without apparent residual effects. It appears that chlorpromazine is clinically a relatively safe drug, and that the therapeutic benefits which may accrue from its use outweigh the risks involved.

FATAL HYPERPYREXIA DURING CHLORPROMAZINE THERAPY

Frank J. Ayd, Jr., M.D.

It is now well established that chlorpromazine in the usual therapeutic doses is a relatively nontoxic compound. It can cause many bothersome side effects that are seldom serious and that subside with continued administration of the drug or may be controlled by the addition of other drugs to the patient's medication. However, this compound is not without its potentially serious side reactions and may even prove fatal. The purpose of this report is to record a fatal reaction to chlorpromazine and to caution against the indiscriminate use of this drug.

CASE REPORT

A 41 year old white man was hospitalized for chlorpromazine therapy for a schizophrenic reaction, unclassified. His past psychiatric history revealed the presence of overt schizophrenic symptomatology for four years. He had been treated with several courses of electroconvulsive therapy that produced a temporary amelioration of his symptoms. Several months prior to admission this patient had been treated with doses of chlorpromazine up to 400 mg./day with some symptomatic improvement. When chlorpromazine was discontinued the patient relapsed.

On admission, physical and neurologic examinations were negative. The psychiatric examination revealed an agitated schizophrenic with paranoid features. This patient was placed on increasing doses of chlorpromazine to a maximum of 2500 mg. on the eighteenth treatment day. On the nineteenth and twentieth treatment days he received 2500 mg. daily. On the twenty-first treatment day he had had 1800 mg. At 6:00 p.m. his temperature was normal. Two hours later he suddenly collapsed. His rectal temperature was 108 F. He had a few epileptiform seizures and lapsed into coma. Intensive treatment of the hyperthermia lowered the temperature to 104 F., but he expired nine hours after his collapse.

NEUROPATHOLOGIC FINDINGS

Unfortunately only the brain of this patient could be obtained for postmortem study. A summary of the gross and microscopic findings suggests an intense process causing profound swelling of neuron cells associated with increasing capillary distention and terminal petechial hemorrhages. The lesions seen would be compatible with intense thermoregulatory disturbance such as would be seen with heatstroke. Anatomic lesions of a destructive nature were not present. The only reliable lesions seen were acute swelling of neurons, particularly in the thalamus and hypothalamus, and intense congestive changes and petechial hemorrhages, which were present throughout the entire brain.

Discussion

Fluctuations of temperature in patients receiving chlorpromazine have been reported. This drug, at any dose level, may cause mild hyperthermia (99 to 101 F.) or hypothermia (96 to 98 F.) in the initial stages of therapy, which subsides as treatment is continued. In a few patients, daily elevations or drops in temperature have been recorded throughout the treatment period. This has occurred most often in patients receiving large doses (500 mg. or more daily).

Chlorpromazine may cause sudden elevations of temperature (up to 105 F.) accompanied by profuse perspiration and some feelings of prostration. This febrile reaction, which subsides after a few hours, is not related to the dosage of chlorpromazine, the route of administration, the climatic environment, or the physical activity of the patient. It may occur once or repeatedly in the first two weeks of treatment, after which time it is rare.

Chlorpromazine also may cause striking hypothermia in the early stages of treatment. The temperature may be as low as 93 F. During this period the patient is lethargic, and the usual defense mechanisms to conserve body heat such as piloerection and vasoconstriction are impaired. Within a few hours the temperature returns to normal. Further treatment with chlorpromazine does not cause a recurrence of hypothermia.

These clinical observations indicate chlorpromazine may affect the function of the hypothalamus, which is the main center for the regulation of body temperature. In cats and monkeys, injury to the rostral part of the hypothalamus causes hyperthermia, while injury to the region dorsolateral to the mammillary bodies results in hypothermia. The hyperthermia and hypothermia produced by chlorpromazine are transient, indicating that this drug in therapeutic doses causes a temporary biochemical impairment of the function of the neurons of the hypothalamus.

The influence of chlorpromazine on the temperature-regulating mechanism may be affected adversely by the environmental temperature. In cold weather many patients taking 300 mg. or more daily report hypersensitivity to freezing temperatures. In hot, humid weather many patients mention a hypersensitivity to the temperature. Some complain that the heat is almost intolerable whenever the temperature rises above 90 F. A few perspire excessively and manifest symptoms of mild heat prostration. This increased sensitivity to heat is not related to the dosage of chlorpromazine, although patients on large doses apparently are more sensitive.

In the case under discussion the fatal hyperpyrexia occurred at a time when the environmental temperature was high. Goldman reports that 8 of his chlorpromazine-treated patients had nonfatal heatstrokes during the torrid temperatures of the summer of 1955. These clinical observations suggest that environmental temperature may enhance the action of chlorpromazine on the thermoregulatory mechanism. This is supported by the experimental studies of Berti and Cima, who found that the toxicity of this drug is accentuated by environmental temperatures. Finally, Ranson and his collaborators in experiments on cats and monkeys found that destructive lesions in the preoptic and supraoptic regions between the anterior commissure and the optic chiasma are followed by hyperthermia when the animal is exposed to a degree of heat that would have little effect on the body temperature of a normal animal.

Although no anatomic lesions in the brain were found that could account for the death of this patient, it is postulated that his demise was due to the toxic action of chlorpromazine on the hypothalamus and that the toxicity of chlorpromazine was accentuated by the environmental temperature.

The above article reports a study conducted early in 1953 before chlorpromazine was commercially available and shortly after its introduction for clinical trials. Since then the author has changed his views. He no longer feels that it is mandatory to hospitalize all patients who are going to be administered large doses of chlorpromazine. Additional clinical experience has convinced him that many patients do respond to large doses of chlorpromazine and that in some instances only large doses are therapeutically effective.

BIBLIOGRAPHY

ACKNOWLEDGMENTS: Thanks are due to the authors, as well as to the publishers, for permission to reprint material from the sources indicated:

The American Journal of the Medical Sciences: "Effects of Chlorpromazine in Psychiatric Disorders," by Irvin M. Cohen, M.D., April, 1955; and "Use of Chlorpromazine in Chronic Alcoholics," by James F. Cummins, M.D., and Dale G. Friend, M.D., May, 1954.

The American Journal of Psychiatry: "The Ataractic Drugs: The Present Position of Chlorpromazine, Frenquel, Pacatal, and Reserpine in the Psychiatric Hospital," by H. Angus Bowes, M.D., Dec., 1956; "Progress in Psychiatric Therapies," by Paul H. Hoch, M.D., Oct, 1955; "A Comparative Study of Various Ataractic Drugs," by Paul E. Feldman, M.D., Jan. 1957; "An Evaluation of Promazine Hydrochloride in Psychiatric Practice," by Stanley Lesse, M.D., May, 1957; "Effects of Chlorpromazine on Chronic Lobotomized Schizophrenic Patients," by Harry Freeman, M.D., and Herbert S. Cline, M.D., Nov., 1956; "Chlorpromazine Treatment of Mental Disorders," by Vernon Kinross-Wright, M.D., June, 1955; "Thorazine and Serpasil Treatment of Private Neuropsychiatric Patients," by Frank J. Ayd, Jr., July, 1956; "Effect of Chlorpromazine and Reserpine on Budgets of Mental Hospitals," by Werner Tuteur, M.D., Jan., 1957; "Azacyclonol (Frenquel) in the Treatment of Chronic Schizophrenics," by Joseph A. Barsa, M.D., and Nathan S. Kline, M.D., Sept., 1956; " The Effect of Meratran on Twenty-Five Institutionalized Mental Patients," by J. W. Schut, M.D., and H. E. Himwich, M.D., May, 1955; "Clinical Studies on a-(2-Piperidyl) Benzhydrol Hydrochloride, a New Antidepressant Drug, by Howard D. Fabing, M.D., J. Robert Hawkins, M.D., and James A. L. Moulton, M.D., May, 1955; "The Use of Chlorpromazine Hydrochloride in the Treatment of Barbiturate Addiction with Acute Withdrawal Syndrome," by William Brooks, M.D., Lawrence Deutsch, M.D., and Robert Dickes, M.D., March, 1955; "Complications of Chlorpromazine Therapy," by Irvin M. Cohen, M.D., Aug., 1956; "Complication During Reserpine Therapy," by C. H. Cahn, M.D., July, 1955; "Recurrent Thorazine Induced Agranulocytosis," by Benjamin Pollack, M.D., Dec., 1956; "Fatal Acute Aseptic Necrosis of the Liver Associated with Chlorpromazine," by R. N. Elliott, M.D., A. H. Schrut, M.D., and J. J. Marra, M.D., May, 1956; and "An Appraisal of Chlorpromazine," by N. William Winkelman, Jr., M.D., May, 1957.

American Journal of Psychotherapy: "Psychotherapy and Ataraxics," by Stanley Lesse, M.D., July, 1956.

A.M.A. Archives of Dermatology: "Meprobamate (Miltown) as Adjunct in Treatment of Anogenital Pruritus," by Oscar J. Sokoloff, M.D., Oct., 1956.

A.M.A. Archives of Internal Medicine: "Hematemesis and Melena Complicating

Treatment with Rauwolfia Alkaloids," by Leo E. Hollister, M.D., Feb., 1957.

A.M.A. Archives of Neurology and Psychiatry: "Some Observations on the Use of Tranquilizing Drugs," by Thomas S. Szasz, M.D., Jan., 1957; "The Use of Reserpine in an Acute Psychiatric Treatment Setting," by Garfield Tourney, M.D., Emil M. Isberg, M.D., and Jacques S. Gottlieb, M.D., Sept., 1955; "Reserpine in Hospitalized Psychotics, A Controlled Study on Chronically Disturbed Women," by Arthur Lemon Arnold, M.D., and Harry Freeman, M.D., Sept., 1956; "Behavioral Changes of Chronic Schizophrenics in Response to Reserpine," by Roy E. McDonald, M.D., Robert B. Ellsworth, Ph.D., and Jane Eniss, R.N., June, 1956; "Effect of Reserpine and Open-Ward Privileges on Chronic Schizophrenics," by Allen S. Penman, Ph.D., and Thomas E. Dredge, M.D., "A Controlled Study of Reserpine on Chronically Disturbed Patients," by M. Duane Sommerness, M.D., Rubel J. Lucero, M.A., John S. Hamlon, M.D., J. L. Erickson, M.D., and R. Matthews, R.Ph., Sept., 1955; "Chlorpromazine, New Inhibiting Agent for Psychomotor Excitement and Manic States," by H. E. Lehmann, M.D., and G. E. Hanrahan, M.D., Feb., 1954; "Chlorpromazine (Thorazine)—Rauwolfia Combination in Neuropsychiatry," by Harold B. Eiber, M.D., July, 1955; and "Chlorpromazine (Thorazine) Treatment of Disturbed Epileptic Patients," by Vincent I. Bonafede, M.D., Aug., 1955.

American Practitioner and Digest of Treatment: "Psychiatric Experience with Chlorpromazine," by Willis H. Bower, M.D., Mark D. Altschule, M.D., and Leonard Cook, Ph.D., Jan., 1955; and "Use of a Chlorpromazine-Dextro-Amphetamine Combination in Anxiety Neuroses," by Thomas M. Hart, M.D., Dec., 1956.

American Professional Pharmacist: "The Ataractic Drugs: Their Uses and Limitations in Psychiatry," by Howard D. Fabing, M.D., May, 1956.

American Psychiatric Association, publishers of *"Psychiatric Research Reports"*: "Use of Reserpine in Chronic Non-Disturbed Psychotics," by James Boudwin, M.D., and Nathan S. Kline, M.D., April, 1956; "Use of Reserpine on an Admission Service," by Ernest Gosline, M.D., and Nathan S. Kline, M.D., July, 1955; "Improved Behavior Patterns in the Hospitalized Mentally Ill with Reserpine and Methyl-Phenidylacetate," by John T. Ferguson, M.D., April, 1956; "The Influence of Chlorpromazine on Psychotic Thought Content and Mechanism," Douglas Goldman, M.D., July, 1955; "Clinical Trial of a New Phenothiazine Compound: NP-207," by Vernon Kinross-Wright, M.D., April, 1956; "Reserpine in the Treatment of Disturbed Adolescents," by George T. Nicolaou, M.D., and Nathan S. Kline, M.D., Feb. 19, 1955; and "The Use of Reserpine (Serpasil) in Three Hundred and Fifty Neuropsychiatric Cases," by Veronica M. Penington, M.D.

British Medical Journal: "A Clinical Trial of Benactyzine Hydrochloride ("Suavitil") as a Physical Relaxant," by Anthony Coady, M.B., M.R.C.P., and Eric C. O. Jewesbury, D.M., M.R.C.P., D.P.M., March 3, 1956.

California Medicine: "Chlorpromazine Alone and with Reserpine: Use in the Treatment of Mental Diseases," by Leo E. Hollister, M.D., Kenneth P.

Jones, M.D., Bernard Brownfield, M.D., and Franklin Johnson, M.D., Sept., 1955; and "Use of Tranquilizers in Diseases of the Skin," by Paul Levan, M.D., and Edwin T. Wright, M.D., Aug., 1956.

The Canadian Medical Association Journal: "The Use of Chlorpromazine and Reserpine in Psychological Disorders in General Practice," by H. Azima, M.D.; and "Psychosis and Enhanced Anxiety Produced by Reserpine and Chlorpromazine," by G. J. Sarwer-Foner, M.D., and W. Ogle, M.D.

Clinical Medicine: "Office Treatment of Pain and Psychic Stress: The Use of a New Tranquilizing Agent," by Jack R. Wennersten, M. D., Dec., 1956.

The Danish Medical Bulletin: "Suavitil in the Treatment of Psychoneuroses," by Olaf Ostergaard Jensen; and "A New Drug Effective on the Central Nervous System," by E. Jacobsen.

Delaware State Medical Journal: "New Drug Therapies in Psychiatry," by F. A. Freyhan, M.D., Patricia Turner, M.D., and Rita Stenzler, M.D., Aug., 1956.

Diseases of the Nervous System: "Evaluation of the Therapeutic Effects of Drugs in Psychiatric Patients," by Lincoln D. Clark, M.D., Sept., 1956; "A Review of the Newer Drug Therapies in Psychiatry," by Vernon Kinross-Wright, M.D., June, 1956; "Large Doses of Chlorpromazine in the Treatment of Psychiatric Patients," by Frank J. Ayd, Jr., M.D., May, 1955; "Frenquel," by Richard C. Proctor, M.D., and Theodore Odland, M.D., Jan., 1956; "Treatment of Depression with Meratran and Electroshock," by Henry E. Andren, M.D., Sept., 1955; "Combination Reserpine-Methylphenidylacetate in Epileptics with Psychosis," by G. Donald Niswander, M.D., and Earl K. Holt, M.D., Jan., 1957; "Ineffectiveness of Chlorpromazine and Rauwolfia Serpentina Preparations in the Treatment of Depression," by Lawrence H. Gahagan, M.D.,; and "Agranulocytosis While Receiving Combined Reserpine-Chlorpromazine Therapy," by Joseph A. Barsa, M.D., and Nathan S. Kline, M.D., March, 1956.

Geriatrics: "Hydroxyzine: A New Therapeutic Agent for Senile Anxiety States," by Mervin Shalowitz, M.D., July, 1956.

GP: "Ataractics in Medical Practice," by Joseph F. Fazekas, M.D., James G. Shea, M.D., and Paul D. Sullivan, Jr., M.D., Dec., 1956.

International Record of Medicine and General Practice Clinics: "Use of the Tranquilizing Properties of Reserpine," by J. Campbell Howard, Jr., M.D., and Frank J. Vinci, M.D., April, 1956; "The Use of Azacyclonol and Pipradol in General Practice," by Thomas G. Allin, Jr., M.D., and Raymond C. Pogge, M.D., April, 1956; "Meprobamate, Its Pharmacologic Properties and Clinical Uses," by F. M. Berger, M.D., April, 1956; "Treatment of Anxiety States with Meprobamate (Miltown)," by Walter A. Osinki, M.D., Sept., 1956; and "Preliminary Study on the Use of Hydroxyzine in Psychosomatic Affections," by Luis Farah, M.D., June, 1956.

Journal of the American Geriatrics Society: "The Treatment of Anxiety, Agitation and Excitement in the Aged," by Frank J. Ayd, Jr. M.D., Jan., 1957.

The Journal of the American Medical Association: "Reserpine (Serpasil) in the

Management of the Mentally Ill," by Robert H. Noce, M.D., David B. Williams, M.D., and Walter Rapaport, M.D., May 7, 1955; "Treatment of Two Hundred Disturbed Psychotics with Reserpine," by Joseph A. Barsa, M.D., and Nathan S. Kline, M.D., May 14, 1955; "A Clinical Study of Mechanics of Action of Chlorpromazine," by Erwin Lear, M.D., Albert E. Chiron, M.D., and Irving M. Pallin, M.D., Jan. 5, 1957; "Chlorpromazine in the Treatment of Neuropsychiatric Disorders," by N. William Winkelman, Jr., M.D., May 1, 1954; "Use of Chlorpromazine and Reserpine in the Treatment of Emotional Disorders," by William W. Zeller, M.D., Paul N. Graffagnino, M.D., Chester F. Cullen, M.D., and H. Jerome Rietman, M.D., Jan. 21, 1956; "Clinical Study of a New Tranquilizing Drug," by Lowell S. Selling, M.D., April 30, 1955; "Therapeutic Process in Electroshock and the Newer Drug Therapies," by Leo Alexander, M.D., Nov. 3, 1956; "Improving Senile Behavior with Reserpine and Ritalin," by John T. Ferguson, M.D., and William H. Funderburk, Ph.D., Jan. 28, 1956; "Use of Meprobamate (Miltown) in Convulsive and Related Disorders," by Meyer A. Perlstein, M.D., July 14, 1956; "Reserpine (Serpasil) in the Management of the Mentally Ill and Mentally Retarded," by Robert H. Noce, M.D., David B. Williams, M.D., and Walter Rapaport, M.D., Oct. 30, 1954; "Adverse Reactions to Meprobamate," by Henry T. Friedman, M.D., and Willard L. Marmelzat, M.D., Oct, 13, 1956; "Inherent Dangers in Use of Tranquilizing Drugs in Anxiety States," by Herman A. Dickel, M.D., and Henry H. Dixon, M.D., Feb. 9, 1957; "Edema and Congestive Failure Related to Administration of Rauwolfia Serpentina," by George A. Perera, M.D., Oct. 1, 1955; "Jaundice Caused by Chlorpromazine (Thorazine)," by Lawrence R. Loftus, M.D., Kenneth A. Huizenga, M.D., Maurice H. Stauffer, M.D., Howard P. Rome, M.D., and James C. Cain, M.D., April 9, 1955; and "Liver Function and Hepatic Complications in Patients Receiving Chlorpromazine," by Irvin M. Cohen, M.D., and John D. Archer, M.D., Sept. 10, 1955.

Journal of the American Osteopatic Association: "Meratran with Reserpine: Adjunctive Use in the Treatment of Parkinson's Disease," by John C. Button, M.D., April, 1956.

Journal of Clinical and Experimental Psychopathology: "Has Chlorpromazine Inaugurated a New Era in Mental Hospitals," by Winfred Overholser, M.D., June, 1956; "Some Considerations on the Use of Chlorpromazine in a Child Psychiatry Clinic," by Herbert Freed, M.D., and Charles A. Peifer, Jr., June, 1956; "Undesirable Effects and Clinical Toxicity of Chlorpromazine," by Irvin M. Cohen, M.D., June, 1956; and "Fatal Hyperpyrexia During Chlorpromazine Therapy," Frank J. Ayd, Jr., M.D., June, 1956.

Journal of Individual Psychology: "Modern Drug Treatment and Psychotherapy," by Alexandra Adler, M.D., Nov., 1957.

The Journal of the Michigan State Medical Society: "What's New and Usable in the Chemical Treatment of Abnormal Behavior," by John T. Ferguson, M.D., Sept., 1956; and "Thorazine in the Treatment of Acutely Disturbed

Psychotic Patients," by Gordon R. Forrer, M.D., July, 1956.

The Journal of Nervous and Mental Diseases: "Prospects in Psychopharmacology," by Harold E. Himwich, M.D., Nov., 1955; "Reserpine in the Treatment of Patients with Chronic Mental Disease, A Controlled Study," by Lawrence Koltonow, M.D., April, 1956; "Promazine Hydrochloride in the Treatment of Chronic Catatonic Schizophrenics," by Clarke W. Mangun, M.D., and Warren W. Webb, Ph.D., June, 1956; "The Use of Chlorpromazine in Psychotherapy," by H. L. Newbold, M.D., and W. David Steed, M.D., March, 1956; and "Chlorpromazine for the Control of Psychomotor Excitement in the Mentally Defficient," by Judith H. Rettig, M.D., Aug., 1955.

Medical Annals of the District of Columbia: "Chlorpromazine and Reserpine," by Francis N. Waldrop, M.D., and F. Regis Riesenman, M.D., May, 1956; "Meprobamate in Anxiety Reactions Involving Depression," by Abraham Ruchwarger, M.D., Oct., 1956; "The Use of Chlorpromazine in the Treatment of Acute Alcoholism," by Salomon N. Albert, M.D., Edward L. Rea, M.D., Cecil A. Duverney, M.D., James Shea, M.D., and Joseph F. Fazekas, M.D., May, 1954; and "Complications and Concomitants," by Otis R. Farley, M.D., May, 1956.

Mental Hospitals: "Drug Therapy—Clinical and Operational Effects," by Benjamin Pollack, M.D., April, 1956.

Military Medicine: "A Case of Corticotropic Hormone-Induced Psychosis Treated with Promazine Hydrochloride," by Lt. Dean J. Plazak, M.C., Feb., 1957.

Modern Medicine: "Pharmacology of the Ataractic Drugs," by Edward B. Truitt, Jr., Ph.D., Jan. 15, 1957.

The New England Journal of Medicine: "A Critique of the Tranquilizing Drugs, Chlorpromazine and Reserpine, in Neuropsychiatry," by Harry Freeman, M.D., Nov. 8, 1956; "Use of Chlorpromazine and Reserpine in Mental Disorders," by Mark D. Altschule, M.D., March 15, 1956; "Experience with the Use of Chlorpromazine and Reserpine in Psychiatry," by George W. Brooks, M.D., June 14, 1956; "Clinical Study of Proclorperazine, a New Tranquilizer for the Treatment of Nonhospitalized Psychoneurotic Patients," by Thomas J. Vischer, M.D., Jan. 3, 1957; and "Use of Chlorpromazine in the Withdrawal of Addicting Drugs," by Charles E. Friedgood, M.D., and Charles B. Ripstein, M.D., Feb. 10, 1955.

New York State Journal of Medicine: "Short-Term Treatment of Psychiatric Patients with Reserpine," by Stephen B. Payn, M.D., and Fred V. Rockwell, M.D., June 1, "Potentiation of Hypnotics and Analgesics," by Robert Wallis, M.D., Jan. 15, 1955; and "Drug-Induced Blood Dyscrasias," by Stuart L. Vaughan, M.D., Sept. 1, 1955.

Northwest Medicine: "Drug Therapy in the Emotionally Disturbed Aged," by Sol Levy, M.D., March, 1956.

Postgraduate Medicine: "The Tranquilizing Drugs," by Morris Fishbein, M.D., May, 1956.

Proceedings of the Rudolph Virchow Society: "Chlorpromazine and Reserpine, and Their Relation to Other Treatments in Psychiatry," by Lothar B. Kalinowsky, M.D., 1956.

Psychiatric Quarterly: "Observations During the Treatment of 175 Psychotic Patients with Reserpine," by Rudolf B. Freund, M.D., July, 1955; and "Preliminary Report on Five Hundred Patients Treated with Thorazine at Rochester State Hospital," by Benjamin Pollack, M.D., July, 1955.

Quarterly Journal of Studies on Alcohol: "Miltown as a Tranquilizer in the Treatment of Alcohol Addicts," by Joseph Thimann, M.D., and Joseph W. Gauthier, M.D., March, 1956.

South Dakota Journal of Medicine: "Ambulatory and Comparative Treatment of the Anxiety Neurosis Syndrome with Chlorpromazine, Phenobarbital and Dimethylane," by Wallace Marshall, M.D., Oct., 1956.

Southern Medical Journal: "Chlorpromazine and Reserpine as Adjuncts in Electroshock Treatment," by Merritt W. Foster, Jr., M.D., and R. Finley Gayle III., July, 1956.

Texas State Journal of Medicine: "Drugs Recently Introduced in the Treatment of Psychiatric Disorders," by Irvin M. Cohen, M.D., Sept., 1956.